Oxford Cases in Medicine and Surgery

Oxford Cases in
Medicine and Surgery

Second edition

Hugo Farne
BMBCh MRCP
Registrar in Respiratory Medicine, London Deanery

Edward Norris-Cervetto
BMBCh MRCEM DPhil
Registrar in Emergency Medicine, Oxford Deanery

James Warbrick-Smith
BMBCh MRCS DPhil
Registrar in Plastic Surgery, Wales Deanery

OXFORD
UNIVERSITY PRESS

OXFORD
UNIVERSITY PRESS

Great Clarendon Street, Oxford, OX2 6DP,
United Kingdom

Oxford University Press is a department of the University of Oxford.
It furthers the University's objective of excellence in research, scholarship,
and education by publishing worldwide. Oxford is a registered trade mark of
Oxford University Press in the UK and in certain other countries

First edition published 2010
Second edition published 2015
Impression:1

Published in the United States of America by Oxford University Press
198 Madison Avenue, New York, NY 10016, United States of America

British Library Cataloguing in Publication Data
Data available

Library of Congress Control Number: 2015942565

ISBN 978-0-19-871622-8 (pbk.)

Printed in Great Britain by
Ashford Colour Press Ltd, Gosport, Hampshire

Foreword to the first edition

There is an abundance of excellent medical and surgical textbooks, written in both traditional and more novel formats. However, in a climate in which the content and mode of delivery of medical education remain in constant flux there remains a need for new resources that stimulate interest in the reader as well as providing the important and relevant facts. *Oxford Cases in Medicine and Surgery* fulfils this need. This book's uniqueness—and its educational value—stems from the way that the authors have approached the learning aspect from direct clinical symptoms, highlighting the most important differential diagnoses but also explaining how to differentiate them. This approach represents the book's real strength, mirroring as it does the integrated systems-based approach that is commonly used by many medical schools.

In my experience as a clinical teacher, course organizer, and examiner over the past decade, this is the first book that has attempted to bring together, and explain from a basic science concept, the reasons for the clinical picture or condition. This will help readers enormously, whether they are undergraduate or postgraduate medical, dental, or nursing students. It is an important book for those who wish to understand the reasons for clinical presentations and their differing management.

Christopher L.H. Chan
Senior Lecturer/Honorary Consultant Surgeon
Barts and The London School of Medicine and Dentistry

Acknowledgements

Dr D. Dennis and Dr T. Lancaster: thank you for your case-based seminars, which inspired this book. We hope to have captured the essence of what you taught us as medical students.

Miss A. Ashcroft, Dr J. Bowen, Miss P.J. Clarke, Dr J. Dwight, Dr R. Graham, Prof A. Handa, Dr T. Lancaster, Dr T. Littlewood, Dr N. Meston, Dr N. Slater, Prof C. Tapper, Dr J. Teh, and Dr T. Walker: thank you, for sharing your invaluable clinical and educational experience with us.

Miss G. Jeffers, Miss C. Connelly, Professor T. Hope, and the staff from OUP: thank you, for believing in our project and your ongoing support.

Emily, Rachel, Annabel, and Èlia: thank you for your patience, yet again.

Students and readers: thank you for your encouragement and feedback after the first edition.

Editorial advisors

Contents

Abbreviations

AAA	abdominal aortic aneurysm	cANCA	cytoplasmic-staining antineutrophil cytoplasmic antibodies
ABC	airways, breathing, and circulation		
ABG	arterial blood gas	CBT	cognitive behavioural therapy
ABPI	ankle–brachial pressure index	CCB	calcium-channel blocker
ACA	anterior cerebral artery	CCK	cholecystokinin
ACE	angiotensin-converting enzyme	CCP	cyclic citrullinated peptide
ACEi	angiotensin-converting enzyme inhibitor	CEA	carcinoembryonic antigen
		CLO	columnar lined oesophagus
ACTH	adrenocorticotropic hormone	CMV	cytomegalovirus
ADH	antidiuretic hormone	CNS	central nervous system
ADP	adenosine diphosphate	COCP	combined oral contraceptive pill
AFP	alpha-fetoprotein	COPD	chronic obstructive pulmonary disease
ALP	alkaline phosphatase		
ALT	alanine aminotransferase	COX	cyclooxygenase
AMA	antimitochondrial antibodies	CRP	C-reactive protein
AMTS	Abbreviated Mental Test Score	CSF	cerebrospinal fluid
ANA	antinuclear antibodies	CT	computed tomography
APTT	activated partial thromboplastin time	CT-KUB	CT of kidneys, ureters, and bladder
		CTPA	CT pulmonary angiogram
ARBs	angiotensin II receptor blockers	CVP	central venous pressure
ARDS	acute respiratory distress syndrome	DCBE	double-contrast barium enema
ASIS	anterior superior iliac spine	DIC	disseminated intravascular coagulation
ASMA	antismooth muscle antibodies		
AST	aspartate aminotransferase	DSM-5	*Diagnostic and Statistical Manual of Mental Disorders*, 5th edition
ATLS	advanced trauma life support		
AV [node]	atrioventricular [node]	DVLA	Driver and Vehicle Licensing Agency
BCG	bacille Calmette-Guérin [vaccine against tuberculosis]	DVT	deep vein thrombosis
		EBV	Epstein–Barr virus
b.d.	twice a day [drug dosing]	ECG	electrocardiogram
BMI	body mass index	EEG	electroencephalogram
BNF	British National Formulary	eGFR	estimated glomerular filtration rate
BP	blood pressure	ELISA	enzyme linked immunosorbent assay
BPH	benign prostatic hyperplasia		
bpm	beats per minute	ENT	ear, nose, and throat
BPPV	benign paroxysmal positional vertigo	ERCP	endoscopic retrograde cholangiopancreatography
BTS	British Thoracic Society	ESR	erythrocyte sedimentation rate
CABG	coronary artery bypass graft	ESWL	extracorporeal shock wave lithotripsy

EUS	endoscopic ultrasound	IM	intramuscular
FAP	familial adenomatous polyposis	INO	internuclear ophthalmoplegia
FATP1	fatty acid transporter protein 1	INR	international normalized ratio
FBC	full blood count	IPAA	ileal pouch–anal anastomosis
FER	forced expiratory ratio	ITP	immune thrombocytopenic purpura
FEV_1	forced expiratory volume in 1 second	ITU	intensive therapy unit
		IV	intravenous
FiO_2	fraction of inspired oxygen	IVC	inferior vena cava
FMTC	familial medullary thyroid carcinoma	IVF	*in vitro* fertilization
FNA	fine needle aspiration	IVP	intravenous pyelogram/pyelography
FOBT	faecal occult blood test	IVU	intravenous urogram/urography
FVC	forced vital capacity	JVP	jugular venous pressure
G6PDH	glucose-6-phosphate dehydrogenase	LABA	long-acting β_2-agonist
GCA	giant cell arteritis	LAMA	long-acting muscarinic agents
GCS	Glasgow Coma Scale	LAD	left anterior descending coronary artery
GGT	γ-glutamyl transferase		
GI	gastrointestinal	LDH	lactate dehydrogenase
GORD	gastro-oesophageal reflux disease	LDL	low-density lipoprotein
GP	general practitioner	LFTs	liver function tests
GTN	glyceryl trinitrate	LHRH	luteinizing hormone-releasing hormone
GUM	genitourinary medicine		
Hb	haemoglobin	LIF	left iliac fossa
HDL	high-density lipoprotein	LMN	lower motor neuron
β-HCG	β-human chorionic gonadotropin	LMWH	low-molecular weight heparin
HDU	high-dependency unit	LNG-IUD	levonorgestrel-releasing intrauterine device
HHS	hyperosmolar hyperglycaemic syndrome		
		LP	lumbar puncture
HiB	*Haemophilus influenzae* B	LPL	lipoprotein lipase
HIT	heparin-induced thrombocytopenia	LUQ	left upper quadrant
HNPCC	hereditary non-polyposis colorectal cancer	LUTS	lower urinary tract symptoms
		MCA	middle cerebral artery
HOCM	hypertrophic obstructive cardiomyopathy	MC&S	microscopy, culture, and sensitivities
HONK	hyperosmotic non-ketotic [coma/acidosis]	MCPJs	metacarpophalangeal joints
		MCV	mean corpuscular volume
HPOA	hypertrophic pulmonary osteoarthropathy	MDT	multidisciplinary team
		MEN	multiple endocrine neoplasia
HR	heart rate	MI	myocardial infarction
HRT	hormone replacement therapy	MMSE	Mini Mental State Exam
IBD	inflammatory bowel disease	MRCP	magnetic resonance cholangiopancreatography
IBS	irritable bowel syndrome		
ICD-10	WHO *International Statistical Classification of Diseases and Related Health Problems*, 10th revision	MRI	magnetic resonance imaging
		MRU	magnetic resonance urogram
		MSU	midstream urine
		MTC	medullary thyroid carcinoma
ICDs	implantable cardioversion devices	NBM	nil by mouth
Ig	immunoglobulin	NG	nasogastric [tube]

NICE	National Institute for Health and Care Excellence	RLN	recurrent laryngeal nerve
NIV	non-invasive ventilation	RUQ	right upper quadrant
NSAID	non-steroidal anti-inflammatory drug	SACD	subacute combined degeneration of the cord
NSCLC	non-small cell lung cancer	SAH	subarachnoid haemorrhage
NSTEMI	non-ST elevation myocardial infarction	SALT	speech and language therapist
NUD	non-ulcer dyspepsia	SC	subcutaneous
NYHA	New York Heart Association	SCLC	small cell lung cancer
o.d.	once a day [drug dosing]	SIADH	syndrome of inappropriate ADH secretion
OGD	oesophagogastroduodenoscopy	SLE	systemic lupus erythematosus
OSCE	Objective Structured Clinical Examination	SOL	space-occupying lesion
$PaCO_2$	arterial partial pressure of carbon dioxide	SSRV	small structured round virus
		STEMI	ST-elevation myocardial infarct
PaO_2	arterial partial pressure of oxygen	SVC	superior vena cava
pANCA	perinuclear-staining antineutrophil cytoplasmic autoantibodies	T_3	tri-iodothyronine
		T_4	thyroxine
PBC	primary biliary cirrhosis	TB	tuberculosis
PCA	posterior cerebral artery	t.d.s.	three times a day [drug dosing]
PCD	primary ciliary dyskinesia	TFTs	thyroid function tests
PCNL	percutaneous nephrolithotomy	TG	thyroglobulin
PCOM	posterior communicating artery	TIA	transient ischaemic attack
PE	pulmonary embolism	TIBC	total iron-binding capacity
PEF	peak expiratory flow	TIPS/TIPSS	transjugular intrahepatic portosystemic shunt
PEFR	peak expiratory flow rate	TMJ	temporomandibular joint
PET	positron emission tomography	TNF	tumour necrosis factor
P_i	inorganic phosphate	tPA	tissue plasminogen activator
PK	pyruvate kinase	TPN	total parenteral nutrition
PMN	polymorphonuclear leucocyte	TRAM	tranverse rectus abdominis myocutaneous [flap]
PPAR	peroxisome proliferator-activated receptor	TSH	thyroid-stimulating hormone
PPI	proton pump inhibitor	TTG	tissue transglutaminase
PSA	prostate-specific antigen	TURP	transurethral resection of the prostate
PSC	primary sclerosing cholangitis	TWOC	trial without catheter
PT	prothrombin time	UC	ulcerative colitis
PTH	parathyroid hormone	U&Es	urea and electrolytes
PTHrP	parathyroid hormone-related peptide	UMN	upper motor neuron
PUJ	pelviureteric junction	UTI	urinary tract infection
q.d.s.	four times a day [drug dosing]	VTE	venous thromboembolism
RAPD	relative afferent pupillary defect	WCC	white cell count
RBC	red blood cell [count]	WLE	wide local excision
RCA	right coronary artery		
RIF	right iliac fossa		

Introduction

Why we wrote this book

The inspiration for this book comes from our time as medical students. The problem we found with existing textbooks was twofold.

First, most books are organized by pathology. For example, they may have chapters on 'cardiology' that then discuss specific conditions, like 'myocardial infarction', in detail. But patients do not present with ready-made diagnoses like 'myocardial infarction'. They present with symptoms, such as 'chest pain', which could be a myocardial infarction—but could also be anything from reflux oesophagitis to aortic dissection.

Secondly, there are also textbooks based around cases rather than pathologies. Our experience is that these tend to skip over the diagnostic approach too quickly, in order to move on to a discussion of the underlying disease. Many give the reader so much information in the initial case presentation that the diagnosis is virtually made for you. For example, a '62-year-old diabetic male with sudden onset, crushing chest pain; tachycardia on examination; ST elevation on his ECG, plus raised troponins' has a myocardial infarction. But by giving so much information upfront, these books neglect to address what many students find most challenging—how do you decide what information to collect in order to make a diagnosis? Patients present with symptoms such as 'chest pain' and it is your job to elicit the key clues on history and examination, and to arrange the key investigations that will confirm that this is a myocardial infarction and rule out other diagnoses.

Knowing what to do when faced simply with 'confusion' or 'abdominal pain' can be daunting and tricky—we know, and that is what motivated us to write this book.

We hope this book will help you start thinking like a diagnostician from your first day on the wards. Thus, we hope you will be able to work out why your patient is short of breath or has abdominal pain in a way that is safe and efficient, and avoids you missing important diagnoses. Even with detailed knowledge of anatomy, physiology, biochemistry, pathology, history-taking, examination skills, and data interpretation, it can be difficult to integrate everything when faced with acutely ill patients on the wards. We benefited greatly from case-based seminars that taught us a hypothesis-driven, logical, step-by-step approach to diagnosis. Our hope is that this book emulates the teaching that we found so beneficial.

Finally, we wanted to write a workbook that students will enjoy using and where even the simplest concepts are clearly explained.

The need for a logical diagnostic approach

Looks like an elephant. Sounds like an elephant. Smells like an elephant. Probably an elephant. Experienced clinicians often use pattern recognition to guide diagnosis. As a student, you will begin to do this rapidly for conditions that you will encounter frequently—chances are that, by now, you easily recognized that the 62-year-old diabetic male mentioned above was having a myocardial infarction. Pattern recognition is useful

Step 1: What could it be?	Step 2: What is most likely? What must I exclude (*)?	Step 3: Key clues on history?	Step 4: Key clues on examination?	Step 5: Key clues on basic investigations?	Step 6: Patient improving with management?
Acute coronary syndrome Pneumothorax Aortic dissection Boerhaave's perforation Peptic ulcer disease Stable angina Musculoskeletal Oesophagitis (e.g. due to reflux) Oesophageal spasm Pulmonary embolism Pleurisy (secondary to infection) Anxiety Myopericarditis Aortic aneurysm Coronary spasm Cholecystitis Pancreatitis	**Acute coronary syndrome*** Pneumothorax* Aortic dissection* Boerhaave's perforation* Peptic ulcer disease **Stable angina*** **Musculoskeletal** Oesophagitis Oesophageal spasm **Pulmonary embolism*** Pleurisy **Anxiety** Myopericarditis Aortic aneurysm Coronary spasm Cholecystitis Pancreatitis	Acute coronary syndrome* Pneumothorax* Aortic dissection* Boerhaave's perforation* Peptic ulcer disease Stable angina* Musculoskeletal Oesophagitis Oesophageal spasm **Pulmonary embolism*** Pleurisy Anxiety Myopericarditis Aortic aneurysm Coronary spasm Cholecystitis Pancreatitis	Acute coronary syndrome* **Pneumothorax*** Aortic dissection* Boerhaave's perforation* Peptic ulcer disease Stable angina* Musculoskeletal Oesophagitis Oesophageal spasm Pulmonary embolism* Pleurisy Anxiety Myopericarditis Aortic aneurysm Coronary spasm Cholecystitis Pancreatitis	Acute coronary syndrome* **Pneumothorax*** Aortic dissection* Boerhaave's perforation* Peptic ulcer disease Stable angina* Musculoskeletal Oesophagitis Oesophageal spasm Pulmonary embolism* Pleurisy Anxiety Myopericarditis Aortic aneurysm Coronary spasm Cholecystitis Pancreatitis	Acute coronary syndrome* **Pneumothorax*** Aortic dissection* Boerhaave's perforation* Peptic ulcer disease Stable angina* Musculoskeletal Oesophagitis Oesophageal spasm Pulmonary embolism* Pleurisy Anxiety Myopericarditis Aortic aneurysm Coronary spasm Cholecystitis Pancreatitis
50-year-old male with chest pain	50-year-old male with chest pain	50-year-old male with sharp, left-sided chest pain, came on suddenly whilst watching TV. Smoker with known COPD. No risk factors for venous thrombosis.	Upper left zone of chest is hyper-resonant with reduced air entry and reduced vocal resonance. Chest not tender to palpation. No signs of DVT in calves.	Chest radiograph shows air in pleural space on left, with lung collapsing away from the upper left apex.	Patient improves after insertion of a chest drain for pneumothorax. Chest pain resolves completely.

Figure 0.1 A stepwise approach to clinical diagnosis.

and efficient, and we have tried to illustrate stereotypical presentations of some diseases in our short cases.

Looks like a crocodile. Sounds like a crocodile. Smells like a crocodile… but is actually an alligator. Pattern recognition is a problem when a disease presents in a way that mimics another disease. For example, patients with oesophageal spasm may describe the same pain as those with an acute coronary syndrome. Such diagnostic puzzles are the stuff that hospital grand rounds and television shows are made of. But misdiagnosis due to (incorrect) pattern recognition can have disastrous consequences—you could inadvertently thrombolyse a patient you thought was having a myocardial infarction but actually had an aortic dissection. This is one reason why it is important to always follow a logical diagnostic approach.

Looks like an elephant. Sounds like a lion. Not sure what it smells like. Must be a… ? You cannot recognize a pattern you have never seen before, an especially big problem for the inexperienced medical student starting a clinical placement. On other occasions, the symptoms may not fit any known pattern, and even experienced clinicians may struggle initially with the diagnosis. This is another reason for having a logical diagnostic approach.

A logical approach to diagnosis

Below is an outline of the diagnostic strategy we have used throughout this book. We recognize that, over time, everyone develops their own diagnostic strategy and that tutors may teach you differing approaches. This is simply one that has worked for us.

'50-year-old male with chest pain'. It is tempting to assume that he is having a myocardial infarction, like the 62-year-old diabetic male mentioned above. However,…

- **Step 1:** Think of all the things that could cause this presentation. Use anatomy, a surgical sieve (e.g. INVITED MD), etc. to come up with as long a list as possible.

- **Step 2:** Highlight from your list the most common causes. For example, acute coronary syndrome is a common cause of chest pain, viral costochondritis is not. Mark the ones that you *must* exclude because they are lethal. In the case of chest pain, Boerhaave's perforation of the oesophagus is important as, if untreated, it carries a 100% mortality.

- **Step 3:** Think of key clues in the patient history for each of the diagnoses. For example, patients with Boerhaave's perforation of the oesophagus invariably give a history of vomiting immediately before onset of the pain. Now take a history that deliberately tries to pick up these clues, rather than just going through a set of 'standard' questions which may miss things. Also consider the patient themselves (e.g. their age, occupation, etc.) and how this affects the relative likelihoods of your differential diagnoses. *Has the patient's history or epidemiological factors made any diagnoses more/less likely?*

- **Step 4:** Think of key clues on examination for your diagnoses. For example, patients with a pneumothorax will have an area of the chest that is hyperexpanded, hyperresonant to percussion, with absent breath sounds. Perform a thorough examination looking for these clues. *Have your examination findings made any diagnoses more/ less likely?*

- **Step 5:** Don't order a set of 'standard' investigations. Think about those investigations that will help confirm or dismiss each diagnosis. Also include those that are relevant for management. Thus urea and electrolytes are necessary if a patient is put nil by mouth and on intravenous fluids, or started on drugs that are renally excreted or potentially nephrotoxic. Try to prioritize investigations into those that are more readily available (e.g. an MRI head scan is not a viable option for everyone who presents with a fall). Also think about which investigations are safe for this patient—is radiation exposure necessary, is the woman pregnant, do they have contraindications to MRI? *Then ask yourself, have your investigation results made any diagnoses more/less likely?*

- **Step 6:** Always try to confirm your diagnosis. *Is the patient getting better with your management for your proposed diagnosis? If not, why not?*

What this book *is* about

✓ **Common acute presentations**: We cover 29 of the most common patient presentations in acute general medicine (internal medicine for our American readers) and general surgery. These reflect both the general medical and surgical syllabus at UK medical schools and those presentations that you are most likely to encounter during clinical attachments.

✓ **Diagnostic strategy**: This book is primarily a diagnostic manual. It should equip the student with a framework for thinking about the most common general medical and surgical presentations.

✓ **Pattern recognition**: The cases are loosely based on real clinical scenarios, although any likeness to a particular patient or individual is unintended. Some cases represent stereotypical presentations of diseases, from which the student may begin to pick up pattern recognition skills. Others illustrate more unusual presentations, and are designed to keep readers on their toes and remind them to keep an open mind at all times.

✓ **Basic management**: For completeness, we include a discussion of the basic management for many of the diseases featured in the cases. Points on management cover the core knowledge expected of a medical student but are necessarily brief. We have tried to highlight areas of contention, and to refer to landmark trials and guidelines where relevant. Some of this is covered under our 'viva questions'.

What this book is *not* about

✗ **Every possible diagnosis:** It is not logistically possible to condense the entirety of the medical and surgical syllabus into a book of this style—indeed, such an attempt would run counter to the aims of this book. Our aim is to cover the most *common* presentations, and in so doing we also cover the most common diagnoses. We are fully aware that many diagnoses are not covered. But our hope is that we have provided a framework that will enable the reader to exclude the more common conditions, and be able to deal intelligently with clinical conundrums. The reader should be equipped to recognize the salient features of the case in question, and know when to ask for specialist help. A case-based book which attempted to cover all possible diagnoses which may be encountered would not only be so long as to be unwieldy, but would also run the risk of suggesting that pattern recognition is a surrogate for a rational diagnostic strategy.

✗ **Basic sciences and clinical skills:** This book does not aim to teach disease pathology or how to take a history, examine a patient, and how to interpret basic investigations (biochemistry, haematology, radiology). However, we believe that this book can be fruitfully read alongside books and teaching about basic science and clinical skills.

✗ **Specialities**: It should also be noted that the cases covered reflect only a selection, albeit a broad one, of the diseases and presentations that a medical student needs to cover. The bulk of the omissions relate to the specialities (e.g. obstetrics and gynaecology, paediatrics, ear, nose, and throat, ophthalmology, etc.) and general practice (family medicine).

✗ **Epidemiology**: This book does not contain detailed epidemiological data on the exact likelihood of diagnoses, because such data are rarely available and hardly memorable. Instead, we consider diagnoses to be either 'common', 'occasional', or 'very rare'. This is based on data, where available, or the cumulative experience of our senior reviewers (all of them consultants of many years' standing).

✗ **Detailed management**: This book does not focus on drug doses, surgical techniques, or other details of management, because these can already be found in other textbooks.

How to use this book

- **A workbook, not a reference text**: This is intended to be an exercise text where you 'learn by doing'. Try to cover up the answers and work through the text (without cheating!) to get the most out of it.

- **Find a presentation**: We have structured this book by presenting complaint, rather than pathology, because patients present with 'chest pain' rather than 'aortic dissection'. For ease of reference there is also an index by disease. Each chapter can be read individually, so the student can read those that relate to the presentation they last encountered or that was most recently discussed. Every chapter contains a core case, short cases, and viva questions, in that order.

- **Core case**: Each core case is a clinical problem that walks you through the diagnostic approach. The information the clerking doctor might receive is provided in an initial box, followed by a question. The answer follows, with another section with clinical information and another question, and so on.

- **Short cases**: The short case 'vignettes' are designed to highlight some of the other conditions that can present in a similar manner (indeed, with the same symptom). They will help develop your 'pattern recognition' of some diseases, but also remind you that pathologies can masquerade as one another, hence the need for a logical approach.

- **Viva questions**: These questions are designed to test aspects of anatomy, pharmacology, physiology, etc. related to the cases. We hope they will prepare the reader for the inevitable quizzing that occurs on teaching ward rounds or in theatres/operating rooms.

- **Single Best Answer questions**: A handful of single best answer (SBA) questions, a format commonly used in medical school written exams, are also included at the end of each chapter.

- **Differential diagnosis**: Font sizes in a differential diagnosis figure illustrate how likely a diagnosis **is** (or isn't).

- **Important points**: Important points are in **bold** text or indicated with this symbol Δ .

Headache

Core cases

Read through the sections in the case boxes, covering up the sections that follow so that you don't see the answer. At the end of each case box, try to answer the question before reading on.

Mr Lennon is a 74-year-old man referred to the hospital by his general practitioner (GP) because of a severe headache.

Headache is a common symptom with many causes. It is essential to rule out the sinister causes first, i.e. those that require urgent investigation and management because if left untreated they cause lasting damage and/or mortality.

What sinister causes must you rule out?

The sinister causes can be remembered using the mnemonic VIVID:

Vascular: subarachnoid haemorrhage (SAH), haematoma (subdural or extradural), cerebral venous sinus thrombosis, cerebellar infarct

Infection: meningitis, encephalitis

Vision-threatening: temporal arteritis,[†] acute glaucoma, cavernous sinus thrombosis, pituitary apoplexy, posterior leucoencephalopathy

Intracranial pressure (raised): space-occupying lesion (SOL; e.g. tumour, abscess, cyst), cerebral oedema (e.g. trauma, altitude), hydrocephalus, malignant hypertension, idiopathic intracranial hypertension

Dissection: carotid dissection

Taking a good history is key to any diagnosis, but particularly so when tackling headache as the symptom is so subjective and examination findings are often unhelpful.

With a mental list of the sinister causes, what questions will you ask first in the history? What 'red flags' will help you exclude the sinister causes?

The approach to headache is the same as that to pain anywhere in the body: you need to start by characterizing the pain. One useful way of doing this is by following another mnemonic, SOCRATES:

Site of pain, and has it moved since it began?

Onset of pain—was it sudden or gradual, and did something trigger it?

Character of pain—throbbing, dull ache, sharp stabbing?

Radiation of pain—has the pain spread?

---

† Note that temporal arteritis is another name for giant cell arteritis, a systemic vasculitis. The term 'temporal arteritis' is more common when headache is the presenting symptom.

Attenuating factors—does anything make the pain better (e.g. position, medications)?

Timing of pain—how long has it gone on for, has it been constant or coming and going? Is it worse at a particular time of the day?

Exacerbating factors—does anything make the pain worse (e.g. lying down, standing up, coughing, fatigue)?

Severity—on a scale of 0 to 10, where 10 is the worst pain ever (e.g. childbirth).

In addition, you should enquire about the presence or absence of the following 'red flags':

- **Decreased level of consciousness.** This is a worrying feature of any medical presentation. Combined with headache, SAH needs exclusion. If there is a history of **head injury**, it could suggest a subdural haematoma (fluctuating consciousness) or extradural haematoma (altered consciousness following a lucid interval). Meningitis and encephalitis can also affect consciousness.

- **Sudden onset, worst headache ever.** Suggests SAH, with blood in the cerebrospinal fluid (CSF) irritating the meninges. It can be informative to ask the patient whether they remember the *exact* moment when the headache started—a very severe headache of almost instantaneous onset is characteristic of SAH. Patients describe it like, for example, 'being hit on the back of the head with a bat'.

- **Seizure(s) or focal neurological deficit** (e.g. limb weakness, speech difficulties). Suggests intracranial pathology, although a migrainous aura can give neurological signs.

- **Absence of previous episodes.** Recurrent episodes are usually less sinister. A new onset of headache suggests a new pathology. In someone over 50 years old, a new-onset headache should raise your suspicions of temporal arteritis.

- **Reduced visual acuity.** Temporal arteritis is more common in older patients. Transient blindness (amaurosis fugax) is usually due to a transient ischaemic attack (TIA), but these rarely produce a headache. In the context of headaches, loss of vision can be due to the causes listed above (using the acronym VIVID). If you are concerned about temporal arteritis, ask about jaw claudication and scalp tenderness. If you are concerned about carotid or vertebral artery dissection, ask about minor neck trauma (e.g. yoga, recent neck chiropractic manipulation).

- **Persistent headache, worse when lying down,** and coupled with **early morning nausea.** Suggests raised intracranial pressure. This is worse when lying flat for prolonged times (e.g. overnight) as our intracranial pressure rises when we lie down, but can even occur when the patient is bending over. Headaches that are worse when standing up suggested *reduced* intracranial pressure and are common after a lumbar puncture (LP), but these are *not* sinister (most resolve with analgesia, time, and lying down during the headache).

- **Progressive, persistent headache.** This could be an expanding SOL (e.g. tumour, abscess, cyst, haematoma).

- **Constitutional symptoms.** Weight loss, night sweats, and/or fever may suggest malignancy, chronic infection (e.g. tuberculosis), or chronic inflammation (e.g. temporal arteritis).

- **Past medical history.** A history of a malignancy that is known to metastasize to the brain (e.g. lung, breast). Also a history of HIV or other immunosuppression (e.g. transplant patients), resulting in a higher risk of intracranial infection (e.g. toxoplasmosis, abscess, tuberculosis).

You start by characterizing Mr Lennon's headache. He tells you the pain is on the right side of his head and hasn't ever moved. It started 4 days ago, since when it has been getting worse. He can only characterize it as intense. He has tried over-the-counter analgesics with no benefit, and when asked specifically, says there is no change with position or time of day.

He has had no changes in consciousness, nor seizures, that he is aware of. When asked about other symptoms, he tells you he has found it hard to eat and open his mouth properly since yesterday because of jaw pain. He has not noticed any constitutional symptoms, and he hasn't noticed any change in vision. He has never had anything like this before.

How does this information help focus the differential diagnosis and your approach?

Mr Lennon gives a good description of his headache. The gradual onset over 4 days makes a number of the more sinister causes less likely, specifically SAH. In addition, one of the red flags is present: a new-onset headache in someone older than 50. In such presentations, particularly given suggestive symptoms like possible jaw claudication, your priority is to exclude temporal arteritis.

You have begun to narrow your diagnosis, but you still want to exclude sinister causes with your examination and investigations.

What signs will you look for on clinical examination?

Basic observations

- **Altered consciousness.** Assess Mr Lennon's Glasgow Coma Scale (GCS) score, although it is likely to already be obvious from the history-taking. The significance of altered consciousness is discussed earlier.
- **Blood pressure and pulse.** Check for malignant hypertension.
- **Temperature.** Fever and headache suggest intracranial infection.

Focal neurological signs

Note that the following list is not exhaustive.

- **Focal limb deficit.** Makes intracranial pathology more likely.
- **Third nerve palsy.** This consists of ptosis (droopy eyelid), mydriasis (dilated pupil), and an eye that is deviated down and out. One cause is an SAH due to a ruptured aneurysm of the posterior communicating artery (PCOM). PCOM aneurysms are a cause of headache.
- **Sixth nerve palsy.** Convergent squint and/or failure to abduct the eye laterally. This nerve can be compressed either directly by a mass or indirectly by raised intracranial pressure. Remember that the sixth nerve has the longest intracranial course and is therefore most likely to get compressed at some point.
- **Twelfth nerve palsy.** Look for tongue deviation. A twelfth nerve palsy can arise from a carotid artery dissection.
- **Horner's syndrome.** Triad of partial ptosis, miosis (constricted pupil), and anhydrosis (dry skin around the orbit). Results from interruption of the ipsilateral sympathetic pathway. In the context of our differential diagnosis, Horner's syndrome should raise suspicions of a carotid artery dissection (ask about neck pain) or cavernous sinus lesion.

Eye inspection

- **Exophthalmos?** This may indicate a retro-orbital process such as cavernous sinus thrombosis.
- **Cloudy cornea? Fixed, dilated/oval pupil?** This may suggest acute glaucoma.
- **Optic disc appearance on fundoscopy.** Look for papilloedema, indicating raised intracranial pressure.

Other

- **Reduced visual acuity.** This can suggest acute glaucoma or temporal arteritis, for example.
- **Scalp tenderness.** Classically seen in temporal arteritis.
- **Meningism.** Check whether the patient has a stiff neck or photophobia, suggesting meningism due to infection or SAH.

On examination, Mr Lennon is not obviously photophobic as he is sitting in a well-lit environment. His heart rate is 84 beats/min (bpm), his blood pressure is 134/81 mmHg, and his temperature 36.5 °C. Examination of his cranial nerves reveals reduced visual acuity in his right eye but not his left, which he previously hadn't noticed. Fundoscopy is normal. The rest of his cranial nerves are intact but you do notice that his right scalp is tender to light touch. There are no limb signs and no neck stiffness.

Mr Lennon is an elderly man with a 4-day history of new-onset right-sided temporal headache, possibly jaw claudication, a right-sided decrease in visual acuity, and a tender scalp.

What is the most likely diagnosis? What is the pathology, and why is it an emergency?

Mr Lennon's history and clinical features are highly suggestive of **temporal arteritis** (aka giant cell arteritis, GCA). This is a disease of unknown aetiology that typically appears in patients over 50 years of age. It is characterized by the formation of immune, inflammatory granulomas in the tunica media of medium/large-sized arteries. The inflammation (or thrombosis or spasm induced by it) can be sufficient to block the lumen of medium-sized arteries affected by this disease. Inflammation of the mandibular branch of the external carotid artery causes jaw claudication. Inflammation of the superficial temporal branch of the external carotid artery causes headache and scalp tenderness. Inflammation of the posterior ciliary arteries causes visual disturbances, due to ischaemia to either the retina (blurring, visual field loss) or the optic motor muscles (double vision = diplopia).

The reason to worry about this presentation is that with visual loss in one eye the other eye is at risk without prompt treatment. Temporal arteritis with visual disturbance is therefore an **ophthalmological emergency** and patients should be referred to the on-call ophthalmologist as soon as possible. Unfortunately, visual loss prior to arrival at hospital is unlikely to be reversible regardless of treatment.

How will you proceed in light of your working diagnosis?

Having taken a full history and examined the patient, you should arrange only first-line investigations that are quick to do—such as blood tests to demonstrate an **elevated erythrocyte sedimentation rate (ESR) and C-reactive protein (CRP)** that would be consistent with a systemic inflammation such as temporal arteritis. Management should then aim to reduce the immune-mediated inflammation that is causing the ischaemia in Mr Lennon's arteries and the best way to do this is using **high-dose corti-costeroids**. The principal reason for urgent treatment of temporal arteritis is to protect the vision in the fellow, unaffected eye, rather than aiming to restore vision to the affected eye.

Once initial treatment is under way, more time-consuming investigations can be arranged to help confirm the diagnosis and rule out alternatives. In this case, a **temporal artery biopsy** could be arranged to help confirm the diagnosis as it may show granulomas in temporal arteritis. However, the interrupted nature of the granulomas means they can be missed on the biopsy. Also, a biopsy is not strictly neces-sary as the American College of Rheumatology guidelines suggest only 3 of the following 5 criteria need be present to diagnose temporal arteritis:

- Age of onset of symptoms >50 years
- New headache
- ESR >50 mm/h
- Clinically abnormal temporal artery (tender or non-pulsatile)
- Biopsy of temporal artery showing mononuclear cell infiltration or granuloma.

As Mr Lennon is over 50 years old, has a new headache and a tender temporal artery, he doesn't strictly need a biopsy to diagnose temporal arteritis.

Mr Lennon's 40-year-old daughter has come to see her father. You have explained that you think he has temporal arteritis, an inflammation of some of the blood vessels supplying his head. Miss Lennon is now worried that she may have the same problem as she also frequently gets headaches.

You ask her to characterize the headache using SOCRATES. She tells you the headaches only affect the right side of her head. They come on over half an hour, and make her feel nauseated and sensitive to bright light and noise. She only finds relief by hiding in a dark room and getting some sleep. They last hours, but less than a day, and are relatively infrequent, occurring three or four times a year since her early twenties. You also ask about the red flags, none of which are present.

The lack of red flags makes a sinister cause of headache unlikely. But there are several non-sinister syndromes that cause headache. These syndromes are not 'benign' because they cause significant morbidity (in the form of pain). However, they are unlikely to cause lasting damage or mortality in the short term.

What different types of non-sinister headache are there?

Causes of non-sinister headache are listed in Figure 1.1.

Tension-type headache
Migraine
Sinusitis
Medication overuse headache

Temporomandibular joint (TMJ) dysfunction syndrome (TMJ syndrome)

Trigeminal neuralgia

Cluster headache

Figure 1.1 Causes of non-sinister headache.

Some of these are 'primary headaches' because the symptom (headache) is primary, i.e. if the headaches were removed there would be no harmful pathology. This is in contrast to 'secondary headaches', where the headache is only one of many possible symptoms that result from pathology such as head trauma, intracranial lesion (e.g. tumour), vascular lesion (e.g. SAH), or infection. The following are secondary headaches: sinusitis, medication overuse headache, and temporomandibular joint (TMJ) syndrome. Sinusitis and TMJ syndrome cannot be diagnosed in the absence of additional symptoms. A diagnosis of medication overuse headache can only be made in patients using analgesic and/or migraine medication.

In addition to the pain history (e.g. SOCRATES), what questions should you ask to characterize non-sinister headaches?

- **Does the patient suffer from different types of headache?** If so, separate histories will be needed for each as they may reflect distinct syndromes. Thus patients with migraine are also vulnerable to medication overuse headaches from the treatment for their migraine.

- **Are there any predisposing (trigger) factors?** Factors such as stress and fatigue are known triggers for tension headaches and migraines. Some migraine sufferers point to certain foods as triggers (e.g. cheese, caffeine), and alcohol can trigger cluster headaches.

- **How disabling are the headaches?** Migraines render many sufferers incapable of performing even the activities of daily living for around a day. Cluster headaches are severely painful and disabling but often occur at night, allowing daytime duties to continue. Tension-type headaches usually allow normal activities to be continued.

- **Does the patient get an 'aura' before the headache?** Auras are usually visual phenomena, although focal neurological deficits (e.g. limb weakness) are sometimes present. About a third of migraine sufferers report auras as a feature of their migraines.

Going back to the list of differential diagnoses in Figure 1.1, what are the key features of each diagnosis in the history?

- **Tension-type headaches.** Very common. Often bifrontal pain. They are episodic, occurring with variable frequency. The pain is described as pressure or tightness around the head like a tightening band. Other than the headache there are no other features (e.g. no photophobia). The headaches last no more than a few hours and are not severely disabling. However, in rare cases they may occur almost daily, in which case they become disabling. Stress and fatigue are well-known trigger factors.

- **Migraine.** Common, although not as common as tension headaches, and twice as common in women as in men. Migraines are stereotyped, i.e. attacks exhibit the same pattern of symptoms and become recognizable to patients. They are typically unilateral (migraine is a corruption of the Latin (*he*)*mi-cranium*). Associated with an aura in about a third of sufferers (**migraine with aura** or **classical migraine**, as opposed to **migraine without aura** or **common migraine**). The pain is described as throbbing or pulsatile. There is sensitivity to light, sound, and even smell, and nausea can also be a feature. Migraines last between 4 and 72 hours, unless successfully treated. Some patients suffer from **aura without migraine**. Such attacks are in the differential for TIAs (particularly in older patients) and epilepsy.

- **Sinusitis.** Patients usually report facial pain coming on over hours to days in conjunction with coryzal symptoms. The pain is tight, as in tension headaches, and is often exacerbated by movement. The headaches last several days, with a time course consistent with the infection. The headaches are moderately severe but not disabling. However, patients with chronic sinusitis may find the headaches frequent enough to interfere with their daily activities.

- **Medication overuse.** Surprisingly common, particularly in women (about fivefold the incidence in men). This is seen particularly with migraine medications and analgesics. The headaches experienced resemble either migraine or tension-type headaches. Most patients will be taking very large quantities of analgesic medication. It is often difficult for patients to accept that the over-treatment of headache is actually the cause of their ongoing headaches. Treatment consists of withdrawal from analgesic use, which often results in a period of exacerbation before improvement occurs.

- **TMJ syndrome.** Most common in individuals aged 20–40, and four times more prevalent in women. As well as headache, patients get a dull ache in the muscles of mastication that may radiate to the jaw and/or ear. Patients also often report hearing a 'click' or grinding noise when they move their jaw.

- **Trigeminal neuralgia.** A rare condition, occurring more often in women, with a typical age of onset around 60–70 years. Patients complain of unilateral stabbing, sharp facial pain involving one or more of the divisions of the trigeminal nerve. The pain lasts only seconds, and can be triggered by eating, laughing, talking or touching the affected area. Although attacks last seconds, there may be several or even hundreds a day and patients can develop a longer-lasting background pain. Patients often avoid known triggers like shaving. Interestingly, attacks rarely occur during sleep, unlike migraine or cluster headaches.

- **Cluster headache.** Predominantly affects men. The headaches occur in 'clusters' for about 6-12 weeks every 1-2 years, hence the name. Attacks tend to occur at exactly the same time every day or night, like an alarm clock going off. The pain is focused over one eye. The pain is intense and causes the patient to wake up and can be so severe that suicide is contemplated, until the pain diminishes, around 20-30 minutes later. They will probably have a red, watery eye, rhinorrhoea, and Horner's syndrome, suggested by the patient noticing a droopy eyelid (ptosis) during attacks. These headaches are very disabling.

> You ask Miss Lennon the additional questions listed earlier. She tells you she sometimes gets 'normal' headaches, which respond to paracetamol, but it is these other headaches that she worries about. When you ask about any 'aura' or visual disturbance, she tells you they are often preceded by seeing a small black spot with bright, zigzagging lines. When she has a headache, she has to stay in bed all day until it goes, but will be fit and well the day after.
>
> **What is the most likely diagnosis, given Miss Lennon's history?**

It may be tempting to dismiss Miss Lennon's headaches as tension headaches, which almost everyone experiences at some point. However, Miss Lennon describes a *unilateral* headache that makes her feel sick, photophobic, phonophobic, and is preceded by a visual phenomena (zigzag lines). It is therefore very likely that Miss Lennon suffers from **migraine with aura**.

Migraine affects about 15% of the population, but many do not seek help as they think there is no treatment. This is not true, as acute abortive treatment including triptans ($5HT_1$-agonists such as sumatriptan), analgesics (aspirin, paracetamol), and antiemetics (metoclopramide) have been shown to be highly effective if the patient takes them as soon as they feel a migraine coming on—something that most migraine sufferers recognize easily. Preventive treatments are only useful with high frequencies of attacks (e.g. fortnightly) and will usually only reduce migraine frequency by 50%.

> **Should you examine Miss Lennon and, if so, what would you look for? Should you order any investigations and, if so, which?**

All of the non-sinister causes of headache are diagnosed on history. However, you should conduct a physical examination, both to provide the patient with reassurance and to look for:

- **Blood pressure,** to exclude malignant hypertension.
- **Head and neck examination** for muscle tenderness, stiffness, or limited movement—which can occasionally mimic tension-type headaches. If present, such findings may need treatment in order to relieve the headache.
- **Focal neurological signs.** The presence of focal neurological signs in somebody with headache should alert you to intracranial pathology.
- **Fundoscopy,** to exclude raised intracranial pressure.

Investigations are only ever indicated where warranted by the history and examination and should not be ordered routinely.

Short cases

Mrs Harrison is a 42-year-old woman who presents to the Emergency Department complaining of a severe headache and nausea. She has a history of migraine attacks but this time she says it is different—it came on suddenly after dinner, without warning, and felt as if someone had hit her on the back of the head. Her husband, annoyed at having to drive her to the hospital in the middle of the night, cynically thinks she is just having 'a bad migraine'.

What is the likely diagnosis? What key investigation should be requested?

Patients know their disease better than any doctor, so if a patient tells you that something doesn't feel like what they normally have (e.g. migraines in this case), take them seriously. You should take a full history and examine the patient for key signs as discussed in the main case (e.g. neck stiffness suggesting meningism). But the history given is classic for a **subarachnoid haemorrhage (SAH)**, so you should arrange an urgent **CT head scan**, looking for blood in the CSF (fresh blood appears bright on CT, for example in the Sylvian fissures). Studies have shown[1] that if the CT scan is performed within 6 hours of onset using a multirow, high-resolution, third-generation CT scanner, the sensitivity and specificity for detecting an SAH are 100%. Older scanners or those done beyond 6 hours risk missing small bleeds, so if the CT scan is negative in such cases one should do an LP at 12 hours post headache looking for xanthochromia (yellow CSF due to bilirubin content from breakdown of subarachnoid blood). Xanthochromia in the CSF remains a reliable test for SAH for up to 12 days post headache (12 hour to 12 day rule).

If the CT confirms an SAH, Mrs Harrison will need urgent referral to a neurosurgical unit. Patients are initially managed with regular **nimodipine** (a calcium channel blocker that reduces spasm of the ruptured cerebral artery, thus preventing ischaemia, i.e. a stroke) and bed rest at 30–45° supine.

If she survives and her symptoms improve, she should receive cerebral angiography to find the source of a bleed—usually a ruptured aneurysm. The neuroradiologist will usually be able to insert a platinum coil to cause the aneurysm to clot, scar, and heal. Coiling has been shown by the **ISAT study**[2] to have fewer complications than surgically clipping the aneurysm via an open craniotomy. The family should be made aware that SAH carries a high risk of mortality and morbidity: 50% of patients die before arriving at hospital; a further 17% die in hospital; another 17% survive but with lasting neurological deficits; and only 17% survive without any sequelae.

Mr McCartney is a 32-year-old salesman who is worried that he might be having repeated 'mini-strokes' (TIAs), like his father. He says that every couple of months he suffers from an attack where he sees a shimmering light in the corner of his eyes and gets a ringing in his ears. This usually occurs towards the end of the day, lasting half an hour. He is fully conscious throughout and never feels dazed or confused afterwards.

Could this gentleman be suffering from TIAs like his father?

TIAs and strokes are caused by areas of the brain ceasing to function due to a lack of blood (because of an embolism or haemorrhage) and are therefore characterized by 'negative', *loss-of-function*, symptoms and signs (loss of vision, numbness, loss of power in muscles). In contrast, epilepsy is caused by over-activation of areas of the brain and thus produces 'positive', *gain-of-function*, symptoms and signs (flashing lights, muscle convulsions, odd sensations in the skin). Migraine can produce both negative and positive symptoms. This gentleman describes clear gain-of-function symptoms (shimmering light, noises) that are more suggestive of epilepsy or migraine.

It could be epilepsy, but seizures tend to be followed by a postictal phase where the patient is exhausted and sometimes confused. It is therefore more likely to be a case of **migraine aura without headache**. A characteristic feature is a slow march of symptoms (e.g. visual disturbance affecting more and more of the visual field) then resolution in a similar fashion. Migraine without aura is an odd condition where patients experience the aura signs of typical migraine patients (e.g. shimmering lights with zigzagging edges, noises) but without the headache. One can reassure the patient that his symptoms are almost certainly not 'mini-strokes' but more likely due to a type of migraine without headaches. The patient may wish to have a trial of antimigraine medication as soon as one of these attacks starts (e.g. sumatriptan) or prophylactic medication to prevent it occurring (e.g. propranolol) and see if they help.

SHORT CASE

Ringo is a 16-year-old who presents with a runny nose and headache. He has been blowing out green mucus from his nose for a few days but has come to see you because the headache, which is located above his eyes, is now very bad. His nasal septum is slightly deviated and his forehead is indeed tender to gentle tapping.

Can we send this patient home on analgesia and rest?

It is possible that this young man simply has a viral rhinosinusitis, but the green mucus and the highly localized pain above his eyes suggest he may have developed an infection of his frontal sinuses.

Sinusitis usually affects the maxillary sinus and resolves spontaneously, occasionally needing a helping hand from antibiotics (e.g. amoxicillin) if it fails to resolve. However, **frontal sinusitis** can be particularly dangerous because it is possible for the bacteria to erode backwards into the brain, causing meningitis or a brain abscess. For this reason, a suspected case of frontal sinusitis should be taken seriously and referred to ear, nose & throat (ENT) specialists who can arrange a CT head scan to check if either frontal sinus is affected. If it is, he will need antibiotics and draining of the frontal sinuses (antral lavage). It is possible that his deviated nasal septum is predisposing him to episodes of sinusitis and, if so, he could benefit from a rearrangement of his nasal septum (septoplasty).

SHORT CASE

A 10-year-old girl is referred to the hospital by her GP for persistent headache in the occipital area that is worse in the morning. The parents have also noticed that she has become clumsy over the last few months. As part of your cranial nerve examination you perform fundoscopy, where you see the result shown in Figure 1.2.

Figure 1.2 Fundoscopic view of the patient's retina.

Reproduced with kind permission of Dr Neda Minakaran, Specialist Registrar in Ophthalmology, Imperial College Healthcare NHS Trust.

What is your next step?

The appearance of the optic disc (poorly defined margins) is suggestive of **papilloedema**, potentially due to raised intracranial pressure. This would be consistent with headaches which are worse in the morning. One cause of raised intracranial pressure is a brain tumour, and in children most brain tumours are found in the posterior fossa that would explain the occipital headache. In addition, the most common type of tumour in children is a medulloblastoma in the cerebellum, which may explain her clumsiness. Thus you must rule out a **central nervous system (CNS) tumour** as the problem in this child. An urgent **head MRI scan** should therefore be requested.

If a tumour is found, the neurosurgeon will use dexamethasone to reduce the brain inflammation (improving the headache) and discuss the surgical options to remove the tumour with the family.

References

1 Perry JJ, Stiell IG, Sivilotti MLA, et al. Sensitivity of computed tomography performed within six hours of onset of headache for diagnosis of subarachnoid haemorrhage: prospective cohort study. *BMJ* 2011;**343**: d4277.
2 Molyneux AJ, Kerr RS, Yu LM, et al. International subarachnoid aneurysm trial (ISAT) of neurosurgical clipping versus endovascular coiling in 2143 patients with ruptured intracranial aneurysms: a randomised comparison of effects on survival, dependency, seizures, rebleeding, subgroups, and aneurysm occlusion. *Lancet* 2005;**366**: 809-817.

Viva questions

What are the main causes of SAH?

The main causes of SAH are:

- **Rupture of an arterial aneurysm,** usually a 'berry aneurysm' at the junction between arteries of the circle of Willis (~45%)
- **Trauma** (~45%)
- **Arteriovenous malformations,** rupture of haemangiomas,' rupture of cerebral vein around the brainstem (~10%)

What is your differential diagnosis for intracranial tumours?

The list of possible intracranial tumours is very long but the most common are:

- **Secondary brain tumours (metastatic).** These are the *most common type of brain tumours* in adults, accounting for ~90% of all intracranial tumours. The five most common sources of primary cancer metastasizing to the brain are lung, kidney, breast, melanoma, and colon.
- **Primary brain tumours.** These can be divided into axial (within the brain parenchyma) and extra-axial:
  - **Axial or neuroepithelial tumours (~50%).** These are tumours of the brain matter itself. They include (the latter three are more common in children):
    Astrocytomas (glioblastoma multiforme is a grade 4 astrocytoma)
    Ependymomas
    Oligodendrogliomas
    Medulloblastomas
  - **Extra-axial:**
    Meningioma (~15%). A slow-growing tumour of the meninges that compresses the brain. Often associated with neurofibromatosis type II (inherited predisposition to schwannomas and meningiomas), these tumours can usually be surgically removed with good prognosis.
    Vestibular schwannoma. Previously and incorrectly called an 'acoustic neuroma', this type of tumour is relatively common in young adults. It may compress cranial nerve VIII (hearing loss) and VII (facial palsy).
    Pituitary adenomas, prolactinomas, and craniopharyngiomas
    Other: choroid plexus papillomas, haemangiomas, pineal gland tumours, etc.

At what level of the spine should you insert a needle during an adult LP? What are the surface anatomy landmarks? What structures do you pass through as you perform an LP?

The spinal cord in adults ends at L1/L2, with peripheral nerves extending beyond that as a loose bundle of nerve fibres floating in CSF (the cauda equina, literally the 'horse's tail'). Modern studies

CONTINUED ➤

CONTINUED

have shown that in children the spinal cord ends only slightly lower (L2/L3) but certainly not as low as many older textbooks claim. A safe place to insert the needle is thus at or below L3/L4. This can be found by tracing a line between the posterior superior iliac crests (Tuffier's line), which marks the L4/L5 space.

The following structures are sequentially traversed as you perform an LP:

- Skin
- Subcutis
- Supraspinous ligament
- Interspinous ligament
- Ligamentum flavum (first 'give' as you push the needle)
- Dura mater (second 'give' as you push the needle)
- Arachnoid space—the destination

What are the indications, contraindications, and risks of an LP?

Indications

- **Diagnostic LP:** looking for oligoclonal bands (e.g. multiple sclerosis), high protein (Guillain–Barré syndrome), blood or bilirubin (e.g. SAH), pathogens (e.g. bacterial meningitis, viral encephalitis), malignant cells (e.g. CNS lymphoma), or a rapid improvement in gait and cognitive function after removal of 30 mL of CSF (e.g. normal pressure hydrocephalus).
- **Therapeutic LP:** intrathecal drug administration (e.g. haematological malignancy in children), temporary reduction in intracranial pressure (e.g. idiopathic intracranial hypertension).

Relative contraindications

- **Raised intracranial pressure** due to an SOL, as the sudden drop in pressure can cause the brain-stem to cone through the foramen magnum. Suspect raised intracranial pressure in a history of early morning headaches, nausea, and vomiting that are made worse by lying down or straining; in anyone with impaired consciousness, papilloedema on fundoscopy, focal neurological signs (e.g. VIth nerve palsy). If there is any doubt about an SOL then imaging should be performed prior to LP.
- **Increased bleeding tendency** (e.g. patient on warfarin, disseminated intravascular coagulation, low platelets).
- **Infection at prospective site of puncture.**
- **Cardiorespiratory compromise.** Deal with this before doing any other procedure.

Risks

- **Headache.** About 30% of patients will get a headache due to the intracranial hypotension. Contrary to conventional wisdom, there is no evidence that hydration status, bed rest after LP or volume/speed of CSF removed makes any difference to the incidence of post-LP headache. However, there is good evidence that using smaller needles with atraumatic tips inserted and removed correctly reduces the incidence of headache. Be sure to take a reasonable volume, as it

CONTINUED ➤

CONTINUED

is better to avoid a second procedure, the volume removed is not associated with post-LP head-ache, and it will be rapidly replaced (we produce ~50 mL an hour!).

- **Nerve root pain.** About 10% of patients will get pain in a lumbosacral nerve root distribution, due to irritation by the needle of one of the nerves that form the cauda equina. This can be minimized by inserting the needle slowly and withdrawing it from the cannula slowly. Provide analgesia and reassure the patient that the pain will gradually subside.
- **Infection at the site of the puncture.**

With regards to raised intracranial pressure, what are (1) its main symptoms and signs and (2) its main causes?

1 The main symptoms and signs of raised intracranial pressure are:
   - **Headache,** often worse when lying down
   - **Nausea,** usually first thing in the morning, after lying down all night
   - **Papilloedema,** a swollen optic disc when visualized by fundoscopy
   - **Visual blurring**
   - **Cushing's reflex,** a paradoxical bradycardia and raised blood pressure, often with irregular breathing
   - **Cushing's peptic ulcer,** causing epigastric pain

2 There are a variety of mechanisms that can lead to raised intracranial pressure:
   - **SOL,** such as a tumour, haematoma, abscess, or cyst
   - **Cerebral oedema,** secondary to trauma or some other lesion
   - **Increased blood pressure in the CNS,** due to vasodilator drugs (glyceryl trinitrate (GTN) spray, Viagra), malignant hypertension, hypercapnic vasodilation, venous sinus thrombosis, or superior vena cava obstruction
   - **Increased volume of CSF (hydrocephalus),** which can be due to obstruction of CSF drainage (e.g. by a tumour), dysfunction of the arachnoid granulations responsible for CSF reabsorption (e.g. SAH or meningitis irritating the granulations, idiopathic intracranial hypertension), or increased CSF production (by a choroid plexus papilloma)

Single Best Answers

1. Which of the following is not an acutely life-threatening cause of headache?

a. Sinusitis
b. Raised intracranial pressure
c. Meningitis
d. Subdural haematoma

2. How would you treat cluster headache acutely?

a. High-flow oxygen and/or nasal or sub-cutaneous triptan
b. Paracetamol, NSAID, and/or opioid analgesia
c. Verapamil
d. Oral triptan
e. All of the above

3. A patient presents with unilateral ptosis and mydriasis. What is the cause?

a. Second nerve palsy
b. Third nerve palsy
c. Fourth nerve palsy
d. Sixth nerve palsy
e. Horner's syndrome

4. A CT is reported as having a ring-enhancing lesion. Which of the following would be consistent with this CT finding?

a. Brain tumour (primary or metastatic)
b. Brain abscess
c. Multiple sclerosis
d. Toxoplasmosis
e. All of the above

5. Normal ventricles look white in which imaging modality?

a. CT without contrast
b. CT with contrast
c. T1-weighted MRI
d. T2-weighted MRI
e. b and d

Confusion

Core case

Read through the sections in the case boxes, covering up the sections that follow so that you don't see the answer. At the end of each case box, try to answer the question before reading on.

Mrs Norman is an 84-year-old woman who is referred by her GP to her local hospital. She attends with her daughter, who reports that her mother is usually forgetful. However, when she visited that day she found that her mother was much worse than when she last saw her 3 days previously, as she was very 'confused' and 'not herself'.

'Confusion' is a very vague term that can refer to various medical syndromes.

What syndromes can cause a patient to appear 'confused'?

- **Delirium**: an acute impairment in cognitive ability together with impaired consciousness.
- **Dementia**: a chronic, progressive impairment in cognitive ability but with intact consciousness. Note that this is different from delirium and that you cannot diagnose dementia from a single mental status assessment.
- **Mental impairment**: a permanent impairment in cognitive ability.
- **Psychosis**: the patient may not be confused, but have a disorder of thought content/perception (e.g. delusions and/or hallucinations).
- **Receptive dysphasia**: the patient may have difficulties comprehending your questions (e.g. due to damage to Wernicke's area of the brain).
- **Expressive dysphasia**: the patient may be cognitively intact but have difficulties verbalizing an answer to your questions (e.g. due to damage to Broca's area of the brain).

Note that these syndromes may coexist in patients, particularly delirium and dementia which are both very common.

It is often difficult to take a good history from a confused patient. However, you should nevertheless try to get some basic information from her.

What questions should you ask of all confused patients?

Remember to start by checking the patient's airway, breathing, and circulation (ABC) and whether they are in any pain that requires analgesia.

To work out what type of confusion this is, you should start by conducting a **quick screen of confusion** because if the patient does poorly in your screen, taking a conventional history may prove unhelpful. For example, you may ask:

- **Are they oriented to time, place, and person? Can they tell you why they are here?** The Abbreviated Mental Test Score (AMTS; see Box 2.1) is a simple 10-question screening tool for assessing confusion where a score of less than 6/10 indicates cognitive impairment. An alternative is the 30-question Mini Mental State Exam (MMSE), where a score of less than 26/30 indicates cognitive impairment. Be aware that there are many other scoring systems in routine use, such as the Confusion Assessment Method (CAM), Montreal Cognitive Assessment (MoCA), etc.

- If their ability to converse is impaired, **can they follow a three-step command? Can they name three common objects?** These questions test for receptive and expressive dysphasia respectively. It will be fairly obvious early in your interaction with the patient whether either of these questions is relevant (they do not need to be asked routinely).

- **Other symptoms?** Are they in pain? (even the most confused patient will complain of pain). You should also ask about breathlessness, cough, and urinary symptoms as a chest or urinary tract infection (UTI) is often the cause of confusion.

Box 2.1 The Abbreviated Mental Test Score

Remember this address: 33 Dorchester Street

Orientation in time

What time is it (nearest hour)?	1 point
What year are we in?	1 point
How old are you?	1 point

Orientation in space

What building are you in?	1 point

Orientation in person

Who am I? Who is that person (e.g. nurse)?	1 point

Long-term memory

What is your date of birth?	1 point
What year did the Second World War end (or alternative date, e.g. particular Olympic Games)?	1 point
Who is the current Prime Minister?	1 point

Short-term memory

Please count backwards from 20 to 1	1 point
Can you remember the address I told you?	1 point

Score < 6/10 = dementia or delirium likely

Reproduced from Hodkinson HM 'Evaluation of a mental test score for assessment of mental impairment in the elderly'. *Age and Ageing*, 1972, **1**, pp. 233–238, with permission from Oxford University Press.

If the patient is accompanied, what collateral history should you try to ascertain from their companion?

If the patient has been accompanied by someone who knows them, try to ascertain:

- Their **normal state.** It may be that they are behaving no differently from how they normally behave, but that it has been mistaken for confusion (e.g. if they have dementia, psychosis, mental impairment, etc.).

- The **time course** of their confusion. An acute onset argues against dementia and in favour of delirium. A **fluctuating course** is also suggestive of delirium.

- Their **drug history (including alcohol).** Any number of drugs can cause confusion. Consider both the introduction and cessation of drugs. This information is particularly important in elderly patients who may have dementia and/or be taking a number of medications which may or may not have changed recently.

Remember that a history of dementia does not exclude an acute confusional state. On the contrary, such patients are at a greater risk of developing confusion in addition to their dementia.

If the patient has scored poorly on your quick screen of confusion and they are unaccompanied, you should move on quickly to the examination as conversation with the patient is unlikely to be productive and multiple questions may be distressing for them. However a collateral history is critical and must be obtained at a later time (e.g. calling the next of kin or GP once you have finished with the patient).

Mrs Norman is drowsy and confused with an AMTS of 5/10, but there is no obvious expressive or receptive dysphasia. She reports that she fell over but otherwise is not sure why she has been brought in. She reports no other symptoms. Her daughter reports that her mother does not drink any alcohol. She takes a thiazide diuretic for hypertension, and is currently taking lactulose for constipation and clotrimazole for thrush.

Before you move on to examine Mrs Norman, you should start formulating an idea as to what might be the cause of her acute confusion (delirium).

What causes of delirium can you think of?
The list is long and you may find using a 'surgical sieve' is helpful.

Which of the diagnoses in your list are most likely in Mrs Norman?

There are a number of different mnemonics for remembering a 'surgical sieve'. The one used here is INVITED MD. The diagnoses more likely in Mrs Norman, given both what is most common and her age, are given in **bold type**.

Infectious (e.g. **chest**, **urinary**, encephalitis, brain abscess, sepsis)

Neoplastic (e.g. brain tumour)

Vascular (e.g. stroke, myocardial infarction causing hypoperfusion)

Immune (e.g. rare conditions such as neuropsychiatric lupus, Hashimoto's encephalopathy)

Trauma (e.g. **subdural haematoma**, extradural haematoma)

Endocrine (e.g. hypothyroidism, hyperthyroidism, diabetic ketoacidosis)

Drugs (e.g. intoxication or withdrawal of alcohol, opiates, or psychiatric medications; or **use of diuretics, digoxin, thyroid medication**). Drug toxicity accounts for ~30% of delirium

Metabolic (e.g. hypoxia, hypercapnia, hypoglycaemia, hypercalcaemia, **sodium or other electrolyte imbalances**, thiamine, folate, or vitamin B_{12} deficiencies)

Degenerative conditions. These will be chronic and will not cause the delirium, but they will predispose patients to becoming delirious

In elderly patients, don't forget that they may be hypothermic.

Note: While the surgical sieve approach is undoubtedly helpful for remembering a broad differential diagnosis, it is important to realize that some diagnoses do not 'pigeonhole' precisely into categories. Hypothermia is a good example.

Before taking a full history you should have checked Mrs Norman's vital signs, to ensure that they are stable. These also provide some diagnostic information.

What vital signs would you be most interested in and why?

The vital signs of particular interest are:

- **Pulse and respiratory rate**: a tachycardia or tachypnoea could occur secondary to infection, for example.

- **Blood pressure**: hypoperfusion of the brain (due to systemic hypotension) decreases patient consciousness. Also consider the relationship between the pulse and blood pressure—is there hypertension and bradycardia? This is known as the Cushing response and is indicative of raised intracranial pressure.

- **Oxygen saturation**: hypoxia also affects consciousness and can be easily measured with a pulse oximeter.

- **Temperature**: fever may indicate an underlying infective process. Alternatively, hypothermia also causes confusion and is not uncommon in older people.

- **Blood glucose**: hypoglycaemia or hyperglycaemia can depress consciousness. In patients with type 1 diabetes mellitus, hyperglycaemia may be associated with ketoacidosis (which also affects the mental state). In type 2 diabetics, extreme hyperglycaemia may indicate a hyperosmolar hyperglycaemic syndrome (**HHS**, or HyperOsmolar Non-Ketotic (HONK) state). A capillary glucose is sufficient at this stage, although any abnormal result should be followed up with a venous blood sample.

Mrs Norman's pulse is 108 bpm, her respiratory rate is 20/min, and her blood pressure 90/60 mmHg. Her oxygen saturation is 96% on room air, her temperature is 37.6 °C and her capillary glucose is 5.6 mM.

Confused patients may be inattentive, drowsy, and/or uncooperative, making a full examination difficult. Given this and the most likely diagnoses in your differential, what are the most important signs to look for?

Even with patients who are difficult to examine, you should be able to do the following:

- **Consciousness**: assess this using the Glasgow Coma Scale (GCS; see Box 2.2). This was developed before head imaging modalities (CT and MRI) were widely available and is a good prognostic indicator. It also enables you to track progression.

- **Septic focus**: look for evidence of a septic focus such as:
  - **Chest**: look for signs of infection on percussion (dull) and auscultation (bronchial breathing, crackles).
  - **Urine**: check for suprapubic tenderness, and if there is a catheter bag check whether the urine is cloudy, perform urinalysis and send off a specimen for microscopy, culture, and sensitivities (MC&S).
  - **Cellulitis**: carefully inspect the skin. In diabetics pay particular attention to the feet, checking between the toes, as these are particularly vulnerable. Also check for any venous or arterial lines that may be a focus for infection.
  - **Meningitis**: check for neck stiffness (suggestive of meningism, from any cause), photophobia, and a purpuric rash (suggestive of meningococcal septicaemia, specifically).

Box 2.2 Glasgow Coma Scale

Best motor response

Moves arms in normal manner (obeys commands)	6
Localizes hands to painful stimulus (e.g. push finger into angle of jaw)	5
Withdraws from painful stimulus (e.g. press hard on fingernails)	4
Flexes all limbs in response to pain	3
Extends all limbs in response to pain	2
No movement in response to pain	1

Best verbal response

Talks fluently	5
Talks, but not fluently	4
Says words but sentences make no sense	3
Makes noise in response to painful stimulus	2
Silent despite painful stimulus	1

Best eye response

Eyes are spontaneously open and blinking naturally	4
Opens eyes in response to verbal command	3
Opens eyes in response to painful stimulus	2
Does not open eyes despite painful stimulus	1

GCS ≤8/15 = Patient may not be able to protect own airway from aspiration and/or obstruction and needs consideration of a definitive airway, i.e. intubation.

Reprinted from *The Lancet*, Vol. 394, Teasdale G and Jennett B, 'Assessment of coma and impaired consciousness: a practical scale', pp. 81–84, Copyright 1974, with permission from Elsevier.

- **Pupils**: check these, looking for symmetry, size, and direct and consensual responses to light. You may find pupils that are dilated and sluggish to react (drug overdose, e.g. cocaine, tricyclic anti-depressants; severe hypoxia; hypothermia; postictal), or pinpoint and sluggish to react (opiate or barbiturate overdose), or asymmetrical pupils (usually a normal variant called anisocoria, but very rarely suggestive of coning secondary to raised intracranial pressure or a third nerve palsy).
- **Focal neurological signs**: look for signs of focal neurological pathology (e.g. suggesting stroke or a space-occupying lesion): dysphasia, visual field defects, nystagmus, tone and reflex symmetry, plantar responses, focal weakness (moving all limbs if not cooperating), ataxia, and sensory or visual inattention.
- **Needle track marks**: suggests intravenous (IV) drug abuse.
- **Asterixis** (metabolic flap): suggests hypercapnia, hepatic encephalopathy, or uraemia as a cause.
- **Breath** for alcohol. Traditional textbooks refer to fetor hepaticus (liver failure), uraemic fetor (renal failure), or fruity (ketones in ketoacidosis) breath but these signs are difficult to reliably assess and distinguish.
- **Bitten tongue** and/or **posterior shoulder dislocation** suggests a convulsive seizure.

You examine Mrs Norman and find that she has a GCS of 12/15 (Eyes = 3, Verbal = 4, Motor = 5). Her lung fields are clear, her abdomen is soft and non-tender, there are no signs of cellulitis or meningism, and she does not have a catheter or any lines in place. There are no signs of focal neurology and her pupils are equal and reactive to light.

What investigations would you request?

It can be difficult to discern the precise cause of delirium in many patients, even if the most common causes in a patient of this age are, statistically, infection or medications. Therefore, you should run a full 'confusion screen' consisting of:

- **Septic screen**: full blood count (FBC), C-reactive protein (CRP), blood cultures, urine dipstick and urine MC&S, chest radiography.
  - **FBC**: the white cell count (WCC) may be elevated if there is a systemic infection. Anaemia could contribute to hypoxia.
  - **CRP**: an elevated CRP points towards an inflammatory picture, although, as with the WCC, it is non-specific regarding the cause.
  - **Blood cultures**: these should be taken to look for infection and, if positive, to identify the organism and its sensitivity and resistance to various antibiotics. However, they take time to come back so are of more relevance in management than diagnosis.
  - **Urine analysis**: it is important that this is performed on a midstream urine (MSU) sample, in-out catheter sample, or suprapubic catheter sample because the first part of a micturition stream will always be contaminated. A combination of both positive leucocyte esterase and positive nitrites are highly suggestive of a UTI. The positive predictive value for a UTI if only nitrites are positive is higher than if only leucocytes are positive, but either in isolation is much less predictive of a UTI than when both are positive. A combination of positive glucose and ketones suggests diabetic ketoacidosis. A midstream sample can also be taken to look for specific bacteria.
  - **Urine MC&S**: as with the blood cultures, these should be taken to look for the offending organism if there are signs of infection on the urine dipstick.
  - **Chest radiograph**: consolidation is seen in a chest infection. An enlarged heart would be suggestive, although not diagnostic, of heart failure, which could be the cause of cerebral hypoperfusion.
- **Metabolic screen**: arterial blood gas (ABG), urea and electrolytes (U&Es), calcium, thyroid function, liver enzymes, thiamine, folate, vitamin B_{12}:
  - **Blood gas**: This would provide further information about hypercapnia and acid–base balance. Uraemia, diabetic ketoacidosis, and some toxins can cause metabolic acidosis. A venous gas is perfectly adequate if the patient is not hypoxic on oxygen saturation monitoring or drowsy with hypercapnia a possible cause.
  - **U&Es** (including **calcium**, which in some hospitals is part of a 'bone profile'): a variety of different electrolyte imbalances can cause an acute confusional state (e.g. low sodium, high calcium), as can uraemia in renal failure.
  - **Thyroid function tests (TFTs)**: if clinical signs or the history suggests hypo- or hyperthyroidism, you should investigate T_3/T_4 and TSH levels. In some hospitals this is routinely performed as a first-line investigation in confused patients.
  - **Liver enzymes**: liver failure can result in a hepatic encephalopathy and is suggested by deranged liver enzymes. Abnormal levels, in particular a disproportionately raised gamma-glutamyl transferase (GGT), may point to alcohol abuse.
  - **Thiamine, folate, and vitamin B_{12} levels**: if you suspect the patient is malnourished, e.g. a homeless patient, an alcohol or drug abuser, or an elderly patient living alone who appears cachexic (such patients may live on a minimal 'tea and toast' diet), then look for a deficiency in thiamine, folate, and vitamin B_{12}. Again this is part of the routine confusion screen in some hospitals, as these deficiencies are treatable.
- **Toxicology screen**: Contrary to popular perception, there is no such thing as a 'tox screen' which will assay blindly for medications, toxins, and recreational drugs. Urine testing kits are available that will tell you if a patient has consumed a variety of *specific* recreational drugs in the recent past,

but as they tell you nothing about whether the consumption was today or several days ago, nor the amount involved, they are of no value diagnostically in confused patients. Testing for actual and current levels of a specific drug in the patient's blood is possible but most labs only routinely do this for some prescription medications and alcohol. In an elderly patient like Mrs Norman, alcohol and prescription medications are likely candidates, whereas recreational drugs are unlikely.

- **Electrocardiogram (ECG)**: an ECG should be done to exclude ischaemia or arrhythmia leading to a low-output state and hypoperfusion.

> Mrs Norman's investigations were requested and she was found to have a raised WCC and ++ leucocyte esterase and +++ nitrites in her urine. Her other investigations were unremarkable.
>
> **In light of the history, examination, and investigations, what is the diagnosis?**

The urine analysis confirms that Mrs Norman has a **UTI**, even though clinically she had no suprapubic tenderness. It is not unusual for UTI to present without fever, especially in elderly people who often have difficulty regulating their temperature. Moreover a significant number of patients routinely take antipyretic medications such as paracetamol or steroids, masking infections. It may appear odd that a 'simple' UTI could cause confusion, but you should think of how your own mental ability drops when you have a bad cold with a good-going fever. That same drop in mental performance in someone who is already old and frail explains why infections that may appear relatively trivial to young adults can cause acute confusion in older people. However, it is important to remember that UTIs are common in older people and may be coincidental. Therefore you must keep an open mind and be prepared to review the diagnosis if there is no response to treatment.

> **How would you manage Mrs Norman acutely?**

- **Resuscitation**: as with any acute presentation, you must first assess the need for resuscitation by examining the ABC.
- **Antibiotics**: check your local guidelines for which antibiotics to use for a UTI, as there are different patterns of resistance from common infective organisms (e.g. *Escherichia coli*) depending on where you practice. Avoid unnecessary catheterization and cannulation as these increase the risk of infection.
- **Confusion**: there are a number of conservative measures you should take in confused patients:
    - Ensure confused patients are not left unattended. Ideally they should be cared for by the same staff day after day, as this helps them orientate themselves in an alien environment.
    - Where possible, put them in a quiet side room.
    - If relevant, ensure they have their glasses and hearing aids, and that they are working.
    - Discontinue non-essential medications as these may be contributing to the confusion.
    - Promote good sleep hygiene, e.g. by avoiding late-night prescriptions.
    - Consider providing fluids and nutrition, as they may be unable or unwilling to maintain a balanced intake. If you suspect thiamine deficiency secondary to alcoholism or malnutrition, you **must** treat (e.g. with thiamine or Pabrinex, a cocktail of B vitamins). Thiamine deficiency rapidly causes irreversible cerebral damage and if you wait for the results of your investigations it may already be too late.
- **Sedation**: If the patient becomes aggressive and is considered a risk to themselves or others, you may have to resort to sedating them. However, this should be a **measure of last resort** (as these drugs

can exacerbate the confusional state). Usually it is possible to calm someone down either by talking to them or by other means, e.g. arranging a dedicated nurse to stay with them. If such measures prove unsuccessful, you may have to give them:

- Haloperidol. This takes about 30–60 minutes to take effect and can have extrapyramidal side effects; use with caution in patients with Parkinson's or Lewy body dementia.
- Lorazepam. This acts more quickly, taking 5–10 minutes, and is useful in restoring sleep.

In the longer term, the management of the confused patient involves treating the underlying cause of their confusion—in this case the UTI. Be wary of non-compliance in confused patients, particularly if they appear not to be responding to treatment (check the drug charts to see the patients are taking their medications).

Short cases

Mr Nash is a 44-year-old man on the cardiac care unit who becomes confused and aggressive 4 days after suffering a myocardial infarction. Looking at his notes, you find nothing unusual in his observations (pulse, blood pressure, temperature, blood glucose, oxygen saturation), drug history, or blood tests (including inflammatory markers, electrolytes, and liver enzymes). However, you see in his initial clerking that he admitted to drinking 50–60 units a week and has a history of alcoholism.

What should you consider as a first step in this patient? What is the most likely diagnosis? What should you prescribe immediately? What must you consider in the medium- to long-term?

- **First step**: aggressive patients pose a risk to themselves, healthcare workers, and other patients. You should initially consider how to calm him down; if necessary, he may need sedation. However, you should be cautious about prescribing tranquillizers too readily, particularly given the potential cardiac side effects in a patient with ischaemic heart disease. Never put yourself at risk, and call security for help if a patient is aggressive.
- **Diagnosis**: having dealt with the immediate danger, you should proceed with investigating his confusion. The investigations already documented eliminate a number of possibilities. In a man with a history of alcoholism and a 4-day hospital stay, **alcohol withdrawal** is the most likely candidate (severe cases are termed 'delirium tremens' and are associated with a high mortality). Such patients are at high risk of developing Wernicke's encephalopathy due to thiamine deficiency, and this may potentially progress to permanent brain damage.
- **Immediate prescription**: alcohol withdrawal is a medical emergency and can lead to fits and even death. Chlordiazepoxide should be prescribed in accordance with local guidelines, many of which advocate the use of the Clinical Institute Withdrawal Assessment (CIWA) scale to guide dosage and frequency over the first 24 hours, followed by reducing doses over the next days. You should also prescribe thiamine to prevent irreversible brain damage.
- **Medium- to long-term**: do not forget that this man must be counselled about his alcohol intake and referred to specialist services as relevant.

Mr McMurphy is a 65-year-old man who is found to be confused on the ward round the day after resection of his colorectal cancer. His observations and investigations prior to the operation were all normal. There are no signs of infection on inspection of the wound site and he does not look or feel hot or sweaty. His peripheral pulses are present (if a little weak), lung fields are clear, his heart sounds are normal, and there are no obvious signs of infection elsewhere. He is not connected to a pulse oximeter, ECG, or blood pressure monitor so you ask for this to be done, and also request some investigations.

Given his history, what are the possible causes of his confusion that you should be thinking about?

Postoperative patients are commonly confused; this can be for any number of reasons related to their operation:

- **Hypoxia**: due to any combination of:
  - anaemia from significant blood loss in surgery
  - opiate analgesics leading to a depressed respiratory rate
  - pulmonary embolism reducing gas exchange
  - basal atelectasis due to inadequate analgesia which prevents the patient from deep breathing
- **Opiates**: direct effect of opiate analgesics on their mental state
- **Electrolytes**: derangement due to:
  - intra- and postoperative fluid replacement
  - renal failure caused by hypoperfusion
- **Infection**: although there are no focal signs this is possible; it becomes much more likely if the patient is febrile, tachycardic and/or tachypnoeic.
- **Sleep loss**: hospitals are noisy and it is even harder to sleep if you are in pain.
- **Alcohol withdrawal**: patients who consume large volumes of alcohol are at significant risk of withdrawal symptoms, and these are often most pronounced a couple of days into their admission. Careful history-taking and appropriate use of alcohol detoxification regimes should prevent this from occurring.

SHORT CASE

Mrs Murdoch is a 47-year-old woman who is brought in by ambulance after her neighbour went around to check on her and found her 'out of sorts'. You try asking Mrs Murdoch some questions and find her speech is unintelligible. Her neighbour says she lives alone and is self-sufficient, so there is no one to provide any detail as to how long this has been going on. She does, however, say that Mrs Murdoch is a regular churchgoer and is abstinent of alcohol.

Mrs Murdoch's pulse is 72 bpm, blood pressure 131/83 mmHg, oxygen saturations of 98% on room air, respiratory rate of 13/min, her temperature is 37.3 °C. On examination, she is thin but not overly dishevelled, has no signs of a septic focus, and no asterixis. Her pupils are equal and reactive to light. A neurological examination reveals an intention tremor in both hands and significant ataxia such that she can barely stand or walk. Her GCS is 13/15 (Eyes = 4, Verbal = 3, Motor = 6).

You manage to speak to her daughter, who confirms her mother does not drink. She also tells you that she has suffered with bipolar disorder for over 20 years, for which she takes lithium. She is on no other medications.

You request a full set of bloods, including a metabolic screen, and ask the nurses to conduct a urinalysis when she next passes water. Her blood glucose is 4.2 mM. Her results show:

Haematology		Biochemistry			
Hb	117 g/L	Na	132 mM	Corrected Ca	2.58 mM
WCC	4.1×10^9 cells/L	K	4.2 mM	ALP	32 U/L
		Urea	12.3 mM	AST	23 U/L
		Creatinine	103 µM	TSH	1.35 mU/L

A CT head scan shows no evidence of haemorrhage or any SOL.

What other blood result would you like to know? What is the most likely diagnosis? What other mechanism(s) might be contributing to her confusion?

The differential diagnosis could still include an ischaemic stroke, less easily detected on CT than MRI, but given her relatively young age and the fact that she takes lithium, you should certainly order a **lithium serum level**.

Lithium toxicity could account for her confusion. Her renal impairment may be due to **dehydration**, which is most likely acute as indicated by the raised urea; remember that urea rises out of proportion to creatinine initially because urea is normally reabsorbed in the proximal tubule, whereas creatinine is not. Mrs Murdoch also has mild hyponatraemia, but this is not sufficient to cause her confusion. Her lithium levels come back and are 3.7 mEq/L (normal range 0.5–1.2).

Your priority should be to maintain her renal function while monitoring her lithium levels until they return to normal. In the longer term, her lithium dose may need changing, although you will also want to investigate her compliance (e.g. was she taking more than her usual dose because she felt down?).

SHORT CASE

Mrs Barnes is a 54-year-old woman who is brought in by ambulance in the early hours of the morning after she was found by her husband wandering the streets. Her husband has come with her, although in her confused state she does not recognize him. She was reportedly behaving aggressively towards the paramedics but is now happy to be in the hospital. You find that she is not oriented in time and scores 5/10 on an AMTS. Her husband tells you that normally she is intellectually very capable (a crossword champion, no less!). He says she was perfectly fine when she went to bed and is distressed at the sudden turn of events. When you ask him, he recalls that she had a headache before going to sleep for which she took paracetamol. She is otherwise fit and well and takes no regular medications. She has never smoked, is not diabetic or hypertensive, has no family history of note (both her parents died in old age), and is not known to have raised cholesterol.

Mrs Barnes's pulse is 109 bpm, blood pressure 121/78 mmHg, oxygen saturations are 98% on room air, respiratory rate 12/min, and her temperature is 40.3 °C. On examination, she is alert with a GCS of 14/15 (Eyes = 4, Verbal = 4, Motor = 6). There is no dysarthria or impairment of sensation, limb movement, or vision, although she is photophobic and you therefore cannot perform fundoscopy. Her lungs are clear, there is no cellulitis, and no neck stiffness, rash, or herpetic lesions.

A CT is requested and shows no signs of haemorrhage or raised intracranial pressure. A lumbar puncture is then performed which shows an opening pressure of 28 cm, glucose 1.8 mM, protein 3.2 g/L, WCC 1120/mm^3 (90% neutrophils), red cell count 2/mm^3, and Gram-positive intracellular diplococci.

What is the diagnosis?

Why were you interested in whether she smoked, was diabetic, hypertensive, had any family history, or high cholesterol?

Mrs Barnes has **meningococcal meningitis**, based on the results of the lumbar puncture (very high WCC primarily neutrophils, Gram-positive intracellular diplococci, protein >1 g/L, and CSF:blood glucose ratio <0.5, assuming blood glucose is in the normal range of 3.5–5.5 mM). Hers is an atypical presentation (mild headache and photophobia without neck stiffness or rash), but serves as a reminder that meningo-encephalitis can present in a variety of ways.

Based on the history and examination (i.e. before you got the lumbar puncture results), a stroke was a possibility so you were interested in her risk factors as they inform about the likelihood of this. The lack of focal neurology makes a stroke less likely (and confusion is not a typical feature of stroke), and the CT helps exclude a haemorrhagic stroke.

SHORT CASE

Mr Babbitt is a 59-year-old man who is brought in by his son because he is 'not himself'. You try asking him some simple questions but find his speech is unintelligible. His son tells you his father has his own business as an independent property lawyer and is usually 'compos mentis'. They have dinner together once or twice a week, the last time being before the weekend, 3 days ago, when he was perfectly fine. His medical history is notable for lung cancer, for which he is under the care of a multidisciplinary team. His son says it has spread to the adrenals and that the prognosis is not good. He also comments that his father seems to have lost his appetite, which he attributes to a combination of the cancer and his medications, and has been increasingly tired, which he attributes to his low calorie intake. He cannot remember which medications his father takes. He says his father does not drink or smoke, but used to smoke 20 a day for 40 years.

His vital signs are: pulse 96 bpm, blood pressure 98/58 mmHg, oxygen saturations 99% on room air, respiratory rate 12/min, temperature 37.5 °C. On examination, he is alert with a GCS of 14/15 but confused (Eyes = 4, Verbal = 4, Motor = 6). You note he has a dry tongue and no peripheral or pulmonary oedema. Chest and abdominal examination are otherwise unremarkable. There are no signs of focal neurology.

A bedside blood glucose and urinalysis are unremarkable. His bloods come back shortly after and show:

Haematology		Biochemistry			
Hb	134 g/L	Na	112 mM	Corrected Ca	2.49 mM
		K	6.2 mM	ALP	32 U/L
		Urea	9.1 mM	AST	15 U/L
		Creatinine	78 µM	TSH	pending
		CRP	3 mg/L		

How should you investigate a patient with hyponatraemia?

Hyponatraemia is a common cause of acute confusion. Assuming Mr Babbitt's confusion is due to hyponatraemia, what is the likely underlying cause(s)? What should you be wary of when treating him?

Mr Babbitt has **hyponatraemia**, a common cause of confusion (particularly in patients on diuretics and/or with an element of renal failure). The investigation of hyponatraemia is outlined in the flow chart (Figure 2.1).

You should start by excluding pseudohyponatraemia by measuring the patient's serum osmolality:

- High or normal serum osmolality indicates a 'pseudohyponatraemia', i.e. a low-sodium result as an artefact. If the sodium is low, you would expect the overall osmolality to be low (given that sodium is the dominant ion that determines osmolarity). Some machines that measure sodium concentrations in laboratories assume a constant volume of water. If the serum is very concentrated, e.g. with protein or glucose, there will be less water in the vial and therefore less dissolved sodium. This gives rise to an artefactually low sodium reading. Curiously, blood gas analysers, such as those found on many acute wards, are *not* affected by this artefact.

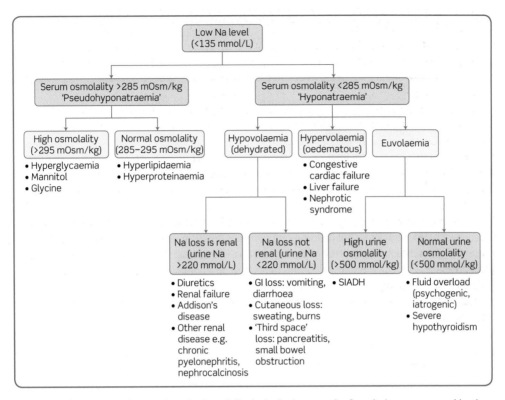

Figure 2.1 Investigating hyponatraemia. Osmolality is the ionic strength of a solution as measured by the lab, osmolarity is the calculated surrogate based on the concentrations of ions.

Based on a diagram by Dr N. Meston, John Radcliffe Hospital, Oxford, with permission. Data from Marshall WJ et al., *Clinical Chemistry*, 7th edition, 2012, Elsevier.

- If the patient has a low serum osmolality, i.e. a true hyponatraemia, you should work out whether they are hypervolaemic, euvolaemic, or hypovolaemic (this distinction is made largely on clinical findings):

  - Hypervolaemic patients have signs of fluid overload, specifically peripheral and pulmonary oedema and a raised jugular venous pressure (JVP). Hypervolaemic hyponatraemia occurs in many conditions, including congestive cardiac failure, hepatic failure, and nephrotic syndrome.

  - Hypovolaemic patients are dehydrated and have the corresponding signs, e.g. low urine output, tachycardia, low blood pressure, dry mucous membranes, and decreased skin turgor. Hypovolaemia results in hyponatraemia as it stimulates secretion of antidiuretic hormone (ADH) in an attempt to retain fluid, thereby diluting sodium levels. A urine sodium will identify the site of sodium loss as the kidney or elsewhere:

  - Urine sodium <220 mM indicates that the kidneys are responding normally to a drop in circulating volume by concentrating the urine. This suggests an extra-renal source of sodium loss, e.g. from the gut (vomiting, diarrhoea), skin (sweating, burns), or into the peritoneal cavity (pancreatitis, small bowel obstruction);

  - Urine sodium >220 mM implies the kidneys are unable to concentrate urine normally and that salt is being lost in this manner. Causes include diuretics, renal failure, and mineralocorticoid insufficiency (Addison's disease).

- Patients who have neither the clinical signs of hyper- or hypovolaemia should be considered euvolaemic. Measuring their urine osmolality will identify whether this is due to:
  - the Syndrome of Inappropriate ADH secretion (SIADH), where excess ADH allows water to re-enter the serum in the distal tubules impairing the ability of the kidneys to concentrate the urine, leading to a high urine osmolarity (>500 mmol/kg). Note that there are a number of other criteria that must be met before you can make a diagnosis of SIADH; or
  - fluid overload (psychogenic polydipsia or iatrogenic), which would be acute; or
  - severe hypothyroidism (rare).

In Mr Babbitt's case, while lung cancer often causes SIADH (due to ectopic secretion of ADH by small cell lung cancers), the cause is more likely to be **Addison's disease**. First, the hyponatraemia is hypovolaemic (low blood pressure, heart rate at the upper end of normal, no oedema). Although a urinary sodium has not been performed, his high potassium suggests this is due to a failure of the Na/K exchange mechanism in the distal tubule. This happens in adrenal insufficiency (Addison's disease), where a lack of mineralocorticoid (aldosterone) synthesis results in reduced Na/K exchange in the distal tubule with subsequent poor Na and water retention. The adrenals are a common site of metastases from the lungs, although it is unusual for this to result in an Addisonian picture.

You can confirm your hypothesis with a Synacthen test which, if he has Addison's disease, will show no increase in cortisol after stimulation with adrenocorticotropic hormone (ACTH). It is important you perform a brief neurological examination on admission, including fundoscopy to look for signs of papilloedema due to raised intracranial pressure from brain metastases, which could cause his confusion and may coexist with hyponatraemia.

The management of hypovolaemic severe hyponatraemia is a *slow* infusion of normal saline. You should be wary of correcting his hyponatraemia too rapidly, as this can cause central pontine myelinolysis and death. Thus, you should measure his serum sodium every 2–4 hours and, given this appears to have happened acutely (in the last 3 days), aim to increase his sodium by <2 mM/hour, and by no more than 10 mM/day. You can stop the infusion once he improves symptomatically, usually around 120 mM—there is no need to reach a sodium of 135 mM.

SHORT CASE

Miss Robertson is a 16-year-old student who is brought in by her parents, having woken up sweating and confused. You talk to her and find she is disoriented in person, place, and time, with an AMTS of 4/10. Her speech is slightly slurred. Her parents tell you that she was recently diagnosed with insulin-dependent diabetes. The family was finding this difficult, particularly the repeated injections and getting the glucose control right. You explain that you must ask about the possibility of recreational drugs and they tell you that as far as they know, she drinks a little but takes no illicit substances. You additionally ask if there were any other symptoms the night before (e.g. complaints of headache or visual problems), but they say she seemed perfectly normal.

You assess her vital observations. Her pulse is 98 bpm, blood pressure 120/71 mmHg, oxygen saturations 100% on room air, respiratory rate 13/min, temperature 37.6 °C. You also do a bedside glucose test which gives a level of 2.1 mM.

What is the cause of Miss Robertson's confusion? How should she be treated? What are the risks if she does not receive treatment?

Miss Robertson's confusion (and slurred speech) is caused by **hypoglycaemia**—normal glucose levels are 3.5–5.5 mM. Note that the sweating and rapid pulse rate are due to adrenergic overactivity, which is a consequence of hypoglycaemia. Severe hypoglycaemia, involving seizures or coma, is relatively common in childhood insulin-dependent diabetes, with nearly a third of patients having had at least one severe hypoglycaemic episode. This is particularly common in recently diagnosed diabetics who are still working on their glucose control and who are vulnerable to iatrogenic hypoglycaemia from an insulin overdose. Nonetheless, drug toxicity (specifically alcohol) is the most common cause for teenagers to present to the Emergency Department as confused or unconscious and you should take care to exclude drugs.

You should take a blood glucose sample to confirm the diagnosis, as capillary glucose sticks only provide an estimate. However, hypoglycaemia is a medical emergency so she needs glucose immediately—don't wait for a blood sample to confirm the result before treating, as hypoglycaemia is *much* more likely to kill a patient acutely than hyperglycaemia, so you won't do her any harm by giving glucose. Given that she is able to eat and drink, she should immediately be given a sweet drink or glucose tablets and monitored. As her glucose levels rise her consciousness should also improve. If she were not able to eat or drink (e.g. if she was unconscious), you could give her any of:

- Dextrose in gel form rubbed into her mouth (e.g. Hypostop)
- 50 mL of 20% glucose or 250 mL of 10% glucose IV, repeated up to two times if no recovery after 10–15 minutes, then consider a 10–20% glucose infusion (50% glucose is effective in improving glucose levels but can cause phlebitis when given via a peripheral vein)
- glucagon intramuscularly (IM; children who struggle with hypoglycaemic episodes may have an IM glucagon pen at home).

Note that hypoglycaemia in known diabetics on a long-acting insulin preparation or oral hypoglycaemic agent should be treated with a glucose infusion (rather than a bolus of glucose IV).

You should check Miss Robertson's blood glucose again after 10–15 minutes. If she has recovered, give her a carbohydrate-based snack (e.g. toast, banana, cereal). If she has not yet recovered, continue treatment and reassess her blood glucose in another 10–15 minutes.

In the longer term, Miss Robertson should be referred for specialist review of her glucose control.

As mentioned earlier, **seizures** or **coma** may occur in hypoglycaemia.

Viva questions

What functions are tested in the MMSE?

The MMSE tests the following cognitive functions: orientation in space and time, short- and long-term memory, attention, language (comprehension and expression), calculation, and visuospatial ability.

What do you understand by the term 'acute confusional state'?

Acute confusional state is defined in the Diagnostic and Statistical Manual of Mental Disorders (DSM) as an observable state of relatively sudden impaired attention, awareness, and cognition (including perception) that tends to fluctuate during the course of the day. There should be evidence that this disturbance is caused by a medical condition, intoxicating substance, medication, or combination of causes. It is interchangeable with the term 'delirium'.

Which diabetics get ketoacidosis and why? What clinical signs would you expect to see in ketoacidosis?

Ketogenesis is inhibited by even tiny amounts of insulin, so only type 1 diabetics become ketoacidotic. Clinically, signs and symptoms could include:

- polyuria, polydipsia, and a decreased mental state due to hyperglycaemia
- nausea, vomiting, abdominal pain, fatigue, shortness of breath, or Kussmaul breathing due to acidosis
- hypotension and tachycardia due to dehydration
- ketotic or 'fruity' breath (much talked about at medical school but rarely seen in practice nowadays, as patients with diabetic ketoacidosis (DKA) are usually treated before this late sign can develop).

Confusion and Kussmaul breathing are late signs and should be taken particularly seriously.

How would you distinguish an opiate overdose from a tricyclic antidepressant or cocaine overdose?

- **Opiates**: people take opiates to 'chill out'. An overdose will cause pinpoint pupils and respiratory depression. Needle track marks may be visible.
- **Cocaine**: people take cocaine for a 'buzz' because it has *sympathetic*-like effects. In an overdose, key signs include dilated pupils, sinus tachycardia, hypotension, and pyrexia. Patients may also have respiratory depression and urinary retention.
- **Tricyclics**: tricyclics, on the other hand, have both *sympathetic* stimulatory *and parasympathetic* inhibitory effects, the former particularly on the heart and central nervous system. Patients present with signs of sympathetic stimulation (dilated pupils, sinus tachycardia, brisk reflexes, urinary retention) and parasympathetic inhibition (dry mouth, drowsiness). They may also have upgoing plantar reflexes.

What treatment would you give someone presenting with confusion and a history or suspicion of alcohol abuse, and why?

All such patients should be given thiamine (e.g. Pabrinex, which also contains other B vitamins). They should be started on this immediately as prophylaxis for Wernicke's encephalopathy—a complication of alcohol abuse. Wernicke's classically presents as a triad of confusion, ataxia, and ophthalmoplegia, and is potentially reversible in the early stages which is why treatment should be started immediately. Failure to do so results in irreversible damage, known as Korsakoff's syndrome, characterized by amnesia and confabulation. Confabulation is when patients fill in gaps in their memory with fabricated stories.

Traditionally it is said that glucose should *not* be given as it can allegedly exacerbate Wernicke's, although there is little evidence to support this.

In an adult with a head injury, what are the indications for a CT scan? Why do we not scan every patient?

Head injuries can result in life-threatening pathology which can be difficult to detect by other means. For example, patients with an extradural haematoma often have a lucid interval after the incident that precedes progressive neurological deterioration. However, it would be inappropriate to give every patient with a head injury a CT scan, mainly because of the large dose of radiation exposure (there are also resource constraints to consider).

The 2014 NICE guidelines outline the indications for a CT head post-head injury (see Figure 2.2).

Criteria for immediate CT head:

- GCS < 13 on arrival at ED
- GCS < 15 at 2h post incident
- Post traumatic seizure
- Focal neurological deficit
- Vomiting > 1
- Suspected skull fracture

Criteria for urgent CT head (within 8 hours):

- Any head injury on warfarin
- Loss of consciousness or amnesia plus
    - Age > 65
    - Fall > 1m
    - Fall > 5 stairs
    - Pedestrian vs vehicle
    - Bicycle vs vehicle
    - More than 30min amnesia before injury

Figure 2.2 Indications for a CT head post-injury.

Data from National Institute for Health and Care Excellence (NICE) (2014) CG176. Head injury: Triage, assessment, investigation and early management of head injury in children, young people and adults. London: NIC, Available from: <http://publications.nice.org.uk/head-injury-cg176>.

A woman is brought into the ED by two friends because she is confused after getting drunk and taking an overdose. She says she took 'everything that was in the cabinet' and you are told by the paramedics that her bathroom cabinet and bins contained empty packets of amitriptyline, paracetamol, and zopiclone. You ensure she does not need immediate resuscitation and consult ToxBase online for advice on how to manage this overdose. You decide to put a cannula in place, perform an ECG (which is normal) and take bloods which reveal that her paracetamol levels are high enough to warrant treatment with intravenous *N*-acetylcysteine. As you explain this to the patient, who is sobering up and is by now less confused, she tells you she doesn't want you to proceed. You explain carefully admitting her and giving *N*-acetylcysteine will potentially save her life, but she continues to refuse.

What should you do?

There are two conflicting ethical principles in this scenario: the obligation on the doctor to do what is best for the patient (beneficence) and the patient's right to choose their own treatment (patient autonomy). Except in the case of life-threatening conditions or where the patient has been assessed as lacking the competence to make their own decisions, adult patients can refuse any treatment. Thus, this woman is entitled to refuse treatment if you are convinced she is mentally competent. However, she will need to prove competence as per the Mental Capacity Act 2005 which stipulates that she must convince the clinician that at that particular moment in time she is able to:

(a) understand the information given to her that is relevant to the decision

(b) retain that information long enough to be able to make the decision

(c) use or weigh up the information as part of the decision-making process

(d) communicate that decision to you.

Assessing someone's mental capacity can be done by any clinician experienced in this process, and does not automatically warrant a psychiatric opinion. The consultant from the Emergency Department interviewed the patient and felt that although she understood the potentially fatal consequences of refusing treatment and admission, her current state of inebriation and emotional crisis made it doubtful that she was able to weigh up the information given to her appropriately. She was therefore held and treated under the Mental Capacity Act 2005. This approach is in line with advice from both the College of Emergency Medicine and the Royal College of Psychiatrists. As is often the case, by the next day the patient was grateful for the care she was receiving and consented to complete her treatment and engage with the mental health liaison team prior to discharge for support.

Single Best Answers

1. Which of the following is a cause of confusion?

a. Hypothermia
b. Pneumonia
c. Stroke
d. Hyponatraemia
e. All of the above

2. A patient is referred to you with stroke. On examination you notice they have a receptive dysphasia (amongst other findings). Damage to which part of the brain causes a receptive dysphasia?

a. Broca's area
b. Wernicke's area
c. Brodmann's area
d. Primary auditory cortex
e. Primary motor cortex

3. A young man is brought into hospital with pinpoint pupils. There is concern that he may have taken an overdose. Which of the following drugs can give you pinpoint pupils?

a. Cocaine
b. Tricyclic antidepressants
c. Opiates
d. Amphetamines
e. All of the above

4. You diagnose a confused patient as suffering from alcohol withdrawal. Which of the following drugs must you prescribe to prevent irreversible brain damage (Wernicke–Korsakoff syndrome)?

a. Haloperidol
b. Lorazepam
c. Chlordiazepoxide
d. Saline
e. Thiamine

5. A confused elderly woman with a 4-day history of severe diarrhoea is brought to the Emergency Department. Which of the following biochemical states is she most likely to be in?

a. Pseudohyponotraemia
b. Euvolaemic hyponatraemia
c. Hypovolaemic hyponatraemia
d. Hypervolaemic hypernatraemia
e. Hypernatraemia

Blackout

Core case

Read through the sections in the case boxes, covering up the sections that follow so that you don't see the answer. At the end of each case box, try to answer the question before reading on.

Mr Williams is a 19-year-old student who is brought in by ambulance after collapsing while at a university ball. A friend who witnessed the collapse has accompanied him to hospital and confirms that he lost consciousness.

What are the commonest causes of a transient loss of consciousness?

Note that the terms 'syncope' and 'loss of consciousness' are not interchangeable as loss of consciousness can be due to either syncopal or non-syncopal causes. Syncope is a form of loss of consciousness in which hypoperfusion of the brain is the cause (from the Greek *syn* (together) and *kopein* (to cut), referring to the fact that the blood flow that joins the brain together with the rest of the body has been cut).

Syncopal causes can be subdivided by mechanism as follows:

- **'Reflex':** this is believed to involve activation of a primitive reflex that leads mammals to 'play dead' when faced with danger. Their heart rate slows and their blood pressure drops temporarily, reducing cerebral perfusion and leading to syncope. Some people appear to have a low threshold for activating this reflex in specific situations—for example after standing still for a long time, after seeing something frightening (e.g. blood, needles), or when straining (micturition, defecation).

- **'Cardiac':** pathologies causing a reduction in cardiac output (such as arrhythmias or outlet obstruction) can also lead to syncope.

- **'Orthostatic':** orthostatic hypotension basically means low blood pressure on sitting or standing (as opposed to lying flat). When we stand up there is a sudden drop in blood pressure that we compensate for by vasoconstriction, particularly of the 'capacitance' veins in the legs. This reduces the intravascular space, enabling us to maintain the pressure. However, this vasoconstriction takes a few seconds, so to prevent a transient fall in blood pressure every time we stand, there is a temporary increase in heart rate. Patients with reduced intravascular volume (e.g. from dehydration) and/ or in whom the normal autonomic response (transient tachycardia and peripheral vasoconstriction) to standing is blunted (e.g. due to drugs or autonomic neuropathy) are vulnerable to blackouts.

- **'Cerebrovascular':** these are non-cardiac structural causes of reduced cerebral perfusion, i.e. obstructions to the blood flow between the heart and the brain. They are relatively uncommon.

The main causes of a transient loss of consciousness are summarized in Figure 3.1, with the most common in large font. You should also remember that patients may believe they have lost consciousness when in fact they haven't. Such patients may have a non-epileptic ('psychogenic') 'seizure' or transient global amnesia (rare!).

SYNCOPAL

Reflex causes

Vasovagal syncope

Carotid sinus hypersensitivity

Situational syncope (e.g. micturition)

Cardiac causes

Arrhythmias

Structural cardiac pathology causing outflow obstruction
(e.g. aortic stenosis, hypertrophic obstructive
cardiomyopathy – HOCM)

Orthostatic causes

Drugs (anti-hypertensives, anti-sympathetics)

Dehydration

Autonomic instability

Baroreceptor dysfunction (in hypertensive patients)

Cerebrovascular causes

Vertebrobasilar insufficiency

Subclavian steal

Aortic dissection

NON-SYNCOPAL

Intoxication (e.g. alcohol, sedatives)

Head trauma

Metabolic (mainly hypoglycaemia)

Psychogenic (non-epileptic) seizure

Epileptic seizure

Narcolepsy

Figure 3.1 Main causes of transient loss of consciousness.

The age of any given patient makes particular causes of loss of consciousness much more likely than others.

What is the main cause of loss of consciousness in a patient:

(1) **aged 25 years?**

(2) **aged 55 years?**

(3) **aged 85 years?**

1   In **young patients**, the commonest cause of loss of consciousness is **vasovagal syncope**. Patients describe a warning or presyncopal sensation—an odd sensation in the stomach, going pale and clammy, and knowing they are going to lose consciousness.

2   In **middle-aged patients**, the most common causes of loss of consciousness are **vasovagal syncope** (see earlier) and **cardiac arrhythmias**. This is because cardiac arrhythmias are usually secondary to ischaemic heart disease, itself more common as patients age and accumulate an increasing burden of atherosclerotic lesions. By this line of reasoning, one would expect cardiac arrhythmias to account for most episodes of lost consciousness in elderly patients as well, but in reality many of the patients who have sufficient ischaemic heart disease to cause arrhythmias in middle age will

succumb to an atherosclerosis-related death (usually cardiac or stroke) before reaching 'old age'. Patients typically describe losing consciousness without any warning, while playing sport or without any obvious trigger (e.g. suddenly passing out while sitting in front of the television). Arrhythmias are important as there is a high risk of fatal arrhythmia.

3   In **elderly patients**, the most common cause of loss of consciousness is **orthostatic hypotension caused by medications**. These include diuretics and angiotensin-converting enzyme (ACE) inhibitors (reduced blood volume and vasodilatation), β-blockers (inability to increase heart rate on standing), α-blockers (inability to vasoconstrict the major capacitance veins), and calcium channel blockers (inability to vasoconstrict and some are negatively inotropic/chronotropic). Many elderly patients are on a number of these drugs simultaneously and find it hard to maintain adequate blood pressure. Patients typically describe losing consciousness after standing up, because their body is unable to compensate for the sudden drop in blood pressure. The condition carries a significant morbidity (from broken bones, loss of confidence and independence) and mortality (from head injuries but also from venous thromboembolic disease and infections acquired as a consequence of prolonged bed rest after a fall).

> Now that you have your differential diagnosis and some idea of what is most common in a person of Mr Williams' age, you can move on to the history.
>
> **What questions should you ask about the episode of loss of consciousness itself?**

In the history, from both the patient and a witness (if available), you should get a detailed description of what happened before, during, and after the episode. Specifically:

Before

- **Was there any warning?** If there was no warning, there is most likely a cardiac cause (e.g. cardiac arrhythmia, aortic stenosis) or, more rarely, a cerebrovascular cause (e.g. subclavian steal syndrome). Note that sometimes arrhythmias are preceded by palpitations. Patients with other causes of blackout tend to have some warning (e.g. aura preceding an epileptic seizure, dizziness preceding a vasovagal episode).

- **Were there any precipitating factors** (e.g. exercise, straining, standing up, fear, pain)? Postural triggers suggest orthostatic hypotension. Other precipitating factors are consistent with a vasovagal episode. Loss of consciousness caused by head turning suggests carotid sinus hypersensitivity. Blackout while sitting or lying down is suggestive of a cardiac arrhythmia. Passing out when exercising suggests a primary cardiac pathology such as aortic stenosis, cardiomyopathy (e.g. HOCM) or cardiac channelopathy (e.g. long QT syndrome). Symptoms immediately following vigorous arm activity may suggest subclavian steal.

- **Was there any recent head trauma?** This may seem obvious, but patients will not always associate head trauma with an episode of loss of consciousness, especially if there is some delay between the two. Be wary of subdural haemorrhages (particularly in elderly people and alcoholics) which may be precipitated by head trauma days or weeks earlier and may be associated with subsequent seizures.

During

- **How long was the patient unconscious—seconds or minutes?** Blackouts due to a vasovagal episode or an arrhythmia are short-lived, lasting seconds.

- **Did they bite their tongue or move their limbs, or were they incontinent of urine or faeces?** Note that tongue-biting is virtually pathognomonic of an epileptic seizure, whereas twitching and incontinence can be features with other causes, e.g. vasovagal.

After

- **Did they recover spontaneously? If not, how long did it take them to recover? Were they confused after recovery?** A spontaneous recovery argues against a metabolic or neurological cause (other than epilepsy). A slow recovery with confusion suggests an epileptic seizure.

These points are summarized in Table 3.1.

Table 3.1 Summary features of episodes of loss of consciousness

	Epilepsy	Vasovagal (i.e. a faint)	Arrhythmia
Before	May have stereotyped aura (partial seizure); or no warning (general seizure)	Vagal symptoms (sweating, pallor, nausea). May have a precipitant (e.g. fear)	No warning
During	Can last minutes Stereotyped episodes, same every time Tongue-biting pathognomonic Twitching and incontinence may also occur but not specific	Lasts seconds. May twitch or be incontinent	Lasts seconds. May twitch or be incontinent
After	Slow recovery, confused for 5–30 minutes	Rapid recovery on sitting or lying	Rapid spontaneous recovery

Mr Williams remembers feeling unwell and dizzy before passing out, but seems all right now, half an hour later. His friend tells you that he appeared well earlier in the evening, although he was inebriated. However, immediately before he collapsed his friend says 'the colour drained from his face'. He tells you Mr Williams was unconscious for only a few seconds and was a little surprised but not particularly confused when he came around.

Other aspects of the history can also help in the diagnosis of blackouts.

What would you particularly ask about in the history?

Past medical history

- **Has it happened before?** If it has happened before, you should ask the same questions about previous episodes and if they are increasing in frequency.
- **Diabetes?** This predisposes to vascular disease, hypoglycaemia, polyuria and dehydration, and autonomic dysfunction that can cause orthostatic hypotension.
- **Cardiac illness?** Ask about palpitations and chest pain as well as previous diagnoses. The presence of heart disease is a strong predictor of a cardiac cause of syncope. Arrhythmias may arise

following infarction. Left ventricular outflow obstruction may occur secondary to aortic stenosis, HOCM, etc.

- **Peripheral vascular disease?** Ask about claudication in case the patient is not aware of having peripheral vascular disease. Peripheral vascular disease is associated with coronary artery disease, as both are manifestations of the same underlying pathological process—atherosclerosis. It is also associated with cerebrovascular events (transient ischaemic attacks (TIAs), strokes), but these are very rarely a cause of transient loss of consciousness.

- **Epilepsy?** If they have epilepsy, did this episode resemble one of the patient's typical seizures?

- **Anaemia?** This can contribute to hypoxia. The patient may give a history that suggests a cause for anaemia such as myelodysplastic syndrome, frequent blood transfusions, or melaena.

- **Psychiatric illness?** Panic attacks are associated with hyperventilation and loss of consciousness. Non-epileptic 'seizures' are also more common amongst patients with psychiatric comorbidities.

Drug history

- **Insulin? Oral hypoglycaemics?** These will obviously make patients susceptible to hypoglycaemia—although note this is not the case for diabetic medications that act by increasing sensitivity to (rather than production of) insulin, e.g. metformin.

- **Antihypertensives?** (e.g. diuretics, ACE inhibitors, β-blockers, calcium channel blockers). All can cause hypotension.

- **Vasodilators?** (e.g. glyceryl trinitrate (GTN), isosorbide mononitrate). These can also cause hypotension, particularly in elderly patients.

- **Antiarrhythmics?** These can paradoxically predispose to arrhythmias.

- **Antidepressants?** Hypotension can be a side effect with some antidepressants, e.g. tricyclic antidepressants.

- **Warfarin? Other anticoagulants?** Patients on such medications are more vulnerable to sub-dural haemorrhages, and your threshold for requesting a CT head will be lower if they are taking these drugs.

Social history

- **Alcohol?** Many people who are intoxicated are brought in as 'loss of consciousness of unknown cause', although some might not have lost consciousness but simply have lost the ability to maintain an upright posture.

- **Stimulant recreational drugs?** Drugs such as cocaine and amphetamines stimulate the heart, causing tachyarrhythmias and potentially a drop in cardiac output.

Family history

- **Sudden death in any relations <65 years of age?** Such a history is significant in all cases of unexplained syncope, but is particularly informative regarding exercise-induced syncope. Some cardiomyopathies and arrhythmias are hereditary.

Mr Williams has no significant past medical history of note, only childhood asthma. He is not taking any medications. He sheepishly admits to consuming more than 8 units of alcohol earlier that evening, but no recreational drugs. He has no family history of note.

The history argues in favour of some causes and against others, but you still need to exclude some of the less likely causes as they are potentially very serious.

What signs would you look for on examination?

The examination may be unremarkable, but you should look for the following:

- **Tongue:** a bitten tongue. Make sure you look at the side of the tongue.
- **Dehydration:** signs of dehydration (e.g. dry mucous membranes, tachycardia, hypotension), as this can contribute to hypovolaemia and predispose to cerebral hypoperfusion.
- **Head trauma:** any signs of head trauma (you might expect this to have been mentioned in the history, although perhaps not from this patient if he was overly inebriated!). If there has been head trauma, try to establish whether it came before or after the loss of consciousness, i.e. did they hit their head as they fell?
- **Heart:**
  - A slow or irregular pulse, suggesting heart block or atrial fibrillation.
  - A heart murmur. Aortic stenosis can cause outflow obstructions and cerebral hypoperfusion.
- **Carotid bruits:** suggest carotid artery stenosis (although loudness of the bruit has no relation to severity of the stenosis).
- **Blood pressure:** check for orthostatic hypotension. Take the blood pressure lying down and repeatedly during the first 3 minutes of standing. Orthostatic hypotension is defined as a drop of ≥20 mmHg in systolic blood pressure or ≥10 mmHg diastolic on standing.
- **Focal neurological signs:** look for signs of peripheral neuropathy (e.g. due to diabetes mellitus, chronic alcohol abuse) or parkinsonism that may be associated with autonomic dysfunction (e.g. in multisystem atrophy). In the case of suspected seizures, check that there has been a full neurological recovery.

Mr Williams' examination is unremarkable.

What first-line investigations would you request and why?

You should perform the following investigations on anyone with loss of consciousness:

- **Bloods:**
  - **Capillary blood glucose:** you should exclude hypoglycaemia. You will also be looking for undiagnosed diabetes which can lead to polyuria and dehydration, and which in established diabetics is associated with autonomic dysfunction that can lead to hypotension and blackouts. Although diabetes mellitus is also a risk factor for cerebrovascular disease, strokes and TIAs very rarely cause blackouts.
  - **Full blood count (FBC):** to look for an anaemia that may be a contributing factor.
  - **Urea and electrolytes (U&Es):** check for biochemical evidence of dehydration (raised urea, out of proportion to creatinine), exclude an electrolyte abnormality predisposing to an arrhythmia.
- **Electrocardiogram (ECG):** NICE guidelines (2010) advise that all patients presenting with loss of consciousness should have an ECG. An ECG can be helpful if it shows an abnormality, but if it is

normal it does not exclude a cardiac cause as arrhythmias can be intermittent, particularly if the patient is asymptomatic at the time of the recording. 24–72 hour ambulatory ECG (Holter) monitoring is rarely helpful as few patients have arrhythmias every week and a positive result is just as likely in elderly patients who have experienced a blackout as in those who haven't.

There are a number of investigations you wouldn't carry out initially on everyone with an episode of loss of consciousness, but only if your history and examination suggest certain diagnoses:

- For a structural cardiac abnormality such as a valve lesion, consider an **echocardiogram**.
- For carotid sinus sensitivity, consider a **carotid sinus massage** (see the viva question on this topic).
- For epilepsy, consider a **brain scan** (CT or MRI). This is to look for a structural intracranial abnormality that may precipitate epilepsy (e.g. a brain tumour). 2010 NICE guidance on transient loss of consciousness specifically discourages the routine use of electroencephalography (EEG). Indeed, EEG has a low specificity, thus there is a risk of a false positive result; for this reason it should never be used as a 'rule out' test. Anyone suspected of having epilepsy should be referred to a neurologist, as only they are qualified to make this diagnosis (and by extension, only they should request EEGs).

Mr Williams' blood glucose, ECG, FBC, U&Es, and oxygen saturations are normal.

In light of his age, history, and investigations, what diagnosis is most likely?

Bear in mind that in approximately 50% of cases of loss of consciousness, no diagnosis is made. Given that the patient is young and has an unremarkable history and normal first-line investigations, the most likely diagnosis is **vasovagal syncope**. A cardiac arrhythmia is unlikely given the patient's age and the lack of family history of congenital heart problems. The normal ECG suggests that there is no congenital heart pathology such as Brugada syndrome. Indeed, cardiac arrhythmias in general are unlikely if there is no history of palpitations, no clinical evidence of heart disease, and an entirely normal ECG.

Your consultant agrees that this is most likely a vasovagal attack and decides to discharge Mr Williams.

What advice would you give him on discharge? Does he need to be followed up, and if so, by whom?

Mr Williams has had what is probably a vasovagal attack. You should explain this and give him lifestyle advice—that is, to sit or lie down if he feels like he is going to faint. Now is also a good opportunity to encourage Mr Williams to avoid excessive alcohol consumption. You should advise him to see his GP if he has recurrent episodes, but no follow-up is necessary unless these occur.

Short cases

Mrs Maxwell is a 37-year-old woman who has been referred to neurology outpatients by her GP after several episodes of loss of consciousness. The GP wonders if she has epilepsy. The GP's letter adds that Mrs Maxwell is anxious and has a history of depression. She has come to outpatients with her husband.

You ask her about the attacks. She describes a series of different events. On one occasion, she says she was having an argument with her 8-year-old son and then woke up on the floor. On another occasion, she was out shopping with her husband and son and collapsed. She also says she has ended up on the floor at home without knowing how she got there. Her husband corroborates a number of these episodes. There never appears to be any warning or precipitant.

Her husband tells you the episodes typically last a few minutes. He says that sometimes she twitches, but not always. Afterwards she appears fine, although she sometimes develops a head-ache after the episode. She tells you that she frequently suffers with headaches.

Given the history, what is the most likely diagnosis?

Recurrent and unprovoked losses of consciousness in a woman of this age should raise your suspicion of epilepsy. However, this is a life-changing diagnosis and you should be cautious when mentioning it. Her history is suggestive of **non-epileptic seizures**: the episodes are not stereotyped, her recovery is relatively rapid, and there is no postictal confusion. She also has a background of depression and possibly anxiety, which are commonly seen in patients with non-epileptic seizures. You should consider referral to a neurologist, who will have experience of distinguishing epileptic from non-epileptic (psychogenic) seizures and how best to manage both groups.

Mr Woodward is a 69-year-old man who is brought to his GP by a friend after fainting in the street. Mr Woodward has been visiting family for the past couple of days and has been complaining of 'dizzy spells', although this is the first time he has lost consciousness. When asked what he means by 'dizzy spells', he confirms that he means light-headedness rather than vertigo (i.e. there is no rotational component to the sensation). He says this occurs on standing and only started about a month ago. On the occasion on which he lost consciousness, his friend says he came round a few seconds later. He says he wasn't particularly confused afterwards, other than wondering why it happened. His medical history includes hypertension, angina, and benign prostatic hyperplasia for which he takes aspirin, ramipril, amlodipine, isosorbide mononitrate, and doxazosin. He has been taking these for several years, except the doxazosin which he started a month ago.

What is the most likely diagnosis? What is the physiological basis for this?

Mr Woodward has a history of light-headedness associated with standing that suggests **orthostatic hypotension**. The timing of these symptoms coincides with his new prescription of doxazosin for his prostate problems. This is not uncommon; not all patients (or doctors!) associate the onset of new symptoms (side effects) with the start of a new medication. Mr Woodward has good reason to feel light-headed when he stands up: the ACE inhibitor (ramipril) has several mechanisms of action including reducing salt and therefore water reabsorption, subsequently reducing the circulating volume; the calcium channel blocker (amlodipine) acts on calcium channels in vascular smooth muscle in the arterial walls to reduce contraction (although they do not affect venous smooth muscle); the nitrate (isosorbide mononitrate) promotes nitrous oxide (NO)-mediated dilation of the venous system; added to this, the α-blocker (doxazosin) will further impair the increase in heart rate and vasoconstriction of the large capacitance veins, respectively, when he stands. Therefore Mr Woodward is probably suffering from iatrogenic orthostatic hypotension. This could be confirmed by comparing the lying versus standing blood pressure, looking for a postural drop in blood pressure at any point during the first 3 minutes of standing.

The key to management is to modify his medications by reducing doses to the minimal effective dose, trying different medications altogether (e.g. a different type of α-blocker or a 5α-reductase inhibitor for his benign prostatic hyperplasia), or trying non-medical management of some of his problems (e.g. a transurethral resection of the prostate (TURP) for his benign prostatic hyperplasia).

SHORT CASE

Mr O'Brien is a 42-year-old estate agent who presents to his GP after several episodes of loss of consciousness over the last 2 months. The episodes occurred when he was running or rushing, e.g. to catch a bus. Each was immediately preceded by sweating. He does not recall any palpitations, nausea, chest pain, or shortness of breath. He tells you that some of these episodes were witnessed and he was told that he was only unconscious for a few seconds. He has not bitten his tongue or been incontinent at any time. He says he recovers rapidly and is able to carry on as normal, although he has been taking it a bit easier.

He has no known history of cardiovascular disease, epilepsy, or diabetes, and takes no medications. His pulse rate is 72 bpm and regular. There is a slow-rising carotid pulse. His apex beat is undisplaced and there are no heaves or thrills. Heart sounds I and II are both audible and there is a loud ejection systolic murmur which radiates to the carotids. His examination is otherwise unremarkable. His blood glucose, ECG, and U&Es are normal. In light of his heart murmur, you order an echocardiogram.

What do you think the echocardiogram would show? How might this account for his episodes of loss of consciousness?

Mr O'Brien's echocardiogram showed severe **aortic stenosis**, consistent with his systolic ejection murmur. His cardiac output was significantly reduced as a result of the outflow obstruction caused by his aortic stenosis. It was this that was predisposing him to blackouts.

There are three main causes of aortic stenosis. In a young patient a congenital bicuspid valve is most common. In the elderly, calcification of the valve commonly leads to stenosis. Rheumatic fever is a third cause of aortic stenosis but thankfully is relatively rare in the UK today. Mr O'Brien's echocardiogram showed a bicuspid aortic valve.

An important differential diagnosis in a young patient presenting like this is HOCM, but this would not account for the slow-rising pulse and would have been seen on echocardiography.

Miss Gokhale is a 15-year-old school student who has come to neurology outpatients with her mother following three suspected seizures in the past 4 months. The first occurred during break time at school, after which she was brought to hospital by ambulance. Two subsequent attacks have taken place, one at home and another at school. Miss Gokhale has no recollection of the episodes, although she knows that she is confused for some time after they occur. Her mother, who spoke to witnesses at school, says that during each attack she 'goes tense and shakes vigorously'. She has not bitten her tongue or been incontinent. The attacks last 5–10 minutes, after which her daughter is confused for around 30 minutes.

What is the most likely diagnosis and why?

Given the stereotyped nature, the lack of vagal symptoms before the attacks, and the slow spontaneous recovery with persistent confusion, Miss Gokhale has most likely had **epileptic seizures**. An EEG and brain MRI were performed to try to confirm the diagnosis. Neither showed any abnormality. However, epilepsy is a clinical diagnosis and the neurologist felt there was enough in her history to warrant this diagnosis, so she was commenced on anticonvulsants.

A couple of months later, Miss Gokhale comes back to hospital via ambulance while fitting. The seizure started at a dinner with her friends over half an hour ago and she has not fully regained consciousness at any time.

What complication has happened to Miss Gokhale and how should she be managed acutely? What possible causes are there?

Miss Gokhale is in **status epilepticus**. This is a medical emergency and requires urgent attention. As always, you should start by assessing her airway, breathing, and circulation (ABC). As part of this she should be given high-flow oxygen, have monitoring set up (continuous ECG, pulse oximeter, blood pressure cuff), a blood capillary glucose measurement, and two intravenous (IV) lines put in with bloods taken for an FBC, U&Es, Ca^{2+}, and Mg^{2+}. Levels of anticonvulsant medications are helpful to check concordance (especially while she cannot communicate a history). Two IV lines are useful because IV access can be easily disrupted in patients who are convulsing. If she is hypoglycaemic you should treat her with 250 mL of 10% dextrose immediately.

Having checked her ABC, you should rapidly assess D and E: disability (pupils and Glasgow Coma Scale (GCS) if she has temporarily stopped fitting) and exposure (a quick check for any obvious external signs of injury). Then you should try to end her seizure. Start by giving her a benzodiazepine such as IV lorazepam, IV/PR diazepam, or IV/IM/buccal midazolam. If she is still fitting 10 minutes later, you can repeat this. If 10 minutes after that she is still fitting, you should contact an intensive care consultant and start giving her a phenytoin infusion. Be sure to monitor her ECG and blood pressure when starting the infusion for arrhythmias and hypotension (both are side effects of phenytoin given acutely). By this time the intensive care specialists will have taken over and, if she is still fitting 10 minutes later, may decide to give her a general anaesthetic such as thiopentone to terminate the seizure.

Once the acute situation has been dealt with, you should investigate the cause of her seizure. In particular consider:

- Poor compliance with anticonvulsant medications, or use of additional medications which alter seizure thresholds or levels of serum anticonvulsants
- Metabolic causes (hypoglycaemia, electrolyte imbalance—renal or liver failure are unlikely in this patient, given her age)
- Alcohol or other toxins (e.g. amphetamines, lead poisoning, cocaine)
- Hypoxia
- Infection (intercurrent infection lowering the seizure threshold in a known epileptic, encephalitis/meningitis)
- Hypertensive encephalopathy
- Cerebral (tumour, head injury, or abscess are all possibilities—stroke, arteriovenous malformation, and vasculitis would be unlikely given her age)

In Miss Gokhale's case, the seizure was terminated with the initial dose of lorazepam. She later revealed that she had stopped taking her medications after a month as she had started to gain weight and felt self-conscious. In addition, she had consumed alcohol at dinner, which may have triggered the seizure.

Viva questions

What are Stokes–Adams attacks? How are they treated?

A Stokes–Adams attack is a sudden transient loss of consciousness induced by a slow or absent pulse and subsequent loss of cardiac output.† The underlying problem is either complete (third-degree) heart block or sinoatrial disease. Attacks are not associated with a change in posture or any other trigger. They usually last seconds but if they continue for more than 15-20 seconds twitching may occur due to cerebral anoxia. After an attack the patient becomes flushed as the well-oxygenated blood sat in the pulmonary capillaries during circulatory arrest is pumped around. The treatment is to implant a pacemaker.

†*The term Stokes–Adams attack comes from two physicians who described the condition, but is not used much nowadays, as the terms 'cardiogenic syncope' or 'syncope due to cardiac arrhythmia' are preferred.*

How would you define epilepsy? How are seizures classified?

Epilepsy is defined as a **tendency to have recurrent, unprovoked seizures.** A single seizure is not enough to diagnose epilepsy. A seizure is defined as transient excessive electrical activity with motor, sensory, or cognitive manifestations discernible to the patient or an observer.

Seizures are broadly grouped as generalized or partial, depending on whether the abnormal electrical activity affects the whole brain from the start (generalized) or is focal, at least initially (partial):

- **Generalized seizures** can be further subdivided depending on symptoms during the seizure:
  - **Tonic-clonic ('grand mal'):** patients are initially rigid (tonic phase) and then convulse, making rhythmical muscular contractions (clonic phase)
  - **Absence ('petit mal'):** usually in children, the patient loses consciousness and appears vacant and unresponsive to observers for up to 30 seconds
  - **Atonic:** a brief loss of muscle tone, causing the patient to fall to the ground
  - **Tonic:** like the tonic phase of tonic-clonic seizures
  - **Clonic:** like the clonic phase of tonic-clonic seizures
  - **Myoclonic:** an extremely brief muscle contraction (<0.1 second) seen as a jerky movement
- **Partial seizures** can be divided into those where consciousness is unimpaired (simple) and those where it is impaired (complex). Alternatively they may be classified by the brain area affected, e.g. temporal lobe (*déjà vu/jamais vu*, olfactory/auditory aura, epigastric discomfort), frontal lobe (motor), parietal (sensory), occipital (visual).

An elderly patient presenting to hospital with a loss of consciousness is often seen as an unexciting or unglamorous case, but is in fact a patient who requires rapid, effective multidisciplinary team management. Why is loss of consciousness in older people so important?

Loss of consciousness in an elderly person carries a very high risk of:

- **Morbidity:** elderly patients who lose consciousness and fall are likely to:

CONTINUED ➤

CONTINUED

- Injure themselves seriously. Falling can result in head trauma and subdural haematomas; radial fractures that make washing, cooking, and eating difficult; neck of femur fractures that confine them to bed, etc.
- Lose their confidence. Ask yourself if you would walk confidently down a flight of stairs if the last time you did so you fell down 15 stairs and broke a hip and both ankles. This often leads to significant anxiety or depression, which needs managing.
- Lose their independence. For example, an elderly patient who has fractured a clavicle and radius may go from living alone to being dependent on carers to wash, get dressed, cook, and feed themselves.

- **Mortality:** loss of consciousness in an elderly patient may not sound life-threatening, but if the patient suffers, say, a neck of femur fracture, they may need a prolonged hospital stay. Their immobility while in hospital may lead to a deep vein thrombosis and pulmonary embolus. Or they may get pressure sores, which in turn may get infected. They may get urinary tract infections from indwelling catheters, or pneumonia from the lack of movement and small areas of collapsed lung (atelectasis), leading to poor clearance of mucus. A fractured neck of femur continues to be a major (albeit indirect) cause of death in elderly people in the developed world.

- **Cost:** loss of consciousness in an elderly person, if accompanied by a fracture, can result in a lengthy hospital stay, prolonged physiotherapy, investment to adapt their house for their new immobility, regular (often daily) visits by carers to help with activities of daily living (ADLs), days off work for caring relatives eager to help, and sometimes moving into a nursing home. All of this entails significant cost to the patient, their family, and the state.

Heart block is a common cardiac cause of loss of consciousness. What is the classification of heart block affecting the atrioventricular (AV) node (i.e. not the bundles or fascicles)? How are the different types distinguished on ECG?

- **First-degree (incomplete) heart block:** every atrial contraction is transmitted to the ventricles, but conduction is slower than normal. It is caused by damage to the AV node (e.g. from ischaemic heart disease, fibrosis, inflammation). On ECG the gap between atrial contraction (P wave) and ventricular contraction (QRS complex), the PR interval, is >200 ms (one large square on a normally calibrated ECG). This isn't really a 'block', more a 'slowing down'. In keeping with this, it is usually asymptomatic.

- **Second-degree heart block:** some but not every atrial contraction is transmitted to the ventricles. This can be because of excessive vagal stimulation to the AV node or damage to the AV node or bundle of His. Two subtypes are recognized:

  - **Mobitz type I block:** each heart beat shows a progressively increased PR interval until eventually a QRS complex is missed entirely, as if the AV node block is getting progressively worse and then resetting itself. This pattern on an ECG is called Wenckebach. 'Wenckebaching' can be normal in ultrafit athletes.

  - **Mobitz type II block:** QRS complexes are found to be missing after P waves without a prolonged PR interval prior to the preceding QRS complex or a shortened PR interval before the next QRS. There is often a pattern, with QRS complexes missed after every second (2:1) or

CONTINUED ➤

CONTINUED

third (3:1) P wave. This is usually due to impaired conduction after the AV node. It has a high risk of progressing to complete heart block.

- **Third-degree (complete) heart block:** this results in no conduction at all between the atria and ventricles. On ECG the P waves are unrelated to the QRS complexes, which are broad. While the atria continue to contract at the pace set by the sinoatrial pacemaker, the ventricles rely on spontaneous conduction originating in the bundle of His to contract at a slow rate of about 40 bpm.

What is a tilt table test and what is it used for?

A tilt table test is sometimes used to help determine whether there is a vasovagal cause for blackouts. The patient is placed on a 'tilt table' that swings them from a supine position through 90° to upright. The patient is connected to continuous ECG and blood pressure monitoring and asked to report their symptoms every 3–5 minutes. A baseline is established by monitoring the patient supine for 5 minutes. The patient is then tilted (head up) to between 60° and 90° for between 10 and 60 minutes (a variety of different protocols are used). The test is considered positive if:

- the patient experiences loss of consciousness with a significant fall in blood pressure or heart rate, in which case they are returned to a supine position; or
- symptoms develop.

If an initial test is negative, it can be repeated while infusing drugs that increase the susceptibility to the test by vasodilation (e.g. GTN) or bradycardia (e.g. adenosine), or by performing carotid sinus massage to achieve the same result. This increases the sensitivity but decreases the specificity of the test—under such conditions as many as 45% of control subjects with no history of syncope may have a positive test!

The test is of limited value in patients with situational syncope, e.g. on micturition. It is contraindicated in patients who have orthostatic hypotension.

A false negative rate as high as 30% has been reported, although it is difficult to determine, as there is no gold standard for comparison. Thus a negative test cannot be used to exclude a vasovagal cause.

The low specificity and sensitivity means that this test is not routinely used.

What are the main side effects and interactions of anticonvulsant drugs in general, and specifically: sodium valproate, lamotrigine, carbamazepine, phenytoin?

All anticonvulsants are teratogenic: 2–3% of babies born to patients on one anticonvulsant are affected (around 4–6% if on two or 10% if on three anticonvulsants). Specific drugs are associated with specific defects: sodium valproate with neural tube defects, phenytoin with cleft palate and congenital heart disease. Although the risk of spina bifida from valproate use can theoretically be reduced by high-dose folate supplementation during the first trimester, current NICE advice is to avoid the use of any anticonvulsants during pregnancy where possible.

Carbamazepine and phenytoin interfere with the hepatic metabolism of the contraceptive pill by inducing cytochrome P450, therefore patients on the pill should be advised to double their dose and/

CONTINUED ➤

CONTINUED

or use barrier contraceptives. By the same mechanism they can interfere with warfarin dosing (requiring a greater dose of warfarin for the same target international normalized ratio (INR)).

The specific side effects include:

- Sodium valproate: weight gain, hair loss and curling, nausea, rash, drowsiness, tremor, drug-induced hepatitis
- Lamotrigine: rash (Stevens–Johnson syndrome), headaches, dizziness, insomnia, vivid dreams
- Carbamazepine: rash, nausea, ataxia, diplopia, agranulocytosis, hyponatraemia
- Phenytoin: acne, rash, ataxia, ophthalmoparesis, sedation, gingival hyperplasia

---

What should you, by law, advise patients with an episode of loss of consciousness about driving?

The Driver and Vehicle Licensing Agency (DVLA) have very clear guidelines on this (<http://www.dvla.gov.uk/>). Your actions depend on the cause of the loss of consciousness. For cars and motorcycles:

- If it was a simple faint with prodromal symptoms and a provoking factor can be identified that is unlikely to recur while sitting, there are no driving restrictions and there is no need to advise the DVLA.
- If the loss of consciousness was likely due to a transient loss of blood supply to the brain (syncope) with a *low risk of recurrence*, the patient can drive 4 weeks after the event.
- If the loss of consciousness was likely syncope with a *high risk of recurrence*, the patient can drive 4 weeks after the event if the cause has been identified and treated, or 6 months after if not identified or treated.
- If the loss of consciousness is unexplained and there are no suggestions it was a seizure, the patient cannot drive for 6 months.
- If the loss of consciousness was associated with seizure markers, the patient cannot drive for one (seizure-free) year.

If someone with epilepsy has been on antiepileptic medication for many years and wants to stop (e.g. due to a desire to be pregnant), they cannot drive for 6 (seizure-free) months after they have stopped.

Note that your responsibility as a medical practitioner is to tell the patient that they must inform the DVLA, not to contact the DVLA yourself. Some patients will be reluctant to do so given the lifestyle implications, so you may want to warn them that their insurance is invalid if they continue to drive under such circumstances.

An elderly patient complains of regular episodes of loss of consciousness at the weekend when he wears his tie to church. Your consultant suspects carotid sinus hypersensitivity. What simple bedside procedure can you do to test this? How is it performed?

You may want to consider performing a **carotid sinus massage**, whereby an ECG and blood pressure are monitored for bradycardia and/or hypotension induced by the carotid sinus massage.

Carotid sinus massage must not be done in anybody with possible atherosclerotic plaques in the carotids, as these may dislodge, causing a stroke. For this reason, Doppler ultrasound examination

CONTINUED ➤

CONTINUED

of both carotids is recommended before doing a carotid sinus massage in any patient with a history of stroke, TIA, or with a carotid bruit on auscultation. Patients should be advised that carotid sinus massage always carries a small but real risk of stroke.

Carotid sinus massage should always be done with a patient connected to a 12-lead ECG, with a large IV cannula *in situ* and a resuscitation trolley (with atropine) at hand, in case the massage triggers a cardiac arrest rather than just a transient blackout. Ideally, one needs beat-to-beat blood pressure monitoring, which was traditionally done invasively but can nowadays be done non-invasively.

During the test, pressure is applied in a firm circular motion to one carotid sinus at a time (where the carotid artery meets the angle of the jaw) for about 5 seconds. You should perform the test both with the patient lying down and standing up.

The procedure is considered positive if symptoms are reproduced during or immediately after the massage, in the presence of asystole longer than 3 seconds and/or a fall in systolic blood pressure of 50 mmHg. There are two possible components to the response: bradycardia and/or reduced blood pressure. Only patients with a significant or predominant bradycardic component may benefit from cardiac pacing.

[For budding cardiologists] What are the following (rare) cardiac causes of loss of consciousness, and why are they important: HOCM; long QT syndrome; Brugada syndrome; arrhythmogenic right ventricular dysplasia?

These rare causes of loss of consciousness are important as they are associated with sudden cardiac death in young people and athletes.

- **HOCM** is a genetic mutation, either inherited (autosomal dominant) or sporadic, resulting in non-physiological left ventricular hypertrophy. Left ventricular outflow obstruction is due to asymmetrical septal hypertrophy which occludes the outflow tract during systole. This is exacerbated by systolic anterior movement of the mitral valve anterior leaflet. The outflow tract gradient is exacerbated by exercise.

- **Long QT syndrome** is in fact a collection of disorders with different genetic mutations of cardiac ion channels (sodium and potassium). All of them result in prolonged repolarization and a long QT interval on the ECG, particularly on exertion, and are associated with ventricular tachycardia.

- **Brugada syndrome** is caused by a mutation of the cardiac sodium channel gene, at least in some patients. It is often inherited in an autosomal dominant manner. The ECG findings are a right bundle branch block and saddle-shaped ST elevation in V_1–V_3 (the QT intervals are normal). The condition is associated with ventricular dysrhythmias.

- **Arrhythmogenic right ventricular dysplasia** occurs when the myocardium is partially replaced by fatty or fibrofatty tissue. It occurs primarily in the right ventricle, and results in an arrhythmia, hence the name. The ECG is characterized by T-wave inversion in V_1–V_3 (a non-specific finding), right bundle branch block, and an epsilon wave in 50% of cases (a terminal notch at the end of the QRS complex). In addition there may be ventricular ectopics, which can progress to ventricular tachycardia (VT) or ventricular fibrillation (VF).

An implantable cardioverter defibrillator (ICD) device is the only intervention that can prevent sudden death in all of these patients, although β-blockers have some protective value.

Single Best Answers

1. **Which of the following is not a common cause of loss of consciousness?**

   a. ACE inhibitors
   b. Carotid sinus hypersensitivity
   c. Stroke

   d. Heart block
   e. Hypoglycaemia

2. **A patient presents with episodes of loss of consciousness. The GP's letter includes a list of their medications. Which could likely be responsible for the patient's blackouts?**

   a. Aspirin
   b. Simvastatin
   c. Metformin

   d. Ramipril
   e. c and d

3. **A patient falls off his bike and hits the right side of his head. He is initially alert but loses consciousness an hour later. CT head shows a biconvex, lens-shaped haemorrhage in the right parietal area. Which part of intracranial vasculature is most likely to have been damaged?**

   a. Anterior cerebral artery
   b. Middle cerebral artery
   c. Middle meningeal artery

   d. Bridging veins
   e. Superficial temporal artery

4. **What is the most common cause of aortic stenosis in the elderly population of developed countries?**

   a. Congenital bicuspid valve
   b. Rheumatic fever
   c. Infective endocarditis

   d. Calcification
   e. Connective tissue disorders

5. **A patient is seen in cardiology outpatients after an unexplained episode of loss of consciousness. The consultation reveals a family history of sudden death. Which of the following syndromes would you be concerned about (amongst others)?**

   a. Brugada syndrome
   b. Dressler's syndrome
   c. Eisenmenger syndrome

   d. Leriche's syndrome
   e. Wolff-Parkinson-White syndrome

Neck lump

Core cases

Read through the sections in the case boxes, covering up the sections that follow so that you don't see the answer. At the end of each case box, try to answer the question before reading on.

Note: we deviate slightly from the trodden path of previous chapters in that we present two core cases. The diagnostic pathway differs for lateral and midline neck lumps and thus we use two core cases to clarify and streamline the approach. As such, the first stage when assessing a patient with a neck lump is to determine if the lump is lateral or midline.

Lateral neck lump

> Mr Haversham is a 76-year-old man who presents to his GP with a suspected flare-up of gout in his big toe. While taking a history, the GP notices a lump on the side of Mr Haversham's neck.
>
> **What is your differential diagnosis for a lateral neck lump?**
>
> Try to think of the anatomical structures in the neck, and any pathology that may arise from those structures.

CORE CASE

Considering the anatomy and associated pathology, the lump may represent:

- **Artery**: carotid artery aneurysm, subclavian artery aneurysm, carotid body tumour (i.e. chemodectoma or paraganglioma of the carotid body)
- **Nerves**: neurofibroma, schwannoma
- **Lymphatics**: lymphatic malformations
- **Lymph nodes**: infective, neoplastic (primary or metastatic), granulomatous
- **Salivary glands**: infective, autoimmune, neoplastic
- **Larynx**: laryngocele
- **Pharynx**: pharyngeal pouch
- **Branchial arch remnant**: branchial cyst/sinus/fistula
- **Skin/superficial subcutaneous**: lipoma, epidermal cyst, abscess, dermoid cyst
- **Muscle/cartilage/bone**: sarcomas (e.g. rhabdomyosarcoma, fibrosarcoma, osteosarcoma), cervical rib, torticollis

> **How does the age of the patient influence your differential diagnosis? What are the most common causes of lateral neck lumps in (1) children, and (2) adults?**

The age of the patient has an enormous bearing upon the pathology you should expect to encounter:

- **In children**, about 75% of neck lumps are benign. Congenital and inflammatory lumps are most common. Thus the differential diagnosis will be weighted in favour of branchial cleft cysts, lymphatic malformations, and lymphadenitis. If malignancy is diagnosed in paediatric neck lumps, it is usually a lymphoma or sarcoma, or sometimes a papillary thyroid carcinoma.

- **In adults over 40**, as many as 75% of lateral neck lumps are malignant. Of the malignant neck lumps, about 80% are metastases and the rest are mostly lymphomas. In fact, ▲ **in the absence of signs of infection, a lateral neck mass in an adult is lymphadenopathy due to metastatic carcinoma (usually squamous cell) until proven otherwise.**

What questions should the GP ask about the lump itself?

- **How long has the lump been there?**
  - Less than a few weeks: most likely infective or inflammatory lymphadenopathy, although some patients will present with malignant neck lumps that have only been noticed within the last few days.
  - More than a few weeks: must exclude malignancy.
  - Years, with little change: most likely benign.
  - Note that congenital neck lumps, despite being 'congenital', may only 'appear' later in life as they may fluctuate in size (e.g. following an infection).
- **Has the lump got bigger, smaller, or stayed the same size?** A lump that is gradually increasing in size must be regarded as a malignancy until proven otherwise. Remember that a progressive increase in size of a malignant neck lump may be reported as a sudden appearance by the patient.
- **Is the lump painful?** Most neck lumps are not painful. The only lumps that are classically painful are acute infective lymphadenitis or an infected branchial cyst.
- **Are there any other lumps?** If the patient has noticed other similar lumps elsewhere on their body (for example, groin or axilla) then it is likely that the lump represents either a systemic disease (e.g. HIV, Epstein–Barr virus (EBV) giving rise to infectious mononucleosis) or disseminated malignancy (e.g. lymphoma).

Which associated symptoms should the GP ask about?

Given that most neck lumps in adults are enlarged lymph glands, and the most common underlying causes are infection and malignancy, you should ask:

- **Are there symptoms suggestive of infection?** Ask about malaise, fever, rigors, etc. But note that fever, night sweats, and weight loss are also 'B symptoms' of lymphoma. Therefore the time course of symptoms can be useful—an acute history favours infection whereas a more prolonged history favours malignancy. There may also be more 'local' symptoms of infection, such as pain from a dental abscess or coryzal symptoms from an upper respiratory tract infection.
- **Are there any symptoms suggestive of head and neck cancer?** Head and neck cancers are not usually associated with weight loss or malaise, but there are a number of other suggestive features. Those to enquire about include: dysphonia, stridor (inspiratory noise due to airway obstruction around the larynx), stertor (inspiratory noise due to airway obstruction in the pharynx e.g. snoring), breathing difficulty, dysphagia (difficulty swallowing; see Chapter 6),

odynophagia (painful swallowing), globus (sensation of an oesophageal/tracheal obstruction), cough, haemoptysis (see Chapter 8), otalgia, unilateral hearing loss, nasal discharge, epistaxis, and lumps or ulcers on the head or face that have increased in size or started to bleed. There is unfortunately no symptom or group of symptoms that is strongly correlated with early head and neck cancer—this list is merely a guide. Perhaps the only exception is carcinoma of the glottis, for which a change in voice or hoarseness is a highly sensitive (but non-specific) symptom.

Other than symptoms, are there any aspects of the history that may make an infective or malignant process more likely? Think about risk factors.

- **Infection**: Has the patient had a recent infection (in particular an upper respiratory tract infection)? Is there a history of contact with someone known to have infectious disease? Recent trauma, insect bites, or animal bites/scratches? (Cat scratches or bites can result in cat-scratch fever, due to *Bartonella*.)
- **Malignancy:** Is there a known current or previous cancer, or a family history of head and neck cancer? Has the patient previously had radiotherapy to the neck? Have they ever been a smoker and/or do they have a high alcohol intake?

Why is it important to ask about social history in the context of a neck lump?

Smoking and high alcohol consumption are strong independent risk factors for the development of head and neck cancer, thus you must *always* ask about them.

The GP asks Mr Haversham about the lump in his neck. He explains that it has been there for several months and that he didn't think it was worth going to see his doctor about something so small that was causing him no pain. When specifically asked whether the lump has increased in size, Mr Haversham explains that it has probably doubled, but reiterates that it causes him no bother. He is not aware of any other unusual lumps on his body.

With the exception of his painful big toe, Mr Haversham has felt well recently. He has not been feverish and has not been aware of any insect bites or trauma to his neck. He has not been abroad for over a year and has not been in contact with anyone unwell. The GP runs through a quick checklist of oral, nasal, otological, pharyngeal, and laryngeal symptoms, all of which are absent.

Mr Haversham takes no regular medications and has no known allergies. He enjoys a glass of wine each day, and is a smoker with a 30-pack-year history (i.e. 20 cigarettes a day for 30 years).

The GP explains to Mr Haversham that it would be wise for him to examine the lump on his neck. When approaching the examination of a neck lump, the first stage is to localize the lump.

What specific information should the GP glean about the location of the lump?

There are three key questions to address that will enable the GP to narrow their differential diagnosis considerably:

1 **Is it superficial or deep?** Superficial lumps include lipomas, abscesses, epidermal cysts, and dermoid cysts.

2 **Is it in the anterior or the posterior triangle of the neck** (i.e. in front of or behind the sternocleido-mastoid)? If we only consider deep structures, we can usually allocate lesions to the anterior or posterior triangle as follows:

- **Anterior triangle:** Branchial cyst/sinus/fistula, carotid body tumour (chemodectoma), carotid artery aneurysm, salivary gland, laryngocele, lymphadenopathy. (While we acknowledge that thyroid masses are strictly in the anterior triangle, and that a single nodule in the lateral aspect of a thyroid lobe may present as a lateral lump, we have omitted discussing them in this first case for the sake of simplicity.)
- **Posterior triangle:** lymphatic malformation, cervical rib, pharyngeal pouch, subclavian aneurysm, lymphadenopathy.

3 **What is its relationship to muscle?** Asking the patient to nod their head against resistance will tense the sternocleidomastoid muscle on both sides of the neck (this also demonstrates which triangle the lump is in—see Figure 4.2). Shrugging the shoulder against resistance will contract trapezius. Any lump that is underneath the muscle will be concealed when the muscle contracts.

What other features of the lump should be characterized during palpation?

- **Is it tender and/or warm?** The only neck lumps that are classically tender and/or warm are infected or inflammatory masses. An important exception in at-risk patient groups is tuberculous adenitis. In the acute phase this may present with painless lymphadenopathy and overlying erythema, whereas progressive disease can present with a discharging sinus or a 'cold' abscess.

- **Is it solid or fluctuant?** There are various textbook descriptions of degrees of lump firmness that correspond to different causes of cervical lymphadenopathy, but in practice it can be hard to distinguish a supposedly 'hard' from a 'rubbery' lump. Classically, lumps can be divided into:
  - **Hard lumps:** malignant lymph nodes
  - **Rubbery lumps:** chronic inflammatory lymph nodes (e.g. tuberculosis) or lymphomatous nodes
  - **Soft lumps:** acute inflammatory lymph nodes
  - **Fluctuant lumps:** branchial cysts, cystic hygromas, pharyngeal pouches, laryngoceles, cold abscesses, epidermal cysts, dermoid cysts.

- **Is it pulsatile?** Subclavian or carotid aneurysms are pulsatile. Carotid body tumours are often pulsatile but not necessarily so.

- **Is it mobile?** This question relates principally to lymphadenopathy. The majority of lymph nodes are relatively mobile. Malignant lymph nodes may be tethered to adjacent structures, while tuberculous nodes may appear matted together.

Is there anything other than the lump that the GP should examine?

It is always important to examine the entire neck systematically. For many of the isolated causes of a neck lump (such as a carotid body tumour or pharyngeal pouch), examining the neck and characterizing the lump is likely to be sufficient. However, lymphadenopathy and parotid masses require further assessment. The remainder of the clinical examination will be dictated by the history and examination findings thus far. The following is a possible guide:

- If **infectious lymphadenopathy** is suspected:
  - Examine the throat, paying particular attention to the tonsils.
  - Systematically examine all lymph nodes of the head and neck.

- If **malignant lymphadenopathy** is suspected:
  - Examine the scalp, face, ears, mouth, and nose for a potential squamous cell carcinoma or melanoma. Otalgia in the absence of any pathology detected by otoscopy is suggestive of malignancy (with referred pain to the ear).
  - Systematically examine all lymph nodes of the head and neck.
  - Examine the breasts (in women) and the lungs.
  - Consider palpating for hepatosplenomegaly if lymphoma or chronic lymphocytic leukaemia is suspected.
  - Perform a full abdominal examination if Virchow's node (left supraclavicular node) is palpable.
  - To complete the search for malignancy it will be necessary to use a fibreoptic endoscope to examine the nasal cavity, nasopharynx, oropharynx, and hypopharynx—something usually done by ENT specialists.
- If there is a **parotid swelling:**
  - Examine the integrity of the facial nerve. This nerve sits between the deep and superficial lobes of the parotid, and a palsy may result from an invasive malignant tumour (but not from a benign adenoma, which is non-invasive).
  - Examine the oral cavity for displacement of the soft palate by a tumour involving the deep lobe of the parotid.

The GP examines Mr Haversham's neck. There is a prominent lump in the left anterior triangle. The lump lies just anterior to the superior third of sternocleidomastoid. The lump is not concealed by muscular contraction. It is approximately 4.5 cm × 3 cm in size, elliptical in shape, and has a smooth surface and borders. It is not tender or warm, has a hard consistency, is non-pulsatile and non-mobile, appearing to be tethered to adjacent structures. There are no other palpable lesions in the neck.

Based upon the history and examination findings thus far, what is the likely anatomical origin of this lump?

It is most likely that this swelling represents **lymphadenopathy**. It is not tender or warm, suggesting that it is not an acute inflammation or infection. It is not obscured by muscular contraction, thus it is superficial to the muscles. It is firm, and therefore not a cystic structure or a lipoma. Most worrying is the fact that this firm lump appears tethered to surrounding structures—a 'red flag' sign for a malignant lymph node.

The GP examines Mr Haversham's scalp, face, ears, mouth, and nose, but detects nothing abnormal.

How should the GP proceed? Are there any initial investigations that may help determine the cause of the lymphadenopathy?

This lump must be regarded as **squamous cell carcinoma that has metastasized to the lymph nodes** until proven otherwise. Mr Haversham should be referred urgently to a specialist head and neck cancer clinic.
There are two initial investigations that are routinely used:

- **Ultrasound:** the shape, size, echogenicity, and vascularity of lymph nodes can be used to distinguish pathological nodes from normal superficial nodes. Furthermore, malignant nodes have relatively typical ultrasound appearances.
- **Fine needle aspiration (FNA):** this is used to provide a cytological diagnosis. FNA may be ultrasound-guided. Note that lymphoma may be suggested by FNA, but that core biopsy is usually required to confirm the specific subtype.

FNA of Mr Haversham's neck lump revealed squamous cell carcinoma. A thorough examination of his oral cavity, coupled with fibreoptic nasoendoscopy (FNE), revealed a primary tumour in 'coffin corner' at the posterior tongue/floor of the mouth. It is notoriously difficult to detect tumours in this region, hence the rather macabre nickname.

Midline neck lump

CORE CASE

Mrs Luther is a 53-year-old woman who presents to her GP because she is becoming increasingly self-conscious about a lump in the front of her neck.

What is your differential diagnosis for a midline neck lump?
Split the differential into thyroid and non-thyroid masses (Figure 4.1).

Thyroid	Non-thyroid
Physiological goitre†	Lipoma
Multinodular goitre†	Dermoid cyst
Graves' disease	Epidermal cyst
Hashimoto's thyroiditis	Abscess
Thyroglossal cyst	Lymphoma
Thyroid cyst	
Solitary adenoma	
Carcinoma	
Subacute thyroiditis (de Quervain's, Riedel's)	

Figure 4.1 Differential diagnosis for midline neck lump.
†Goitre simply means an 'enlarged thyroid gland'. Physiological goitre refers to its natural enlargement during puberty and pregnancy. Multinodular goitre refers to areas of focal hyperplacia within the thyroid gland that cause it to enlarge in a nodular manner.

The key when assessing a midline neck lump is to determine whether the lump is of thyroid origin and, if so, whether it is malignant.

Which questions should the GP ask about the lump itself?

- **How long has the lump been there?** The 'sudden' appearance of a midline lump is suggestive of acute haemorrhage into a thyroid cyst or, more rarely, a fast-growing thyroid carcinoma (anaplastic) or subacute thyroiditis. Thyroglossal cysts have often been present for some time but may 'appear' in adults following an episode of infection. Duration is of little help when attempting to distinguish between the remaining benign and malignant thyroid masses.

- **Has the lump got bigger, smaller, or stayed the same size?** Haemorrhage or infection of an existing lump may produce rapid increases in size. The majority of thyroid neoplasms are slow growing, with the exception of anaplastic carcinoma.

- **Is the lump painful?** Most midline neck lumps are not painful. Subacute thyroiditis, infected thyroglossal cysts, or acute haemorrhagic cysts are often painful. Hashimoto's thyroiditis may result in discomfort, particularly when swallowing, but few patients would describe this as pain. Thyroid cancer is usually painless, but anaplastic carcinoma can cause pain due to infiltration of surrounding structures (such as ear pain due to vagus nerve involvement).

- **Are there any other lumps?** A thyroid swelling in association with cervical lymphadenopathy must be regarded as malignant until proven otherwise.

Which associated symptoms should the GP ask about?

- **Are there any symptoms suggestive of hyper- or hypothyroidism?** These are listed in Table 4.1. (Note that the term 'thyrotoxicosis' is interchangeable with hyperthyroidism.)
- **Are there any symptoms suggestive of compression or invasion?** A midline neck lump such as a goitre may become so large that it exerts a pressure effect on adjacent structures and causes symptoms such as stridor, dyspnoea, dysphagia, and/or discomfort during swallowing. Changes in the quality of the voice may be due to malignant invasion of the recurrent laryngeal nerve and/or vocal cords, but are also common in hypothyroidism due to oedema of the vocal cords.
- **Are there symptoms suggestive of infection?** Ask about malaise, fever, rigors, etc.

Table 4.1 Symptoms suggestive of hyper- or hypothyroidism

Hyperthyroid	Hypothyroid
Irritable/nervous/restless	Apathetic/blunting of thought/fatigue
Increased appetite but weight loss	Weight gain
Diarrhoea	Constipation
Heat intolerance	Cold intolerance
Palpitations	menorrahgia
Oligomenorrhoea	

Are there any particular aspects of (1) the past medical history and (2) family history that the GP should enquire about?

1   Past medical history:
   - **Any autoimmune disorders?** Both Graves' disease and Hashimoto's thyroiditis occur more commonly in patients with other autoimmune disorders such as type 1 diabetes mellitus, pernicious anaemia, vitiligo, and Addison's disease.
   - **Known risk factors for thyroid malignancy?** Previous radiation to the neck (e.g. mantle irradiation of Hodgkin's lymphoma) is a risk factor for the subsequent development of papillary thyroid carcinoma.

2   Family history:
   - **Autoimmune disease?** There may be a familial predisposition to such disorders.
   - **Hereditary forms of thyroid carcinoma?** Approximately 25% of medullary thyroid carcinoma (MTC) is familial. Familial MTC may either be inherited in isolation, or as part of a multiple endocrine neoplasia (MEN-2) syndrome.

Mrs Luther comments that the lump has been present for several months. She happened to notice it while putting on her make-up, but explains that it has never been painful. She thinks that it has increased in size since she first noticed it, but feels that she is probably self-conscious to a degree that isn't necessarily warranted by the size of the lump. She is not aware of any other lumps.

The GP asks direct questions about any symptoms of thyroid dysfunction, breathing or swallowing difficulty, change in voice, and fever. Mrs Luther replies that she has none of these symptoms. There is no significant past medical history or family history. She takes no regular medications and has no allergies. She is a non-smoker and enjoys moderate alcohol intake at weekends.

The GP proceeds to examine the lump.

What should the GP determine about the location and characteristics of the lump?

- **Location:**
    - **Superficial lump?** Lipoma, epidermal cyst, dermoid cyst or abscess.
    - **Deep lump?** Thyroid gland.
- **Relationship to other structures:**
    - **Moves on swallowing?** Thyroid gland (attached to pretracheal fascia).
    - **Moves on tongue protrusion (i.e. deglutition)?** Thyroglossal cyst (attached to hyoid bone).
    - **Tethered to neighbouring muscle or skin?** Malignancy or Riedel's thyroiditis.
- **Character of the lump:**
    - **Diffuse, smooth enlargement?** Physiological goitre, Graves', Hashimoto's, or de Quervain's thyroiditis. In the latter it is also tender.
    - **Solitary, solid nodule?** Malignancy more likely.
    - **Solitary, cystic nodule?** Thyroglossal, epidermal, dermoid, or thyroid cysts.
    - **Multiple nodules?** Multinodular goitre (focal hyperplasia) more likely.

Note that it is difficult to distinguish these possibilities accurately from clinical examination, thus some form of imaging is always needed to confirm or refute your impression.

What else should the GP examine?

- **Is there any cervical lymphadenopathy?** This should raise suspicion of thyroid malignancy, but may also reflect infective causes of neck swelling. The thyroid gland drains to lymph nodes along the carotid sheath.
- **What is the extent of any thyroid swelling?** Bear in mind that the enlargement of the thyroid may extend retrosternally. The GP may wish to examine Mrs Luther with her neck extended, to percuss for retrosternal extension of the lump, or to try and elicit Pemberton's sign (elevating the arms above the head results in facial venous congestion and plethora due to thoracic inlet obstruction by a retrosternal mass).
- **Are there any signs of hyper- or hypothyroidism (Table 4.2)?**

Table 4.2 **Signs of hyper- or hypothyroidism**

Hyperthyroidism	Hypothyroidism
Hand signs	
Fine tremor	Bradycardia
Tachycardia/atrial fibrillation	
Sweating	
Palmar erythema	
Thyroid acropachy (clubbing)	
Onycholysis	
Eye signs	
Lid lag	Loss of outer third of eyebrows
Lid retraction	
Exophthalmos (in Graves' specifically)	
Chemosis	
Ophthalmoplegia	
Other	
Thyroid bruit	Slow, deep voice
Wasting/proximal myopathy	Dry, coarse skin
Pretibial myxoedema (in Graves' specifically)	Oedematous-looking face
	Slow reflexes

Mrs Luther has a 2 cm × 3 cm nodule to the left of her trachea, in the lower third of her neck. The lump is deep and moves when Mrs Luther is asked to swallow—thus it appears that this is a nodule in the left lobe of the thyroid gland. The nodule is firm and non-tender to palpation. The right lobe of the thyroid is not palpable, and there appear to be no other nodules. There is no cervical lymphadenopathy and Mrs Luther is clinically euthyroid.

Which simple investigations should the GP request?

Clinical examination has poor sensitivity for thyroid status and thus the GP should request biochemical tests of thyroid function. Mrs Luther's thyroid status will have a considerable influence upon her further investigation and management. Firstly, note that the presence of a goitre (which Mrs Luther doesn't have) says nothing of a patient's thyroid status—they could be hyper-, hypo-, or euthyroid, and thus you must confirm their status in order to manage them appropriately. Secondly, thyroid status is critically important when considering thyroid nodules because patients with malignancy are almost always euthyroid—hence a diagnosis of hyperthyroidism in a patient with a thyroid nodule should be seen as a 'good' sign.

As a first step, the GP should request:

- **Thyroid-stimulating hormone (TSH)**: in all patients with a thyroid lump. Elevated levels are usually consistent with hypothyroidism while suppressed levels are usually consistent with hyperthyroidism.[†] The GP may request additional tests of thyroid function according to the initial TSH result:

- if TSH is low, request **free tri-iodothyronine (T$_3$)** and **free thyroxine (T$_4$)**
- if TSH is high, request **thyroid peroxidase antibodies** (Hashimoto's).

- **Serum calcitonin**: only if there is a significant family history of thyroid cancer (or MEN-2). MTC is a tumour of the calcitonin-secreting parafollicular C-cells, thus calcitonin can be used as a serum marker.

The GP requests a serum TSH, which is later reported as 3.9 mU/L.

Should Mrs Luther be referred to an endocrine surgeon or endocrinologist?

Broadly speaking, if a patient has evidence of altered thyroid function they should be routinely referred to an endocrinologist as thyroid cancer is very rare in this group. By contrast, euthyroid patients with thyroid nodules (either solitary nodules or dominant nodules in multinodular goitres) should be referred to an endocrine surgeon in the first instance. Thus, Mrs Luther should be referred to an **endocrine surgeon**.

Given that Mrs Luther's lump is not rapidly enlarging, and she has no associated lymphadenopathy or changes to her voice, this referral can be non-urgent. Obviously, if she had any degree of stridor associated with her lump then she would need to be seen by the surgical team the same day.

Mrs Luther is referred to an endocrine surgeon. She is euthyroid and clinical examination has revealed a single firm nodule in the left lobe of the thyroid.

What further investigation(s) is the surgeon likely to request?

The first-line test for the investigation of thyroid nodules is FNA. Ultrasound may be used to guide aspirations, and can provide an estimate of nodule size and an assessment of whether the nodule is solid, cystic, or mixed (solid and mixed nodules have a higher likelihood of malignancy).

There is relatively little indication for **radionuclide scanning** nowadays. These scans use isotopes (^{99}Tc or ^{123}I) to indicate whether a nodule is functioning or not. Nodules are thus reported as either being 'hot' (functioning) or 'cold' (non-functioning). Hot nodules are almost always benign, whereas about 5–20% of cold nodules are malignant. However, given that about 90% of scanned nodules are cold, radionuclide scanning has little specificity for detecting malignancy. A serum TSH assay serves much the same purpose.

There is also little indication for **CT** scanning or **MRI** as a first-line investigation in the majority of cases. The exceptions include retrosternal extension of a goitre, invasive tumours, and haemoptysis. As an aside, it is important to avoid the use of iodinated contrast media with CT scans as these can reduce subsequent uptake of therapeutic radio-iodine by thyroid tissue if needed for treatment.

Mrs Luther is examined by a surgeon and an ultrasound-guided FNA of the nodule is performed. The aspirate is reported by the pathologist as a 'follicular lesion/suspected follicular neoplasm'.

Does Mrs Luther have thyroid cancer? How should she be managed?

[†] The relationship of TSH to thyroid status will differ if the abnormality originates at the level of the anterior pituitary or hypothalamus, but these patients would not present with a thyroid mass, and in any case this is very rarely the cause of thyroid disturbance.

There are a number of potential outcomes for FNA of a thyroid nodule:

- Insufficient aspirate to make a diagnosis = Thy1
- Benign (e.g. thyroiditis) = Thy2
- Follicular lesion/suspected follicular neoplasm = Thy3
- Suspicious of malignancy = Thy4
- Diagnostic of malignancy = Thy5

Unfortunately, FNA cannot distinguish between a benign **follicular adenoma** and a malignant **follicular carcinoma**. Thus it is not possible to say whether Mrs Luther has cancer or not. As a consequence, most patients whose pathology shows follicular cells will be discussed by the thyroid cancer multidisciplinary team (MDT) and will be usually treated as if they have cancer (lobectomy ± completion thyroidectomy if the pathology is malignant). There are a number of stages to subsequent management:

1   **Surgery.** Low-risk[†] follicular carcinoma may be treated by thyroid lobectomy whereas high-risk patients are usually offered total or near-total thyroidectomy.

2   **T_3 replacement.** The patient must have replacement thyroid hormone as their thyroid gland has now been removed. However, TSH levels need to be high (hence the patient is hypothyroid) at the time of administration of subsequent radio-iodine (see point 3), because the high TSH stimulates uptake of radio-iodine. We therefore need to stop the administration of exogenous thyroid hormone prior to radio-iodine therapy, so that TSH is released from negative feedback and levels have time to rise. T_3 has a half-life of about 2.5 days and thus can be stopped 2 weeks before radio-iodine therapy. By contrast, if T_4 (which has a half-life of 7–10 days) was used to replace the patient's thyroid hormone, it would need to be stopped about 6 weeks prior to radio-iodine therapy, and the patient would spend longer in an unpleasant hypothyroid state.

3   **^{131}I ablation.** The radio-iodine is selectively taken up by thyroid cells, which are then destroyed by the radiation. This is done for all patients who have undergone total or near-total thyroidectomy as a way of eliminating any malignant cells left behind after surgery. T_3 suppression is stopped 2 weeks before treatment so that any remaining thyroid cells take up the ^{131}I. Some countries are investigating an alternative strategy whereby thyroid hormone replacement does not need to be stopped prior to ^{131}I ablation, and patients are given recombinant TSH to stimulate radio-iodine uptake.

4   **T_4 suppression.** Give a dose sufficient to suppress TSH secretion completely (as TSH will stimulate any remaining, potentially malignant, thyroid tissue to regrow). If thyroglobulin (TG) levels then rise above zero in the presence of T_4 suppression, it suggests a return of the malignant thyroid cells.

5   **Follow-up.** This is usually annual clinical examination with measurement of serum TSH and TG.

Fortunately the prognosis for most differentiated thyroid cancer (follicular or papillary) is very good, and the overall 10-year survival rate is approximately 80–90%.

[†] There are various features that are used to allocate patients with differentiated thyroid cancer to either high-risk or low-risk groups. The principal factors contributing to high risk are older age, male gender, poorly differentiated histological features, tumour size (>4 cm), extrathyroidal invasion, and metastatic spread (but not lymph node involvement, unlike in many other cancers).

Short cases

Mr Fry is a 23-year-old bartender who presents to his GP concerned about a lump in his neck. On further questioning he reveals that he has noticed a very slight swelling in his neck 'above his Adam's apple' for the past few years. However, the lump has approximately doubled in size over the course of the last week. It is not painful and he is aware of no other lumps. He has recently suffered from an upper respiratory tract infection, and had to take one day off work last week, but is otherwise fit and well. He takes no regular medications and has no known allergies. He smokes 10 cigarettes each day, and consumes about 35 units of alcohol (as spirits) each week.

On examination, there is an upper midline neck lesion measuring 2 cm × 2 cm. When Mr Fry is asked to stick his tongue out or swallow, the lump rises up his neck. It does not appear to be attached to the large neck muscles. The lump has well-defined boundaries and a smooth surface. It feels cystic and is non-pulsatile. It is mildly tender to palpation. The overlying skin appears normal. No other lumps are detected on clinical examination.

What is the diagnosis? How do you account for the recent change in the size of the lump?

An upper midline cystic lesion that is attached to the hyoid bone (hence rises when the tongue is protruded) is consistent with a **thyroglossal cyst**.

These are the most common upper midline neck lesions, and can present at any age between approximately 4 months and 70 years, but most present before the age of 30. The vast majority of thyroglossal cysts are midline (about 10% are lateral), and about 75% of these are at the level of the hyoid. The cysts represent abnormalities in the descent of the thyroid gland from the junction of the anterior two-thirds and posterior one-third of the tongue to its normal position inferior to the thyroid cartilage. The thyroid gland travels down the thyroglossal tract, any part of which may remain and form a sinus or cyst.

The sudden increase in size of the cyst represents infection secondary to the patient's recent upper respiratory tract infection (hence the lump is tender to palpation). It is not uncommon for thyroglossal cysts to present in this way.

Treatment is by surgical resection of the cyst ± the mid-portion of the hyoid bone (Sistrunk's procedure). There are three reasons for excision:

1   eliminating the chance of further infection
2   eliminating the (small) chance of carcinoma in the cyst
3   cosmesis.

Mrs Slocock is a 47-year-old woman who presents to her GP with a lump in her neck. She reports that she has recently noticed a slight swelling in the right side of her neck. She first noticed the lump about 6 weeks ago when she happened to feel her neck (for no particular reason) and noted slight asymmetry. She has continued to feel the lump every few days but is unsure whether it has changed in size. The lump is not painful and she is not aware of any other lumps. She reports feeling well, has no significant past medical history, and takes no regular medicines. She has never smoked, but drinks approximately two bottles of wine per week.

On examination there is a 2 cm × 2 cm lump in the deep tissues of the upper right anterior triangle. The lump does not appear to be attached to sternocleidomastoid. It is firm, non-tender, and has a transmitted pulse. It is possible to move the lump from side to side but not up and down.

What is the most likely diagnosis? How should Mrs Slocock be investigated?

The examination findings suggest that Mrs Slocock has a **carotid body tumour** (also known as a chemodectoma). The lump is located in the region of the carotid bifurcation, is mobile from side to side but not up and down (due to its relation with the carotid artery), and has a transmitted pulse. Large vascular carotid body tumours may be truly pulsatile. Carotid body tumours are a type of glomus tumour or paraganglioma (glomus cells are specialized chemoreceptor cells). They are typically slow growing, but large tumours may exert pressure effects resulting in complications such as cranial nerve palsies or Horner's syndrome.

Carotid body tumours require imaging to determine their precise location. Suitable modalities include duplex ultrasound, angiography, and CT/MRI.

Treatment in the majority of patients is surgical excision. However, as these are such slow-growing tumours it is not unusual for conservative management to be adopted in elderly patients.

SHORT CASE

Miss Banfi is an 18-year-old student who presents to her GP with a sore throat, headache, fever, and fatigue. She has felt unwell for 5 days and is concerned that her symptoms have not improved. On further questioning, she has not had a cough and has had no coryzal symptoms. A couple of her peers at college are suffering from the same symptoms. She has otherwise been fit and well. She has recently started using the combined oral contraceptive pill, and has no known allergies. She does not smoke, but drinks approximately 20 units of wine each week. She has never been outside the UK.

On examination, Miss Banfi is febrile. She has enlarged tonsils and multiple palpable lumps in her neck. Miss Banfi was unaware of these lumps until the GP palpated them. There are five firm and tender lumps, all of which are subcutaneous and in the posterior triangle. Three of the lumps are on the left and two are on the right. The lumps are relatively mobile and are not warm or pulsatile. The GP performs an abdominal examination and detects splenomegaly.

What is the likely cause of the neck lumps? Which blood tests could the GP order to clinch a diagnosis? Should the GP prescribe Miss Banfi a course of amoxicillin for her sore throat?

Multiple, firm, subcutaneous lumps in the posterior triangle can be little other than lymph nodes. The fact that they are tender and coexisting with an acute febrile illness makes it highly likely that this is **cervical lymphadenitis**. The combination of sore throat, lymphadenopathy, fever, tonsillar enlargement, and (most importantly) splenomegaly are characteristic of glandular fever (also known as infectious mononucleosis), caused by **Epstein–Barr virus** (EBV). Toxoplasmosis and acute cytomegalovirus (CMV) can also cause lymphadenopathy and splenomegaly, but would not account for the sore throat and swollen tonsils.

The GP could order the following blood tests:

- **Full blood count**: looking for leucocytosis and lymphocytosis.
- **Heterophil antibody tests**: the Paul–Bunnell (monospot) test is based on the fact that an EBV antigen is similar to antigens on the red blood cells of many animals but not humans, so that

mixing blood from an EBV-positive human patient with animal blood causes the animal's red blood cells to aggregate and precipitate out of solution—something that can be readily appreciated under the microscope. More modern tests use enzyme-linked immunosorbent assay (ELISA) to detect the same antibodies. However, both tests rely on anti-EBV antibodies being present and so can be falsely negative during the early stages of infection (the first 2 weeks), before antibodies are produced.

- **Blood film**: looking for lymphocytosis and atypical T-lymphocytes (large with irregular nuclei).

EBV yields a positive result in all three of the above blood tests. A more specific test is to detect IgM towards the EBV viral capsid antigen (although other herpesviruses, e.g. CMV, can induce IgM antibodies to cells that express EBV antigens). This is often combined with testing for IgG towards EBV nuclear antigen, which only appears after some delay but persists lifelong. If positive, this indicates prior exposure and excludes acute infection. EBV DNA levels are sometimes measured using PCR in those with prior infection (now latent) to assess for reactivation, e.g. immunosuppressed transplant patients—but this is not a diagnostic test for glandular fever.

The GP should not prescribe amoxicillin or ampicillin for Miss Banfi's sore throat as both of these antibiotics can precipitate a severe rash in patients with acute EBV infection. There is no specific management for glandular fever, although Miss Banfi should avoid any contact sports for a few months as there is a risk of damage to the enlarged and delicate spleen. Miss Banfi may, however, derive symptomatic benefit from analgesics and throat lozenges.

SHORT CASE

Mr Farquhar is a 22-year-old trainee accountant who presents to his GP with a lump in the left side of his neck. The lump has been present for a couple of weeks and has gradually been increasing in size. Mr Farquhar remarks that he has had a slight swelling in the same place on two previous occasions, but the lump was less prominent and gradually disappeared over the course of a week. On specific questioning, both of these previous episodes corresponded with an upper respiratory tract infection. The last episode was approximately one month ago. His current lump is not painful. His is aware of no other lumps. He is currently well, takes no regular medications, and has no allergies. He is teetotal and has never smoked.

On examination, there is a single palpable lesion in the left anterior triangle, anterior to the junction of the superior third and inferior two-thirds of sternocleidomastoid. The lump does not move when Mr Farquhar is asked to swallow or stick out his tongue. The lump is smooth, non-tender, fluctuant, and non-pulsatile. It measures approximately 2.5 cm × 2 cm and is not mobile.

Which diagnosis is most likely?

It is most likely that Mr Farquhar has a **branchial cyst**—a fluctuant, non-tender lump in the upper third of the neck anterior to sternocleidomastoid. Branchial cysts are congenital epithelial cysts that result from failure of obliteration of the second branchial cleft. Despite being congenital, the cyst may not present clinically until early adulthood. They are usually unilateral, about 60% are in the location described in this case, and about 80% present as a persistent swelling. The remaining 20% that present as intermittent swellings often coincide with upper respiratory tract infections. It is likely that the two previous neck lumps that Mr Farquhar describes represent such phenomena, but it is also possible that the lumps were reactive lymph nodes.

SHORT CASE

Miss Pellegrino is a 23-year-old waitress who presents to her GP with a 2-month history of a lump in her neck. She does not think that the lump has changed in size, and reports that it is not painful. She is not aware of any other lumps. She has otherwise been fit and well, and reports no systemic symptoms. There is no history of trauma to the neck. She has no significant past medical history, and her only regular medication is the combined oral contraceptive pill. She smokes 20 cigarettes a day, and consumes approximately 15 units of wine each week.

Examination reveals a non-midline 1.5 cm × 1.5 cm lump in the left anterior triangle of her neck. The lump has smooth regular borders and is fluctuant. It is non-tender. The lump cannot be moved separately from the overlying skin, but is mobile over deeper tissues. It does not change position when Miss Pellegrino is asked to swallow or when she is asked to stick her tongue out. There is a punctum overlying the lump, but no other skin changes. There is no cervical lymphadenopathy.

What is the most likely diagnosis? What treatment should Miss Pellegrino be offered?

The examination findings are of a cystic (fluctuant) lump within the skin, hence this is likely to be a **dermoid cyst** or **epidermal cyst**. Dermoid cysts are either formed at embryological lines of fusion (hence a neck dermoid would be midline) or following a puncture injury (as an 'implantation' dermoid). Miss Pellegrino's lump is neither in the midline, nor follows any known trauma to the neck. Coupled with the fact epidermal cysts are more common than dermoids, it is most likely that this is an **epidermal cyst**.

Epidermal cysts are formed when sebaceous glands are blocked—hence they are often associated with a punctum. They can occur on any part of the skin other than the palms or soles, since these areas have no sebaceous glands.

Epidermal cysts may be **excised** (according to local funding arrangements for surgical excision of benign masses) for cosmetic reasons. The cyst is excised under local anaesthetic. An incision is made to encompass the punctum, and the cyst is removed with the capsule intact. If the entire cyst is not successfully removed it is liable to recur.

SHORT CASE

Miss Phelps is a 32-year-old lifeguard who presents to her GP with a midline neck lump. The lump has been present for a couple of months, but Miss Phelps is not sure whether it has changed in size. The lump is not painful, and Miss Phelps is not aware of any other lumps. On direct questioning, she reports that she has become rather irritable towards her boyfriend recently. Her appetite has increased, although she has gained no weight. In addition, she reports that her eyes have started to feel rather 'gritty' and wonders whether she may be developing hay fever. Miss Phelps is otherwise well. She has no significant medical history and takes no medications. She smokes about 10 cigarettes daily, but does not drink alcohol. There is no significant family history.

On examination, Miss Phelps has a diffuse midline swelling in the lower third of her neck. The lump measures approximately 6 cm across. It is non-tender, and moves upwards when Miss Phelps is asked to swallow. The lump is smooth and there are no palpable nodules within it. There is no cervical lymphadenopathy.

Miss Phelps' pulse is 105 bpm, regular. Her palms are rather sweaty. The GP notes that she has exophthalmos and is also able to demonstrate lid lag.

What is the likely diagnosis? Would you like to request any investigations? How should Miss Phelps be managed?

Miss Phelps probably has **Graves' disease**. She has a smooth goitre, is clinically hyperthyroid, and also has signs of thyroid eye disease. In the context of hyperthyroidism, eye signs only occur with Graves' disease. Interestingly, smoking increases the risk of Graves' eye disease and thus Miss Phelps should be advised to stop smoking.

The next step should be to confirm Miss Phelps' thyroid status by requesting serum **TSH** and, possibly **free T$_3$** and **free T$_4$**. A suppressed serum TSH level with elevated free T$_3$ and free T$_4$ would support the diagnosis.

Miss Phelps should be referred to a specialist endocrine clinic. There are four broad treatment options available to her:

1 **Antithyroid medication**: drugs such as carbimazole and propylthiouracil are used for control of symptoms for up to about 18 months in the hope of remission. Those who recur need definitive treatment with either radio-iodine or surgery. Patients taking carbimazole need to be warned of the rare but serious risk of agranulocytosis, and must be advised to seek urgent medical attention if they develop signs of infection.

2 **β-Blockers**: remember that thyroxine essentially makes tissues more sensitive to adrenaline and noradrenaline, hence β-blockers counteract the symptoms of hyperthyroidism.

3 **Radio-iodine (^{131}I)**: but about 10% of patients will be rendered hypothyroid within 5 years. In addition, Graves' eye disease is a relative contraindication to radio-iodine, women of child-bearing age must be warned not to become pregnant within 6 months of receiving treatment, and those with household contacts (particularly children) must take contact precautions for up to 2 weeks, depending on dosages used and the ages of the contacts.

4 **Total thyroidectomy** and subsequent lifelong replacement therapy with levothyroxine.

Viva questions

What are the anatomical boundaries of the anterior and posterior triangles of the neck?

The boundaries of the anterior triangle are the inferior ramus of the mandible, the anterior border of sternocleidomastoid, and the midline of the anterior neck. Clinically speaking, lumps superficial, within, or deep to sternocleidomastoid are also considered to be within the anterior triangle.

The boundaries of the posterior triangle are the posterior border of sternocleidomastoid, the superior border of the clavicle, and the anterior border of trapezius (see Figure 4.2).

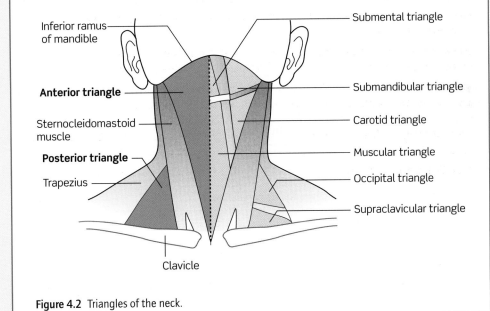

Figure 4.2 Triangles of the neck.

A patient presents with intermittent painful swelling of the parotid gland on one side of his face. Which single question will you ask him about precipitants of the swelling?

The key question is to ask the patient whether the painful swelling is related to eating. This history is typical of sialolithiasis—salivary gland calculi. Calculi may get stuck in the salivary duct(s), causing outflow obstruction. Increased salivary production during eating produces increased back-pressure into the gland which results in painful distension.

What are the characteristic features of the MEN syndromes?

The MEN syndromes represent a predisposition to specific endocrine tumours and are inherited in an autosomal dominant fashion. There are three main syndromes:

1 MEN-1
   - Parathyroid (hyperplasia or adenoma)
   - Pituitary (prolactinoma or growth hormone-secreting tumour)
   - Pancreas (insulinoma, gastrinoma, non-functional)
2 MEN-2A
   - Thyroid (MTC)
   - Adrenal (phaeochromocytoma)
   - Parathyroid (hyperplasia or adenoma)
3 MEN-2B
   - Thyroid (MTC)
   - Adrenal (phaeochromocytoma)
   - Mucocutaneous neuromas

Turner's syndrome (45 XO) is associated with which neck lump?

Cystic hygromas are strongly associated with Turner's syndrome.

Sjögren's syndrome is a risk factor for which neck lump?

Patients are at increased risk of non-Hodgkin's lymphoma.

What is the surface anatomy of the thyroid gland?

The isthmus of the thyroid gland lies inferior to the cricoid cartilage, over the second and third tracheal rings—lower than most people think. The lateral lobes extend superiorly as far as the middle of the thyroid cartilage, and inferiorly as far as the sixth tracheal ring. See Figure 4.3.

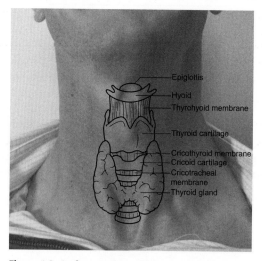

Figure 4.3 Surface anatomy of the thyroid gland.

What is the pathophysiology of (1) Graves' disease and (2) Hashimoto's disease?

1   Graves' disease is an autoimmune non-destructive, stimulatory thyroid disease. The underlying mechanism is antibody-mediated stimulation of the TSH receptor (sometimes referred to as type V hypersensitivity). It presents as **hyperthyroidism and exophthalmos** (due to infiltration of the extraocular muscles by immune cells).

2   Hashimoto's disease is an autoimmune destructive thyroid disease. Antithyroid antibodies are present, including antibodies to the TSH receptor but they are non-pathogenic. The underlying mechanism is T-cell-mediated destruction of the thyroid gland (type IV hypersensitivity). It usually presents as **hypothyroidism.**

Which histological types of thyroid neoplasia are there? Which are most common?

The following are all types of thyroid neoplasia:

- Papillary (~60%)
- Follicular (including Hürthle cell tumours) (~25%)
- Medullary (~5%)
- Lymphoma (~5%)
- Anaplastic (rare)
- Metastases (rare)

What are the indications for prophylactic thyroidectomy?

There is a significant risk of MTC in children with a family history of MEN-2A, MEN-2B, or familial MTC (FMTC). The underlying mutations in the *RET* proto-oncogene are inherited in an autosomal dominant manner (chromosome 10q). In contrast to sporadic MTC, the familial form is more likely to be bilateral and metastasize early. As such, it is recommended that these children undergo prophylactic thyroidectomy and lifelong replacement with levothyroxine therapy. The timing of surgery depends upon the underlying condition. Current British Thyroid Association/Royal College of Physicians guidelines recommend surgery at the following ages:

- MEN-2A: before 5 years
- MEN-2B: before 1 year
- FMTC: after 10 years

More precise indications for age-related prophylactic thyroidectomy are being considered based upon the actual codons inherited.

What are the potential complications of thyroidectomy?

As with any surgical procedure, we can divide complications into those specific to the particular operation, and complications of surgery in general:

1 Potential complications specific to thyroidectomy:

- **Injury to the recurrent laryngeal nerve(s)**. Risk 1 in 100. Unilateral damage produces a weak, hoarse voice. Bilateral damage may require tracheostomy.
- **Injury to the superior laryngeal nerve(s)**. Risk 1 in 20. Damage leads to difficulties adjusting the pitch of phonation—for example difficulty shouting or singing.
- **Transient voice changes**. Risk 1 in 10. Occurring in the absence of nerve injury, and lasting 3–6 months.
- **Transient hypocalcaemia**. Risk 1 in 6. Due to bruising of the parathyroid gland.
- **Hypoparathyroidism**. Risk 1–2 in 100. Due to parathyroid gland damage.
- **Hyperthyroid storm**. Very rare. If hyperthyroid patients are not adequately medicated prior to surgery, large concentrations of thyroid hormones may be released during surgery. Mortality may be as high as 20–30%.
- **Postoperative haemorrhage and airway compromise**. Very rare, but very serious.

2 Potential complications of surgery in general:

- Infection.
- Hypertrophic or keloid scarring.
- Thromboembolism (deep vein thrombosis (DVT) or pulmonary embolism (PE)).
- Anaesthetic complications (e.g. inadequate analgesia, respiratory depression, urinary retention, cardiac depression).

How does the tachycardia seen with hyperthyroidism differ from the tachycardia seen in generalized anxiety states?

The tachycardia associated with hyperthyroidism can be distinguished from anxiety-driven tachycardia in two ways:

1 **Rhythm**: hyperthyroidism is often associated with atrial fibrillation, particularly in older patients.

2 **Timing**: tachycardia due to hyperthyroidism will persist while the patient is sleeping, while tachycardia due to anxiety should disappear.

In euthyroid patients with a solitary nodule on clinical examination, what features of the history and examination will raise your suspicions of thyroid malignancy?

There are a number of features that increase the likelihood that a thyroid nodule is malignant:

1 Demographic factors
- Male sex
- Age <20 years or >70 years

CONTINUED ➤

CONTINUED

2 History
- Rapid growth
- Compression symptoms (e.g. dysphagia, dysphonia, hoarseness)
- Previous neck irradiation
- Family history of MEN or familial MTC

3 Examination
- Firm, hard nodule
- Fixity to adjacent structures
- Cervical lymphadenopathy

Single Best Answers

1. A patient presents to their GP with a neck lump, noted to be in the midline. Which of the following would be on your differential?

a. Pharyngeal pouch
b. Branchial cyst
c. Cystic hygroma

d. Multinodular goitre
e. All of the above

2. An elderly patient presents with a rapidly growing neck lump on the left. Which of the following symptoms would you be most interested in?

a. Dysphonia
b. Cough
c. Dysphagia

d. Otalgia
e. All of the above

3. A female patient presents with a lateral neck lump that you think is a parotid mass. Which of the following is most important in your examination of this patient?

a. Examine the abdomen for hepatosplenomegaly
b. Examine the ears

c. Examine the breasts
d. Examine the facial nerve
e. Examine the throat

4. A hyperthyroid patient is started an carbimazole. What in particular should you warn then about?

a. Nausea and vomiting
b. Infection
c. Headache

d. Palpitations
e. Skin sensitivity

5. Which of the following is not a type of thyroid cancer?

a. Squamous cell carcinoma
b. Follicular
c. Anaplastic

d. Medullary
e. Papillary

Haematemesis

Core case

Read through the sections in the case boxes, covering up the sections that follow so that you don't see the answer. At the end of each case box, try to answer the question before reading on.

> It is 3 a.m. and an ambulance arrives at the Emergency Department carrying Mr Tucker, a 42-year-old man of no fixed abode. He has blood down his chin and over his shirt, but is alert and orientated. The emergency services were called out by the staff of a local night shelter. Mr Tucker was trying to gain access to the night shelter but this was denied due to his intoxication. As he argued with the staff, he began to vomit. The staff saw he was vomiting blood and called for an ambulance. The paramedics state that on the way to the hospital he retched and brought up a few spoonfuls of blood. Mr Tucker is immediately taken to the resuscitation room.
>
> **How will you manage this patient?**

First of all, **call for help.** You cannot manage an emergency alone—it involves teamwork. Call for help and involve your seniors.

Second, this patient has potentially lost a lot of blood. Start with ABCDE—Airway, Breathing, Circulation, Disability, Exposure.

Airway: Ensure it is patent. Can he talk? Is there any gurgling or stridor? Beware of blood in the oropharynx in a patient with haematemesis. If necessary, use suction to remove the blood.

Breathing: Are there any signs of respiratory distress (tachypnoea, use of accessory muscles, low saturations)?

Circulation: Does he have a pulse? Is he in shock (tachycardia, narrow pulse pressure, hypotension, cold peripheries)?

Disability: what is the patient's Glasgow Coma Score (GCS)? Always calculate this in an emergency as a GCS ≤8 (or rapidly dropping towards that point) suggests that the patient may soon require intubation to protect their airway. If you can't remember the components of a GCS in an emergency, use the AVPU score (patient is Alert, responds to Voice, responds to Pain or is Unresponsive), where an avPu score (i.e. a patient who is responding to painful stimuli but not voice) is roughly equivalent to a GCS = 8.

Exposure: The patient may have suffered multiple trauma and/or have various sites of blood loss. Although it is unlikely, what the hostel staff perceived as drunken behaviour may in fact represent behaviour from an unwitnessed assault resulting in significant head injury, and the haematemesis may reflect a stab wound to the chest or abdomen. Always expose the patient or you will be caught out by unsuspected findings.

> Mr Tucker looks dishevelled and is obviously inebriated. He starts to tell you about his days in the army as the team take his vital observations, indicating that his airway is clear and he is breathing. He has a heart rate (HR) of 130 bpm, respiratory rate of 30/min and blood pressure (BP) of 86/52 mmHg (supine). His oxygen saturations are 97% on air. His GCS is 14/15 (M6, V4, E4) and full exposure of his body reveals yellow (old) bruising over his forearms but no other obvious signs of trauma.
>
> **What is your next step?**

Mr Tucker is in **shock,** often defined as a BP <90/60 mmHg. He needs fluid resuscitation:

- Apply high flow **oxygen** (15 L/min).
- **Get intravenous (IV) access:** insert a large-bore (14G–16G) cannula and if you can't do it yourself, ask a senior to help. They may need to resort to ultrasound-guided peripheral vascular access, to intraosseus access or to central venous access.
- **Send bloods for:**
  - **Venous blood gas:** this will give you a rapid estimate of the patient's haemoglobin. Note that it takes time for haemodilution to cause a drop in haemoglobin concentration or haematocrit as both red blood cells and plasma volume are lost equally when bleeding. Venous blood gas analysis will also provide a lactate, which is indicative of the degree of shock: hypoperfused tissues rely on anaerobic respiration with a consequent increase in lactate. As lactate is an acid, this will be reflected in the pH.
  - **Clotting:** to check for a bleeding tendency that may need correcting. Some Emergency Departments now have point-of-care clotting machines that will tell you the INR within 10 minutes, at the bedside, and using only a few drops of blood.
  - **Cross-match four units** of blood.
  - **Full blood count** (FBC) for a more accurate haemoglobin and a platelet count. Low platelets can contribute to bleeding.
  - **Urea and creatinine:** is he hypovolaemic and/or in acute renal failure? Is there an elevated urea to indicate a significant gastrointestinal (GI) bleed (effectively a large protein meal) that happened long enough ago to be digested and broken down into urea?
  - **Electrolytes:** does he have an electrolyte disturbance from vomiting? K^+ may be elevated due to destruction of ingested red blood cells although you will get the K^+ result on the VBG before you get it from the labs.
  - **Liver enzymes, bilirubin, and albumin:** these may suggest chronic liver disease, a major cause of oesophageal varices and therefore of haematemesis (clotting also reflects liver synthetic function).
- **Volume resuscitation:**
  - **Give up to 2 L of warmed crystalloid solution (e.g. Hartmann's, Plasmalyte, normal saline)** as 250 ml aliquots stat (i.e. allowed to go in as rapidly as possible, monitoring HR and BP for response).
  - **Consider giving 1 or 2 units of blood** only if there is fresh blood on digital rectal examination (suggesting ongoing bleeding) or signs of shock despite giving the crystalloid solution. Fluid resuscitation should be first-line treatment for shock as a 2008 UK audit of acute upper gastrointestinal bleeding found that patients receiving a transfusion had higher rates of rebleeding and mortality.

    Haemoglobin levels are less helpful in actively bleeding patients because of the delayed drop in haemoglobin. However, a chronically anaemic patient with a low baseline haemoglobin should have a lower threshold for transfusion.

    In patients who are too unstable to wait for cross-matched blood, use O, Rh-negative blood.

- **Monitoring**: if the patient is shocked (or incontinent), consider inserting a urinary catheter. Patients who are unwell enough to require high dependency unit (HDU) or intensive care unit (ICU) care will additionally require a central venous pressure (CVP) and arterial line.

Two large-bore cannulas are inserted, bloods are taken, and fluid resuscitation commenced. Mr Tucker is observed carefully for 30 minutes. His HR is now 110 bpm and his BP has risen to 100/61 mmHg.

What are the causes of haematemesis? Which are the most common and how might this affect your initial management?

Haematemesis is due to bleeding in the upper GI tract (proximal to the ligament of Treitz that demarcates the boundary between the duodenum and jejunum). Potential causes are given in Figure 5.1.

Oesophagitis/gastritis/duodenitis
Bleeding peptic ulcer (gastric or duodenal)
Oesophageal varices

Mallory–Weiss tear

Oesophageal cancer

Gastric cancer

Arteriovenous malformations

Bleeding diathesis

Trauma to oesophagus or stomach

Vascular angiodysplasia in oesophagus or stomach (e.g. Dieulafoy lesion, scleroderma ('watermelon stomach'), hereditary haemorrhagic telangiectasia) Boerhaave's oesophageal perforation

Haemobilia

Aorto-enteric fistula

Figure 5.1 Causes of haematemesis.

By far the most common causes are oesophagitis/gastritis/duodenitis, ulcers, and varices. If you suspect varices (e.g. a patient with known varices on previous endoscopy, or with known cirrhosis), you should include the following in your initial (pre-endoscopy) management:

- **Terlipressin 1–2 mg 4–6 hourly**: Terlipressin is an ADH agonist that causes splanchnic vasoconstriction thereby reducing mesenteric blood flow and portal pressure. It is associated with improved mortality in variceal bleeding (~33% reduction in mortality).

- **Prophylactic antibiotics**: again found to improve outcomes in patients with cirrhosis and upper gastrointestinal bleeding (21% reduction in mortality in a 2010 Cochrane review of 12 trials and 1241 patients).

Note that there is no evidence for the use of proton pump inhibitors pre-endoscopy (but very good evidence for their use post-endoscopy if ulcers are seen).

The consultant asks you to calculate Mr Tucker's Blatchford score.

What is the Blatchford score and how does this differ from the Rockall score?

The Blatchford score (Table 5.1) stratifies patients presenting to hospital with haematemesis into high and low risk groups, and can be used to help guide which patients may be managed as outpatients and which may require urgent intervention. Patients with a score of zero are regarded as low risk and may be suitable for outpatient management. By contrast, patients scoring 6 or more are high risk and the majority will require intervention.

The Rockall score was developed to predict the risk of rebleeding and mortality in patients with upper GI haemorrhage, but is often used as an indicator for severity that helps guide urgency of endoscopy. The advantage of Blatchford as an initial assessment score is that it is independent of endoscopy findings. The scoring systems are given in Tables 5.1, 5.2, and 5.3.

The criteria in Table 5.2 are used to calculate the initial Rockall score, which is based on clinical findings alone. In addition, there are criteria based on findings at endoscopy that serve to calculate the final Rockall score (a combination of pre- and post-endoscopy findings) (Table 5.3).

Table 5.1 The Blatchford score

	1 point	2 points	3 points	4 points	6 points
Urea (mmol/L)		6.5–7.9	8–9.9	10–25	>25
Hb men (g/L)	120–129		100–119		<100
Hb women (g/L)	100–119				<100
Systolic BP (mmHg)	100–109	90–99	<90		
Other markers	Pulse ≥100 Melaena	Syncope Hepatic disease Cardiac disease			

Reprinted from *The Lancet*, Vol. 356, Blatchford O, Murray WR, Blatchford M, 'A risk score to predict need for treatment for upper gastrointestinal haemorrhage', pp. 1318–1321, Copyright 2000, with permission from Elsevier.

Table 5.2 The initial Rockall scoring system (pre-endoscopy)

	0 points	1 point	2 points	3 points
Age	<60 years	60–79 years	≥80 years	
Shock		HR >100 bpm	Systolic BP <100 mmHg	
Comorbidities		Heart failure, ischaemic heart disease, any major comorbidity	Renal failure, liver failure, disseminated malignancy	

Reproduced from *Gut*, TA Rockall, RF Logan, HB Devlin, TC Northfield, 'Risk assessment after acute upper gastrointestinal haemorrhage', 38, 3, pp. 316–321, Copyright 1996, with permission from BMJ Publishing Group Ltd.

Table 5.3 Additional elements to calculate the final (post-endoscopy) Rockall score

	0 points	1 point	2 points	3 points
Stigmata of recent haemorrhage			Blood in the upper GI tract, adherent clot, visible, or spurting blood vessel	
Diagnosis	Mallory–Weiss tear, no lesions identified	All other diagnoses	Malignancy of upper GI tract	

Reproduced from *Gut*, T A Rockall, R F Logan, H B Devlin, T C Northfield, 'Risk assessment after acute upper gastrointestinal haemorrhage', 38, 3, pp. 316–321, Copyright 1996, with permission from BMJ Publishing Group Ltd.

Haematemesis carries an overall mortality of 10% and is therefore a very serious condition. You need to establish whether Mr Tucker is a candidate for emergency endoscopy.

What are the indications for an emergency endoscopy in a patient with haematemesis? What other investigations would you request?

NICE guidelines simply suggest emergency endoscopy 'in unstable patients with severe acute upper gastrointestinal bleeding immediately after resuscitation', although practice varies between hospitals. Suspicion of continuing upper GI bleeding and/or a Blatchford score of ≥6 suggest the need for urgent endoscopy. Although rare, the patient with an aortic graft (particularly a recent graft) may also require an urgent endoscopy to exclude aorto-enteric fistula.

In addition to an oesophagogastroduodenoscopy (OGD), you should consider the following investigations for patients with haematemesis:

- **Erect chest radiograph.** A perforated peptic ulcer may cause both haematemesis and a pneumoperitoneum (although peptic ulcers tend to either bleed or perforate, but rarely do both). You may also see a left-sided pleural effusion if there has been a Boerhaave's perforation, although these are more likely to present with pain and vomiting that isn't haematemesis.

- **CT scan of the chest–abdomen.** All patients with a known aortic graft (e.g. to repair an aortic aneurysm) require a contrast CT aortogram to rule out an aorto-enteric fistula, provided they are haemodynamically stable enough to be transferred to CT.

To determine if Mr Tucker qualifies for an emergency endoscopy, you take a history. You are interested in trying to establish the aetiology of his haematemesis and, in particular, whether he has oesophageal varices.

What questions will you specifically ask on the history?

Presenting complaint and systemic enquiry

- **How much blood has the patient vomited?**
- **What exactly was the character of the vomit?** Fresh blood suggests an upper GI bleed. 'Coffee grounds' suggests blood that has been partially digested by stomach acids but might be confused with faeculent vomiting, as may occur with small bowel obstruction.
- **Melaena (tarry black stools) or frank blood in stool?** Melaena is due to an upper GI haemorrhage and digestion of the blood during GI transit. Haematochezia is fresh blood in the stools. It is usually due to lower GI haemorrhage but can be due to an upper GI haemorrhage if the bleeding is profuse or the GI transit time fast (note that blood can act as a cathartic, reducing transit time).
- **Did forceful vomiting trigger the haematemesis?** Suspect a Mallory–Weiss tear or Boerhaave's perforation.
- **Recent weight loss?** Suspect upper GI malignancy.
- **Problems swallowing?** Suspect oesophageal malignancy.
- **Easy bruising, distended abdomen, puffy ankles, lethargy?** Suspect liver failure. This could explain a bleeding tendency and/or, if the liver is cirrhotic, explain oesophageal varices.
- **Epigastric pain?** Gnawing epigastric pain suggests gastric carcinoma, whilst episodic dyspepsia suggests gastro-oesophageal reflux disease (GORD).

Past medical history

- **Previous upper GI haemorrhage?** How was it managed?
- **Heartburn or epigastric pain?** Suspect a bleeding peptic ulcer or bleeding oesophagitis/gastritis/duodenitis.
- **History of GORD?** If no diagnosis of GORD, history of reflux or waterbrash? Chronic GORD causes oesophagitis and, ultimately, Barrett's oesophagus and adenocarcinoma.
- **Aortic repair with grafts?** Suspect an aorto-enteric fistula until proven otherwise.
- **Bleeding tendency?** Suspect a clotting problem that needs correcting.
- **Chronic liver disease?** Suspect both a bleeding tendency and oesophageal varices.

Drug history

- **Anticoagulants** (e.g. warfarin, rivaroxaban)? Suspect a clotting problem.
- **Regular non-steroidal anti-inflammatory drugs (NSAIDs), aspirin, clopidogrel, steroids, or bis-phosphonates?** Suspect peptic ulcer disease.
- Remember that many drugs can cause liver toxicity long term **(e.g. methotrexate, amiodarone)**.
- **β-Blockers** may mask the signs of shock by preventing a tachycardia in a patient who is hypovolaemic.

Social history

- **Excessive alcohol consumption?** Increases the risk of cirrhosis leading to oesophageal varices, gastritis, and peptic ulcer disease.
- **Smoking?** Increases the risk of peptic ulcer disease and upper GI malignancy.
- **IV drug use? Tattoos?** Suspect chronic viral hepatitis leading to liver cirrhosis.

Mr Tucker is unsure whether the vomiting triggered the haematemesis or whether it was haematemesis from the very beginning. He tells you that he had drunk four 2 L bottles of cider that day and admits that he drinks about two 2 L bottles of cider every day. He frequently has heartburn but denies any reflux. He smokes 'as much as [he] can' and admits to having taken illicit drugs in the past, saying 'you name it, I've done it'. He has never had any surgery and there's been no change in his stools or weight. He does not take any regular medications.

What will you look for on examination?

Look for the following in particular:

On inspection

- **Tattoos? Needle track marks? Piercings?** All are risk factors for chronic viral hepatitis which can cause cirrhosis (in turn causing a bleeding tendency and/or oesophageal varices).
- **Signs of liver disease**: jaundice, scratch marks (jaundice is itchy), bruising, spider naevi (more than four), palmar erythema, Dupuytren's contracture of the palm, gynaecomastia, ascites, ankle oedema, caput medusae? Suspect liver cirrhosis.

- **Purpura?** Suspect thrombocytopenia (e.g. immune thrombocytopenic purpura (ITP), chronic liver disease).
- **Thoraco-abdominal scar?** Has the patient had an abdominal aortic aneurysm (AAA) repair with a graft?
- **Cachexia?** Suspect malignancy.

Abdominal palpation

- **Hepatomegaly?** Can occur in liver disease (although cirrhotic livers are often shrunken).
- **Splenomegaly?** Suspect portal hypertension (usually, but not always, due to liver cirrhosis).
- **Epigastric tenderness?** Suspect peptic ulcer disease or gastritis/duodenitis.
- **Epigastric mass? Supraclavicular lymphadenopathy (Virchow's node)?** Suspect malignancy.

Digital rectal examination

- **Haemorrhoids?** Suspect portal hypertension. Remember that internal haemorrhoids are not palpable.
- **Melaena or haematochezia?** Confirms a GI bleed. Melaena is due to upper GI bleeding. Haematochezia is usually a lower GI bleed but can rarely be due to upper GI bleeds and a rapid GI transit time.

Mr Tucker is jaundiced, has signs of recent IV drug use, and several tattoos. He is thin, but not cachectic. He has palmar erythema and at least 10 spider naevi over his chest and shoulders (see Figure 5.2). A digital rectal examination is unremarkable.

Figure 5.2 Spider naevi on the chest.

CONTINUED ➤

CONTINUED

The erect chest radiograph and blood results become available. The erect chest radiograph is normal. The blood results show:

Haematology			Biochemistry			
Hb	127 g/L	Na	136 mM	Albumin	20 g/L
RBC	3.2×10^{12} cells/L	K	4.1 mM	Bilirubin	62 µM
WCC	5×10^9 cells/L	Urea	10.1 mM	ALT	105 U/L
Platelets	105×10^9 cells/L	Creatinine	102 µM	AST	94 U/L
MCV	112 fL			ALP	230 U/L
				GGT	230 U/L
				Amylase	56 U/L

Clotting	
PT	21.5 seconds
APTT	52 seconds

What do these blood results suggest? Are there any further investigations you will request in light of his history, examination, and initial blood results?

Mr Tucker's blood results show:

- **Macrocytic anaemia**: the high MCV is consistent both with alcohol consumption (although the mechanism by which this causes macrocytosis remains unclear) and vitamin B_{12} or folate deficiency anaemia. Note that the haemoglobin is borderline low. Haemorrhage causes a proportional loss of blood volume and blood contents, so the concentration of red cells and haemoglobin may not change during an acute haemorrhage, by which stage the kidneys will have retained fluid but red blood cells will not yet have been replaced. The very slight anaemia is more likely due to malnutrition—this patient is homeless and therefore at high risk of malnutrition and deficiency of folate and/or vitamin B_{12}.

- **Low albumin**: this is most likely due to chronic liver disease but could be due to malnutrition (insufficient protein in diet), malabsorption, or renal nephrotic syndrome (losing albumin via kidneys).

- **Raised liver enzymes** (ALT, AST) suggesting damage to hepatocytes, which would be consistent with alcohol abuse and liver cirrhosis.

- **Raised bilirubin**. This explains the jaundice.

- **Raised GGT**, particularly in the absence of any changes to ALP, is consistent with alcohol abuse.

- **Prolonged clotting times**: clotting factors II, VII, IX, and X (which mainly affect the PT but also the APTT) are made by the liver, hence prolonged clotting times are consistent with liver disease. More importantly, it suggests a bleeding tendency which may cause, and will certainly exacerbate, any upper GI bleeding.

- **Raised urea**: in the presence of normal renal function (e.g. normal creatinine), this is known as 'pre-renal uraemia'. In this case, it is probably a reflection of increased protein ingestion due to blood in his GI tract.

You should arrange for the following investigations:

- **Viral hepatitis and HIV serology.** Given Mr Tucker's tattoos and evidence of IV drug use, he should be screened for viral hepatitis and HIV. He should be informed you are screening for this.
- **Urinalysis.** Mr Tucker has low albumin so you should rule out proteinuria, which would suggest a nephrotic syndrome (losing protein via the kidneys).

What will you tell the gastroenterology registrar about Mr Tucker's need for an urgent endoscopy?

Mr Tucker is a 42-year-old man of no fixed abode and significant alcohol abuse who presented with haematemesis. He is haemodynamically stable following fluid resuscitation, and shows no overt signs of ongoing upper GI bleed. He has a Blatchford score of 8 due to a HR >100 mmHg at presentation, Hb 127, urea >10 and signs of liver failure (spider naevi, palmar erythema). There is also a suspicion of oesophageal varices due to chronic liver disease (high alcohol intake, jaundice, caput medusae, IV drug use, tattoos). Because of this, he may need an **emergency endoscopy**.

The gastroenterology registrar agrees that an emergency endoscopy is required.

It is difficult to accurately identify the aetiology of haematemesis until endoscopy is performed.

How would you manage any haematemesis patient whilst they await endoscopy? Is there anything you would do differently or in addition in the case of Mr Tucker, and why?

All patients awaiting endoscopy for haematemesis should be managed as follows:

- **Regular observation.** Hourly to begin with. Every 30 minutes if ↓BP or ↑HR.
- **Nil by mouth.** The patient must remain nil by mouth for 6 hours prior to the endoscopy. If the endoscopy is not going to occur within 6 hours then the patient should remain on clear fluids. Stomach contents will obstruct the view at endoscopy and carry a significant risk of aspiration into the lungs during the procedure.
- **Fluids.** All patients will need ongoing IV fluids as they are nil by mouth and potentially still bleeding.
- **Pro-kinetic** 1 hour pre-endoscopy, e.g. erythromycin 250 mg IV or metoclopramide 10 mg IV. This empties the stomach to help the endoscopist get better views.
- If ongoing active bleeding, **consider correcting coagulopathy and/or platelets**. Specifically, transfuse platelets if active bleeding and a count of <50 × 10^9/L, and fresh frozen plasma to patients who have either a fibrinogen <1 g/L or an INR >1.5.

Finally, given Mr Tucker's history of alcohol abuse and potential malnourishment, you should consider:

- **Thiamine.** To prevent Wernicke's encephalopathy in someone who is potentially malnourished.
- **Monitoring for alcohol withdrawal symptoms.** As he is a chronic alcoholic, he will start to withdraw during his admission. He should be written up for a regular, reducing dose course of chlordiazepoxide with extra doses PRN (as required).

What forms of imaging could be used if endoscopy failed to reveal the source of bleeding?

- **Angiography.** A femoral catheter is sited and used to inject a contrast agent into the coeliac axis and superior mesenteric artery. In this way, actively bleeding vessels can be visualized.

- **Laparotomy**. In some cases (especially with posterior peptic ulcers), it is necessary to proceed to laparotomy to visualize and stop the bleeding.

> The endoscopy is performed and reveals a bleeding, distended oesophageal vein in the distal oesophagus.
> **How will the gastroenterologist manage the bleeding oeosphageal varix?**

The gastroenterologist needs to **stop the bleeding** (Figure 5.3). This can be done by:

- **Endoscopic band ligation**. This is the preferred method for stopping a bleeding oesophageal varix. Rubber bands are placed on the end of the endoscope and used to ligate the bleeding vessel and any other obviously distended vessels.
- **Endoscopic sclerotherapy**. This is usually not performed as first-line treatment in oesophageal varices as it can induce necrosis of the oesophageal mucosa and is less effective than banding.
- **Balloon tamponade**. A tube is passed down into the stomach. A terminal balloon is inflated in the stomach to keep the tube in place and the stomach is aspirated of its contents. A second balloon along the length of the tube is inflated to apply pressure to the bleeding vein and induce haemostasis. This technique is associated with a rebleed rate of 50% and serious complications (oesophageal ulceration and aspiration pneumonia) in 15–20%. Thus it is reserved for when endoscopic band ligation has failed or is not possible because of blood obstructing the view.

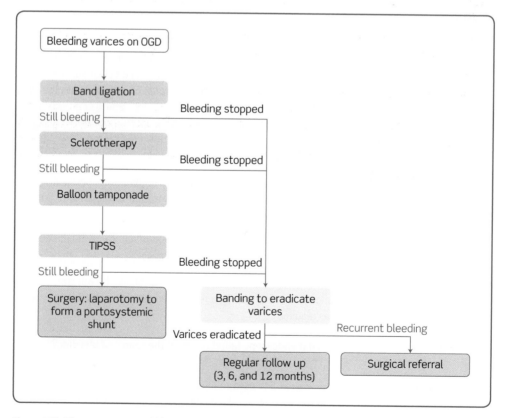

Figure 5.3 The management of bleeding oesophageal varices.

- **Transjugular intrahepatic portosystemic shunt (TIPS or TIPSS)**. This complex procedure involves passing a catheter down the jugular vein and creating a shunt from a hepatic vein to the portal vein to relieve the portal hypertension. If this is not possible, a portosystemic (aka portocaval) shunt can be placed surgically.

- **Portocaval (portosystemic) shunt**. This surgical technique involves placing a shunt between the portal and systemic circulation, thus bypassing the liver and reducing the portal hypertension that is causing the oesophageal varices. Remember that a major role of the liver is to metabolize many substances absorbed by the gut into the portal circulation ('first-pass metabolism') so that the blood is 'detoxified' before entering the systemic circulation. By placing a shunt that bypasses the liver, many toxins absorbed by the gut will enter the systemic circulation and can trigger an encephalopathy. Because of this, portocaval shunts are now rarely performed.

What long-term management might be offered to Mr Tucker for his portal hypertension?

- **Lifestyle advice.** It is essential that you offer to refer him for help to stop drinking alcohol and smoking (he is very unlikely to manage to quit either addiction without professional and ongoing help). Although the likelihood of success in changing such deeply embedded habits is small, the recent dramatic events may help Mr Tucker to realize the need for such changes, particularly if the advice is given by a doctor.

- **Keep his BP low.** This minimizes the chances of oesophageal varices rebleeding. Typical agents used include propranolol or isosorbide mononitrate (especially if β-blockers are contraindicated, e.g. in asthma).

- **Antibiotics.** A 1-week course of antibiotics (e.g. ciprofloxacin) should be considered in patients with liver cirrhosis and upper GI bleeding, as 50% of them will develop sepsis.

- **TIPS/TIPSS.** See previous question.

- **Treat encephalopathy.** The liver usually removes lots of dietary toxins from the blood before they reach the systemic circulation. If this filtering does not occur due to liver failure or portosystemic shunts, the patient is at risk of encephalopathy. If patients develop encephalopathy, they can be placed on a very low protein diet and given lactulose or enemas to decrease GI transit time and minimize GI absorption. Lactulose also reduces the pH in faeces, making the environment more hostile to ammonia-producing bacteria.

Short cases

Figure 5.4 is a clerking for a patient in the Emergency Department.

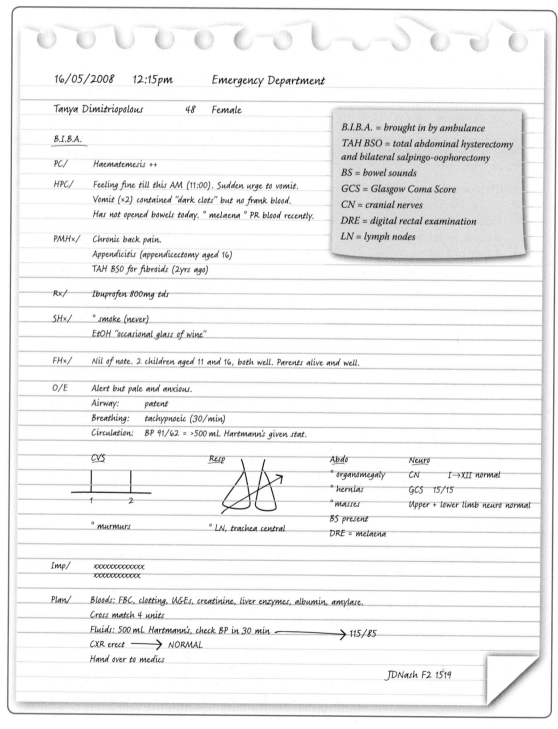

16/05/2008   12:15pm   Emergency Department

Tanya Dimitriopolous   48   Female

B.I.B.A.

PC/   Haematemesis ++

HPC/   Feeling fine till this AM (11:00). Sudden urge to vomit.
Vomit (×2) contained "dark clots" but no frank blood.
Has not opened bowels today. ° melaena ° PR blood recently.

PMH×/   Chronic back pain.
Appendicitis (appendicectomy aged 16)
TAH BSO for fibroids (2yrs ago)

Rx/   Ibuprofen 800mg tds

SH×/   ° smoke (never)
EtOH "occasional glass of wine"

FH×/   Nil of note. 2 children aged 11 and 16, both well. Parents alive and well.

O/E   Alert but pale and anxious.
Airway: patent
Breathing: tachypnoeic (30/min)
Circulation: BP 91/62 = >500 mL Hartmann's given stat.

CVS   Resp   Abdo   Neuro
° organomegaly   CN   I→XII normal
° hernias   GCS   15/15
° masses   Upper + lower limb neuro normal
BS present
° murmurs   ° LN, trachea central   DRE = melaena

Imp/   xxxxxxxxxxxx
xxxxxxxxxxx

Plan/   Bloods: FBC, clotting, U&Es, creatinine, liver enzymes, albumin, amylase.
Cross match 4 units
Fluids: 500 mL Hartmann's, check BP in 30 min ———————> 115/85
CXR erect ———> NORMAL
Hand over to medics

JDNash F2 1519

Sidebar notes:
B.I.B.A. = brought in by ambulance
TAH BSO = total abdominal hysterectomy and bilateral salpingo-oophorectomy
BS = bowel sounds
GCS = Glasgow Coma Score
CN = cranial nerves
DRE = digital rectal examination
LN = lymph nodes

Figure 5.4 Clerking notes for a 48-year old woman with haematemesis.

SHORT CASE

The presence of 'dark clots' in vomit is strongly suggestive of blood that has been modified by stomach acid, and thus of an upper GI bleed. This would also explain the melaena (dark faeces due to blood modified during intestinal transit). The most likely diagnosis for any upper GI bleed in someone who takes regular ibuprofen and has heartburn is a **bleeding peptic ulcer**. However, as was stated in the core case, note that it is difficult to diagnose the aetiology of upper GI bleeds accurately until endoscopy is performed.

An OGD was performed and revealed an actively bleeding peptic ulcer in the fundus of the stomach. The bleeding was stopped using an endoscopic fibrin sealant and adrenaline injection around the ulcer, and an infusion of omeprazole (a proton pump inhibitor) was started after the endoscopy to reduce the risk of rebleeding. Biopsies were taken and revealed that the ulcer was positive for *Helicobacter pylori*. Mrs Dimitriopolous was discharged on a course of triple therapy (a proton pump inhibitor and a combination of two antibiotics) for eradication of *H. pylori*. She was asked to stop taking ibuprofen and was instead started on regular paracetamol, with a view to adding codeine if her back pain was not controlled.

What is the *most likely* diagnosis?

SHORT CASE

Mr Doherty is a 28-year-old man who presents to his local Emergency Department with haematemesis and chest pain. He celebrated his 'stag do' the previous night with his friends. After a particularly spicy vindaloo, they went clubbing and consumed copious alcohol. They were kicked out of a club when Mr Doherty started to throw up. His friends find this hilarious but Mr Doherty looks pained. He tells you that his chest hurts a lot and that he has vomited 'at least six times' since they left the nightclub. The last two times he has vomited blood and that is why he has come to hospital, much to the disappointment of his friends who seem keen to continue the party in the hospital until security turns up and asks them to leave.

Mr Doherty's past medical history is unremarkable and he takes no regular medications. He smokes 'socially' but is adamant that he only drinks at weekends, although he admits this is frequently 'more than is healthy'. He denies taking any illicit drugs. He has not had any epigastric pain, heartburn, or noticed any changes in his bowel habit.

On arrival at the Emergency Department, his ABCs are checked and found to be stable. A chest radiograph was normal. Indeed, the only findings of note are his obvious inebriation, a purple appearance to his face due to burst superficial capillaries from vomiting, and persistent chest pain.

What diagnosis should you consider in Mr Doherty's case?

Mr Doherty has presented with chest pain and haematemesis after many episodes of forceful vomiting. A **Mallory–Weiss tear** of the oesophageal mucosa, or the rare but more serious diagnosis of Boerhaave's perforation of the oesophagus, should be considered. Given that his observations and chest radiograph were normal in the Emergency Department, a Boerhaave's perforation is less likely. Ultimately, an OGD will be needed to confirm or exclude the diagnosis.

SHORT CASE

Mrs Jones-Harcourt, a 42-year-old woman, presents to the Emergency Department because she is vomiting copious amounts of blood. She was at a cocktail party with some friends when one of them noticed a trickle of blood coming out of her left nostril. She then began to vomit blood and is now very distressed, as her clothes are covered in blood. She continues to bring up blood as the emergency staff attend to her. A large-bore IV cannula is inserted into each antecubital fossa, bloods are taken for investigations, and 500 mL aliquots of normal saline are given stat until her BP normalizes. Once her observations are stable, she is given water to wash out her mouth and her face is wiped clean. The attending doctor asks her to lean forward and notices that blood is still coming out of her left nostril.

What is the cause of this lady's haematemesis? How should it be managed?

The presence of blood coming out of this lady's nose should make you strongly suspect a **nosebleed (epistaxis)**, with most of the blood falling back into the pharynx where it is causing vomiting. (Figure 5.5 shows a diagram of the blood supply to the nose.)

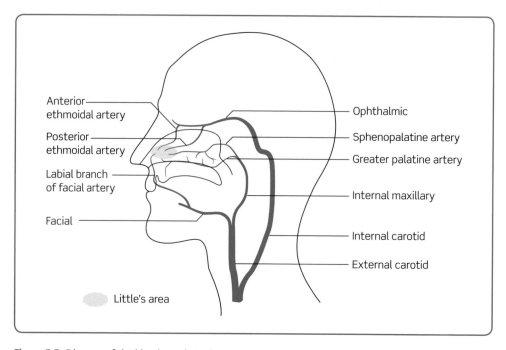

Figure 5.5 Diagram of the blood supply to the nose.

Anterior nosebleeds from Little's area account for 90% of epistaxis but rarely cause haematemesis. These can often be resolved by asking the patient to sit up with her head leaning forward (this prevents blood flowing back into the pharynx) and pinch the front of the nose firmly for 10 minutes ('Trotter's method'). If this fails it is worth trying to spray the nose with a phenylephrine-containing spray or to insert an adrenaline-soaked gauze, and then reapply pressure for 10 minutes in the hope that the vasocontriction from the phenylephrine or adrenaline, pressure, and time can stem the bleeding. If this also fails, the next step is to pack the nose for 12 hours with a specialized nasal pack (they expand on contact with moisture, thus applying pressure to the nasal mucosa from within) and admitting the patient under the care of ENT for the pack to be removed the next day. Once an anterior nasal bleed has been stopped, one should look for stigmata of bleeding that may be amenable to cautery (with silver nitrate sticks) under local anaesthetic spray, in an attempt to reduce further bleeds. Irrespective of cautery, patients should be discharged with either Naseptin or petroleum jelly (Vaseline) ointment to be applied to the nose for the next few days and advice to avoid hot drinks (which cause vasodilatation in the nose) for the next 24 hours to reduce recurrence.

Posterior nosebleeds from branches of the sphenopalatine artery are less common but more serious and more likely to result in haematemesis, as the blood is more likely to drip back into the pharynx. These can sometimes be stopped using a urinary catheter with a balloon inserted via the nose into the oropharynx, where the balloon is inflated and the catheter then pulled back to apply pressure to the posterior nose. They should all be referred to ENT urgently for further management.

Viva questions

What are the main risk factors for peptic ulcer disease?

- *Helicobacter pylori*
- Smoking
- Alcohol
- NSAIDs and aspirin
- Blood group O
- Hypercalcaemia
- Physiological stress (not psychological stress)
- Burns (Curling's ulcers) or brain trauma (Cushing's ulcers[†]).

[†] Remember that Harvey Cushing was a neurosurgeon.

Why are alcoholics particularly vulnerable to haematemesis?

Alcoholics have a tendency to suffer haematemesis for several reasons:

1 **Anatomy**. As their liver becomes damaged and fibrosed, blood flows through less freely. Consequently, the circulation must find ways that bypass the liver. These are called portosystemic anastamoses (links between the hepatic/portal and systemic circulations). They occur at:
   - the oesophagus, giving rise to oesophageal varices
   - the umbilicus, giving rise to caput medusae
   - the rectum, giving rise to rectal varices
   - the diaphragm, and
   - the retroperitoneum.

2 **Physiology**. Alcoholics are at risk of cirrhosis. This impairs the liver's ability to function, including its ability to synthesize clotting factors. Consequently, alcoholics can develop an impaired clotting function and a tendency to bleed. Alcohol is also an irritant to the oesophageal and gastric mucosa, thus predisposing alcoholics to oesophagitis, gastritis, and peptic ulcers.

3 **Behaviour**. Alcoholics are more prone to vomiting and therefore to Mallory–Weiss tears, Boerhaave's perforation, and tearing an oesophageal varix.

What is the Child–Pugh score used for?

The Child–Pugh score is used to assess the severity of liver cirrhosis. It is prognostic: those with a score of 5-6 (class A) have a 100% one year survival vs 45% for those with 10-15 points (class C). The higher the score, the more likely it is that the patient has portal hypertension, oesophageal varices, and ultimately, haematemesis.

Can you draw a simplified clotting cascade?

A good way of drawing the clotting cascade is to start from the bottom—this is the most important part, the easiest to remember, and this way you are less likely to get tied up in detailing which factors activate which other factors. The clotting cascade can be activated by the extrinsic pathway (measured as the PT and affected by warfarin and liver disease) or the intrinsic pathway (measured as the APTT and affected by heparin, haemophilias, and von Willebrand disease). Figure 5.6 shows a simplified diagram of the blood clotting cascade.

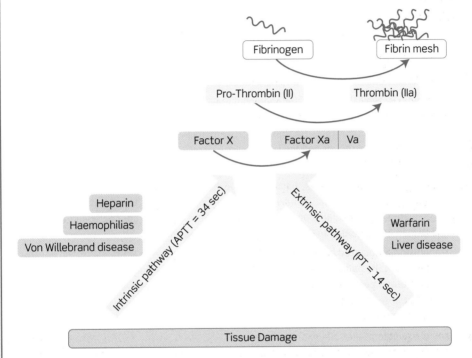

Figure 5.6 Simplified diagram of the blood clotting cascade.

What are the indications for a packed red cell ('blood') transfusion in adults?

Repeat audits across the UK indicate that about 25% of packed red cell transfusions are unnecessary (and thus difficult to defend medico-legally should a complication arise). The main indications for a packed red cell transfusion in an adult are listed below. It is important to use single-unit transfusions where possible, to aim only for the transfusion threshold haemoglobin (e.g. Hb 70 g/L rather than a normal Hb of 130 g/L) and to reassess after each transfusion.

- **Catastrophic haemorrhage,** such as that seen in major trauma and amputations, with associated hypotension. These patients will also require other blood products as per a massive tranfusion protocol as they will be losing clotting factors and platelets in addition to red cells.
- **Hb <70 g/L** *plus* signs of compromise (tachycardia, syncope, dyspnoea). If there are no signs of compromise, try to address the underlying cause without tranfusion (e.g. is there an iron deficiency anaemia that can be corrected?).
- **Hb <80 g/L** *plus* signs of compromise in patients >65 years or who have ischaemic heart disease or severe respiratory disease.

What are the risks and complications associated with blood transfusions?

Blood transfusions carry significant risks and any complication should be reported to the hospital's transfusion practitioner so that it can be investigated and reported to the UK's Serious Hazards Of Transfusion (SHOT) committee.

Immune-mediated complication

- **Acute transfusion reaction:** due to the immune system attacking foreign platelets, white cells, or serum proteins. The patient becomes febrile and/or develops an urticarial skin rash (erythema, hives, and itching). Treatment involves confirming the blood transfusion is correct (patient details, blood group), temporarily stopping the transfusion, giving paracetamol and/or antihistamines, and resuming the tranfusion at a slower rate if the patient is stable. Staff should then monitor the patient carefully for any signs of deterioration suggesting either anaphylaxis or bacterial contamination of the sample (bacteraemia).

- **Anaphylaxis:** typically due to immunoglobulin A (IgA)-deficient patients who have anti-IgA antibodies attacking the IgA in the transfused blood. The patient becomes breathless and hypotensive. Potentially fatal, treatment is with adrenaline (0.5 mg intramuscularly (IM)), chlorphenamine, corticosteroids and fluids.

- **Haemolytic transfusion reaction:** due to mismatch of ABO blood group alleles. The patient rapidly becomes cold, feverish, nauseated, and has chest and/or flank pain. They may also develop dark red urine from the haemolysis. Stop the blood transfusion, anticipate shock and disseminated intravascular coagulopathy (DIC), involve intensive care early and use IV fluids and IV mannitol (diuretic) to flush out the products of haemolysis.

- **Transfusion-associated lung injury (TRALI)**: Thought to be due to antibodies in the transfused blood causing the patient's white blood cells to aggregate and clog up the pulmonary capillaries. The patient becomes severely breathless. Treatment is with respiratory support.

- **Delayed haemolytic reaction:** due to mismatch of alleles of non-ABO blood groups (e.g. Duffy, Kell, Kidd, etc.). Patient slowly develops malaise, jaundice, and fever. Treatment is supportive and the symptoms are self-limiting.

- **Alloimmunization:** Cross-matching blood involves ensuring the recipient's serum lacks antibodies against blood groups A/B, Rhesus, and other rarer blood groups (e.g. Duffy, Kell). Blood is matched based on the ABO and Rhesus antigens for all patients because these blood groups are common. However, other blood groups are rare so unless the patient has antibodies against them, a Duffy-negative patient may be given Duffy-positive blood. In the acute setting, this causes no problem but the patient may develop anti-Duffy (or anti-Kell, etc.) antibodies that will prevent future transfusions with that type of blood. The more transfusions a patient has, the more likely they are to develop antibodies to rarer blood groups and the harder it becomes to find blood that is compatible with the patient's serum antibodies.

- **Post-transfusion purpura:** the mechanism for this acute, self-limiting reaction is unclear. It appears that the recipient develops antibodies against residual platelets in the red cell transfusion and these antibodies then go on to destroy the patient's own platelets. This leads to non-blanching haemorrhages in the skin (purpura). Treatment is by intravenous immunoglobulin (IVIG) infusion (to overwhelm the disease causing antibodies, effectively diluting them in a sea of random antibodies) or plasmapheresis to remove the offending antibodies. More likely in women who have given birth and thus potentially been exposed to platelets with different antigens (from the baby).

CONTINUED ➤

CONTINUED

Non-immune complications

- **Transfusion-associated circulatory overload (TACO):** typically in elderly patients, due to unnecessary overtransfusion and overly aggressive fluid resuscitation.
- **Coagulopathy:** massive transfusion of red blood cells can dilute clotting factors and platelets to the point where the blood is unable to clot. Treated by transfusing platelets and/or fresh frozen plasma.
- **Transfusion-transmitted infection:** Thankfully rare, this can present acutely as septicaemia and septic shock. Stop the transfusion (and send it back to the lab for testing) and treat as for any other severe sepsis patients with IV antibiotics, IV fluids and oxygen as necessary. Infection with viral hepatitis, HIV, Creutzfeld–Jakob disease (CJD) prion, etc. are all possible but thankfully rare with modern transfusion services. HIV and viral hepatitis are screened for but CJD prion is currently not screened for.

Christine is a 57-year-old woman who presented to her local Emergency Department with haematemesis. She was found to have oesophageal varices secondary to advanced alcoholic cirrhosis. After a long consultation with the hepatologists, she enrolled in a programme to stop drinking alcohol and is on a waiting list for a liver transplant. She visits her GP for a follow-up appointment and says that she has been abstinent of alcohol for the last 2 months. The GP notices that her latest blood results show a slight rise in her GGT level and asks if Christine has been drinking anything at all. She bursts into tears and confesses that she had a bottle of wine over the weekend to celebrate her husband's birthday.

Is Christine still eligible for a liver transplant?

The demand for healthy livers for transplantation far exceeds supply, despite advances in hepatology that have allowed a single liver to be divided and donated to multiple recipients. The general perception is that liver transplants should be prioritized so that patients with liver pathology that is 'out of their control' (e.g. primary biliary cirrhosis) get priority over patients whose 'chosen lifestyle' has damaged their liver (e.g. alcoholism, viral hepatitis C from IV drug use). This is not a moral judgement but relates to the likelihood of the transplanted liver being damaged.

For this reason, many liver transplant services require that patients with cirrhosis from alcohol abuse enrol in a programme of alcohol cessation and must be abstinent for a certain period of time (typically 3–6 months). Patients unable to meet these criteria are felt to be unlikely to comply with immunosuppressive therapy post-transplant or to come to outpatient follow-up, with a higher risk of rejection and post-transplant complications—when of course the donated liver could go to someone else. However, there is little evidence that patients with alcohol dependence who complete a 3–6 month abstinence programme have significantly lower rates of post-transplant alcoholism than patients who do not complete these programmes. Nonetheless, the consensus is that a patient who is unable to abstain from alcohol for 3–6 months prior to a liver transplant should not be eligible for a new liver.

It is important to distinguish between a 'slip' and a 'relapse'. It is possible that Christine has had a one-off slip that has not occurred before and will not occur again, in which case one could argue that she is still eligible for a liver transplant. It is also possible that she has in fact relapsed into alcohol abuse, in which case she would no longer be suitable for a liver transplant. It would perhaps be suitable to reassess this patient in a few weeks' time with repeated blood tests for alcohol levels and GGT (carbohydrate-deficient transferase is sometimes also measured, although this is more useful in heavy alcohol consumption). If she is still drinking, she will have to be removed from the transplant list. If not, the GP will have to use their professional judgement about whether to report the one-off 'slip' in her alcohol abstinence.

Single Best Answers

1. Which of the following is not an element of the Rockall score?

a. Pulse
b. Comorbidities
c. Alcohol history

d. Age
e. Blood pressure

2. Why is it important to know if a patient with haematemesis is taking β-blockers?

a. They can cause a coagulopathy
b. They mask the signs of shock
c. They cause peptic ulcers

d. They cause cirrhosis
e. It is not important

3. Which of the following is true of spider naevi (and therefore helps distinguish them from other skin lesions)?

a. Spider naevi blanch with pressure
b. Spider naevi refill from the outside towards the centre

c. Spider naevi are found in the distribution of the IVC (inferior vena cava) ✗ SVC
d. Spider naevi always suggest pathology
e. None of the above

4. Which procoagulant clotting factors are made by the liver?

a. IV
b. V
c. VI

d. VII
e. All of the above

5. A known alcoholic presents with haematemesis. A full blood count is requested. Given the history, what result would you expect?

a. Microcytic anaemia
b. Normocytic anaemia
c. Macrocytic anaemia

d. All of the above
e. None of the above

Dysphagia

Core case

Read through the sections in the case boxes, covering up the sections that follow so that you don't see the answer. At the end of each case box, try to answer the question before reading on.

Mrs Sweeney is a 76-year-old retired greengrocer who presents to her GP because she is having difficulty swallowing.

Different patients mean different things when they say 'swallowing difficulty'. What could Mrs Sweeney mean?

When a patient says 'swallowing difficulty', they could mean:

- **Dysphagia:** difficulty swallowing. If they really mean dysphagia, try to understand when/where exactly it feels as though the food 'gets stuck'. Those with high dysphagia (oropharyngeal and upper oesophageal) describe difficulty initiating a swallow or immediately upon swallowing. Those with low dysphagia (lower oesophageal) feel the food getting stuck a few seconds after swallowing.

- **Odynophagia:** painful swallowing. Odynophagia may be due to malignancy, but is more commonly a feature of infection such as candidiasis.

- **Globus:** the common sensation of having a lump in the throat without true dysphagia. Globus is very common and its aetiology is poorly understood—however, only a small proportion of affected patients will seek medical help and it is an entirely benign condition.

What is your differential diagnosis for dysphagia?

Dysphagia is an impairment of swallowing and thus can involve any structure between the mouth and the lower oesophageal sphincter. Try to organize your differential *anatomically* into 'high dysphagia' (oropharyngeal and upper oesophageal) and 'low dysphagia' (lower oesophageal), and think about whether the underlying mechanism is *structural* or *functional* (Figure 6.1).

Which diagnoses are the most common?

Broadly speaking, high dysphagia is more likely to be due to generalized/systemic neuromuscular disease, whereas low dysphagia is more likely to be due to a local obstructing lesion.

	Functional	Structural		
		Luminal	Mural	Extrinsic
High dysphagia	Stroke Parkinson's disease Myasthenia gravis Multiple sclerosis Myotonic dystrophy Motor neurone disease Inadequate saliva production (2ary Sjogrens, anticholinergics etc)		Cancer Pharyngeal pouch Cricopharyngeal bar	
Low dysphagia	Achalasia Chagas disease Nutcracker oesophagus Diffuse oesophageal spasm Limited cutaneous scleroderma (CREST) Infective oesophagitis Eosinophilic oesophagitis	Foreign body	Cancer Stricture (caustic or inflammatory) Plummer-Vinson syndrome Schatzki ring Congenital atresia* Post-fundoplication	Mediastinal mass Retrosternal goitre Bronchial carcinoma Thoracic aortic aneurysm Pericardial effusion Ortner's syndrome Dysphagia lusoria*

Figure 6.1 Causes of dysphagia.
Common conditions are depicted in a larger font.
These are congenital conditions that would therefore present at any early age.

In a patient of Mrs Sweeney's age, is there any particular diagnosis that you must rule out?

New-onset dysphagia in middle-aged to elderly patients is carcinoma until proven otherwise.

What questions would you like to ask specifically about the swallowing?

- **What is the duration of the symptoms?** This is a key question: a food bolus stuck in the oesophagus will typically appear immediately during a meal; cancer typically presents with a short history of days to weeks (not because the cancer has appeared in such a short space of time, but because it has reached a size where symptoms rapidly become apparent), whereas chronic motility disorders such as achalasia present with symptoms lasting months to years.

- **Is the dysphagia progressive or intermittent?** Progressive dysphagia is highly suggestive of a stricture (benign or malignant), whereas intermittent symptoms are more characteristic of motility disorders.

- **Is the dysphagia to solids, fluids, or both?** If the patient is able to swallow fluid as normal but has difficulty with solid food items (which feel as if they are sticking[†]) this points towards a mechanical obstruction, i.e. a stricture (benign or malignant). Of course, as the stricture becomes more severe, then the dysphagia may start to involve fluids as well. If the dysphagia is initially more pronounced for fluids than for solids, this suggests a motility disorder (e.g. achalasia or a neuromuscular condition). Many patients will have tried changing their diet before seeing a doctor, in more extreme cases restricting themselves to liquids. Absolute dysphagia to solids, liquids, and saliva is typical of a food bolus being stuck in the oesophagus, occasionally because of an underlying stricture or malignancy, but in most cases simply due to a large piece of poorly chewed meat. The latter, benign cause tends to be a one-off event (patients rarely make the mistake twice—a mother's warning to chew food before swallowing and take small bites only goes so far, but being in the Emergency Department unable to swallow even saliva is very persuasive). An underlying stricture or malignancy will cause food to get repeatedly stuck.

What associated symptoms should you also ask about in the history?

- **Is there any coughing and if so, is it related to eating?** Coughing that occurs immediately after swallowing (i.e. **choking**) suggests that there is a problem with the coordination of swallowing events and thus points towards disorders such as stroke and Parkinson's disease. By contrast, if coughing occurs some time after a meal, this implies regurgitation of food retained within a pharyngeal pouch, aspiration of food remaining within a dilated oesophagus above the gastro-oesophageal junction (e.g. achalasia), or gastro-oesophageal reflux disease. Nocturnal cough, when most people are lying flat and not eating, is more suggestive of achalasia.

- **Do they suffer with halitosis?** This embarrassing symptom is a feature of conditions where food remains lodged in the oropharynx such as Zenker's diverticulum, also known as a pharyngeal pouch.

- **Is there any gurgling or dysphonia?** Patients with a pharyngeal pouch can often be heard to make gurgling noises if they attempt to speak soon after eating or drinking. It may also be possible to see a visible bulging of the neck. **Hoarseness** on the other hand may be related to vocal cord dysfunction due to involvement of the recurrent laryngeal nerve, e.g. if compressed by a tumour.

- **Is there heartburn or waterbrash?** The presence of these two symptoms suggests the dysphagia is related to reflux disease, with or without a stricture. Remember that chronic dyspepsia can predispose to oesophageal cancer. In addition, ~40% of patients with achalasia complain of retrosternal burning.

- **Weight loss:** this is the cardinal 'red flag' for oesophageal cancer, although of course any cause of dysphagia will ultimately result in weight loss if the dysphagia is sufficiently severe and prolonged.

[†] Note that patients may be able to describe foods becoming stuck at a particular level of their oesophagus, but that this reported level often correlates poorly with the true level of the obstruction.

- **Neurological symptoms** should be enquired about in any patient who has features suggestive of a functional dysphagia, e.g. difficulty coordinating swallowing, slow eating, extra effort required to eat/chew, tiredness after eating, and early dysphagia for liquids.
- **Rheumatological symptoms** may be relevant in the context of limited cutaneous scleroderma (previously known as CREST syndrome), in which patients may suffer from a combination of Calcinosis, Raynaud's, (o)Esophageal dysmotility (the E in CREST refers to the American spelling of oesophagus), Sclerodactyly, and Telangiectasia.

Why is past medical/surgical history relevant?

The two key medical conditions to enquire about are **gastro-oesophageal reflux disease (GORD)** and **peptic ulcers**. However, the patient may not have a proven diagnosis of either of these conditions and may simply complain of a combination of dyspepsia and/or waterbrash. GORD and peptic ulcers are directly implicated in the aetiology of two of the most common causes of dysphagia:

- **GORD** predisposes to oesophageal adenocarcinoma and non-malignant strictures of the oesophagus. A history of GORD due to a sliding hiatus hernia is also significant if the patient has had a fundoplication operation to tighten the lower oesophageal sphincter. Postoperative dysphagia is a potential complication of such a procedure if the wraps are made too tight.
- **Peptic ulcers** can also lead to scarring and strictures around the gastric cardia and lower oesophagus.

There may also be a history of a progressive neurological disease such as multiple sclerosis or Parkinson's disease.

Why is a detailed drug history of particular importance when investigating dysphagia?

Drugs can contribute towards dysphagia in two main ways:

1 Drugs such as calcium channel blockers and nitrates, which relax smooth muscle, can cause or exacerbate reflux symptoms by decreasing oesophageal tone.

2 Drugs such as non-steroidal anti-inflammatory drugs (NSAIDs), aspirin, steroids, and bisphosphonates predispose to peptic ulceration.

On further questioning, Mrs Sweeney describes how she has had progressive difficulty swallowing solid foods—particularly meat—over the past 3 weeks. She says that the chunks of food feel as if they are getting stuck midway down her throat, but she has no difficulty with the actual chewing movements.

She has not suffered from any coughing or choking after eating. She has not noticed any changes in her voice or any gurgling after eating or drinking.

When asked directly about any weight loss, she says that she has probably lost some weight (a few kilograms) as her clothes feel somewhat loose, but says that she is not surprised at this because she feels that she is able to eat so little.

Her past medical history is significant for GORD, for which she takes regular omeprazole, and polymyalgia rheumatica, for which she takes daily low dose prednisolone. Her GP has also prescribed calcium, vitamin D, and a bisphosphonate to be taken as bone-protecting therapy as she is on long-term steroids.

The GP examines Mrs Sweeney. What are the relevant aspects of the physical examination?

There is relatively little that can be gained from the examination of a patient with dysphagia, but there are five features that are particularly relevant:

1   **Cranial nerve pathology**: this is particularly important if there are features in the history that suggest a functional dysphagia as the patient may have bulbar palsy for example.

2   **Signs of gastrointestinal (GI) malignancy**: patients with oesophageal carcinoma may be markedly cachectic, and may have a palpable Virchow's node. If there is an oesophageal carcinoma extending into the cardia of the stomach this may be palpable in thin patients. GI malignancies can metastasize to the liver and so it is worth palpating for hepatomegaly, in case of a large metastasis (although this is uncommon).

3   **Neck mass**: It may be possible to palpate a large pharyngeal pouch in thin patients, and this may even gurgle on palpation. A goitre may also be palpable, causing the dysphagia by extrinsic compression.[‡] Head and neck cancers can cause cervical lymphadenopathy and upper (oropharyngeal) dysphagia.

4   **Features of CREST syndrome** (described above).

5   **Koilonychia**: suggests severe iron deficiency anaemia, which may be associated with Plummer–Vinson syndrome (oesophageal webs). This is exceedingly rare!

> Mrs Sweeney has a cachectic appearance. Examination reveals a palpable lymph node in the left supraclavicular fossa but is otherwise unremarkable.
>
> **What is the most likely diagnosis to account for Mrs Sweeney's dysphagia?**

The short history of a progressive dysphagia that is more pronounced for solids than fluids, occurring on a background of GORD in an elderly patient, and coupled with examination findings of cachexia and lymphadenopathy, is highly suggestive of **oesophageal carcinoma**. This is statistically more likely to be adenocarcinoma given that this subtype accounts for about 65% of oesophageal carcinoma in the UK.

> The GP refers Mrs Sweeney urgently to an upper GI surgeon.
>
> **What are the different types of investigation used for dysphagia, and what are the indications for each?**

There are four main investigations for dysphagia and you should be aware of the indications for each:

1   **Barium swallow:**
   - This is a cineradiographic study which monitors the passage of a bolus of barium contrast medium from the upper to the lower oesophageal sphincter of a supine patient. Various lesions have characteristic appearances on barium swallow (see Figures 6.2–6.5). Patients may also be asked to swallow an effervescent agent to produce a double-contrast study that is better at visualizing mucosal lesions. Note that a barium swallow is not the same thing as a barium meal—the latter follows the passage of barium through the stomach and into the duodenum.
   - Barium swallow is useful in investigating patients who may have a high lesion. During endoscopy this region is intubated blindly, and in the presence of a pharyngeal pouch or high oesophageal cancer there is a risk of injury or perforation. It is also indicated in patients with features suggesting achalasia (e.g. intermittent symptoms, difficulties with fluids and solids).

---

‡ Note that there are various other conditions that can cause dysphagia by extrinsic compression of the oesophagus, such as Ortner's syndrome or bronchial carcinoma, but it would be unusual to search for signs of such conditions in the first instance. It is more likely that these would be retrospective diagnoses made once a barium swallow shows extrinsic compression.

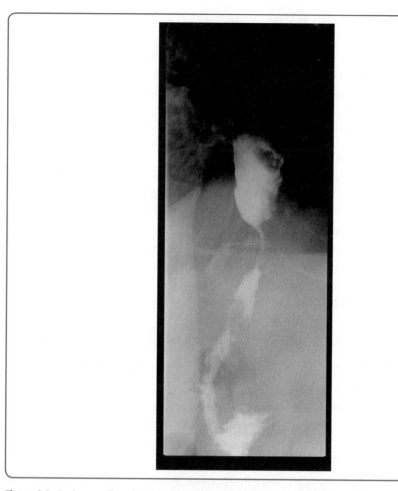

Figure 6.2 Barium swallow showing a mid-oesophageal stricture consistent with oesophageal cancer.

2 **Endoscopy:**
   ■ Allows visualization of luminal and mural lesions, as well as the opportunity to biopsy and treat lesions. Various procedures, such as stricture dilatation, stent insertion, laser coagulation, and Botox injections can all be carried out endoscopically.
   ■ Endoscopy is a more sensitive and specific test than double-contrast barium swallow and is often the first-line investigation for low dysphagia.

3 **Videofluoroscopy:**
   ■ Essentially a modified form of barium swallow in which upright patients are given barium in liquid, solid, or semi-solid form. A speech therapist modifies the swallowing technique throughout the study.
   ■ Most suited to patients with a functional high dysphagia.

4 **Manometry:**
   ■ Assesses the pressures in the lower oesophageal sphincter and the peristaltic wave in the rest of the oesophagus.
   ■ Manometry is the key investigation for diagnosing a motility disorder and distinguishing between the different types of motility disorders (e.g. achalasia and nutcracker oesophagus). It is indicated when barium swallow and/or endoscopy are unremarkable, suggesting a cause other than mechanical obstruction.

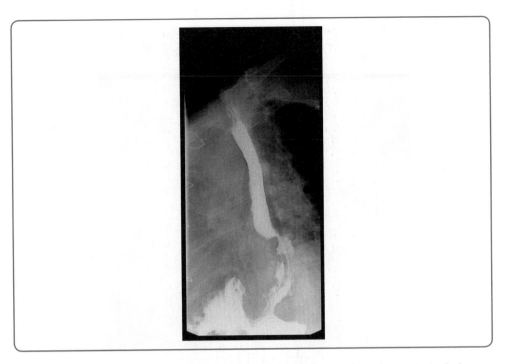

Figure 6.3 Barium swallow showing extrinsic compression of the lower oesophagus by an extraluminal mass.
Reproduced with kind permission from Dr R. Graham.

Figure 6.4 Barium swallow showing the classic 'bird's beak' appearance of oesophageal achalasia.

Figure 6.5 Barium swallow (anterior–posterior projection) showing a pharyngeal pouch.
Reproduced with kind permission from Dr R. Graham.

Mrs Sweeney was seen by an upper GI surgeon within a fortnight. An outpatient oesophagogastroscopy was performed and an irregular ulcerative lesion on a background of 'velvety' epithelium was seen in the distal 5 cm of oesophagus. Multiple biopsy samples were taken. Histology revealed high-grade dysplastic columnar epithelium, with penetration of the basement membrane.

What is the diagnosis and how should Mrs Sweeney be managed?

Mrs Sweeney has oesophageal **adenocarcinoma** on a background of **Barrett's oesophagus** (hence the velvety epithelium in the distal oesophagus). She should be referred to a specialist multidisciplinary cancer team made up of surgeons, pathologists, radiologists, oncologists, and specialist nursing support.

The first thing to do with a cancer patient is to grade and stage the malignancy. Remember that you grade the tumour histopathologically (the more the cells deviate from normality, the higher the grade) and stage the patient by determining how far the cancer has spread anatomically.

The team will assess the stage of Mrs Sweeney's cancer to establish whether the tumour is operable and whether she is fit for surgery. Oesophagectomy is associated with the highest mortality of any elective surgical procedure, and about two thirds of patients are deemed unsuitable for surgery due to advanced disease or comorbidity. Various imaging modalities may be required for **staging:**

- **Spiral CT chest/abdomen:** is the principal modality for initially staging the tumour. If the scan reveals inoperable or metastatic disease then there may be no advantage in further assessment of the primary tumour.

- **Positron emission tomography (PET) scanning** may also be used, e.g. to further assess whether an equivocal lesion or lymph node seen on CT is 'hot' (avidly uptakes fluorodeoxyglucose (FDG), a marker of metabolic activity) or 'cold'. Increasingly, CT and PET are combined into a single PET-CT investigation.

- **Endoscopic ultrasound (EUS):** if there is no evidence of metastatic disease on CT/PET and the patient is a candidate for surgery, EUS is performed as it is the most accurate modality for locoregional staging (consistently better than CT, PET, or MRI). It provides particularly useful information about intramural versus transmural disease and local lymph node involvement.

- **Laparoscopy:** if there is no evidence of metastatic disease on CT/PET (i.e. radical treatment is still an option) and the patient has a distal oesophageal tumour, laparoscopy may be used to exclude peritoneal deposits. Such deposits are notoriously difficult to diagnose on imaging, but their presence would be a relative contraindication to aggressive treatment. However, most laparoscopies are negative.

If the tumour is judged to be suitable for radical treatment, it is necessary for the anaesthetist to also perform a **fitness assessment** for surgery with a combination of lung function tests, electrocardiogram (ECG), exercise tolerance test ± echocardiogram.

Surgery is the definitive treatment modality for early-stage oesophageal adenocarcinoma. Adjuvant chemotherapy (after the surgery) is poorly tolerated, but there is a role for neoadjuvant chemotherapy (before the surgery) to shrink the tumour preoperatively. The majority of patients (~60–70%) diagnosed with oesophageal cancer are unsuitable for surgery at diagnosis (either because of the advanced tumour stage or patient comorbidities) and therefore may either be offered endoscopic mucosal resection/ablation (if localized disease) or multidisciplinary palliative care.

What is Mrs Sweeney's prognosis?

The overall prognosis for oesophageal cancer is usually poor. As with other cancers, prognosis is stage-dependent. For the minority of cancers that are caught at stage 1 (no invasion of muscularis propria and no nodal involvement) the 5-year survival is about 80%. Unfortunately 70% of patients present with lymph node involvement, and in these patients 5-year survival is about 15% even with modern treatments.

Short cases

> **SHORT CASE**
>
> Miss Agarwal is a 27-year-old lawyer who presents with a 2-year history of mild dysphagia to both solids and liquids. She says that she has no problems with coordinating swallowing in her mouth, but feels that food and drink are sticking on their way down to her stomach. She has not noticed any choking or gurgling related to eating and is not aware of any weight loss.
>
> She has visited her GP twice in the last year, complaining of heartburn and a nocturnal cough. These were attributed to GORD and asthma, respectively, and she was offered acid-suppressing medication and a bronchodilator inhaler. Neither of these therapies has eased her symptoms, however. She takes no other medications and is otherwise fit and well.
>
> Given Miss Agarwal's dysphagia to liquids, her GP performs a thorough examination of her peripheral nervous system and cranial nerves, but nothing abnormal is noted. Abdominal and neck examinations are also unremarkable.
>
> The GP refers Miss Agarwal for a barium swallow. This shows a dilated oesophagus with a beak-like terminal narrowing. Manometry is also performed and shows an elevated lower oesophageal sphincter pressure with incomplete relaxation of the sphincter and aperistalsis in the body of the oesophagus.
>
> What is the most likely diagnosis? What are the treatment options for Miss Agarwal?

The history, examination, and investigation findings suggest **achalasia**. Compare this presentation of a young patient, with no loss of weight, and a long history of symptoms, with the classical cancer presentation of an older patient with weight loss and rapidly progressive dysphagia. The bird's beak appearance on barium swallow is classical for achalasia, but it is necessary to perform manometry to distinguish achalasia from other motility disorders such as nutcracker (hypertensive) oesophagus.[§]

It is likely that both Miss Agarwal's 'GORD' and 'asthma' were symptoms of her achalasia, hence the lack of response to medications.

There are a number of treatment options available to Miss Agarwal, although it is important to appreciate that no treatment can restore peristaltic function to her oesophagus and thus her swallowing will never completely return to normal. Treatments are aimed at loosening the lower oesophageal sphincter:

- **Pneumatic balloon dilatation** achieves good results in the majority of patients, and about 60% are free of dysphagia at 5 years. Most patients will require repeat treatments. The main risk is of oesophageal perforation (5%).

- **Surgical (Heller's) myotomy** (longitudinal incision of the muscle fibres of the distal oesophagus) tends to produce better short- and long-term relief of dysphagia, but risks the development of GORD in about 10% of patients. For this reason, there is debate as to whether to perform simultaneous Nissen fundoplication (wrapping the stomach around the lower oesophagus to prevent reflux).

- **Botox injections** produce good results that last up to 1 year, and may be favoured in patients unsuited to interventional therapy.

[§] Note that there are two other small-print diagnoses which may produce identical investigation findings to achalasia: Chagas disease (endemic to Central and South America and due to *Trypanosoma cruzi* infection) and 'pseudo-achalasia' due to an oesophageal carcinoma which infiltrates the myenteric plexus. Endoscopy is required to identify the latter, and should be suspected if there is a <6-month history in an older patient with weight loss.

- **Drugs** such as calcium channel blockers and/or nitrates may relax the lower oesophageal sphincter sufficiently to produce relief of symptoms, but are often ineffective and therefore not first-line therapies. They are primarily reserved for patients unsuitable for surgery or dilatation who fail Botox treatment.

SHORT CASE

Mr Gan is a 64-year-old retired restaurateur who presents to his GP with a 5-week history of progressive dysphagia to solids. He describes how it feels as if food items are getting stuck halfway down his throat. He denies any choking, gurgling, heartburn, or waterbrash. He has, however, suffered from increasing dyspnoea over the past 2 months, and has been coughing for a couple of weeks. The coughing occurs both day and night, and has recently been associated with episodes of haemoptysis. Mr Gan thinks that he has lost about 4 kilos in the past couple of months and describes feeling increasingly lethargic.

He has no significant past medical history and takes no regular medications. He does not drink, but has a 40-pack-year history of cigarette smoking.

On examination, Mr Gan is cachectic. There is hepatomegaly and palpable lymph nodes in his left supraclavicular fossa. Percussion and auscultation of Mr Gan's chest is unremarkable, as is a neurological exam.

In light of Mr Gan's haemoptysis and prolonged dyspnoea, his GP refers him for an urgent chest radiograph. This shows a widened mediastinum and hilar lymphadenopathy. A subsequent CT of his chest and abdomen reveals a mediastinal mass (see Figure 6.6) and bronchoscopic biopsies come back as small cell lung cancer.

Figure 6.6 CT showing mediastinal mass compressing left main bronchus and oesophagus.

What is the mechanism of Mr Gan's dysphagia?

Mr Gan's dysphagia is caused by **extrinsic compression** of the oesophagus by the lung cancer and associated mediastinal lymph nodes. He would be offered palliative care to try and minimize the degree of dysphagia suffered (which may include chemotherapy and oesophageal stenting) but his prognosis, sadly, is poor.

Viva questions

What is Barrett's oesophagus? How common and worrying is this condition?

Barrett's is metaplasia of the squamous epithelium of the lower oesophagus into columnar epithelium (also known as CLO or columnar lined oesophagus). It is usually associated with inflammation and ulceration of the distal oesophagus, and may be endoscopically visible as an area of 'velvety' epithelium. Barrett's is caused by persistent irritation of the squamous epithelium by GORD; both stomach acid and bile are implicated in the aetiology.

The significance of Barrett's is that it is a precursor lesion to adenocarcinoma, increasing the relative risk 30–40-fold. About 1% of the UK population has Barrett's (although only about 5% of these patients are diagnosed). The incidence of adenocarcinoma developing in these Barrett's patients is approximately 1 per 100 person years. Regular endoscopic surveillance is recommended for patients with known Barrett's; the role of lifelong acid-suppressing therapy (proton-pump inhibitors) and antireflux surgery are controversial, although there is reasonable evidence for endoscopic mucosal resection, radiofrequency ablation and photodynamic therapy for high-grade disease.

What are the risk factors for oesophageal cancer?

There are two main types of oesophageal cancer—squamous cell carcinoma and adenocarcinoma (carcinoid, small-cell carcinoma, and leiomyoma are very rare). In recent years there has been a relative decrease in the incidence of squamous cell carcinoma and a corresponding increase in the incidence of adenocarcinoma. Risk factors for these cancers are:

- Squamous cell carcinoma:
    - Alcohol
    - Smoking
    - Dietary nitrosamines (found in pickled/mouldy foods) and nitrates (found in Chinese, Iranian, and South African diets)
    - Aflatoxins
    - Achalasia
    - Plummer–Vinson syndrome (see below)
    - Hereditary tylosis[†]
    - Coeliac disease

- Adenocarcinoma:
    - Barrett's oesophagus (hence any factor which predisposes to reflux oesophagitis)
    - Smoking and alcohol intake are not as important as they are for squamous cell carcinoma

[†] Hereditary tylosis is a very rare autosomal dominant condition, also known as focal non-epidermolytic palmoplantar keratoderma. It manifests as symmetrical keratosis of the palms and soles of the feet.

What is Plummer–Vinson syndrome?

This is a rare collection of features including atrophic glossitis (smooth tongue), cheilosis (cracks at the corner of the mouth), koilonychia, and dysphagia that is associated with iron deficiency anaemia. The dysphagia is due to the development of a postcricoid web of hyperkeratinization. Correction of the iron deficiency may lead to a dramatic improvement in the degree of dysphagia, but persistent dysphagia may require balloon dilatation. The syndrome is most common in middle-aged to elderly women and is premalignant for cricopharyngeal carcinoma.

The condition is also known as Paterson–Brown-Kelly syndrome (Plummer and Vinson described the condition in America, while Paterson and Brown-Kelly described it independently in the UK).

What is the pathophysiology of achalasia?

Achalasia is caused by an absence of ganglion cells in the myenteric plexus (Auerbach's plexus) of the oesophagus. The consequence is a failure of relaxation of the lower oesophageal sphincter, and aperistalsis in the oesophageal body. The underlying cause of these changes in achalasia is unknown. Chagas disease results in an identical pathophysiology, and infiltrating carcinoma can also produce a 'pseudo-achalasia' by invasion of the myenteric plexus. A congenital absence of myenteric plexus ganglion cells also underlies Hirschprung's disease (megacolon) of the intestine.

A dysphagic patient presents with a hoarse voice and bovine cough. Can you think of any pathologies that may account for all these symptoms?

A hoarse voice and bovine cough are characteristic of **recurrent laryngeal nerve pathology**.

There are two main ways in which **dysphagia** may be connected with such a palsy (but more ways in which one can get such a palsy without dysphagia):

1 The nerve may be infiltrated by a primary malignancy of the oesophagus or a mediastinal malignancy that is causing dysphagia by extrinsic compression.

2 Ortner's syndrome describes the situation in which the recurrent laryngeal nerve is compressed by the cardiovascular system—most commonly left atrial dilatation secondary to mitral stenosis. Sufficiently severe left atrial enlargement can also cause dysphagia by extrinsic compression.

A patient with oesophageal adenocarcinoma is judged to be an unsuitable candidate for surgery. What palliative treatments may be available for such a patient?

There are various treatment modalities which may be used to provide symptomatic relief from malignant dysphagia, including:

- Intubation with a rigid silastic endoprosthesis or expandable metal stent
- Endoscopic resection
- Ablation with laser or argon beam plasma coagulation
- Chemotherapy
- Radiotherapy
- Psychological and social support.

How can oesophageal cancer present? What are the most common symptoms?

Oesophageal cancer, although still relatively rare, is now the eighth most common cancer in the UK with around 7000 new cases a year. The most common symptoms are:

- Dysphagia (~75%)
- Weight loss (~60%)
- GI reflux (~20%)
- Odynophagia (~20%)
- Dyspnoea (~10%)

   Less common symptoms include GI bleeding, fatigue due to anaemia, hoarseness (due to involvement of the recurrent laryngeal nerve), cough, facial flushing due to superior vena cava (SVC) obstruction, and breathlessness due to malignant pleural effusion.

What are the specific complications after an oesophagectomy?

Removal of the oesophagus and refashioning of a gullet using the stomach is a major operation. The major complications for a junior doctor to be aware of are:

- **Breakdown of the anastomosis** due to poor blood supply (e.g. tight sutures, tension on the anastomosis), infection, and patient factors (e.g. smoking, diabetes mellitus, old age).
- **Pneumonia** due to poor ventilation secondary to pain, this can be minimized using specialist analgesia (e.g. high thoracic epidural blocks by specialized anaesthetists) and encouraging ventilation (physiotherapy).
- **Cardiac arrhythmia**. Manipulation of the tissue near to the heart predisposes patients to intra-operative and postoperative cardiac arrhythmias.
- **Recurrent laryngeal nerve injury.**
- **Chylothorax/chyle leak** resulting from injury to the thoracic duct.

Single Best Answers

1. What is meant by odynophagia?

a. The sensation of a lump in the throat
b. Painful swallowing
c. Difficulty swallowing

d. Painful chewing
e. Difficulty breathing

2. Which of the following causes functional (rather than structural) dysphagia?

a. Oesophageal cancer
b. Plummer–Vinson syndrome
c. Ortner's syndrome

d. Dysphagia lusoria
e. Limited cutaneous scleroderma (CREST syndrome)

3. Which of the following investigations is not routinely used to grade and stage oesophageal cancer?

a. Oesophagogastroduodenoscopy (OGD)
b. Endoscopic ultrasound (EUS)
c. Manometry

d. PET-CT
e. Laparoscopy

4. What is the most common histological type of oesophageal cancer in the UK?

a. Lymphoma
b. Adenocarcinoma
c. Squamous cell carcinoma

d. Small-cell carcinoma
e. Leiomyoma

5. Which of the following is not a treatment option for achalasia?

a. Calcium channel blockers
b. Oesophagectomy
c. Botox injections

d. Heller's myotomy
e. Pneumatic balloon dilatation

Cough

Core case

 Read through the sections in the case boxes, covering up the sections that follow so that you don't see the answer. At the end of each case box, try to answer the question before reading on.

Mrs Virginia is a 78-year-old woman who presents with a persistent cough.

What specific questions should you ask her in the history?

First, ask open questions about the cough itself:

- **Acute or chronic?** The British Thoracic Society (BTS) defines acute as <3 weeks and chronic as >8 weeks. Between 3 and 8 weeks the cough may be due to recovering acute illness or developing chronic illness.
- **Constant or intermittent?** A cough that is intermittent may suggest an extrinsic trigger (e.g. if the patient only coughs at work there may be an allergy to something in the workplace). A cough that is constant suggests an intrinsic cause.
- **Productive or dry?** The presence of sputum indicates inflammation and/or infection. Patients with chronic obstructive pulmonary disease (COPD) have chronically inflamed airways and often produce white or clear sputum. Patients with infection have yellow or green sputum. Particularly large volumes of sputum, often green or rusty coloured, may be coughed up in bronchiectasis and lung abscesses.
- **Blood?** More specifically:
    - Blood-streaked sputum? Suggests infection or bronchiectasis.
    - Pink and frothy sputum? Suggests pulmonary oedema.
    - Frank blood (haemoptysis)? See Chapter 8. Suggests tuberculosis (TB), lung cancer, pulmonary embolus, bronchiectasis, or other rarer causes (e.g. granulomatosis with polyangiitis (GPA, formerly known as Wegener's granulomatosis), or Goodpasture's syndrome).
- **Timing?** Asthma is classically worse at night and early hours of the morning. Pulmonary oedema or gastro-oesophageal reflux disease (GORD) can also be worse at night due to the positional effects of lying flat. Patients often report sleeping propped up on pillows to mitigate these effects. Trigger factors such as pets, cold weather, or exercise indicate asthma, as does a worsening in spring/summer.
- **Character?** A wheezy cough suggests airway obstruction due to asthma or COPD. A bovine cough (breathy) is characteristic of vocal cord paralysis. A dry cough is suggestive of a bronchitis (usually viral) or interstitial lung disease. A gurgling/wet cough is suggestive of bronchiectasis. Pertussis infection causes a 'whooping' cough.

Second, ask directed questions about factors that might be triggering the cough:

- **Environmental irritants**: Smoking? Occupation? Pets? Change of house, office, etc?
- **Past medical history**: Asthma? GORD? Rhinitis/sinusitis? Heart failure? Recent chest infection?
- **Drug history?** Angiotensin-converting enzyme (ACE) inhibitors in particular can cause a cough.
- **Travel?** The patient may have visited an area of the world where TB is highly prevalent (e.g. Asian subcontinent, central Asia, sub-Saharan Africa).
- **Close contacts?** Ask the patient if household members and work colleagues have had a noticeable cough. This is particularly relevant for TB, where prolonged, close contact is usually required for transmission meaning that TB is most commonly acquired from household members and close contacts.

Third, ask about factors that might be associated with the cough and give you clues about the underlying cause:

- **Fevers, night sweats, rigors, weight loss?** These suggest malignancy, TB, or another severe infection.
- **Breathlessness,** particularly on exertion? This would be in keeping with asthma, COPD, pneumonia, or pulmonary oedema but rarer in lung cancer.
- **Chest pain, particularly pleuritic chest pain?** This may indicate pneumonia, pneumothorax, pulmonary embolism, or viral pleurisy. Equally, it may be due to muscle strain secondary to vigorous coughing, or a fractured rib if there has been any trauma.
- **Wheeze?** This suggests obstruction of the airways such as that found in asthma, COPD, or tumours compressing an airway.
- **Frequent throat clearing and/or rhinorrhea?** Symptoms suggestive of rhinitis.

Mrs Virginia says that she has had a cough for months but that over the last few days she has been 'coughing more, and more muck has been coming up'. She says that the sputum is yellow-green, but there has been no blood. There appear to be no triggers or periodicity.

In her history she reveals that she is a long-term smoker (60 years smoking 10 a day = 30 pack years) and has a diagnosis of COPD. She says she walks a mile a day to the shops and back, and has no history of asthma, allergies, or reflux. She uses inhalers for her COPD ('a dry powder one, a blue spray, and a brown spray') but is not on home oxygen and takes no other medications. Reassuringly, she has had no night sweats, rigors, or weight loss, and is no more breathless than usual. However, she says she has felt a little hot over the last day. She has not been abroad 'since a school trip to France', although she went on a Saga holiday to Eastbourne the previous summer.

What is the differential diagnosis of cough? Try thinking about conditions which present acutely or chronically, and whether the cough would be dry or productive (Figure 7.1).

Which of these are most likely given this patient's presentation?

Mrs Virginia's complaint is an acute worsening of her productive cough. This therefore narrows the differential down to an infectious cause. Of those, the absence of constitutional features (e.g. weight loss, night sweats) or foreign travel makes TB unlikely.

	Dry	Productive
Acute	Asthma Rhinitis/sinusitis with post-nasal drip Upper respiratory tract infection (pharyngitis, laryngitis, tracheitis) Drug induced, e.g. ACE inhibitors Smoke/toxin inhalation Inhaled foreign body Lung cancer (causing obstruction of a major bronchus) Pulmonary oedema (secondary to heart failure)	Lower respiratory tract infection (pneumonia, bronchitis) COPD TB
Chronic	Asthma GORD Post-nasal drip Smoking Lung cancer Drug induced COPD Pulmonary oedema (secondary to heart failure) Non-asthmatic eosinophilic bronchitis Recurrent aspiration (due to impaired swallow) Psychogenic	Bronchiectasis TB Lung cancer Recurrent aspiration (due to impaired swallow) (If congenital: cystic fibrosis or primary ciliary dyskinesia)

Figure 7.1 Differential diagnosis of cough.

What specific signs should you look for on physical examination that would be consistent with an infectious cause? What other signs might you see, given her COPD?

With regard to her likely infection, you should look for:

- **Systemic features**: Is she febrile? Is she sweating? Is she tachycardic?
- **Respiratory distress**: Is her respiratory rate increased? Is she having difficulty breathing—can she complete sentences, is she using her accessory muscles? Is she peripherally cyanosed? Is she confused? (you can assess confusion with an Abbreviated Mental Test Score (AMTS); see Chapter 2). These give an idea of the severity of her condition.
- **Tender cervical lymphadenopathy**: in a patient with a cough, this suggests infection in the upper respiratory tract.
- **Lungs**: reduced chest expansion, breath sounds (reduced in effusion, bronchial sounding in pneumonia), and vocal resonance (increased in consolidation, reduced in pleural effusion).

Given her COPD, you should also note any:

- **Chest wall deformities** (e.g. hyperexpansion or 'barrel chest').
- **Intercostal recession**: a sign of severe COPD.

- **Signs of right heart failure** due to her COPD ('cor pulmonale'), such as peripheral oedema, raised jugular venous pressure (JVP), a parasternal heave, a loud or palpable P_2 heart sound, or tricuspid regurgitation.
- **Asterixis:** even though some COPD patients are chronic CO_2 retainers, asterixis can be seen if COPD deteriorates and CO_2 levels rise significantly.

On examination, Mrs Virginia looks sweaty and unwell. She is cachectic and has a 'barrel chest'. Her fingers are tar-stained. She is tachycardic and tachypnoeic with a pulse of 107 bpm and a respiratory rate of 22/min. Her oxygen saturations are 89% on air. Her temperature is 38.5 °C. She has poor chest expansion, an expiratory wheeze, hyperresonant percussion note throughout but with dullness at the right lung base, and bronchial breath sounds in the same place. Vocal resonance is increased over the area of percussion dullness. You find no lymphadenopathy in the neck. She is not confused, with an AMTS of 9/10.

What investigations would you like to request?

Blood tests:

- **Arterial blood gas (ABG):** you will want to assess her gas exchange to monitor her progress and ensure she doesn't develop respiratory failure. Keep in mind that she has COPD and that her baseline may therefore be different from a 'normal' baseline, e.g. slightly elevated CO_2 levels may be normal for her.
- **Full blood count (FBC):** the white cell count should be raised in infection, with a neutrophilia if it is a bacterial infection.
- **C-reactive protein (CRP):** will also be raised if there is an underlying infective process.
- **Urea and electrolytes (U&Es):** the patient's U&Es may be deranged if she is dehydrated and consequently hypoperfusing her kidneys. Urea is an indicator of severity in pneumonia and influences prognosis.
- **Blood cultures:** This patient has signs of systemic inflammatory response syndrome (SIRS) that suggest an infective process. If a patient is likely to require antibiotics, you should take blood cultures before you start these. That way, if the patient fails to respond to antibiotics, you stand a higher chance of having an organism identified in the lab, as well as its sensitivities to various antibiotics. Remember that it usually takes >24 hours to get a positive blood culture result.

Imaging

- **Chest radiograph:** this may reveal areas of consolidation, potentially in a lobar pattern.
- **Electrocardiogram (ECG):** you must perform this to rule out ischaemia or atrial fibrillation secondary to pneumonia. It may also show right heart strain in some patients with COPD.

Microbiology

- **Urinary antigens:** Urine can be tested for pneumococcal and legionella antigens in patients with a clinical diagnosis of pneumonia who are admitted to hospital. A positive test helps confirm the diagnosis and can guide antibiotic therapy (as *Legionella* will be treated with different antibiotics than those used for *Streptococcus pneumoniae*).
- **Sputum cultures** are rarely useful as the sputum will contain all the commensal flora that is normally found in the upper respiratory tract. However, the chest physiotherapist may be able to help you obtain an induced sputum and/or non-bronchoscopic bronchoalveolar lavage (NBAL) sample,

both of which have a higher yield. Bronchial washings may also be obtained bronchoscopically to get a sputum sample free of the upper airways flora and thereby identify the offending organism, but this is only done if a pneumonia does not respond to conventional antibiotic treatment suggesting infection with an atypical organism.

Mrs Virginia's chest radiograph is shown in Figure 7.2.

How would you interpret this radiograph?

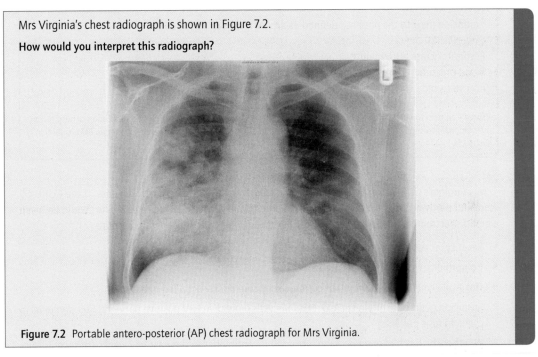

Figure 7.2 Portable antero-posterior (AP) chest radiograph for Mrs Virginia.

Mrs Virginia's chest radiograph shows an area of dense opacity in the right side of her chest. The dense pattern confined to a discrete area of lung is in keeping with consolidation. Given that the right hemidiaphragm is still visible but the right heart border has been obscured this is therefore likely to represent consolidation in the right middle lobe—which is consistent with the clinical findings on examination.

Mrs Virginia's test results are as follows:

Haematology		Biochemistry		ABG (on 28% oxygen)	
Hb	117 g/L	Na	142 mM	pH	7.42
WCC	15.7 × 10⁹ cells/L	K	4.7 mM	pO_2	12.4 kPa
		Urea	9.2 mM	pCO_2	6.2 kPa
		Creatinine	122 µM	HCO_3	32 mM

An ECG showed sinus tachycardia but no other changes.

In light of the history, examination, and investigations, what is the diagnosis? What is the CURB-65 score (see Box 7.1), what is it used for, and how is it calculated? How should she be managed?

Mrs Virginia has a pneumonia exacerbating her COPD. Her mild hypercapnia should not be a cause of concern as her pH is within the normal range, suggesting the CO_2 retention is chronic and therefore unlikely to be clinically significant.

> **Box 7.1 The CURB-65 score**
>
> The **CURB-65** score can be used to calculate severity of pneumonia and therefore determine the need for hospitalization. CURB-65 is an acronym for the constituent prognostic factors; the presence of any one scores 1 point, up to a maximum of 5. Patients with a score of 2 or more should be admitted to hospital.
>
> Confusion (new to the patient), defined as an AMTS of ≤8/10
> Urea >7 mM
> Respiratory rate >30/minute
> Blood pressure <90 systolic and/or <60 diastolic
> >65 years old
>
> Reproduced from *Thorax*, W S Lim et al., 'Defining community acquired pneumonia severity on presentation to hospital: an international derivation and validation study', 58, 5, pp. 3773–82, Copyright 2003, with permission from BMJ Publishing Group Ltd.

Mrs Virginia's CURB-65 score is 2. She should therefore be admitted, partly because of the CURB-65 score and partly because elderly patients with pneumonia can deteriorate rapidly. She should be given a broad-spectrum antibiotic in line with local protocol, which should take into account:

- Severity, as assessed by the CURB-65 score
- Comorbidity with COPD
- Hospital-acquired (nosocomial) infection versus community-acquired infection
- Suspicion of unusual organism (e.g. *Pneumocystis jirovecii* in HIV-positive patients, *Pseudomonas* in cystic fibrosis patients)
- Whether she has had any pneumonia treated by antibiotics in the past few weeks (this would suggest the antibiotics did not work properly, so you may need to use different ones)
- Whether or not a particular antibiotic is deemed to predispose to infections such as *Clostridium difficile* colitis.

Short cases

A week after discharge, Mrs Virginia attends the Emergency Department again, this time with breathlessness. She is agitated but does not complain of any chest pain. She says the breathlessness came on suddenly while she was sitting in her chair at home. An ECG taken in the ambulance showed sinus tachycardia but no other changes. Her oxygen saturations are 92% (on 35% oxygen), her respiratory rate is 28/min, her heart rate 112 bpm, her blood pressure 135/89 mmHg, and her temperature is 37.3 °C. On examination, she has unilaterally decreased chest expansion and an area of hyperresonant percussion, and reduced breath sounds throughout her left lung anteriorly and posteriorly. Her trachea is not deviated.

What are the complications of pneumonia? What is most likely to have happened in this case?

The complications of pneumonia include:

- **Spread of infection**: pleural effusion, empyema, abscess, septicaemia
- **Damage to local structures**: bronchiectasis, pneumothorax

Her breathlessness, apyrexia, and examination suggest a **pneumothorax**. Pneumothorax is an uncommon complication of pneumonia but she also has COPD, which could have left her with bullae in her lungs that are prone to rupture (e.g. after a particularly vigorous cough). You should look for signs of the pneumothorax being a tension pneumothorax by checking for tracheal deviation and hypotension on examination.

Mrs Virginia had no tracheal deviation and was stable. The signs on physical examination indicated a pneumothorax in her left lung, which was consistent with her chest radiograph. It can be difficult to distinguish a large bulla from a pneumothorax on a single chest radiograph, so in this case a comparison was made with the radiograph from her previous admission. If a previous radiograph is not available for comparison, CT of the chest will distinguish between the two. Mrs Virginia's pneumothorax was decompressed using a chest drain.

Miss Lambert is a 33-year-old nurse who has been referred to the respiratory clinic by her GP with a 3-month history of a dry cough. The GP's letter notes that she has never smoked and has no previous history of respiratory illness, reflux, or any allergies, but has a high body mass index (BMI).

You take a history in which Miss Lambert confirms all of this. She adds that her cough got worse in the spring, but can think of no other exacerbating factors. She says that sometimes she wakes up at night coughing. She has not had a fever, night sweats, or rigors. She has had no chest pain. She does not have a wheeze, is no more breathless than usual on exertion, and is not breathless at rest.

What diagnoses are most likely? If you are seeing her in outpatients, what investigations would you conduct and what would you be looking for?

The three most common causes of chronic cough in a non-smoker are **asthma**, **postnasal drip**, and **GORD**. Asthma is a likely cause in this woman, despite the lack of allergies or atopy (e.g. eczema) and her age (asthma is most common in children and older people).

As such, in addition to listening to her lungs, you should perform spirometry (or peak flow measurement if spirometry not available) to assess her lung function. National guidelines for diagnosing asthma emphasize the importance of clinical assessment (see Table 7.1): where the clinical features indicate a high probability of asthma, the guidelines recommend proceeding to a trial of treatment. Where there is a low probability, they advise seeking and treating an alternative diagnosis. Only for those patients with an intermediate probability of asthma do they counsel using the ratio of the forced expiratory volume in 1 second (FEV_1) to the forced vital capacity (FVC). The convention is that a ratio of <0.7 argues in favour of an obstructive airways disease, such as asthma or COPD.

Previous guidelines suggested taking serial peak expiratory flow (PEF) measurements to look for variability, or looking for an improvement in FEV_1 after administration of a bronchodilator. However, PEF measurements are notoriously unreliable (in both those with and without asthma), effort dependent, and thus not particularly helpful. The use of FEV_1 with reversibility testing to diagnose asthma has fallen out of favour as it has a low sensitivity. This is particularly the case for the many patients with normal (or near-normal) spirometry between symptomatic episodes, who have little room for improvement with bronchodilators. In those patients, tests of airway hyper-responsiveness and/or inflammation may prove more useful in future. Figure 7.3 shows PEF in normal adults.

It is often useful to request a chest radiograph, to exclude any unusual but more serious causes such as lung cancer, but we would not expect to see any abnormality indicating asthma.

On examination, Miss Lambert's lungs sound clear, with no added sounds. Bedside spirometry in the clinic yields an FEV_1 of 2.8 L (93% predicted) with an FVC of 3.5 (101% predicted), ratio >0.70. However, this history is suggestive of possible asthma, so she is started on a trial of salbutamol inhalers.

Table 7.1 Clinical features in the diagnosis of asthma

Features suggestive of asthma	Features suggestive of an alternative diagnosis
>1 of: wheeze, breathlessness, chest tightness and cough, particularly if: • worse at night/early morning • triggered by exercise, allergen exposure, cold air or after taking aspirin or β-blockers	Normal physical examination and/or FEV_1/PEF when symptomatic
History of atopic disorder	Prominent dizziness, light-headedness, peripheral tingling (possible hyperventilation syndrome)
Family history of asthma and/or atopy	Chronic productive cough without wheeze or breathlessness (more consistent with another cause of chronic cough)
Wheeze on auscultation	Symptoms with colds only (possible rhinitis)
Otherwise unexplained low FEV_1, PEF, or serum eosinophilia	Voice disturbance (possible vocal cord dysfunction)
	Significant smoking history e.g. >20 pack years (possible COPD)
	Cardiac disease

Data from the BTS/Sign guidelines, available at: <http://www.sign.ac.uk/pdf/sign101.pdf>.

Postnasal drip is still a possibility but is largely a diagnosis of exclusion, confirmed by a trial of treatment. If inhalers do not work after a trial period, you may wish to try antihistamines and/or nasal decongestants. Finally, reflux (GORD) is still also a possibility, particularly given her high BMI, although she does not give any history of heartburn or regurgitation. In your letter to her GP you may want to add that if treatment for asthma and postnasal drip do not work, Miss Lambert could try antacids, histamine H_2 antagonists, or proton pump inhibitors.

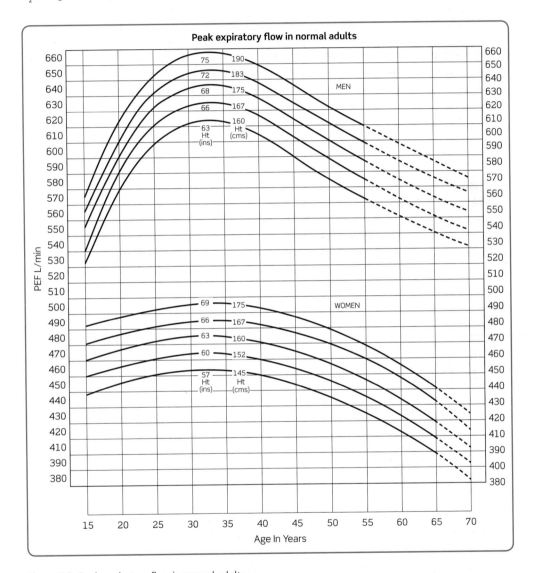

Figure 7.3 Peak expiratory flow in normal adults.

Adapted from Nunn AJ and Gregg I, 'New regression equations for predicting peak expiratory flow in adults'. *British Medical Journal*, 298, pp. 1068–1070, Copyright 1989, with permission from BMJ Publishing Group Ltd.

SHORT CASE

Mr Dunhill is a 48-year-old office worker who comes to his GP complaining of a chronic dry cough. He has had it for the last few months and thought it was a cold, but has come in as it hasn't resolved and is annoying his work colleagues and wife. His coughing spells occur throughout the day and night, with no predictable triggers. On questioning, he comments that he often has heartburn and wakes up with a sore throat.

He is a non-smoker, drinks about 15 pints of lager a week, and has a high BMI. His past medical history includes an inguinal hernia repair and childhood asthma, although he has not had to use an inhaler since he was a teenager. He has no allergies. He has no new pets or other recent changes to his environment (new job or house). He does not have a history of diagnosed GORD despite his heartburn. His only recent travel was to Spain, and he has had no fevers, night sweats, rigors, or weight loss. His examination is unremarkable and spirometry is normal.

What diagnosis is most likely? How would you test your hypothesis?

Mr Dunhill's cough is dry and chronic, and he is a non-smoker. Normal spirometry is not inconsistent with asthma, but his high BMI and heartburn should make you suspicious that his cough is caused by **gastro-oesophageal reflux** irritating his larynx, despite the lack of a formal diagnosis. You could start a **therapeutic trial** with a proton pump inhibitor for GORD and arrange a follow-up appointment in clinic. You should also advise weight loss, as this may bring symptomatic relief. Mr Dunhill was started on such a trial and after 3 months his cough had resolved.

SHORT CASE

Mrs Benson is a 52-year-old woman who complains of a cough during a follow-up visit to her GP. Her GP has recently diagnosed her with hypertension. She has had the cough for a few weeks, but has had no sputum or haemoptysis, fever, breathlessness, chest pain, or wheeze. She has never smoked and does not have a history of asthma or GORD. She has no allergies. She takes enalapril for her hypertension and alendronate, calcium, and vitamin D for osteoporosis prevention because she had a hysterectomy and bilateral salpingo-oopherectomy when she was aged 43. Examination of her respiratory system is entirely normal.

What is the most likely cause of Mrs Benson's cough?

Mrs Benson has had a non-productive cough for the past few weeks. She has also recently been diagnosed with hypertension and started on enalapril. In the absence of any clues in the history or examination to suggest an alternative diagnosis, it is most likely that her cough is due to the ACE inhibitor (enalapril) that she is taking, as ACE inhibitors can cause a dry cough in 10–20% of patients. This is thought to be because ACE is also responsible for breaking down the inflammatory bradykinins in the lungs. Thus, inhibition of ACE leads to a build-up of bradykinins and lung inflammation, triggering cough. Incidentally, this is the same mechanism by which ACE inhibitors can cause facial angioedema—indeed, they are responsible for 20–40% of cases of angioedema presenting to the Emergency Department, although this is often misdiagnosed as an anaphylactic reaction to some unknown allergen.

Her GP changed her prescription from enalapril to an angiotensin II receptor blocker (e.g. losartan, candesartan, valsartan), which offer the same antihypertensive and renal protective effects without causing a dry cough, presumably because they act downstream of ACE and therefore do not interfere with bradykinin levels. Mrs Benson's cough had disappeared by the time she was next seen by her GP a few weeks later.

SHORT CASE

Mr Hedges is a 78-year-old retired man who presented at his GP's surgery with a persistent cough. He says he has had a smoker's cough for 40 years, but that in the last few months it has got worse. He had gone to his GP because his wife was being kept awake by his coughing at night. The cough is non-productive and he has had no fever, chest pain, night sweats, or any significant weight loss that he is aware of—although he admits that he is thin anyway and never weighs himself. He is not known to be asthmatic, has no known allergies, and does not suffer from reflux. He is on no medications and jokes that 'the cigarettes keep me healthy'. He has smoked 20 a day since he joined the army for national service. He is partial to a beer or two but rarely goes to the pub these days (less than once a week).

Mr Hedges' pulse is 80 bpm, blood pressure 130/82 mmHg, respiratory rate 13/min, temperature 37.3 °C. On examination, he is thin but does not appear cachectic, and is comfortable at rest. He appears well perfused with a capillary refill time of <2 seconds. There is no cervical lymphadenopathy or any other peripheral stigmata of respiratory disease, although there is heavy tar staining of the fingers of his right hand. Chest expansion, percussion, and auscultation are all unremarkable.

The GP refers Mr Hedges to the hospital for a chest radiograph and respiratory opinion. The chest radiograph is shown in Figure 7.4.

What is the most likely diagnosis?

Figure 7.4 Chest radiograph for Mr Hedges.

Mr Hedges most likely has **lung cancer**. Although he has had a (smoker's) cough for a long time, the recent change should alert you to possible pathology. Given that the cough is non-productive and that on examination he is afebrile and has no respiratory signs, an infective process appears unlikely. In light of his history of lifelong smoking, lung cancer is a definite possibility. This is made even more likely by the chest radiograph. Although cough is not the most common presentation of lung cancer, tumours can cause a cough if they are situated in the larger, more proximal airways where cough receptors are more widespread.

Assuming a diagnosis of lung cancer is confirmed by biopsy, it will most likely be a **squamous cell carcinoma** because of the hilar location. This will be investigated in more detail by the specialist team. The GP was right to be suspicious and request a chest radiograph.

SHORT CASE

Mr Butler is a 27-year-old retail manager who is referred to the respiratory clinic for investigation of his persistent cough. His referral letter documents an episode of pneumonia 7 weeks ago, which was treated by the GP with antibiotics. He made a good recovery, but the cough became dry and persisted. The cough does not vary with time of day and is not associated with exercise or any other triggers. There is no history of asthma, allergies, or gastro-oesophageal reflux. He has never smoked and takes no regular medications.

Mr Butler's pulse is 64 bpm, blood pressure 120/72 mmHg, oxygen saturations 98% on room air, respiratory rate 11/min, temperature 36.8 °C. There are no peripheral stigmata of respiratory disease and chest expansion, percussion, and auscultation are all unremarkable. Bedside spirometry performed in the respiratory clinic is normal.

What is the most likely cause of his persistent cough? What are the treatment options?

Patients with pneumonia, particularly viral pneumonia, can have a persistent postinfectious cough some time after the infection has subsided. Judging from the history and the negative findings on examination and lung function testing, this looks to be the most likely cause.

A number of treatment options are available:

- **Antitussives (cough suppressants)?** If an underlying cause cannot be identified, these may offer symptomatic relief (e.g. if sleep is being disrupted). These operate via two mechanisms: (1) depressing the brainstem 'cough centre', e.g. codeine, pholcodine (opiates), dextromethorphan (non-opioid); (2) reducing peripheral receptor sensitivity, e.g. benzocaine (a local anaesthetic). Unfortunately, there is currently no high-quality evidence to suggest that cough suppressants actually work, despite their widespread use. Furthermore, the opiate cough suppressants are associated with side effects such as constipation, particularly with codeine but less so with pholcodine, and may be associated with dependence.

- **Inhaled corticosteroids or oral antihistamines?** The evidence is mixed on the efficacy of these agents. It is thought that in some patients chronic cough is associated with airway inflammation, even in the absence of asthma, and that corticosteroids and/or antihistamines suppress this inflammation.

- **Inhaled ipratropium bromide?** This is an anticholinergic that blocks the efferent limb of the cough reflex, and may also decrease stimulation of cough receptors. This has been shown to be of benefit in patients with persistent cough after an upper respiratory tract infection.

Viva questions

How might your management have been altered if Mrs Virginia had a history of weight loss, night sweats, blood-streaked sputum, and had recently returned from Pakistan, where she had lived most of her adult life working as a teacher?

Such a history would make you suspect a diagnosis of **pulmonary TB**. TB is contagious, airborne, difficult to treat, and potentially fatal. Patients suspected of having active pulmonary TB are isolated in a negative pressure side room until they are either deemed non-infective following three negative sputum samples (these patients may or may not have TB, but are not an infection risk to the public) or, following a smear positive sputum sample, have completed 2 weeks of treatment.

Which patients should not necessarily be given 100% oxygen and why?

Patients with COPD are at risk of becoming hypoxaemic for a number of reasons:
- The airways contain significant amounts of mucus that impairs ventilation.
- The lungs are hyperinflated, making them less efficient at moving air.
- The hypoxic vasoconstriction mechanism is blunted. This usually ensures that areas of lung that are poorly ventilated are supplied with less blood, so that gas exchange only occurs in well-ventilated areas. If this mechanism no longer works well, blood travels through poorly ventilated areas of the lung and is not well oxygenated.

When COPD patients become hypoxic, it is tempting to administer 100% oxygen. However, in a subset of COPD patients, it has been observed that administration of 100% oxygen to combat hypoxaemia can be detrimental, leading to patients developing hypercapnia (high CO_2) which obtunds them and can eventually make them comatose. Traditional teaching states that this is because some COPD patients no longer rely on detecting high CO_2 levels to stimulate breathing (as is normally the case in people without COPD) but rather rely on low O_2 levels ('hypoxic drive'). Giving too much oxygen in these cases can actually remove the stimulus to breathe.

However, experiments suggest this is not the case, as hypercapnia develops in COPD patients given O_2 without any significant drop in ventilation rate, so clearly their stimulus to drive is not reduced. One hypothesis is that too much oxygen further diminishes the hypoxic vasoconstriction effect that usually prevents poorly ventilated areas of lung being perfused with blood. In other words, it is believed that giving too much oxygen results in blood being diverted ('shunted') to areas of the lungs that in COPD patients are incapable of efficient gas exchange, thus diverting blood from the areas of lung that are still able to exchange gas efficiently.

For this reason, COPD patients who become hypoxaemic are administered oxygen using 'Venturi' masks, which allow oxygen to be delivered at safer, smaller, fixed ratios (from 24% to 40%) such that the lungs are better ventilated, but not so much so that the COPD patient can become hypercapnic. Please remember however that the appropriate initial treatment in an acute resuscitation scenario (whether the patient has COPD or not) is high flow oxygen.

You see a patient in clinic with lung cancer who has a bovine cough. Can you explain this symptom?

It is likely that this patient has a **recurrent laryngeal nerve (RLN) palsy**. Such a palsy is more common on the left than the right. The left branch of the RLN loops around the arch of the aorta and thus has a longer intrathoracic course (and hence is more likely to be affected by chest pathology) than the right branch—which loops around the right subclavian artery. Damage to the RLN is most commonly due to malignancy (e.g. a Pancoast apical lung tumour) or surgery (e.g. neck surgery).

Single Best Answers

1. **You are asked to examine a patient with long-standing chronic obstructive pulmonary disease (COPD) and cor pulmonale. What might you expect to find?**

   a. Hyperexpanded chest
   b. Peripheral oedema
   c. Raised JVP

   d. Loud P2 heart sound
   e. All of the above

2. **As part of your assessment of a patient with cough and breathlessness, you take an arterial blood gas (ABG). The results show the patient has a Pao$_2$ of 10.2 kPa. How would you interpret this?**

   a. The patient is hypoxic
   b. The patient is becoming hypoxic
   c. The patient's ventilation is impaired

   d. The Pao$_2$ is meaningless without knowing the Paco$_2$
   e. The Pao$_2$ is meaningless without knowing the Fio$_2$

3. **A 38-year-old patient presents with clinical features of pneumonia. Their chest radiograph is reported as having 'widespread patchy infiltrates in both lung fields with air bronchograms visible; in addition there is a 3 cm round area of consolidation in the right upper lobe with a fluid level.' What is the most likely causal organism?**

   a. *Mycoplasma pneumoniae*
   b. *Streptococcus pneumoniae*
   c. *Aspergillus*

   d. *Staphylococcus aureus*
   e. Adenovirus

4. **Which of the following is not a treatment for gastro-oesophageal reflux disease?**

   a. Proton pump inhibitors (PPIs)
   b. H$_1$ receptor antagonists
   c. Magnesium carbonate

   d. Aluminium hydroxide
   e. Alginates

5. **Which of the following is a risk factor for spontaneous pneumothorax?**

   a. Marfan's syndrome
   b. Smoking
   c. Cystic fibrosis (CF)

   d. HIV/AIDS with *Pneumocystis jiroveci*
   e. All of the above

Haemoptysis

Core case

Read through the sections in the case boxes, covering up the sections that follow so that you don't see the answer. At the end of each case box, try to answer the question before reading on.

Mr Morris is a 72-year-old retired electrician who presents to his GP after coughing up blood. He is not coughing up any blood at present, appears well, and is able to talk calmly about what has happened.

The first step should be to establish if this is truly haemoptysis.

What might haemoptysis be confused with by the patient? How will you tell if it really is haemoptysis?

You need to ensure that you are not mistaking haemoptysis with:

- **Haematemesis:** brownish-red blood that is vomited from the gastrointestinal (GI) tract.
- **Epistaxis (nosebleed):** particularly a posterior nosebleed.
- **Bleeding gums:** combined with a cough, this may be confused with true haemoptysis.

To tell if it is really haemoptysis, you can ask the patient where they think the blood is coming from (they may say it initially dripped from their nose), its colour (darker, coffee-ground appearance suggests partially digested blood), any history of nosebleeds, nausea, vomiting, gastric disease, or alcoholism. For the latter, asking if he is an alcoholic is unlikely to yield a valid response. Instead, you can try the TACE questions to detect alcohol dependence[*]:

Does it **T**ake more than three drinks to make you feel high?

Have you ever been **A**nnoyed by people's criticism of your drinking?

Are you trying to **C**ut down on drinking?

Have you ever used alcohol as an **E**ye-opener in the morning?

A positive response to the first question scores 2 points and a positive response to each of the rest, scores 1 point each. A positive response to two of these four questions is considered to indicate possible alcohol abuse or dependence as does a total score of two or more points.

Why should you worry particularly about haemoptysis?

---

[*] Data from Sokol RJ, 'Finding the Risk Drinker in Your Clinical Practice', In: Robinson G and Armstrong R (eds), Alcohol and Child/Family Health: Proceedings of a Conference with Particular Reference to the Prevention of Alcohol-Related Birth Defects, Vancouver, BC., 1988.

Haemoptysis should always be investigated thoroughly for two reasons:

1   It may be the presenting symptom for life-threatening lung disease.

2   Massive haemoptysis, variably defined as anything from >100 mL to >1000 mL over 24 hours, may be life-threatening itself, usually through asphyxiation but potentially also shock.

Haemoptysis is thus a 'red flag' symptom and any patient with haemoptysis requires a thorough diagnostic work-up.

What diagnoses should you be concerned about?

These can be grouped together under a 'surgical sieve'—we have used INVITED MD:

Infective: pulmonary tuberculosis (TB), bronchitis, pneumonia, lung abscess, mycetoma

Neoplastic: primary lung cancer, metastatic lung cancer

Vascular: pulmonary embolism, left ventricular failure, bleeding diathesis (i.e. a bleeding tendency e.g. coagulopathy, severe thrombocytopenia), arteriovenous malformation, vascular–bronchial fistula

Inflammatory: granulomatosis with polyangiitis (formerly called Wegener's granulomatosis), Goodpasture's syndrome, systemic lupus erythematosus, hereditary haemorrhagic telangiectasia (Osler–Weber–Rendu syndrome), polyarteritis nodosa, microscopic polyangiitis

Traumatic: iatrogenic (post-lung biopsy or intubation), wounds (rib fracture, stab injury)

Endocrine: (none)

Degenerative: bronchiectasis

Metabolic: (none)

Drugs: warfarin (bleeding diathesis), crack cocaine use

The most common causes are infective, but these should never be assumed to be the cause. Lung cancer is a 'must exclude' diagnosis in a presentation of haemoptysis.

Note that up to a third of cases of haemoptysis have no identifiable cause.

What questions should you ask Mr Morris about the haemoptysis?

- **What is he coughing up?**
    - **Frank blood**: this is suggestive of a vascular problem such as erosion of a blood vessel (invasive cancer, bronchiectasis, TB), a ruptured arteriovenous malformation, or a vascular–bronchial fistula.
    - **Blood-streaked sputum**: any infection of the lungs can cause this; however, in the context of chronic production of large volumes of sputum this would suggest bronchiectasis.
    - **Frothy sputum**: this suggests pulmonary oedema (secondary to, for example, left ventricular failure or severe mitral stenosis). This is sometimes described as 'pink' but is rarely so, although it may occasionally be bloodstained.
- **How much is he coughing up?** Try to help the patient quantify this by comparing with amounts they might know—a teaspoon, a tablespoon, an eggcup, or more—especially as even a small amount of coughed-up blood will be alarming and seem like a lot to many patients.
- **How suddenly did it start, and has it got worse progressively?** Sudden onset is consistent with pulmonary embolism (PE) or erosion of a cancer into a pulmonary blood vessel. Gradual onset argues for a progressive condition such as bronchiectasis.

Mr Morris tells you he has been coughing up frank blood. He feels it is a lot. When you try to quantify it, he tells you that he has found blood spotting on his handkerchief throughout the day, but he finds it difficult to quantify how much. It seems to have developed fairly rapidly, although he has had a smoker's cough for years. You are also able to confirm that the blood is bright red and almost certainly from the lungs.

What symptoms apart from coughing up blood might you ask Mr Morris about? Think of key clues that would help you narrow your differential diagnosis.

- **Cough productive of sputum?** Indicates lower respiratory tract infection (pneumonia, bronchitis, TB), or bronchiectasis.
- **Fever?** More commonly associated with a lower respiratory tract infection. Night sweats may indicate TB.
- **Weight loss?** This is associated with lung cancer and TB. You should consider whether the weight loss was planned or not, but significant weight loss in a relatively short period is rarely the result of dieting and exercise and should therefore be investigated.
- **Pleuritic chest pain?** Pleuritic chest pain can arise following a PE or pneumonia that has spread to the pleura.
- **Shortness of breath?** Try to quantify this in terms of exercise tolerance: How far can they walk before they get breathless? Can they climb a flight of stairs without getting breathless? Sudden-onset shortness of breath can be caused by PE, whereas a more gradual time course would be consistent with heart failure.
- Has he had **haematuria and/or oliguria?** There are a number of *rare* conditions that can affect both the lungs and kidneys (causing a 'pulmonary–renal syndrome'). The main causes of this are:
  - Goodpasture's syndrome, an autoimmune condition where autoantibodies attack the lungs and the glomeruli in the kidneys. This is important to identify early since the patient progresses rapidly to irreversible renal failure
  - Vasculitides, e.g. granulomatosis with polyangiitis (formerly Wegener's), microscopic polyangiitis, polyarteritis nodosa
  - Systemic lupus erythematosus.

Mr Morris has had a cough for years, but it is only productive when he is unwell. He has not been unwell recently, although he notes that he has unintentionally lost weight—he estimates a stone (about 6.5 kg) in the last 6 months. He has no pleuritic chest pain, but gets breathless after climbing just one flight of stairs at home. He attributes this to his age, and lack of exercise. He has had no urinary symptoms.

What features about Mr Morris' past history will help you narrow your differential diagnosis even further?

- **Smoking history?** Smoking is the most significant risk factor for lung cancer. Quantify how much he smokes or smoked using the average number of cigarettes smoked a day and the number of years smoked, i.e. when he started and, if relevant, quit. Someone who smoked 10 cigarettes a day for 30 years is said to have smoked for 15 pack years (10 cigarettes = 0.5 packs; and 0.5 × 30 years = 15 pack years).
- **Exposure to asbestos or other inhaled industrial substances?** For example silica (i.e. stonecutter's dust), coal, radon, arsenic, haloethers, polycyclic aromatic hydrocarbons. Such exposure is a risk factor for lung cancer and, in the case of asbestos, mesothelioma.

- **Prior lung disease?** This may indicate a chronic condition, such as TB or bronchiectasis, or a vulnerability to repeated infections (e.g. pneumonias) that you may wish to investigate further.

- **Did he grow up abroad or travel recently?** If yes, which country? Has he been vaccinated for TB? TB is endemic in many countries, particularly the Asian subcontinent and southern African states, and has reappeared in many eastern European countries since the collapse of the Soviet Union. Patients with TB can be relatively asymptomatic for extended periods of time.

- **Does he have risk factors for a deep vein thrombosis (DVT)/pulmonary embolus (PE)?** These include prolonged stasis (bed rest or long-haul flight), blood vessel damage from recent trauma or surgery, malignancy causing hypercoagulable blood, other clotting abnormalities, or a history of previous venous thromboembolism. Also ask about a painful swollen limb, particularly leg, which could be a DVT leading to a PE.

- **Is he on anticoagulant medications or does he have a known bleeding diathesis?** These can increase the risk and/or magnitude of internal haemorrhage.

Mr Morris is a smoker with a 50-pack-year history, having started when he did his national service in the navy and was given cigarettes each week as part of his rations (a common story in his generation). As a retired electrician, he has almost certainly had some exposure to asbestos, but denies ever having worked too closely with it as he was primarily concerned with residential housing. He has no history of lung disease. He has not travelled beyond the UK 'for many years' and has not been immunized against TB. He has no risk factors for a DVT/PE other than his smoking history. He is not taking aspirin or warfarin.

The GP conducts a full physical examination, beginning by simply inspecting Mr Morris. The GP then examines his hands, head, neck, and chest. The examination is completed by checking his abdomen and his neurological status. Think of how the diseases mentioned in your differential might manifest during the examination:

What signs should the GP particularly look out for on examination of this man?

- General inspection from the end of the couch:
  - **Hoarse voice**: ?invasion of recurrent laryngeal nerve by cancer
  - **Cachexia**
  - **Purpuric rash** or **petechiae**: ?vasculitis affecting lungs
- Hands:
  - **Clubbing**: ?lung cancer, lung abscesses, bronchiectasis
  - **Tar stains**: ?smoker
  - **Wasting of the dorsal interossei**: ?invasion of T1 nerve root by apical lung cancer (Pancoast tumour)
- Arms:
  - **Hypotonic, hyporeflexive, weak arms**: ?hypercalcaemia due to bone metastases from lung cancer
- Face:
  - **Swollen face**: ?obstruction of superior vena cava by tumour
  - **Bleeding from oral or nasal mucosa**: ?source of blood, i.e. not true haemoptysis
  - **Saddle nose**: ?granulomatosis with polyangiitis (Wegener's)
  - **Horner's syndrome** (miosis, ptosis, and anhydrosis, i.e. ispilateral constricted pupil, droopy eyelid, and lack of facial sweating): ?invasion of the sympathetic supply to the face by apical lung cancer

- - **Jaundice**: ?liver cancer which has spread to the lungs or vice versa
  - **Focal neurology**: ?brain metastases from lung cancer
- Neck:
  - **Cervical lymphadenopathy, non-tender**: ?TB, bronchial carcinoma
  - **Left supraclavicular lymphadenopathy (Virchow's node)**: ?GI malignancy which may have metastasized to the lungs
  - **Tracheal deviation**: ?pleural effusion due to cancer?lung collapse secondary to a large mass such as a tumour or abscess
- Chest:
  - **Asymmetrical lung expansion**: ?lung pathology in side of reduced expansion
  - **Dullness to percussion**: ?pneumonia, lung abscess, malignant pleural effusion
  - **Stridor**: ?tumour or foreign body obstructing bronchus
  - **Crackles**: ?pneumonia, left ventricular failure, bronchiectasis
  - **Pleural rub**: ?mesothelioma, pleuritis from pneumonia
- Abdomen:
  - **Hepatomegaly**: ?liver malignancy which can spread to the lungs, and vice versa
- Legs:
  - **Unilateral signs of DVT**: A DVT may have caused a PE. Look for a unilaterally inflamed leg, unilateral pitting oedema, tenderness over the deep veins or distended, non-varicose superficial veins.

Mr Morris's pulse is 78 bpm, his blood pressure is 132/66 mmHg, his respiratory rate is 14/min and his temperature is 36.5 °C.

The positive findings on examination of Mr Morris include tar stains on his hands and a palpable liver edge 2 cm below the ribs. There were no abnormal findings on examination of Mr Morris' respiratory system.

Mr Morris is referred to the respiratory clinic as an outpatient. He is referred urgently because of his haemoptysis, weight loss, and hepatomegaly. You are the registrar at this clinic and you confirm the history and examination findings obtained by the GP.

Which investigations should you request and why?

- **Oxygen saturations**, which form part of the vital observations and help you to understand the severity of the underlying pulmonary disease.
- **Blood tests:**
  - **Full blood count (FBC)** looking for anaemia, which reflects the magnitude and duration of bleeding or which may be a manifestation of an underlying malignancy. You are also looking for a raised white cell count indicating an infectious or inflammatory process.
  - **C-reactive protein (CRP)** which will be raised in infection, inflammation, and some cases of malignancy.
  - **Clotting screen**, for a bleeding disorder which may be exacerbating if not directly causing the haemoptysis.
  - **Urea and electrolytes (U&Es)** for renal involvement, as in Goodpasture's syndrome or granulomatosis with polyangiitis (Wegener's), which can affect the kidney and the lung.
  - **Calcium, phosphate, and alkaline phosphatase (ALP)** for bone metastasis from a primary lung cancer.
  - **Liver enzymes** for liver involvement of a cancer.

- **Urine test:** urinalysis looking for haematuria, suggesting pulmonary–renal syndrome.
- **Imaging:** chest radiograph

Note: if TB is suspected, strenuous efforts should be made to obtain specimens or tissue from which to culture the organism (particularly given the growing prevalence of resistant strains). The skin sensitivity tests (Heaf, Mantoux) and newer T-cell based assays (e.g. Quantiferon, ELIspot) are only useful to determine latent TB infection and tell you nothing about disease activity. As many people are infected but not diseased, these tests are of little diagnostic value. They are used in contact tracing to see if somebody who has been exposed to open TB has become infected at some stage, but don't tell you whether they have successfully got rid of the infection or are still actively diseased.

What signs would you be looking for on chest radiograph?

- **Mass lesion/nodule(s):** carcinoma, TB, abscess, vasculitides, e.g. granulomatosis with polyangiitis (Wegener's)
- **Diffuse alveolar infiltrates:** pulmonary oedema
- **Hilar lymphadenopathy:** carcinoma, infection (if accompanying infiltrates), TB
- **Lobar or segmental infiltrates:** pneumonia, infarction due to PE, TB, adenocarcinoma causing malignant consolidation (if the tumour is in the airway)
- **Patchy alveolar infiltrates:** bleeding disorders, Goodpasture's syndrome, idiopathic pulmonary haemosiderosis
- **Lobar collapse:** obstructing carcinoma

Mr Morris' oxygen saturations are 95% on room air. His bloods include:

Haematology		Biochemistry	
Hb	145 g/L	Urea	5.8 mM
WCC	4.6 × 10⁹ cells/L	Creatinine	68 µM
		Ca (corrected)	2.54 mM
		CRP	<2 mg/L

Urinalysis is unremarkable.

In light of his history and examination, CT pulmonary angiogram (CTPA) and a skin test for TB are not requested. His chest radiograph is shown in Figure 8.1.

What is the most likely diagnosis? What should your next step be?

Figure 8.1 Chest radiograph for Mr Morris.

The chest radiograph shows a mass lesion, sometimes called a 'coin lesion', in the patient's left hilum. This, in combination with his history (smoker, haemoptysis, and weight loss) and examination (hepatomegaly), is strongly suggestive of **lung cancer** (although there is a broader differential diagnosis for a coin lesion; see the Viva questions).

You need to confirm and classify the diagnosis with **cytology of sputum and bronchoscopic washings**, and ideally a tissue biopsy. This may be obtained either via **CT-guided percutaneous fine needle biopsy** (if it is peripheral) or on **bronchoscopy** (if it is more central, either endobronchial or transbronchial biopsy depending on whether it protrudes into the airway lumen). The reason is that cancer is ultimately a pathological diagnosis: clinical features can make you strongly suspect malignancy, but only a pathological sample will confirm it.

You also need to **stage** the cancer with a **CT scan**, looking for local spread and lymph node involvement, and a **bone scan**, looking for bone metastases.

What features make the other diagnoses listed at the start less likely?

- TB
  - No history of chronic productive cough, fevers, or night sweats. However, he has unintentionally lost weight. He has not travelled abroad for years (although he may have latent TB that has become active).
  - On examination, he is apyrexic. There is no evidence of consolidation or a pleural effusion.
  - White cell count and CRP within the normal range.
  - No features on chest radiography suggesting TB (e.g. apical cavity or calcified nodule).
- Pneumonia
  - No history of fever or cough productive of sputum. No pleuritic chest pain. Does not account for weight loss.

- On examination, resonant percussion note and clear lung fields (no crackles), no tachycardia or tachypnoea, plus good saturations on room air.
- White cell count and CRP within the normal range.

- Bronchiectasis
  - No history of chronic cough productive of sputum, as in classic bronchiectasis, although this does not exclude bronchiectasis. No wheeze and no dyspnoea at rest although, as mentioned, his exercise tolerance is poor. No history of recurrent respiratory illness. Not typically associated with weight loss.
  - On examination, no clubbing, no crackles or wheeze.

- PE
  - No history of sudden-onset pleuritic chest pain or breathlessness, although his exercise tolerance is poor. The only risk factor is smoking; he has not had a swollen limb recently, been immobile for a prolonged period, had trauma or surgery recently, has no previous history of venous thromboembolism or any clotting disorder and, although we didn't ask, is almost certainly not on the contraceptive pill or hormone replacement therapy! He may have a malignancy based on his chest radiograph (and thus a risk factor for PE) but this has not been confirmed yet.
  - Examination findings no tachycardia, the commonest finding in PE, confirmed by a normal electrocardiogram (ECG). While not 100% sensitive for PE, this is consistent with an alternative diagnosis for the haemoptysis.

If the chest radiograph had not shown anything, what further investigations might you have considered?

If risk factors for cancer are present, e.g. male, over 40 years of age, significant smoking history, you may wish to consider a **CT scan**. If this is still inconclusive, you may also consider further tests including PET and fibreoptic bronchoscopy.

How should Mr Morris be managed, both acutely and in the longer term?

As always, you should check his need for resuscitation (**airway, breathing, circulation, ABC**). From the examination we know that he is in a stable condition. Were his haemoptysis more serious, the priority would be stopping the haemorrhage (e.g. with the help of an interventional radiologist identifying and embolizing the bleeding point).

In the longer term, having had his diagnosis confirmed and his tumour staged, on an outpatient basis, Mr Morris should be referred to the multidisciplinary team (MDT) for management. Management will depend on the results from histology (grade), the stage (spread) of the tumour and the patient's wishes as discussed in the Viva questions.

Short cases

Mr Johnson is a 55-year-old engineer who presents to the Emergency Department with haemoptysis. He has coughed up a teaspoonful of blood, which was a dark red colour, on each of the last 3 days. He has not had fever, weight loss, or breathlessness. However, he has had some chest pain on deep inspiration over the last day, which is not reproduced by pressing on his ribs. He does not recall any trauma to his ribs. He has never smoked, has had no exposure to industrial antigens, or previous lung disease. He grew up in Scotland and has never been outside Europe. He recalls having a sore, swollen calf a few days ago but it resolved on its own so he did not go to the GP. His only risk factor for venous thromboembolism is stasis on the long bus journeys he is making every week back home to Scotland.

On examination, his pulse is 94 bpm and regular, his blood pressure 122/64 mmHg, his respiratory rate 12/min and his temperature 35.9 °C. His oxygen saturations are 94% on room air. There are no signs of cyanosis or stigmata of respiratory disease. His calves are soft and non-tender. His bloods show:

Haematology		Biochemistry	
Hb	152 g/L	Urea	6.1 mM
WCC	5.2×10^9 cells/L	Creatinine	58 µM
		Corr Ca	2.45 mM
		CRP	<2 mg/L

Urinalysis is normal and an ECG confirms a sinus tachycardia with no other abnormalities.

In light of these results, what diagnoses would you like to exclude? Is there a clinical algorithm or scoring system that would help?

Mr Johnson's history and examination do not clearly point to any diagnosis, but the long bus journeys may have predisposed to a DVT (which would explain the swollen calf) and the chest pain and tachycardia suggest a PE, which you should try to exclude.

When you suspect PE based on the history (the clinical examination will rarely show anything more than a tachycardia and/or mild fever), you should refer to the **Wells criteria** to determine, based on your clinical findings, the best investigation. The criteria are listed in Table 8.1, with their scores. A score of ≥4 merits a CTPA (or perfusion scan) to investigate further; a score of <4 only justifies a D-dimer test to *exclude* a PE. The reason for this approach is that patients with a Wells score ≥4 have a ~30% risk of PE but a negative D-dimer is not 100% specific at ruling out a PE, so if the risk of PE is very high, one needs to use a better test than a negative D-dimer to rule out a PE.

It is worth noting that the Wells criteria have been criticized because one of the weightier elements is subjective: whether PE is the most likely diagnosis. This can be the difference between low and moderate risk. An alternative clinical prediction tool has been recently developed, the revised Geneva score (2006), which does not rely on the clinician's judgement, although NICE continues to advocate the use of the Wells score.

Table 8.1 The Wells criteria for PE

Criteria	Points
Clinical signs and symptoms of DVT	3
PE is the most likely diagnosis	3
Heart rate >100 bpm	1.5
Immobilization >3 days or surgery in the last 4 weeks	1.5
Previously diagnosed DVT or PE	1.5
Haemoptysis	1
Malignancy diagnosed in the last 6 months	1

From *Annals of Internal Medicine*, Wells PS et al., 'Use of a Clinical Model for Safe Management of Patients with Suspected Pulmonary Embolism', **129**, 12, pp. 997-1005. Copyright © 1998 American College of Physicians. All Rights Reserved. Reprinted with the permission of American College of Physicians, Inc.

Mr Johnson has a Wells score of 4 (symptoms of a DVT and haemoptysis). Following NICE guidelines, a D-dimer was not performed and the patient proceeded directly to CTPA which confirmed a PE. He was prescribed a prolonged course of anticoagulants and discharged.

SHORT CASE

Miss Gautam is a 19-year-old woman who presents with haemoptysis. She tells you she suffered from a lot of chest infections when she was growing up in Bangladesh. However, she has come to you because in the last week her sputum has become stained with bright red blood. There has been no more than an egg-cupful of blood at most. She has not had coryzal symptoms or felt feverish, but has felt 'not 100%' and had night sweats. She has also lost around a stone [about 6.5 kg] in weight in the last 6 months, although she says she has been dieting and exercising. She denies any chest pain or shortness of breath.

She is a non-smoker, has no history of exposure to industrial agents, or diagnosed lung disease. She grew up in Bangladesh until the age of 16, when she moved to the UK with her family. She has not received the BCG vaccine. She is on the combined oral contraceptive pill but is taking no other medications, and has no other risk factors for venous thromboembolism.

On examination, she has a temperature of 37.2 °C, a pulse of 102 bpm, blood pressure of 109/66 mmHg, respiratory rate of 12/min, and oxygen saturations of 96% on room air. There are no peripheral stigmata of respiratory disease. Her chest expansion is slightly reduced on the right hemithorax, and percussion over the right lower hemithorax is dull. Auscultation of the right upper lung field reveals reduced breath sounds, some crackles, and increased vocal resonance.

Her bloods come back:

Haematology		Biochemistry	
Hb	103 g/L	Urea	5.6 mM
WCC	7.2 × 10⁹ cells/L	Creatinine	47 μM
		Ca (corrected)	2.38 mM
		CRP	11 mg/L

Urinalysis is normal and an ECG confirms a sinus tachycardia.

You send off blood cultures and request a chest radiograph. While you are waiting for the results, your consultant asks you to present the case with your working differential diagnosis and management plan.

What is the diagnosis you are most concerned about? Given this, what specific actions should your management plan consider?

With her history of growing up in the Indian subcontinent and chronic cough (in the absence of smoking), haemoptysis, night sweats, and weight loss, you should be most concerned about **pulmonary TB**, although pneumonia is also a possibility. The suspicion of TB is reinforced by examination and investigation findings consistent with an infection (tachycardia, raised white cell count, and CRP) and consolidation (reduced expansion, dullness to percussion, reduced breath sounds, crackles, increased vocal resonance). The mild anaemia suggests a chronic disease process. This is likely a reactivation of the TB or post-primary infection. Reactivation of TB typically (although not always) affects the upper lobes because *Mycobacterium tuberculosis* is a highly aerobic bacterium and the apices are the most oxygenated part of the lungs.

In addition to reviewing her need for resuscitation (ABC), you need to:

1 Ensure that microbiology know to look for acid-fast bacilli (i.e. using a Ziehl–Nielson or silver stain). Bear in mind that *M. tuberculosis* is a very slow-growing bacterium and it can therefore take many weeks before a positive result is obtained on culture (this is changing with the increasing use of molecular diagnostics).

2 TB is a notifiable disease so you must notify the authorities for contact tracing. They may screen contacts for latent and active TB, and treat as appropriate.

3 Place the patient in isolation to prevent further spread.

4 Test her for HIV, as although she most likely acquired TB during her childhood she may have acquired it more recently secondary to HIV infection which has implications for prognosis and management.

5 Look for signs of spread to other organs. Check particularly for meningeal irritation, bone or joint pain particularly in weight-bearing joints (e.g. Pott's fracture in the spinal column), dysuria or pelvic pain (genitourinary infection), or abdominal pain.

6 If the diagnosis is confirmed, refer the patient to the TB service, which offers specialized care for such patients.

First-line treatment for TB will depend on the likelihood of a drug-resistant strain and the longer-term results of culture and sensitivities. However, the initial approach (as per the NICE guidelines on TB) is with a long-term regimen of four antibiotics: rifampicin and isoniazid for the first 4 months, pyrazinamide and ethambutol for the first 2 months. It is prudent to warn all patients starting rifampicin treatment that their urine will turn a rich orange colour. In addition, all women of childbearing age should be warned that rifampicin can render the oral contraceptive pill less effective and thus other means of contraception should be considered.

Note that long treatment leads to poor compliance. This is a problem that is leading to multidrug-resistant TB, and explains why in some jurisdictions (e.g. New York City, USA) social workers may come to check that patients are taking their medications.

SHORT CASE

Mr Frick is a 28-year-old man who is attending the respiratory clinic at his hospital. He has recently had several episodes of haemoptysis. He is well known to the respiratory physicians, who have managed him since he was a child. He has chronic rhinitis and has suffered for most of his life from a rattly cough which is frequently productive of green sputum. He suffered from many episodes of serous otitis media as a child. He still suffers from frequent episodes of sinusitis and has recently been referred to a fertility clinic by his GP because he and his wife have not been able to conceive a child after 18 months of trying. A recent chest CT showed dilated bronchi with thick walls extending to the peripheries of both lungs (see Figure 8.2).

What diagnosis could explain the constellation of symptoms that Mr Frick has suffered during his life? How would you confirm such a diagnosis? How do you think Mr Frick is being managed?

Mr Frick has a history of recurrent cough productive of green sputum and occasional haemoptysis that is highly suggestive of **bronchiectasis** (*bronchos* = airway; *ektasis* = stretched out). His chest CT (see Figure 8.2) does indeed reveal dilated bronchi. In bronchiectasis, the bronchi are chronically inflamed as the lungs struggle to clear irritant mucus for any of a variety of reasons, e.g. obstruction, thickened mucus, poor ciliary function of the epithelia. The consequence of chronic inflammation is the laying down of scar tissue in the interstitial tissue. Remember that scars shrink, therefore the airway walls are pulled back and the airways expand. The mucus is often green due to the constant presence of neutrophils and macrophages fighting pathogens growing in the retained mucus. As neutrophils and macrophages die, they release an enzyme called myeloperoxidase which is green (and closely related

Figure 8.2 CT chest of Mr Frick. Note the dilated bronchi with thick walls (like a white 'O') with pulmonary artery branches next to them (white dot) forming what is known as the 'signet ring sign' that is typical for bronchiectasis.

to enzymes which give the spicy *wasabi* sauce favoured in Japanese cuisine its green colour). In addition, Mr Frick has suffered from many episodes of sinusitis and serous otitis media (glue ear), both of which suggest an inability to clear mucus.

The inability to clear mucus in various organs of the body is highly suggestive of **primary ciliary dyskinesia (PCD)**. This is an autosomal recessive disorder that affects the protein machinery used by epithelial cells to rhythmically beat their cilia and by spermatozoa to rhythmically beat their tails. The typical consequences of PCD are:

- Bronchiectasis, due to an inability to clear mucus from the lungs.

- Rhinitis and sinusitis, due to an inability to clear mucus from the nasal sinuses.

- Otitis media (both secretory and acutely infective) due to an inability to clear mucus from the middle ear, down the eustachian tube.

- Male infertility, due to sperm immotility. Females are usually fertile because passage of the oocyte along the fallopian tubes is more dependent on peristalsis of the fallopian tubes than on the movement of the cilia that line these tubes.

- Situs inversus. The rhythmical beating of cilia is thought to play an important part in setting up the usual pattern of body asymmetry during embryogenesis. Many patients with PCD have their organs on the 'other side' (e.g. dextrocardia).

Patients with PCD who show the clinical triad of bronchiectasis, sinusitis, and situs inversus may be said to have Kartagener's syndrome or Kartagener's triad.

Investigation of suspected PCD involves a biopsy of the nasal mucosa and examination under a microscope, looking for abnormal beating of the ciliated epithelia. Microscopy of spermatozoa of PCD males often reveals immobile spermatozoa.

Management of PCD involves:

- Regular physiotherapy, to help clear the lungs of mucus.

- Regular or prophylactic antibiotics, to prevent recurrent chest infections and sinusitis.

- Mucolytics, which can help clear mucus in the lungs and sinuses more easily in some patients.

It is worth knowing that patients with PCD tend to show an improvement of symptoms by their early thirties and that many patients lead near normal adult lives.

SHORT CASE

Miss Bonprat is a 31-year-old primary school teacher urgently referred to the respiratory clinic of her local hospital because of sudden haemoptysis. She describes feeling unwell and lethargic for the past few weeks and thinking she had 'caught something off the children'. She developed a cough that morning but was alarmed when she noticed she had coughed up some specks of blood onto her handkerchief. She smokes a pack of 'light cigarettes' every day and has not travelled abroad recently. Systems enquiry is unrevealing. Her past medical history is remarkable for hypothyroidism, for which she takes levothyroxine every day.

Examination of Miss Bonprat reveals only that her blood pressure is 160/110 mmHg and that her urinalysis is positive for protein (+) and blood (+++). A midstream urine sample is sent off to the laboratories, who later that day confirm the presence of red cell casts on urine microscopy.

What diagnosis should you be concerned about?

Miss Bonprat has presented with haemoptysis. She also has hypertension, haematuria, and proteinuria on urinalysis suggesting inflammation of her kidneys (glomerulonephritis) that is manifesting as a nephritic syndrome. The presence of red cell casts (clumps of red cells that have squeezed through damaged glomeruli) is indicative of glomerular damage. The combination of haemoptysis and glomerulonephritis should alert you to the possibility of a **pulmonary–renal syndrome**.

Viva questions

Name several causes of clubbing.

There are many of these and you should structure your answer somehow—for example, by physiological system:

- Cardiovascular
    - Infective endocarditis (subacute bacterial endocarditis)
    - Congenital cyanotic heart disease
    - Atrial myxoma
    - Axillary artery aneurysm
    - Brachial arteriovenous fistula
- Respiratory
    - Pulmonary fibrosis
    - Suppurative lung diseases: abscess, empyema, cystic fibrosis, bronchiectasis
    - Bronchial carcinoma, mesothelioma (although these patients do not always survive long enough to become clubbed)
    - TB
- Gastrointestinal
    - Inflammatory bowel disease
    - Cirrhosis
    - Malabsorption, e.g. coeliac disease
    - Gastric lymphoma
    - Liver abscess
    - Liver or bowel cancer
- Other
    - Congenital clubbing
    - Thyroid acropachy

In the context of a pleural effusion, what is the difference between a transudate and an exudate? What are the causes of each?

The fluid from a pleural effusion can be defined as a transudate or an exudate depending on the protein content.

- A transudate is defined as having <25 g/L of protein. Transudates are low in protein because they are the result of fluid alone squeezing into the pleural space, either due to increased hydrostatic pressure in the lung vasculature (heart failure, fluid overload, constrictive pericarditis) or due to reduction in the oncotic pressure which usually keeps fluid in the vasculature (reduced serum protein due to liver failure, malabsorption/malnutrition, nephrotic syndrome).
- An exudate is defined as having >35 g/L of protein. Exudates are rich in protein because they are the result of cells in the pleural space: either pathogens (infection), inflammatory cells, or malignant cells.

CONTINUED ➤

CONTINUED

- If the pleural fluid protein is between 25 and 35 g/L, Light's criteria should be used to differenti-ate exudates from transudates. These state that the fluid is an exudate if any of the following applies:
  - Pleural fluid protein divided by serum protein >0.5
  - Pleural fluid lactate dehydrogenase (LDH) divided by serum LDH >0.6
  - Pleural fluid LDH more than two-thirds the upper limit of normal serum LDH

How are lung neoplasms classified? How do they respond to treatment?

As for all neoplasms, lung neoplasms can at first be divided into benign (e.g. a hamartoma) and malig-nant (i.e. cancerous). Malignant tumours in turn can be classified as primary or secondary. Broadly speaking, the primary malignant lung cancers are then classified in two groups based on histology:

1 **Non-small cell lung cancer** (NSCLC, 80%)
   - Subdivided into **adenocarcinoma** (30-40%), **squamous** (20-30%), **large cell carcinoma** (10%), and others (5%)
   - If localized, attempt to remove surgically or treat with radiotherapy
   - Otherwise responds poorly to chemotherapy and has poor prognosis if disseminated

2 **Small cell lung cancer** (SCLC, 20%)
   - Responsive to chemotherapy, although rapid relapse is common. Chemotherapy is given mainly because it improves symptoms rather than mortality
   - Early metastasis therefore surgery is rarely the therapy of choice

Haemoptysis is more common in squamous cell carcinoma, which usually affects lung tissue closer to the hilar region and thus the blood has relatively little distance to travel before being coughed up.

Which cancers most commonly metastasize to the lungs?

Secondary lung cancers are most commonly the result of metastasis from the following primary cancers:

- Colorectal
- Breast
- Renal
- Female genital tract: cervix, ovary

Note that metastatic lung cancers rarely cause haemoptysis as they are spreading haematog-enously and therefore tend to be deep in the interstitium rather than endobronchial.

List extrapulmonary manifestations of lung cancer and how they might manifest in terms of signs and symptoms.

- Bone metastases causing bone pain.
- Hypertrophic pulmonary osteoarthropathy (HPOA)—dull, aching, swollen wrists/ankles. Rare.

CONTINUED ➤

CONTINUED

- Ectopic adrenocorticotropic hormone (ACTH) secretion, resulting in Cushingoid features, muscle weakness, oedema and skin hyperpigmentation.
- Hypercalcaemia secondary to bone metastases or PTH-related peptide (PTHrP)-secreting lung cancer. Can result in confusion, polyuria, polydipsia, hypotonia, hyporeflexia, and muscle weakness.
- Eaton–Lambert syndrome, a rare neuromuscular disorder most commonly seen in patients with small cell lung cancer. Characteristically there is proximal muscle weakness that improves on repetition (unlike myasthenia gravis).

What ectopic endocrine secretions are associated with which lung cancers? What symptoms do they cause?

Small cell lung carcinomas are derived from endocrine cells in the lung and therefore have the potential to synthesize and secrete hormones or hormone-like substances. The substances secreted by small cell lung cancers are **antidiuretic hormone (ADH)**, resulting in hyponatraemia, and **ACTH**, resulting in Cushing's syndrome.

  Squamous cell carcinomas may not have the cell machinery to produce cholesterol-based steroids, but they can produce peptides including **PTHrP**. This causes hypercalcaemia.

What extrapulmonary sites does TB most commonly affect? What does it cause in each?

TB can affect virtually any organ. Some of the more common manifestations include:
- Lymph nodes (often cervical or mediastinal)
- Bone: osteomyelitis, septic arthritis, Pott's disease (in the spine)
- Neurological: meningitis, intracranial granulomas
- Renal: granuloma

  TB less commonly affects the heart, skeletal muscles, pancreas, thyroid, or adrenals (causing Addison's disease). Indeed, TB was found on autopsy in 70–90% of Dr Addison's patients in his original description of the eponymous syndrome (this figure is lower in larger, more recent studies).

Give a differential for a solitary coin lesion on a chest radiograph.

A coin lesion could be:
- Parenchymal tumour: benign, primary lung cancer, secondary lung cancer
- Lymph node: lymphoma
- Granuloma: TB, sarcoidosis
- Abscess
- Hamartoma
- Foreign object

What is the doctrine of double effect? How is this relevant to a lung cancer patient being treated with opiates for pain relief?

The doctrine of double effect applies when a treatment has two (or more) effects. The primary (intended) effect is to relieve the symptoms. But a secondary effect, which is foreseen but *not* intended, in some way hastens death. In legal terms, although the treatment is bringing about mortality, as its primary (intended) effect is beneficial it is viewed as distinct from euthanasia.

This applies directly to the lung cancer patient being treated with opiates. As well as providing analgesia, reducing the sensation of breathlessness and suppressing the cough reflex (and hence the likelihood of haemoptysis), opiates can cause respiratory depression if given in sufficiently large doses. However, the benefits are considered to outweigh the drawbacks, particularly given that the doses are usually insufficient to cause respiratory depression (making this a somewhat theoretical point). Thus, opiates are commonly used in terminally ill patients suffering with chronic pain.

Single Best Answers

1. **A patient presents with haemoptysis and haematuria. Bloods are taken for autoantibodies. The results include: pANCA positive, cANCA negative, ANA negative. What is the most likely diagnosis?**

   a. Goodpasture's syndrome
   b. Granulomatosis with polyangiitis (Wegener's)
   c. Systemic lupus erythematosus (SLE)
   d. Microscopic polyangitis (MPA)
   e. Polyarteritis nodosa (PAN)

2. **Which of the following industrial antigens does not cause pulmonary fibrosis?**

   a. Silicon
   b. Coal
   c. Asbestos
   d. Arsenic
   e. Radon

3. **A patient presents with haemoptysis on their return from Bangladesh. You suspect tuberculosis. Which of the following tests would be diagnostic of active tuberculosis disease?**

   a. Heaf test
   b. Mantoux test
   c. Interferon gamma-release assay (IGRA) e.g. Quantiferon, ELIspot
   d. Sputum or biopsy cultures
   e. All of the above

4. **Warfarin use results in an initial, paradoxical increase in clot formation. This is because depletion of which anticoagulant factor(s) occurs faster than that of the vitamin K-dependent clotting factors?**

   a. Protein C and S
   b. Antithrombin III
   c. Factors II, VII, IX and X
   d. Von Willebrand's factor
   e. Thrombomodulin

5. **Which of the following investigations can be used for grading lung cancer?**

   a. CT
   b. Bone scan
   c. Cytology (of sputum, bronchoscopic washings, or fine needle aspirate)
   d. a and b
   e. All of the above

Chest pain

Core case

 Read through the sections in the case boxes, covering up the sections that follow so that you don't see the answer. At the end of each case box, try to answer the question before reading on.

Mr Shepherd is a 67-year-old man who was referred to the Emergency Department by his GP after a 2-hour history of severe chest pain.

What are the most common causes of acute chest pain in an individual of this age?

A good way to come up with a list of causes is to visualize the anatomy of the affected area and think of what could go wrong. Thus, in chest pain, there may be pathology of the heart, aorta, lungs, pulmonary vessels, oesophagus, stomach, thoracic nerves, thoracic muscles, or ribs.

The main causes of acute chest pain in an individual aged over 60 include are listed in Figure 9.1.

Musculoskeletal inflammation†
Acute coronary syndrome
Pulmonary embolism (PE)
Stable angina
Pleurisy (secondary to infection)
Oesophagitis (secondary to gastro-oesophageal reflux disease or hiatus hernia)
Pneumothorax
Anxiety
Peptic ulcer disease or gastritis
Myopericarditis (including stress-induced (Takotsubo) cardiomyopathy)
Cholecystitis
Acute pancreatitis
Thoracic aortic dissection
Thoracic aortic aneurysm
Coronary vasospasm (e.g. secondary to cocaine)
Oesophageal spasm
Boerhaave's perforation of the oesophagus

Figure 9.1 Causes of acute chest pain in adults presenting to the Emergency Department.

† *Most commonly this will be a sprained muscle (e.g. due to coughing), but other causes include Coxsackie B infection (Bornholm's disease), idiopathic costochondritis (Tietze's syndrome), and Varicella zoster infection (causing neuropathic pain restricted to a dermatome(s)).*

> How would your differential change if the patient were a 20-year-old woman on the combined oral contraceptive pill?

A younger patient is less likely to be suffering from diseases of old age, such as:

- Acute coronary syndrome
- Stable angina
- Myopericarditis (usually post-infarction)
- Thoracic aortic dissection
- Thoracic aortic aneurysm

A younger female patient on the combined oral contraceptive pill is more likely to be suffering from:

- PE (the combined oral contraceptive pill is thrombogenic)
- Pneumothorax (especially if tall and thin)
- Cocaine-induced coronary spasm (still rare, but particularly unusual in older people).

> When a patient arrives with chest pain, you need to be thinking about the conditions that present with chest pain that are potentially fatal and require immediate management.
>
> **Which diagnoses fall into this category? What features are going to alert you to these conditions?**

The following diagnoses require immediate management and should be kept in mind:

- **Acute coronary syndrome** (unstable angina, or myocardial infarction (MI))
- **Aortic dissection**
- **Pneumothorax**
- **PE**
- **Boerhaave's perforation**

The key features of each are listed below.

1   **Features of acute coronary syndrome**
   - History of sudden-onset, central, crushing chest pain radiating to either/both arms, neck or jaw, usually lasting a few minutes to half an hour (longer if there is ongoing infarction). Have a higher index of suspicion in those with a previous history of angina on exertion or MI and/or cardiovascular risk factors (smoking, hypertension, hypercholesterolaemia, diabetes mellitus, family history).
   - Signs of hypercholesterolaemia: cholesterol deposits in small skin lumps on the back of the hand or bony prominences like elbows (xanthomata), in creamy spots around the eyelids (xanthelasma), or a creamy ring around the cornea (arcus). Note that arcus is a normal finding in older people.
   - Signs of peripheral (atherosclerotic) vascular disease: weak pulses, peripheral cyanosis, cool peripheries, atrophic skin, ulcers, bruits on auscultation of carotids.
   - Signs of brady- or tachyarrhythmia. An arrhythmia is relevant for two reasons. First, it may be the cause of the ischaemia as both brady- and tachyarrhythmias can cause a drop in cardiac output and subsequently reduced cardiac perfusion and ischaemia. Secondly, arrhythmias most commonly arise in or around scarred myocardium, both from old infarcts and sometimes following an acute infarct (e.g. heart block, ventricular tachycardia—although the latter would normally present with shock rather than chest pain). Thus the presence of an arrhythmia offers a clue as to what might be wrong with the patient.

2   **Features of aortic dissection**
  - History of sudden-onset tearing chest pain radiating to the back. The pain is classically most intense from the very onset.
  - Absent pulse in one arm (due to occlusion of the root of the brachiocephalic trunk or left subclavian artery by the dissection flap).
  - Hypertension (in about 50% of cases) or hypotension (in about 25% of cases).
  - A difference in blood pressure between arms >20 mmHg (about a third of cases).
  - New-onset aortic regurgitation (manifesting as e.g. an early diastolic murmur). This is caused by the new lumen tracking down to the aortic valve and making it incompetent.
  - Pleural effusion, usually on the left. This is due to irritation of the pleura by the dissecting aorta.
  - History of hypertension (most important risk factor); smoking and atherosclerosis (e.g. previous ischaemic heart disease or peripheral vascular disease) are also risk factors, as is a recent aortic valve replacement.

3   **Features of pneumothorax**
  - History of sudden-onset pleuritic chest pain with breathlessness—but beware, it may present as painless breathlessness.
  - A hyperinflated chest wall with impaired expansion. Normally the lack of air in the pleural space creates a vacuum that holds the lungs to the chest wall. If air gets into the pleural space, unopposed elastic recoil of the chest wall will cause it to pop out, while at the same time the lungs will shrivel up. (Note this is different from lung collapse, in which a bronchus is obstructed and the air trapped distally in that segment is gradually absorbed into the blood.)
  - Hyper-resonant percussion over the affected area.
  - Absent breath sounds over the affected area. The crumpled up area of lung will not have any air getting in or out.
  - Tracheal deviation. In **tension pneumothorax**, a flap of pleural membrane acts as a valve so that the pleural space gets increasingly inflated with air. It eventually starts to deviate the mediastinum, and can compress the heart leading to cardiopulmonary arrest. Therefore, a trachea that deviates away from a suspected pneumothorax is an emergency requiring urgent insertion of a large-bore cannula in the midclavicular line just above the third rib to allow the air trapped in the pleural space to escape.

4   **Features of PE** (due to **deep vein thrombosis (DVT)**):
  - History of sudden-onset shortness of breath (seen in 73% in the Prospective Investigation Of PE Diagnosis (PIOPED) study) and/or pleuritic chest pain (66%) and/or haemoptysis (13%) in someone with an inflamed limb and/or risk factors for blood clots (e.g. recent surgery, recent stasis, or hypercoagulable blood due to the oral contraceptive pill or malignancy).
  - Tachycardia: this is the most common finding on examination in patients with a PE.
  - Signs of hypoxia. In practice, most patients with a PE show no signs of hypoxia as you need a very large PE to become hypoxic. Some patients do desaturate on exertion but the majority show no changes in saturations or blood gases.
  - Note that this can be a difficult diagnosis as the frequency of the 'characteristic' symptoms and signs listed above is similar in those with and without a PE. Thus PE should be considered when there is no other explanation for the chest pain. You should refer to the Wells criteria (see Table 8.1) for diagnosis of PE if you suspect this.

5   **Features of Boerhaave's perforation**: note that this is very rare, but it is associated with a high mortality and hence is included.
  - History of sudden-onset severe chest pain immediately *following* an episode of vomiting. Shortness of breath and pleuritic pain may develop shortly afterwards due to subsequent pleurisy and effusion.

- Signs of a pleural effusion after some hours—dullness to percussion, absent breath sounds, decreased vocal resonance.
- Subcutaneous emphysema is present in a minority of cases.
- Abdominal rigidity, sweating, fever, tachycardia, and hypotension are often present as the illness progresses but are non-specific.

Bearing in mind all these possibilities, you take a history from Mr Shepherd. You find that he localizes the pain to his sternum. He says it came on 2 hours earlier in the afternoon as he was gardening and has been there since. He describes it as like 'wearing a shirt two sizes too small' and says it has not moved since it came on. The pain was not exacerbated by breathing, and was not position dependent. He does not have a cough but his pain improved minutes after he was given a glyceryl trinitrate (GTN) spray sublingually in the ambulance, going from 8/10 severity to 3/10 now.

He is a smoker with a 40-pack-year history, has hypertension that is managed with a calcium channel blocker, and hypercholesterolaemia for which he takes a statin. His father died of stroke in his seventies and his mother of 'old age' in her late eighties. He is not known to be diabetic.

On examination, Mr Shepherd appears relatively comfortable (after pain relief), with arcus but no other peripheral signs of cardiovascular disease. His pulse and blood pressure are taken in both arms and found to be equally regular, 84 bpm and 145/90 mmHg. His oxygen saturation is 98% on room air. Both heart sounds are audible with no added sounds and his chest wall is not tender on palpation. Carotid bruits can be heard bilaterally on auscultation. His lungs have normal resonance to percussion, good air entry, and no abnormal sounds on auscultation. His trachea is central. His limbs show no signs of inflammation and he is not febrile.

In light of Mr Shepherd's history, risk factors, and examination, a particular diagnosis for his chest pain appears increasingly likely.

What investigations would you like to request? Think particularly of how you can confirm your expected diagnosis and how you can rule out the 'must exclude' diagnoses listed above.

Electrocardiogram (ECG)

Perform ECGs on anyone with suspected cardiac disease, either two ECGs 30 minutes apart or, if the patient has continuing chest pain, every 10–15 minutes until the diagnosis is made. If the patient is admitted, ECGs should be performed daily for 3 days thereafter, as changes may take 24 hours or more to develop. In the context of chest pain, you are particularly looking for signs of ischaemia and arrhythmias. If you suspect PE, you should also look for signs of right heart strain, although tachycardia is the most common ECG finding in PE. Any guide to reading ECGs will explain these signs. Note that it is particularly important to look for signs of ST segment elevation or new-onset left bundle branch block (LBBB), as the management protocol for individuals with an ST elevation myocardial infarction (STEMI) differs from that for suspected non-ST elevation myocardial infarction (NSTEMI).

Blood tests

- **Troponin:** this should be measured on admission and at 3 to 12 hours (depending on the local test and protocol used) from the onset of pain or the time when the pain was worst. Troponin levels are extremely useful because of their high sensitivity and specificity for damage to cardiac muscle. The drawback is the minimum 3-hour delay in increased troponin levels. An alternative is **CK-MB**, an isotype of the enzyme creatinine kinase, which is released more rapidly following damage but which is less specific for cardiac damage. CK-MB levels fall back to normal within 2–3 days whereas troponin levels remain high for >7 days. Thus, CK-MB levels that are elevated >4 days after an MI suggest that there has been a reinfarction. *Note: troponin levels are specific for cardiac damage but not 100% specific for acute coronary syndrome—you need to consider the context. Other conditions causing a raised troponin include: coronary artery spasm (e.g. from cocaine), aortic dissection causing ischaemia, myopericarditis, hypertrophic cardiomyopathy, severe heart failure, cardiac trauma from surgery or road traffic accident, and PE. Also, remember that troponins are renally excreted so a raised troponin in someone with renal failure should be taken with caution and may need repeating to look at its trend: a rapidly rising trend over time would support acute cardiac damage.*

- **Serum cholesterol:** hypercholesterolaemia is another risk factor for cardiovascular disease that is often undiagnosed and that can be treated. It is worth noting that an MI will result in a decrease in total cholesterol, low-density lipoprotein (LDL), and high-density lipoprotein (HDL) within about 24 hours of the infarct, and that levels will not return to normal (for that patient) for 2–3 months post-infarct. Thus, cholesterol levels should be measured as soon as possible if they are to guide future therapy.

- **Full blood count (FBC):** anaemia from any cause is common and will exacerbate any deficiency in cardiac perfusion, resulting in ischaemic heart disease.

- **Urea and electrolytes (U&Es):** pay particular attention to the potassium, as this may be the cause of an arrhythmia.

- **Inflammatory markers:** The white cell count (WCC) from the FBC and a C-reactive protein level are both measures of inflammation. Accordingly these are elevated in inflammatory processes such as pericarditis and Bornholm's disease (inflammation of intercostal muscles due to Coxsackie B virus infection), but will also be elevated following aortic dissection and MI, which cause inflammation of the affected tissues.

- **Capillary glucose:** there is a significant increase in the risk of cardiovascular disease with diabetes mellitus, particularly if untreated. Type 2 diabetics typically suffer from the complications of diabetes prior to becoming symptomatic for the diabetes itself, and as many as 50% may be undiagnosed. Critically, diabetics are more likely to present with 'silent infarcts'—that is, an MI in the absence of chest pain.

- **Amylase:** It is not uncommon for patients with acute pancreatitis to present with severe, central chest pain and nil epigastric tenderness, so consider measuring an amylase level in patients with risk factors for pancreatitis (alcohol consumption, known gallstones or risk factors for gallstones) or severe chest pain that cannot be explained. Some hospitals will use serum lipase in preference to amylase.

Imaging

Erect chest radiograph: this should be done to help exclude a pneumothorax and aortic pathology (aneurysm or dissection, giving a wide mediastinum). Note that it is possible to have a normal chest radiograph in aortic dissection. If Boerhaave's perforation of the oesophagus is suspected, a chest radiograph will typically show air around the heart shadow (pneumomediastinum), a pleural effusion, and/or a pneumothorax.

Second line

D-dimer levels: elevated D-dimers are simply symptomatic of breakdown of a fibrin clot due to any cause such as recent surgery or trauma, and are therefore *not* diagnostic of DVT or PE specifically.

However, low D-dimer levels can help *rule out* a DVT or PE as these are unlikely to occur without any fibrin breaking down (although a small proportion with PEs will have a false negative result; about ~2% of negative D-dimer results). D-dimers are not done as standard in chest pain but to exclude PE in patients with suspected PE and a Wells score <4. A negative D-dimer combined with a Wells score <4 has a 92% sensitivity at excluding PE.

Mr Shepherd's ECG is shown in Figure 9.2. Comment on any abnormalities.

Figure 9.2 Mr Shepherd's electrocardiogram (ECG).

Mr Shepherd's ECG shows ST depression and prominent R waves in V_1–V_3 but no signs of ST elevation.

He begins to complain of pain once the analgesia wears off. His troponin is 6 ng/mL on admission, (normal range given by the lab <0.4 ng/mL). His chest radiograph is normal.

In light of the history, examination, and investigations, what is the diagnosis? How else might this condition present?

Mr Shepherd is a 40-pack-year smoker with hypertension and hypercholesterolaemia who has presented with central crushing chest pain. This picture is typical for **MI**. He has elevation of cardiac troponin levels, suggesting MI.

His ECG shows ST depression in leads V_1–V_3 which would be consistent with an **anterior NSTEMI**. Remember that transmural infarctions normally result in ST elevation on an ECG and are hence referred to as STEMIs. However, in the case of posterior wall transmural infarctions, the fact that the ECG chest leads are on the opposite side of the chest wall results in ST depression in leads V_1–V_3 rather than ST elevation. Thus, this could also represent a **posterior infarct**, which is treated like a STEMI despite the lack of ST elevation.

MIs present in many different ways and you should have a low threshold for suspecting it in anyone with cardiac risk factors. Ultimately, diagnosis depends on an elevated troponin or rapidly raising troponin trend. Chest pain is not always a feature, particularly in elderly people and long-standing diabetics who frequently have neuropathy and dulled pain sensation. ECG readings are also non-diagnostic, as changes may not be present in infarction.

> **What features of the history, clinical examination, and investigations helped you rule out your other 'must exclude' diagnoses?**

- **Aortic dissection?** Mr Shepherd's pain was not tearing and did not radiate to his back. His pulse and blood pressure were equal in both arms and chest radiography did not suggest a wide mediastinum. Ultimately, the way to rule out aortic dissection if you strongly suspect it is to do CT angiography of the chest or transoesophageal echo, looking for a false lumen.

- **Pneumothorax?** Mr Shepherd did not have areas of the chest that were expanded and hyper-resonant, with decreased air entry. His trachea was not displaced and his chest radiograph is normal.

- **PE?** This was never suspected clinically. The ST depression on ECG, and the large rise in troponin provide a valid alternative diagnosis of the chest pain (NSTEMI). A D-dimer level was not requested but may in any case have been raised as a result of his infarction.

- **Boerhaave's perforation of the oesophagus?** Mr Shepherd did not give a history of vomiting before the onset of his pain. A perforated oesophagus is a very rare diagnosis and even less likely without previous vomiting. Ultimately, the way to rule it out if you strongly suspect it is to perform a chest radiograph after swallowing a water-soluble contrast agent such as Gastrografin.

> **How will the medical team manage Mr Shepherd acutely? How does the management differ between full-thickness infarcts (STEMI and posterior infarcts) and partial-thickness infarcts (NSTEMI)?**

Having assessed the need for resuscitation (airway, breathing, and circulation, ABC), you should consider Mr Shepherd's immediate management. Given that your differential includes life-threatening conditions, treatment should be started in tandem with your diagnostic screen. The longer-term management should consider secondary prevention of further cardiovascular events.

Acutely, all patients with any acute coronary syndrome (STEMI, posterior infarcts, NSTEMI, unstable angina) are started on a cocktail of drugs that can be remembered by the mnemonic MONABASH:

> Morphine, for analgesia, and an antiemetic such as **m**etoclopramide (although there is some evidence that for patients with no gastrointestinal (GI) disturbance there is no benefit in giving an antiemetic)
>
> Oxygen—but **only** if required in order to keep saturations at 94% as there is increasing evidence that hyperoxaemia can worsen outcomes in acute myocardial infarctions and strokes
>
> Nitrates (e.g. GTN, isosorbide mononitrate infusion), for vasodilation
>
> Antiplatelets: aspirin plus other agents such as ADP receptor blockers (clopidogrel, prasugrel, ticagrelor)
>
> Beta-blockers, to reduce myocardial oxygen demand. These are contraindicated if the patient is in heart block, has asthma, or has any signs of acute heart failure

ACE inhibitors, for multiple reasons including attenuation of post-infarct ventricular remodelling that can cause arrhythmias, reduction of angiotensin II-induced vasoconstriction improving cardiac blood flow and reducing after-load, and beneficial effects on endothelial function

Statins, which in addition to reducing cholesterol levels are thought to improve endothelial function, modulate inflammatory responses (e.g. reduce CRP), maintain atherosclerotic plaque stability, and prevent thrombus formation; there is evidence to support their use in the acute setting

Heparin (low molecular weight heparin, LMWH), or similar mechanism drugs such as fondaparinux, to prevent coronary thrombosis

STEMI patients (including posterior infarcts) should also receive either **primary angioplasty** or **thrombolysis** within 12 hours of the onset of pain, the sooner the better, and ideally within 1 hour of the onset of symptoms. Angioplasty is superior to thrombolysis if both are equally available, but rapid treatment is even more important so you should not delay thrombolysis if angioplasty is not likely to be achieved within 1 hour of the onset of the symptoms (e.g. patients in a remote location). Thrombolysis carries significant risks and therefore there are clear indications and contraindications with which you should familiarize yourself before referring a patient for thrombolysis. Realistically, in the UK, paramedics suspecting a STEMI (based on an ECG) will take the patient directly to the nearest primary angioplasty centre. Occasionally such patients will present directly to the Emergency Department; if the hospital in question does not offer primary angioplasty, the Emergency Department doctors should arrange urgent transfer to the nearest tertiary centre.

NSTEMI patients do not receive thrombolysis, as this does not appear to be effective in them. However, NSTEMI patients are candidates for immediate angioplasty if they are haemodynamically unstable, have severe left ventricular dysfunction, ongoing chest pain despite maximal medical management, new mitral regurgitation or ventricular septal defect, or sustained ventricular arrhythmias. The remaining NSTEMI patients should be risk stratified, and those at high risk should have early angioplasty (same admission, usually within 72 hours). The GRACE score provides a schema for stratifying such patients (see Table 9.1). There are numerous online calculators and smartphone apps that will calculate the score for you and with it the in-hospital mortality. Local protocols may set a threshold score above which patients should be admitted and/or reviewed by cardiology.

> Mr Shepherd's consultant decided that the prominent R waves on the ECG were more likely to represent a posterior infarct than an anterior NSTEMI. A right-sided ECG confirmed this and Mr Shepherd received primary angioplasty.
>
> **What advice and medications should Mr Shepherd be discharged on?**

Secondary prevention is important in patients with ischaemic heart disease. Mr Shepherd should be given the following advice and medication (lifelong):

- **Lifestyle changes:** smoking cessation, low-salt diet, exercise, and weight loss. All patients should additionally be offered a cardiac rehabilitation programme with an exercise component, as meta-analyses have shown these reduce mortality.

- **Risk factor control with medications**
  - Blood pressure control: ACE inhibitors if the patient is <55 years and white, calcium channel blockers (CCB) or thiazide diuretics if the patient is >55 years or non-white. A mixture of these three classes of drug may be prescribed if the blood pressure cannot be controlled with one drug alone.
  - Cholesterol reduction: statins, or fibrates if statins are not tolerated.

Table 9.1 **GRACE score**

Variable	Value	Score
Age	≤30	+0
	30–39	+8
	40–49	+25
	50–59	+41
	60–69	+58
	70–79	+75
	80–89	+91
	≥90	+100
Heart rate	90–109	+5
	110–149	+24
	150–199	+38
	≥200	+46
Systolic BP (mmHg)	120–139	+34
	140–159	+24
	160–199	+10
	≥200	+0
Creatinine (μmol/litre)	106.1–141.3	+10
	141.4–176.7	+13
	176.8–353.7	+21
	>353.8	+28
Congestive heart failure	Killip class	
	I	+0
	II	+20
	III	+39
	IV	+59
Cardiac arrest at admission		+39
ST segment deviation		+28
Elevated cardiac enzymes		+14

Reproduced by permission of the GRACE Coordinating Center, Center for Outcomes Research, University of Massachusetts Medical School.

- Diabetic control: tight glucose control is important for cardiovascular risk, although far less important than blood pressure control in diabetics as shown by the United Kingdom Prospective Diabetes Study (UKPDS) trial.
- **Reduced thromboembolic risk:** low-dose aspirin for life and an ADP receptor inhibitor (e.g. clopidogrel, ticagrelor) for a period of 1 year.

- **Secondary prevention:** studies have shown that **ACE inhibitors** (or angiotensin receptor blockers (ARBs) where ACE inhibitors are not tolerated) reduce mortality post-MI. They should be up-titrated to the maximum tolerated dose for the full benefit in terms of secondary prevention and continued indefinitely. There is also some evidence that β-**blockers** reduce mortality post-MI, although this is less clear cut. Thus β-blockers should be given for 12 months post-MI if there is no left ventricular dysfunction, or indefinitely otherwise. If there is severe left ventricular dysfunction, i.e. an ejection fraction <35% on echocardiogram, there is evidence of a mortality benefit from **aldosterone antagonists** (spironolactone, eplerenone).

If there is evidence of severe left ventricular dysfunction (ejection fraction <35%) and a conduction block on ECG (broad QRS complex >120 ms), then the patient is at an increased risk of ventricular arrhythmia and death and is therefore a candidate for an implantable cardioversion device (ICD). These detect the onset of ventricular arrhythmias and shock the heart to stop the arrhythmia.

Short cases

Mr Shepherd undergoes angioplasty to an occluded circumflex artery and is discharged. Four weeks later he presents again with chest pain. However, he says it is different from his previous pain. This time it radiates to his left shoulder, is worse on deep inspiration, and is aggravated by lying down. You note that he has a fever.

What are the complications of an MI, and what has probably happened to Mr Shepherd? How should Mr Shepherd be managed on this admission?

The common complications of MI are covered in the mnemonic DARTH VADER:

Death

Arrhythmia

Rupture (either of the septum or the outer walls)

Tamponade

Heart failure

Valve disease

Aneurysm

Dressler's syndrome (autoimmune pericarditis 2–10 weeks after MI; note that simple post-MI pericarditis is more common than Dressler's syndrome, presenting within 2–4 days)

Embolism

Reinfarction

Given the timing, fever, and pleuritic and positional aspects of the pain, Mr Shepherd has most likely presented with **Dressler's syndrome.**

As in the management of any patient, you should first assess Mr Shepherd's need for resuscitation (ABC), then confirm his diagnosis. A FBC will show leucocytosis and an ECG may show diffuse saddle-shaped ST elevation across a number of leads without reciprocal ST depression, and may also show PR depression. An echocardiogram may show a pericardial effusion; this may also be visible on chest radiograph. The ECG and chest radiograph will additionally help exclude a reinfarction or pulmonary pathology, respectively. Troponin levels should also be measured on this admission for the same reason.

Having requested the relevant investigations, Mr Shepherd should immediately be started on analgesia. Large doses of anti-inflammatory drugs such as aspirin, other non-steroidal anti-inflammatory drugs (NSAIDs) and/or colchicine may be given and are usually sufficient. Patients may require proton pump inhibitors (e.g. omeprazole) to prevent gastric irritation from the high dose aspirin or NSAIDs. If there is a significant pericardial effusion, it can be aspirated (pericardiocentesis) to relieve pressure on the heart. Mr Shepherd's renal function will need close monitoring if he is started on the combination of an ACE inhibitor and NSAIDs.

SHORT CASE

Mrs Thompson is a 62-year-old woman with known angina who has been referred by her GP following increasing frequency in her episodes of chest tightness. She says she usually suffers from angina two or three times a month, but that over the last 2 months her attacks have become more frequent. Some of these episodes are now occurring at rest, often following meals. They are partly alleviated by the GTN spray she has been using for her angina. She is a heavy smoker, blood pressure 163/94 mmHg, and cholesterol 6.5 mM. She had an angiogram 2 years earlier showing mild stenosis of the left circumflex artery. Her other medical history includes reflux disease, but no other conditions. Notably she has no history of gallstone disease and reports no change in stool or urine colour. On admission her examination and investigations are normal, including the ECG, 8-hour troponin levels, and temperature. The team has a high suspicion of a worsening of her angina and perform a repeat angiography, which is unchanged from her previous angiogram.

What diagnoses should you be considering? Which investigations will help you determine the correct one?

Attacks of chest pain of increasing frequency and at rest should trigger alarm bells for the progression of her angina from stable to unstable. At the same time, the fact that her angiogram is unchanged should arouse your suspicion of another diagnosis. The insidious course rules out acute conditions such as infarction or pericarditis. The chronic nature of the problem makes acute pancreatitis or acute cholecystitis unlikely. The important diagnoses to exclude are oesophageal spasm and biliary colic.

Gallstones causing biliary colic can be diagnosed on ultrasound. Oesophageal spasm may be detected by barium swallow and oesophageal manometry, although a normal result does not exclude it. Ultimately the diagnosis may come down to a therapeutic trial. Mrs Thompson was prescribed a proton pump inhibitor for presumptive **oesophageal spasm** secondary to reflux. She responded positively, confirming the diagnosis.

If all else had been excluded, you may have considered a diagnosis of coronary artery spasm (sometimes called variant or Prinzmetal angina) or coronary syndrome X. These are diagnoses of exclusion; they are extremely hard to demonstrate and are, in any case, rare in the absence of underlying coronary artery disease. It is best to avoid such 'dustbin diagnoses' until all other causes have been excluded.

SHORT CASE

Mr Heyward is a 38-year-old man with increasingly severe chest pain that began during an evening in the pub. The pain has not radiated, and was not alleviated by GTN administered in the ambulance. He has a strong family history with both his father and brother suffering heart attacks in their fifties, and is a heavy smoker with a 50-pack-year-history. He is not known to have diabetes, hypertension, or high cholesterol. He has no other significant medical history, although you note that he had what sounds like a viral upper respiratory tract infection 3–4 days ago. On examination of his cardiovascular system you find no abnormalities. An ECG taken at the hospital is shown in Figure 9.3. His other investigations were normal apart from mildly elevated inflammatory markers.

Figure 9.3 Mr Heyward's electrocardiogram (ECG).

With kind permission from Dr J. Dwight.

What does the ECG show? What is the most likely diagnosis?

The ECG shows ST elevation in leads I, II, aVL, V_1–V_5, i.e. throughout most leads, and slight PR segment depression. Acute coronary syndromes typically respond to vasodilators such as GTN. In addition, MI causes ECG changes which are reciprocal (i.e. ST elevation in some leads, ST depression in opposite anatomical leads). This is therefore unlikely to be an acute coronary syndrome, although troponin levels at admission and 3–12 hours after the onset of pain should be checked for confirmation.

Pericarditis is the most likely diagnosis despite the atypical sounding pain and lack of a pericardial friction rub, which can be intermittent. A therapeutic trial of NSAIDs was prescribed which diminished the pain. The patient was treated with analgesia as an inpatient for a few days and was discharged once pain free.

SHORT CASE

Mr Bromley is a 28-year-old, tall, thin man with a sudden onset of severe chest pain. He has recently been on a flight from Egypt and had knee surgery 1 month ago. Otherwise he says he has been fit and well, with no previous medical history. He is not known to have Marfan's syndrome, although it has not been investigated, and there is no family history of note. He is a non-smoker with no risk factors for cardiovascular disease. On examination he is pale, sweaty, and breathless. His pulse is weak and thready, but otherwise his examination is normal.

What diagnoses are most likely? Which first-line investigations will help you determine the correct one?

In a tall, thin, young individual you should immediately be thinking of pneumothorax or Marfan's syndrome predisposing to a dissected thoracic aorta/dissected aortic aneurysm. His recent air travel, although only a short trip, and surgery should alert you to the possibility of a PE. All of these conditions are associated with high mortality and so you must act fast. In your assessment of his ABC you should pay particular attention to his blood pressure—patients with an aortic aneurysm are often hypertensive but can become hypotensive if they dissect back into the pericardial space and develop cardiac tamponade (along with muffled heart sounds and distended neck veins). If they rupture into the chest cavity they tend to exsanguinate before they make it to hospital. An urgent chest radiograph will rule out a pneumothorax (although you should have detected this when percussing, and auscultating his chest) and will show a widened mediastinum in most cases of aortic dissection (~80%). His Wells score for PE is >4 (suspicion of PE and recent surgery) so there is no point in doing a D-dimer: NICE guidelines are very clear that one should proceed to CTPA.

Mr Bromley was hypotensive (80/46) but there was no difference in the blood pressure in each arm. His bedside chest radiograph suggested a widened mediastinum. As he was not haemodynamically stable it was felt unsafe to transfer him for a CTPA and a transthoracic echocardiogram was ordered at the bedside. This showed an **aortic dissection** near the aortic root and a pericardial effusion. Any dissection involving the ascending aorta, such as this one, is classed as a Stanford type A and is a surgical emergency. Dissections of the descending aorta, with no involvement of the ascending aorta, are called type B and are managed medically. However, surgery in type B is indicated if medical treatment fails and complications develop.

SHORT CASE

Mr Perkins is a 32-year-old investment banker who presents with chest pain. It came on while he was at a party in a bar with friends. He has a family history of cardiovascular disease but no other cardiovascular risk factors. He is normally fit and well, although he says he has had a cold and fever for the past couple of days. His ECG shows >2 mm ST elevation in leads V_1–V_4 and, as he is at a hospital with the necessary resources, he is scheduled for primary angioplasty. However, no coronary artery occlusion was seen on his angiogram.

What is the most likely diagnosis? Which question(s) in particular should you ask on the history?

Chest pain and fever suggest an acute inflammation due to, for example, myocarditis/pericarditis but the ECG does not support this (it would classically show saddle-shaped ST elevation in a number of leads not conforming to the territory of a single coronary artery). Normal angiography ruled out coronary artery disease. The most likely diagnosis is **coronary spasm due to cocaine usage**. You should specifically ask about recreational drugs in order to investigate this possibility.

SHORT CASE

Mr Daniels is a 52-year-old man who presents to the Emergency Department with a 4-hour history of chest pain associated with nausea and vomiting. His cardiac risk factors include a 15-pack-year history of smoking, although he quit 10 years ago, and a father and brother who had heart attacks in their fifties. He has no other medical history of note and reports no symptoms of reflux disease, but drinks 20 units of alcohol a week. On examination he appears uncomfortable and dyspnoeic. The rest of his examination is unremarkable except for mild consolidation at his left lung base.

His ECG and troponin on admission are normal. A chest radiograph confirms a small effusion on the left.

What are the most likely diagnoses? If his 8-hour troponin levels are normal, does this change your differential? What complications should you be particularly wary of?

Nausea and vomiting are commonly associated with inferior MIs. However, the small unilateral pleural effusion should alert you to the possibility of **Boerhaave's syndrome**—a perforation in the oesophagus. This was indeed the case with this patient, whose 8-hour troponin levels proved to be normal. Note that the vomiting should precede the onset of pain in Boerhaave's: contrast this with MI (pain precedes vomiting), as it is the vomiting that causes the perforation (whereas in infarction, it is the post-infarct inflammation that irritates the diaphragm). Not unusually, this patient could not recall which came first.

Patients with Boerhaave's are prone to develop a pleural effusion, pneumomediastinum, and/or pneumothorax, perhaps followed by infection with gastrointestinal flora (mediastinitis and sepsis). Treatment consists of prompt antibiotic therapy and surgical repair of the oesophagus with mediastinal washout. Prognosis is grim, with a 30% mortality if surgical intervention is initiated within 24 hours, rising to 50–65% if surgery is delayed beyond 24 hours. Although it is a rare diagnosis it is important to be aware of, as early diagnosis is critical in increasing the chances of survival.

SHORT CASE

Mrs Peacock is a 74-year-old woman 9 days post-op (carotid endarterectomy following an ischaemic stroke) who has been referred to the medical team by her GP for an episode of chest pain that began half an hour ago. She is a type 2 diabetic, for which she takes metformin and gliclazide. She is also treated for hypertension and hypercholesterolaemia, but has never smoked and has no family history of cardiovascular disease. She usually takes warfarin for atrial fibrillation, but this was stopped prior to her operation. She says the pain is always there but is not severe. On examination she appears unwell lying at 30° in bed, with shallow and rapid breathing. Her lung fields are clear on auscultation. Her pulse is weak and irregularly irregular, but her heart sounds are normal, and her examination is otherwise unremarkable. Her oxygen saturation is 98% on room air. The chest radiograph is normal. Her ECG shows atrial fibrillation but no ST elevation or other abnormalities. Her baseline troponin levels are not elevated.

What is the most likely diagnosis? What investigation would you order next to investigate this?

Mrs Peacock is presenting with an episode of chest pain and breathlessness, on a background of cardiovascular risk factors. Left heart failure secondary to myocardial ischaemia is a possibility, particularly given her risk factors (atrial fibrillation and recent stroke), with the breathlessness due to pulmonary oedema. However, if that were the case you would expect bibasal crackles on auscultation of her lungs. The chest radiograph, ECG, and troponin levels also fail to show signs of left heart failure or myocardial ischaemia although a 3–12 hour troponin (depending on local test and protocol) will be needed to rule out an MI if this is still suspected.

Her recent surgery and reduced mobility following her stroke are both risk factors for a **PE**, which would explain her breathlessness. Mrs Peacock was started on low molecular weight heparin to prevent further pulmonary emboli; had an 8 hour troponin which was negative and was sent for CTPA which found multiple small clots in both lungs. She was started on appropriate anticoagulation and made a good recovery.

Viva questions

Why do some but not all patients with acute MIs get nausea and vomiting?

This is called the Bezold–Jarisch reflex. Infarction of the inferior myocardium irritates the diaphragm, resulting in vomiting. It is not uncommon for this to happen during angiography (and worth warning patients undergoing angiography about!). Patients with infarcts in other territories will not irritate their diaphragm.

How can occlusion of the different coronary arteries be distinguished on ECG?

There are four main patterns of infarction, resulting from occlusion of each of the main coronary arteries (see Figure 9.4).

- **Anterior infarct**: ST elevation in leads V_2, V_3, and V_4 indicates infarction of the anterior surface of the left ventricle, supplied by the left anterior descending artery (LAD).

- **Right/inferior infarct**: ST elevation in leads II, III, and aVF indicates infarction of the inferior surface, supplied by the right coronary artery (RCA).

Figure 9.4 Electrocardiogram (ECG) showing the coronary artery territories. The *anterior/septal leads* correspond to the portion of the heart supplied by the left anterior descending artery. The *right inferior leads* correspond to the portion of the heart supplied by the right coronary artery. The *left lateral leads* correspond to the lateral wall of the left ventricle, supplied by both the left anterior descending and the circumflex arteries.

CONTINUED ➤

CONTINUED

- **Lateral infarct**: ST elevation in leads V_5 and V_6 indicates infarction of the lateral surface of the left ventricle and may be involved in a circumflex (Cx) or LAD lesion.
- **Posterior infarct**: ST depression in V_1–V_3 with tall R waves is indicative of circumflex occlusion, i.e. a true posterior infarct. This can be difficult to distinguish from LAD territory ischaemia: look particularly for a dominant R wave in V_1 and inferior lead ST elevation in infarction.

What are the earliest biochemical changes in MI? Why do we use troponin levels if they are only reliable after a few hours (exact timings depend on the assay)?

Troponin levels are used because they have a very high specificity and sensitivity for cardiac damage. Other biochemical markers rise earlier, specifically myoglobin and CK-MB, one of the isomers of the enzyme creatinine kinase. However, these are far less specific for cardiac damage.

Compare the mechanism of action of aspirin, clopidogrel, abciximab/tirofiban, and bivalirudin.

All of these are antiplatelet agents with different mechanisms of action:

- **Aspirin** is an irreversible inhibitor of the enzyme cyclooxygenase (COX), which synthesizes inflammatory mediators including the platelet aggregator thromboxane A2. Platelets have no nuclei so cannot synthesize new COX enzymes to compensate for this irreversible inhibition. Aspirin's action is reversed on synthesis of new platelets.
- **Clopidogrel (and prasugrel and ticagrelor)** irreversibly blocks the adenosine diphosphate (ADP) receptor on platelet cell membranes that prevents them binding to fibrinogen and hence inhibits platelet aggregation.
- **Abciximab** and **tirofiban** reversibly block fibrinogen binding to the glycoprotein IIb/IIIa receptors on platelet cell membranes that mediate platelet aggregation (abciximab is a monoclonal antibody, tirofiban a small molecule).
- **Bivalirudin** is a direct thrombin inhibitor (DTI) and is sometimes used as an alternative to heparin (an indirect thrombin inhibitor).

A patient attends the Emergency Department with central crushing chest pain. Investigations reveal a normal ECG and normal troponins. All other investigations and examinations are normal, and a presumptive diagnosis of new-onset angina is made.

What investigations should you request for a patient such as this presenting with new-onset angina?

Exercise tolerance test. An exercise tolerance test may be performed to investigate the possibility of coronary artery disease and therefore the potential benefit to be derived from angioplasty. A patient's ECG and blood pressure are monitored during increasing amounts of exercise (e.g. on a treadmill). ST depression of ≥2 mm, typical symptoms of exertional angina, or ST elevation ≥1 mm usually indicate stenosis of the coronary arteries. A fall in blood pressure during the test is a poor

CONTINUED ➤

CONTINUED

prognostic sign. It is worth noting that this test only has an 80% sensitivity and 70% specificity for detecting ischaemic heart disease (i.e. 30% of positive results will be false positives).

Stress echocardiogram. Some patients cannot perform an exercise tolerance test, for example due to an inability to walk from severe arthritis, severe peripheral vascular disease, or COPD. In these cases a stress echocardiogram can be conducted. The patient is given dobutamine to simulate 'stress' while their cardiac function is assessed by echocardiogram. A normal heart shows increased motility when stressed, whereas ischaemic myocardium is hypokinetic.

Myoview scan. This is an alternative to the tests above and provides a way of looking directly at blood flow within the heart muscle either during exercise (e.g. on an exercise bike) or under medically induced stress. Patients are injected with a radioactive contrast agent (thallium) and a picture taken with a gamma camera. Pictures at rest and immediately after exercise/stress are compared. Areas of the myocardium with good perfusion appear as 'warm' spots on the scan.

CT coronary angiography: Increasingly, patients are having CT scans of their hearts, with images synchronized with their heart beat (which should be 60 beats per minute or lower to give good-quality images), and contrast given to view the coronary arteries in detail. Calcium, from calcified atherosclerotic plaques, can be seen in the lumen of the coronary arteries and a calcium score calculated reflecting the degree of atherosclerosis.

Angiography/angioplasty. If any of the tests above are positive, the patient is suitable for diagnostic angiography to identify if there is stenosis of a coronary artery. If significant coronary artery disease were found, most centres would undertake coronary angioplasty although if more than one coronary vessel is affected, or if there is a valve lesion(s) suitable for surgery, bypass surgery (with or without valve replacement(s)) can be considered.

What ECG abnormalities would you expect in a patient who suffered a full-thickness inferior MI 2 years previously? What is the basis for these changes?

Old infarcts are visible on ECGs as the infarcted tissue no longer conducts electrical impulses. If they are full thickness, they can be thought of as a window. Thus an electrode positioned next to an area of full-thickness infarct will look through the window of infarcted tissue and pick up the electrical impulses passing through the myocardium on the other side of the heart. This is evident in the ECG in the form of deep, so-called pathological, Q waves (>2 mm deep).

Describe the progression of ECG changes you would expect to see over 7 days in a patient presenting with acute STEMI.

Classically you see the following changes:

1 Tented T waves in the affected leads within minutes of the occlusion (due to localized hyperkalaemia following myocyte ischaemia)

2 ST elevation in the affected leads with ST depression in the reciprocal leads, lasting 24–48 hours

3 T wave inversion, developing in 1–2 days and persisting for weeks or months unless the MI is treated

4 Q waves, developing within days and remaining permanently

What are the Wells criteria for PE?

The Wells criteria establish the pre-test probability of someone having a PE based on several factors (Table 8.1). A cut-off of 4 (out of a possible 7 points) is used to determine the probability of a PE. The combination of a low probability on the Wells criteria (or any other criteria, e.g. Geneva score) and a D-dimer <500 ng/mL predicts with 98% certainty that a patient will not have a PE (but 2% still will). If a D-dimer >500 ng/mL and a PE is still suspected, start LMWH and perform a CTPA.

If there is a high probability, as per the Wells or another score, then LMWH should be started and a CTPA requested. A negative D-dimer in this setting is unhelpful, and may even provide false reassurance - the probability of a PE with a negative D-dimer but high probability Wells score is 19-28%!

Treatment for a CTPA-verified PE is to start anticoagulant therapy (warfarin or rivaroxaban). How long to continue with anticoagulation depends on the cause of the PE and the patient's risk factors for future emboli, but will usually be a minimum of 3 months.

Single Best Answers

1. Which of the following causes of chest pain is life-threatening?

    a. Tietze's syndrome

    b. Bornholm's disease

    c. Boerhaave's syndrome

    d. Oesophagitis

    e. None of the above

2. A patient presents with central crushing chest pain. Their ECG shows ST elevation in leads V_2–V_4. Which coronary artery is most likely to be occluded?

    a. Right main stem (LMS)

    b. Right coronary artery (RCA)

    c. Left main stem (LMS)

    d. Left anterior descending (LAD)

    e. Circumflex (Cx)

3. You are about to start treatment for a patient with a STEMI. Their past medical history includes diabetes, hypertension, asthma, and mild renal impairment with a creatinine between 130–140µmol/L over the past few months. Which medication should they not be treated with?

    a. Aspirin

    b. Statin

    c. ACE inhibitor

    d. β-Blocker

    e. Morphine

4. You have a hyperlipidaemic patient who is intolerant of statins. Which of the following alternatives could you consider?

    a. Abciximab

    b. Clopidogrel

    c. Dipyridamole

    d. Ezetimibe

    e. Tirofiban

5. A 68 year old man has been admitted with a STEMI and has had two drug-eluting stents placed in his left anterior descending (LAD) coronary artery. What drugs should the patient be discharged on, providing there are no contraindications?

    a. Aspirin and a statin.

    b. Aspirin, a statin and an ACE inhibitor.

    c. Aspirin, a statin and a β-blocker.

    d. Aspirin, a statin, an ACE inhibitor, a β-blocker, and a second antiplatelet agent (e.g. clopidogrel)

    e. Aspirin, a statin, an ACE inhibitor and a second antiplatelet agent (e.g. clopidogrel)

Core case

Read through the sections in the case boxes, covering up the sections that follow so that you don't see the answer. At the end of each case box, try to answer the question before reading on.

Mrs Finnegan is a 78-year-old widow who presents to your clinic complaining of increasing shortness of breath. She describes that for the past 4 months she has gradually become increasingly short of breath when she walks back up the hill to her bungalow after going to the shops. She is finally seeking medical help because she now finds herself short of breath when she does her gardening. Her sister (a lifelong smoker) died of lung cancer aged 73, and given that Mrs Finnegan used to smoke, she is especially concerned that she may have lung cancer.

In broad terms, what pathological processes could cause shortness of breath?

Shortness of breath essentially means either that not enough oxygen is getting around the body or that there is a cause for increased respiratory drive. This could be due to many causes, as shown in Figure 10.1:

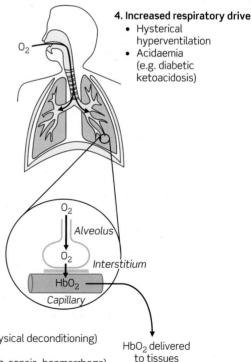

1. Insufficient O_2 getting into the lungs
- Obstructed airways (e.g. asthma, COPD, obstructing tumour, airway oedema in anaphylaxis)
- Decreased lung volume
  - Intra-thoracic (e.g. pneumothorax, pleural effusion)
  - Extra-thoracic (e.g. kyphoscoliosis)
- Decreased volume of 'functioning' lung (e.g. bullous/cystic disease, scarred or fibrosed lung in interstitial lung disease)
- Inability to inflate the lungs
  - increased work to do so (e.g. obesity, increased stiffness in interstitial lung disease)
  - weak respiratory muscles in neuromuscular disorders (e.g. Guillain-Barre, myasthenia gravis)
  - already hyperinflated (COPD)

2. Insufficient O_2 getting into the blood
- Damage to alveolar membrane
  - Emphysema
  - Fibrosis (interstitial lung disease)
- Fluid between the alveolar wall and capillary
  - Oedema (e.g. heart failure)
  - Inflammatory (e.g. pneumonia)
- Disrupted blood supply e.g. pulmonary embolus

3. Insufficient O_2 getting around the body
- Reduced cardia output (e.g. heart failure, aortic stenosis, physical deconditioning)
- Anaemia
- Shock (i.e. blood pressure <90/60 mmHg from any cause, e.g. sepsis, haemorrhage)

4. Increased respiratory drive
- Hysterical hyperventilation
- Acidaemia (e.g. diabetic ketoacidosis)

O_2

O_2

Alveolus

O_2
Interstitium

HbO_2
Capillary

HbO_2 delivered to tissues

Figure 10.1 Mechanisms that can result in the sensation of breathlessness.

Good history-taking begins with listening to whatever the patient has to tell you, followed by open questions to avoid leading the patient's answers. You can then move on to specific questions that can help narrow your differential diagnosis.

What specific questions might you ask someone who presents with shortness of breath?

About the shortness of breath

- **Timing of onset?** This is crucial because vascular (e.g. PE) and mechanical (e.g. pneumothorax, foreign body) pathologies present suddenly. At the other end of the spectrum, it may take weeks or months before diseases such as lung cancer or pulmonary fibrosis cause sufficient dyspnoea for the patient to present.
- **Alleviating or exacerbating factors?** Most shortness of breath will be worse on exertion. However, heart failure will also be worse on lying flat; asthma will usually be worse at certain times of the year (e.g. due to pollen allergy, cold climate), in certain places (e.g. in dusty environments, or when the pets are around), during intense cardiovascular exercise (e.g. running), or in the early hours of the morning. Psychogenic hyperventilation will be worse at times of anxiety and stress.

Risk factors

- **Smoking?** Never forget to ask about smoking and to quantify this in terms of 'pack years' smoked (1 pack = 20 cigarettes; 20 cigarettes a day for a year = 1 pack year).
- **Pets?** The patient may be allergic to pets, especially new ones.
- **Occupational history?** Ask about jobs—there are still lots of people who have been exposed to asbestos, silica dust, and coal particulates in past jobs and who are at risk of pneumoconioses.
- **Medications?** Certain drugs can cause hypersensitivity pneumonitis (previously called extrinsic allergic alveolitis, a type of interstitial lung disease), e.g. nitrofurantoin, amiodarone, methotrexate, bleomycin.
- **Past medical history?** Autoimmune conditions such as rheumatoid arthritis and systemic lupus erythematosus can cause interstitial lung disease and pleural effusions.

Associated symptoms

- **Cough?** A cough points strongly towards a respiratory pathology. The nature of the cough is important: *Is it productive? What colour is the sputum? Is there any blood? When does the cough occur? What does the cough sound like?* A persistent, productive cough over the last few days suggests pneumonia; a persistent, productive cough on most days of the past 3 months and spanning years suggests chronic bronchitis; a dry cough present mainly during the episodes of shortness of breath or at night suggests asthma, but may also be a feature of left ventricular failure; bloodstained sputum may suggest a PE, lung cancer, or a cavitating pneumonia. Certain pathologies are associated with characteristic-sounding coughs—for those of you with a veterinary bent, croup is said to sound like a barking seal (but is a disease almost exclusive of young children), whereas recurrent laryngeal nerve palsy (sometimes associated with lung cancer) can produce a bovine cough.

- **Chest pain?** If there is chest pain, is it pleuritic? Pleuritic chest pain can suggest pneumonia, a PE, or a pneumothorax, because these often involve the parietal pleura. Non-pleuritic chest pain could indicate a cardiovascular pathology.

- **Muscular weakness or fatigue?** Neuromuscular diseases (e.g. Guillain–Barré syndrome, myasthenia gravis, Lambert–Eaton syndrome, polymyositis, motor neuron disease) will usually be accompanied by muscular weakness elsewhere.

- **Tender limbs?** Pulmonary emboli can originate from anywhere in the venous system. Patients usually only notice deep vein thrombosis (DVT) if it occurs in a limb as this will usually cause inflammation—a swollen red, tender, warm, shiny looking limb.

- **Weight loss? Loss of appetite? Night sweats?** These are 'red flag' signs that suggest that a highly metabolic, systemic inflammatory process is going on—often a cancer.

- **Loss of blood?** Anaemia can cause or exacerbate shortness of breath, so ask about heavy menstrual bleeding (in women), fresh rectal bleeding, and melaena.

How would the speed of onset influence your differential diagnosis?
Think of which pathologies present over seconds to minutes, hours to days, and weeks to months.

Which of these conditions must you exclude, due to their need for urgent treatment or poor prognosis?

Shortness of breath can present over various timescales. Figure 10.2 shows the diagnoses that you must exclude in **bold**. Rare diagnoses are in a smaller font.

Seconds to minutes	Hours to days	Weeks to months
Bronchospasm (acute asthma or COPD)	Pneumonia	COPD
Anaphylaxis	Heart failure	Chronic asthma
Laryngeal oedema (secondary to burns or chemical irritation)	Pleural effusion	Heart failure
	Post-operative atelectasis	Pulmonary fibrosis
PE	Chronic pulmonary emboli	Anaemia
Pneumothorax	Altitude sickness	Bronchiectasis
Flash pulmonary oedema*	Guillain–Barré syndrome	Physical deconditioning
Hysterical hyperventilation	Myasthenia gravis	Obesity
Inhaled foreign body	**Acute Respiratory Distress Syndrome (ARDS)**	Pulmonary hypertension
Tension pneumothorax	Lung collapse (e.g. secondary to bronchial carcinoma)	Mesothelioma
Acute epiglottitis/supraglottitis		Pulmonary tuberculosis
		Kyphoscoliosis
		Ankylosing spondylitis
		Motor neuron disease

Figure 10.2 Differential diagnoses for shortness of breath.

* Flash pulmonary oedema refers to pulmonary oedema that develops suddenly, for example, due to a myocardial infarction causing a sudden drop in cardiac function.

We already know that Mrs Finnegan's dyspnoea has developed over several months.

What key clues on history and examination will help you differentiate between the potential diagnoses? Try to think of key clues for the most common diagnoses in the 'weeks to months' column in Figure 10.2.

- COPD
  - Remember that COPD is a bracket term encompassing chronic bronchitis and emphysema.
  - History of chronic bronchitis (a clinical diagnosis, based on the presence of a cough, productive of sputum (~10 mL daily), on most days of 3 months for 2 consecutive years) and permanent, largely irreversible, shortness of breath.
  - Presence of risk factors suggesting a cause for COPD:
    - Smoking (usually more than 20 pack years)
    - Occupational exposure to lung irritants, e.g. in coal miners, tunnel workers
    - α_1-Antitrypsin deficiency (liver failure, family history).
  - Signs of COPD:
    - Hyperexpanded chest
    - Breathing through pursed lips
    - Reduced air entry/chest expansion
    - Prolonged expiratory phase
    - Hyper-resonant percussion note.
- Chronic asthma
  - History of wheeze, breathlessness, chest tightness and/or cough, often worse at night/early morning, during exercise, or when exposed to allergens or cold
  - Presence of associated atopic conditions personally or in family members (eczema, hayfever, allergies, nasal polyps)
  - Symptoms may be exacerbated by drugs such as non-steroidal anti-inflammatory drugs (NSAIDs), aspirin, β-blockers (including those in eye drops used for glaucoma)
  - Wheeze on auscultation of the lungs.
- Interstitial lung disease
  - History of exposure to asbestos, silica, or coal (pneumoconioses causing interstitial lung disease), exposure to drugs (e.g. methotrexate, amiodarone)
  - Signs on examination include:
    - Clubbing (in usual interstitial pneumonitis)
    - Reduced air entry/chest expansion
    - Late inspiratory, fine crackles (may be heard at either the bases or the apices depending on the aetiology).
- Heart failure
  - History of shortness of breath on exertion, orthopnoea (breathless when lying flat), paroxysmal nocturnal dyspnoea (waking up short of breath), swollen ankles (if right as well as left heart failure)
  - Presence of risk factors suggesting a cause for heart failure:
    - Ischaemic heart disease (smoking, diabetes mellitus, hypercholesterolaemia, hypertension, south Asian descent, strong family history)
    - Other atherosclerotic disease (e.g. stroke, transient ischaemic attack (TIA), limb claudication)
    - Hypertension (can cause heart failure in the absence of ischaemic heart disease)

- Valvular disease (e.g. aortic stenosis)
- Cardiomyopathy
- Signs on examination include:
  - Displaced apex beat
  - Third and fourth heart sounds (often difficult to hear in practice)
  - Crackles in both lung bases
  - Raised jugular venous pressure (JVP), hepatomegaly, peripheral oedema (ankles, sacrum).

- Anaemia
  - History of bleeding (e.g. menorrhagia, melaena). Fatigue as well as shortness of breath on exertion.
  - Signs of peripheral (fingers) or central (tongue) cyanosis. Specific signs such as koilonychia, glossitis, and angular stomatitis (all rare). Checking for conjunctival pallor is routinely done but is unreliable.
- **Bronchiectasis** would be suggested by a history of productive cough and recurrent chest infections, or a history of cystic fibrosis.
- **Obesity, kyphoscoliosis, ankylosing spondylitis** can be excluded on inspection.
- **Physical deconditioning** is a diagnosis of exclusion.

Your history-taking reveals that Mrs Finnegan is a retired office worker who is diabetic and takes 'aspirin, a pill for the diabetes, and a water tablet for blood pressure'. Her past medical history is significant for an anterior myocardial infarction (MI) 5 years ago, after which she underwent coronary artery bypass grafting (CABG). Her parents 'died of old age' and her only sister died of lung cancer. She smoked about 10 cigarettes a day from her early twenties until her late sixties. She has slept propped up with several pillows for the last few years as this is 'more comfortable'. She becomes short of breath when gardening or walking uphill, but feels much better if she stops to catch her breath for a minute. She has not had any cough, chest pain, or dark or bloody faeces or urine. She has not lost any weight, had any night sweats, or noticed any change in appetite. However, she is worried that she may have lung cancer like her sister and was hoping you might be able to do a test to rule that out.

On examination, there are no signs of cyanosis or anaemia. Her blood pressure is 155/80 mmHg and her heart rate is 85 bpm and regular. There is no cervical lymphadenopathy. Her JVP is elevated to 6 cm above the angle of Louis and her apex is most prominent lateral of the midclavicular line, in the sixth intercostal space. There is a median sternotomy scar from her CABG 5 years ago. There are no heaves or thrills, and auscultation reveals no murmurs. Chest expansion is symmetrical and resonant to percussion. The trachea is central and breath sounds are heard throughout both lungs, albeit with crackles in both lung bases. Her liver is not enlarged or tender but there is pitting oedema up to her shins bilaterally. Abdominal examination is normal. Neurological examination is also normal.

Mrs Finnegan's history and examination are consistent with a particular diagnosis for her shortness of breath, but this should be confirmed or refuted with basic investigations.

Given the history and examination, what is the most likely cause of Mrs Finnegan's shortness of breath?

Mrs Finnegan is an elderly woman with shortness of breath and significant risk factors for both cardiovascular disease (ex-smoker, hypertension, diabetes mellitus, previous MI) and respiratory disease (>20 pack years of smoking). However, she gives a clear history of predictable shortness of breath on exercise that is relieved by rest. She has orthopnoea, and has a displaced apex beat, pulmonary oedema, and pedal oedema. Put together, this all suggests that Mrs Finnegan likely has **congestive heart failure** that is causing reduced cardiac output, pulmonary oedema, and peripheral oedema.

> **What investigations would you like to arrange?**

Bloods

- **Full blood count (FBC):** looking for anaemia.
- **Blood cholesterol, glucose, and HbA1c:** abnormal cholesterol levels (total >5 mM, low-density lipoprotein (LDL) >3 mM or high-density lipoprotein (HDL) <1 mM) and abnormal glucose levels (random >11.1 mM or fasting >7 mM) will give clues about risk factors for ischaemic heart disease, the main cause of heart failure. Mrs Finnegan is a known diabetic, so her HbA1c level will be useful as this is a measure of her glucose control over the preceding 60 days (non-diabetic HbA1c <6.5%).
- **Thyroid function tests (TFTs):** hyperthyroidism can cause a tachyarrhythmia and high-output cardiac failure.
- **Urea and electrolytes (U&Es):** if you think the patient might have excess fluid and therefore there is a chance you might start diuretics to offload some fluid, you need a baseline of electrolyte levels and renal function. It is best to take all the bloods now, both to avoid putting a needle in the patient twice and because an earlier baseline is better.
- **Brain natriuretic peptide (BNP):** a hormone that is released by ventricular cells in heart failure. It has high negative predictive value (i.e. a negative value makes heart failure unlikely, the exact percentage varying with the assay and cut-off used), but low specificity. Modest rises may be seen in other causes of heart strain (e.g. PE, cor pulmonale in severe lung disease) and other diseases (e.g. renal failure).

Imaging

- **Chest radiograph:** looking for signs of heart failure, pneumonia, pleural effusion, bronchiectasis, or fibrosis (pneumothorax and collapse are unlikely given the examination findings).
- **Electrocardiogram (ECG):** the ECG is nearly always abnormal in patients with heart failure (indeed, an entirely normal ECG has a negative predictive value for heart failure of about 98%). An important cause of heart failure is necrosis to areas of the heart caused by MI. Diabetics often have 'silent infarcts', which are not noticed by the patient. The presence of pathological Q waves or a bundle branch block on the ECG would suggest a previous, full-thickness MI.

Other

If the history were suggestive of lung pathology (rather than cardiac pathology) as the cause of breathlessness, you might consider performing:

- **Peak expiratory flow rate (PEFR).** This can be used to stratify the severity of an asthma attack in chronic asthma.
- **Spirometry.** This is used to distinguish between obstructive and restrictive lung disease. In obstructive airways disease (e.g. asthma, COPD, bronchiectasis), the bronchi are narrowed by mucus such that less air can be forcibly exhaled during a single second (forced expiratory volume in 1 second; FEV_1 <70%

of predicted), but the total lung capacity is not reduced (forced vital capacity; FVC >70%). Note that in severe COPD, the FVC may be reduced as patients are unable to fully expire (due to airways obstruction) in the time before they need to take another breath. In restrictive airways disease (e.g. pulmonary fibrosis), the total lung volume is reduced (FVC <70%) but the amount of air that can be exhaled in the first second remains the same (FEV$_1$ >70%).

Mrs Finnegan's chest radiograph is shown in Figure 10.3.

Figure 10.3 Mrs Finnegan's erect postero-anterior (PA) chest radiograph.

What does it show?

Remember to go through radiographs systematically.

- Check the patient details are correct: none are shown here for confidentiality.
- Check the radiograph is technically adequate: full coverage, good penetration, not rotated, adequate inspiration. This radiograph is rotated to the right.
- Present your findings logically. Mrs Finnegan's radiograph shows a reticular pattern of opacification throughout both lung fields, which is much denser in the lower zones bilaterally. There is upper lobe diversion of the pulmonary veins in both lung fields. The heart shadow is significantly enlarged. There are faintly visible sternal sutures (from her CABG) and a small amount of fluid in the transverse fissure.

Mrs Finnegan's ECG shows pathological Q waves in leads V$_1$–V$_4$. Her FBC is normal. Her glucose is 6.2 mM and her HbA1c is 6.8%. Her total cholesterol = 6.2 mM, LDL = 3.1 mM, and HDL = 1.1 mM.

What is the diagnosis for Mrs Finnegan? Can you identify any risk factors for this diagnosis in her history and investigations?

Mrs Finnegan is probably suffering from **congestive cardiac failure** as she has signs of both left ventricular failure (bibasal crackles suggestive of pulmonary oedema, and a displaced apex beat as well as a chest radiograph showing bilateral pulmonary oedema) and right ventricular failure (peripheral oedema and a raised JVP).

Heart failure is a syndrome, not a true pathological diagnosis. Mrs Finnegan's heart failure could be due to any number of causes (e.g. hypertension, valvular disease, alcohol-induced cardiomyopathy) but it is important to remember that the most common cause of heart failure is ischaemic heart disease and that this patient has significant risk factors for this pathology:

- She smoked 10 cigarettes (half a pack) every day for 40 years = 20 pack years.
- She has diabetes mellitus.
- Her total cholesterol (6.2 mM) and LDL (3.1 mM) are elevated.
- Her hypertension is not well controlled (155/80 mmHg). The NICE guidelines recommend a target blood pressure of <140/85 mmHg for most people, <130/80 mmHg for diabetics or <125/75 mmHg for patients with proteinuria.

The absence of angina in Mrs Finnegan does not exclude ischaemic heart disease since patients with diabetes mellitus may have 'silent' ischaemia.

> **How does Mrs Finnegan's diagnosis explain her symptoms (shortness of breath on exertion, orthopnoea) and signs (displaced apex beat, crackles in the lungs, peripheral oedema, raised JVP)?**

- **Shortness of breath.** The failing heart can't pump enough blood out. This is especially true if venous return to the heart is increased (e.g. exercise, lying down) and the heart is forced to work harder (e.g. exercise). Back pressure forces fluid out from the pulmonary vasculature into the alveoli, causing 'wet lungs' and a feeling of shortness of breath (some patients will say it feels like drowning). A combination of decreased lung compliance, decreased gas exchange, and airways obstruction are the important drivers of dyspnoea in most left ventricular failure patients.

- **Orthopnoea.** Lying down increases venous return to the heart, which is already struggling to pump out all the blood reaching it. This makes congestion of blood in the pulmonary vessels even worse, forcing more fluid out into the lungs and therefore causing shortness of breath. This is why patients with heart failure often sleep propped up with pillows.

- **Displaced apex beat.** The failing heart can't pump out all of the blood reaching it, so it gradually but inexorably dilates, leading to a displaced (and weak) apex beat. This can be thought of as a volume-overloaded heart. Do not confuse this with hypertrophy, which is caused by hypertension or aortic stenosis. Here, the heart has to pump harder and thus grows concentrically, leading to an undisplaced but forceful or heaving apex beat. This can be thought of as a pressure-overloaded heart. Ultimately, a pressure-overloaded heart can also dilate and fail, but this occurs later in the disease process.

- **Crackles in the lungs.** The build-up of blood in the pulmonary vessels forces fluid out of the vasculature into the alveoli. The alveoli are usually kept open by surfactant, but the interstitial fluid dilutes this and results in increased alveolar surface tension, leading to collapse of the alveoli. As the patient breathes in deeply, the alveoli eventually 'pop open'—the crackles you can hear with the stethoscope.

- **Peripheral oedema.** This is caused mainly because the failing heart cannot pump all of the blood reaching it (venous return), so one gets back pressure in the venous system. This is further compounded by salt and water retention due to activation of the renin–angiotensin–aldosterone system by a low cardiac output. The resultant pressure in the venous system can manifest itself as a raised JVP and/or a tender, enlarged liver. The increased blood pressure in the venous system also forces fluid out into the surrounding tissues, particularly in places where the venous pressure is highest, i.e. the dependent parts of the body (ankles in someone who has been standing, sacrum in someone who has been in bed). A raised JVP and hepatomegaly are not always clinically apparent.

What second-line investigations should be arranged for Mrs Finnegan?

- **Echocardiography** to assess ventricular function and confirm low cardiac output and heart failure, assess valve patency, and look for areas of dyskinesia.
- **Coronary angiography** if you suspect this heart is failing because of coronary artery disease. This is quite likely in Mrs Finnegan's case given her history of previous MI and risk factors for atherosclerotic disease. If there is a narrowing(s) in the coronary arteries that is amenable to revascularization (either angioplasty/stenting or bypass grafting), this will offer her the best chance of improving her ventricular function.

Mrs Finnegan went for echocardiography. This showed anterior akinesia and a left ventricular ejection fraction of 30%. Coronary angiography showed patent graft vessels but an occluded left anterior descending artery, plus severe stenosis of the right coronary and circumflex arteries. Based on this, it is fair to proceed based on a working diagnosis of congestive heart failure secondary to ischaemic heart disease.

What drug treatments would you offer this patient? Don't worry about specific drugs. Try to think what types of drug might help with: (1) her symptoms (too much fluid in lungs and limbs), (2) the pathological mechanism involved in heart failure, and (3) the underlying cause of the problem (atherosclerosis, in her case).

---

1   **Symptomatic relief**: her symptoms are largely due to her left ventricular failure (pulmonary oedema). You should treat this as follows:
   - In those patients presenting with acute pulmonary oedema (i.e. not our patient)—sit upright, give oxygen, and reduce cardiac preload with **vasodilators** such as nitrates and furosemide. Morphine has traditionally been used as well and is very effective in reducing the sensation of breathlessness, but studies have shown it increases mortality in patients with acute heart failure. Haemofiltration to remove fluid is also an option, as is continuous positive airway pressure (CPAP) ventilation.
   - Chronically—with a loop **diuretic** such as furosemide, which may be combined with a potassium-sparing diuretic aldosterone receptor antagonist (e.g. spironolactone, eplerenone).

2   **Pathophysiological mechanism**: reduced cardiac output activates two physiological systems that actually worsen the situation in heart failure: the sympathetic and the renin–angiotensin systems. Greater sympathetic activation increases heart rate and contractility via β-adrenergic receptors. This increases the heart's oxygen demand, which may already be compromised in heart failure (particularly if secondary to ischaemic heart disease), and at higher heart rates filling time and therefore cardiac output may be further reduced. Activation of the renin–angiotensin system (due to hypoperfusion of the kidneys, that incorrectly assume the

reduced perfusion is due to reduced vascular volume) results in increased water retention, leading to fluid overload. Addressing the unhelpful response of these two systems is associated with improved mortality:

- **Reduce the oxygen demand of the heart**: heart failure is usually due to not enough blood reaching the hard-working myocytes, which start to die. One way of treating this is to use a β-blocker which slows the heartbeat, although β-blockers must never be used if patient is in acute LVF. The patient may not like it initially (as a slower beating heart will make them feel tired and lethargic) but the many double-blinded, randomized controlled trials have shown that the patient will live longer. The trick is to start with a small dose of β-blocker and increase it very slowly.

- **Inhibit the renin–angiotensin–aldosterone system**: angiotensin-converting enzyme (ACE) inhibitors limit activation of the renin–angiotensin–aldosterone pathway, thus reducing reabsorption of sodium and water from the kidneys. Several double-blinded, randomized controlled trials have now shown that ACE inhibitors reduce mortality in heart failure. Angiotensin II receptor blockers (ARBs) may be used as an alternative to ACE inhibitors. NICE guidelines suggest that aldosterone antagonists such as spironolactone should also be used in those with moderate to severe heart failure (left ventricular ejection fraction <35%).

3 **Underlying cause**: the most common cause of heart failure is **atherosclerosis** of the coronary arteries and you should consider addressing this. Angiography may reveal the potential for revascularization which, if the myocardium is still viable (as assessed by cardiac MRI, thallium scan, or dobutamine stress echocardiogram), offers the greatest potential for improving ventricular function. In addition, there are various ways of preventing atherosclerosis getting worse (and maybe even helping the body start to reverse it): **statins** to reduce cholesterol levels and prevent progression of the atheroma; **aspirin** to reduce the risk of thrombosis leading to heart ischaemia or infarction; and **medication for diabetes mellitus** if the patient is diabetic, as uncontrolled diabetes leads to hyperglycaemia which accelerates atherosclerosis.

In advanced heart failure, treatments can include digoxin, cardiac resynchronization therapy (biventricular pacemakers), implantable cardioversion devices (ICDs), mechanical assist devices, or heart transplantation.

Also, in addition to drug treatments, your management should include conservative measures, such as advice to stop smoking, adopt a healthy (low-salt) diet, minimizing alcohol intake, and taking regular exercise.

> Mrs Finnegan told you that she was concerned she may have lung cancer, because she used to smoke and her sister died of lung cancer.
>
> **Can you reassure Mrs Finnegan that she does not have lung cancer?**

It is important to address a patient's concerns and expectations. If these issues are not addressed, patients will go away unsatisfied and worried. This is not only unethical, as you could prevent the unnecessary agitation, but potentially uneconomical, as they may seek a second opinion.

Mrs Finnegan does not give a history suggesting any warning signs for lung cancer (dry cough, haemoptysis, hoarse voice, loss of weight, poor appetite, night sweats). Head and neck examination revealed no lymphadenopathy or Horner's syndrome. Her chest radiograph showed no 'coin lesions' that could indicate a tumour. But despite all this, it would be unwise to categorically inform the patient that 'she does not have lung cancer' because one cannot be 100% sure that she doesn't have a small tumour which we simply haven't picked up. Given her 20-pack-year smoking history, it is probably wiser to explain that although she is at an increased risk of lung cancer because of her previous smoking, you could not see any tumours on her current chest radiograph nor were there any signs in her history or examination that are suggestive of cancer. Explain that you cannot rule out cancer 100% with any tests, but that you have found no evidence of it at the moment and her current symptoms are much more likely to be due to heart failure.

Short cases

Mr Humbolt is a 52-year-old man who underwent a partial hepatectomy for primary hepatic carcinoma 24 hours ago. On the ward round, Mr Humbolt complains of a 'painful, rattling cough'. His pulse is 105 bpm regular, blood pressure 125/75 mmHg, respiratory rate 18/min and temperature 37.1 °C. Chest expansion is reduced bilaterally and there are crackles in both lung bases. The base of the right lung is dull to percussion and has reduced breath sounds on auscultation.

What reasons can you think of for this patient's breathlessness? What is the most likely diagnosis in this patient?

There are many reasons for breathlessness postoperatively:

- **Atelectasis (alveolar collapse).** Pain sometimes prevents patients from breathing adequately and expectorating any mucus in their lungs. The mucus eventually plugs the bronchioles, preventing air entry, and areas of lung collapse as the trapped air is gradually absorbed into the surrounding tissues. Incentive spirometers and early mobilization with the help of hospital physiotherapists help minimize these problems.

- **Pneumonia.** This is fairly common postoperatively for a combination of factors largely because of poor clearance of mucus due to pain and a somewhat weakened immune response from the physiological stress of surgery.

- **Pulmonary oedema.** This can be due to heart failure and, quite often, due to excessive fluids perioperatively.

- **PE.** DVT is not uncommon after surgery due to the combination of trauma and immobility, and classically occurs 10 days post-operation. Large DVTs can be prevented by using anticoagulant medication (e.g. low molecular weight heparin, factor Xa inhibitors), mobilizing patients as early as possible and using compression stockings for the legs.

- **Anaemia.** Patients may be anaemic if there was significant blood loss during surgery.

- **Pneumothorax.** This should always be considered if the patient has had any interventions near the chest either during the surgery or around the time of surgery (e.g. insertion of central venous line, intercostal anaesthetic block).

The 'rattling cough' is highly suggestive of mucus trapped in the lungs. The reduced chest expansion, crackles, and dull percussion all suggest a collapse of a segment of lung, most notably on the right. This picture would fit with **postoperative atelectasis**, caused by the patient not breathing out deeply enough to clear his lungs of mucus. This can be prevented with adequate analgesia, incentive spirometry, and early mobilization with the help of hospital physiotherapists. Nonetheless, it is important to confirm this diagnosis and exclude the others listed above. A chest radiograph is particularly useful in this regard (looking for collapse, consolidation from pneumonia, oedema, or a pneumothorax). Blood tests are less useful at this stage as inflammatory markers will be raised postoperatively.

The most important treatment for postoperative atelectasis is physiotherapy (most hospitals will have a 24 hour on-call physiotherapy service for this very reason), analgesia, and oxygen.

SHORT CASE

Maggie is a 16-year-old student referred to the respiratory physicians for her recurrent shortness of breath. She describes how she has found herself getting short of breath over the last few months. This mainly occurs in the evenings, and is often associated with a dry cough. In between these episodes, she describes herself as being fine, although she admits that she feels 'a bit unfit because I'm breathless when I go for even a gentle run with my dad'. She denies any weight loss, fevers, dark faeces, or changes in menstruation. She thinks her father suffers with eczema, and is sure that her brother and father have mild hay fever, as does she. She lives at home with her family, none of whom smoke, and a pet dog.

What is the most likely cause of Maggie's shortness of breath? How can this be confirmed? What long-term management will she require?

Maggie has intermittent episodes of shortness of breath that are worse in the evenings and on exercising. Some episodes are associated with a dry cough but in between episodes she is apparently fine. She also has a family history of atopic individuals, with several members including herself having hay fever and/or eczema. The picture of reversible, intermittent shortness of breath and cough in someone with a family history of atopy is strongly suggestive of **asthma**.

Asthma is a disease caused by a hypersensitive immune reaction in the bronchi, which leads to excessive mucus production and bronchoconstriction. The combination leads to an **obstructive airways disease** which can be **confirmed on spirometry**. This should show a relatively normal FVC but a significantly reduced forced expiratory ratio (FER)—as the problem is not lung capacity but obstruction affecting the speed at which air can get out of the lungs (for the precise diagnostic criteria see Chapter 7).

Management of asthma is based on three different mechanisms:

1 **Avoidance of trigger(s)**. These can include smoke, allergens (e.g. dust mites, pollen, pets), or exercising in cold air, but often no obvious trigger is known.

2 **Bronchodilation**. Dilatation of the bronchi can be achieved by either increasing sympathetic stimulation to the lungs (e.g. β_2-agonists or phosphodiesterase inhibitors = theophyllines) or decreasing parasympathetic stimulation to the lungs (e.g. antimuscarinics). These compounds can be inhaled in short-acting forms for acute attacks, or in long-acting forms for prophylaxis. β_2-Agonists and theophyllines can also be given intravenously (IV) if needed.

3 **Reduction of immune response in lungs**. This can be achieved using inhaled or, in severe cases, oral corticosteroids. There are also newer agents that target specific parts of the immune response (e.g. montelukast, a leukotriene receptor antagonist, and omalizumab, an anti-IgE antibody).

SHORT CASE

Mr Marley is a 67-year-old retired musician. He has been referred to the respiratory physicians by his GP because of persistent shortness of breath and recurrent chest infections. You enter the room to find him standing with his arms propped against the edge of the table. His breathing is laboured and he has a rattling cough. He finally sits down and explains that he always feels short of breath, and his wife has noticed that he often wheezes. He coughs up phlegm every day, and says he has been doing so for at least 2 years, although it is worse in winter. He knows this is all because of his lifetime habit of smoking—he has smoked about 30 cigarettes a day for over 40 years.

On examination, you find there is peripheral and central cyanosis. His breathing is laboured, with intercostal recession and an audible wheeze. His chest appears hyperinflated. The rest of the examination is normal.

Spirometry in the clinic reveals FEV_1 = 65% of predicted and FVC = 70% of predicted.

What is the likely diagnosis? How should this be managed?

Mr Marley is a patient with >20 pack years of smoking who has had a productive cough every day for >3 consecutive months a year for at least 2 years (chronic bronchitis) and hyperinflated lungs (suggesting emphysema). The combination of chronic bronchitis and emphysema in a lifelong smoker is highly suggestive of **COPD**. This is a disease caused by the persistent toxicity of smoke, which leads to goblet cell hyperplasia (and thus excessive mucus production), damaged ciliated epithelial cells (which usually clear mucus), and inhibition of α_1-antitrypsin (and thus active trypsin, which degrades the interstitial matrix proteins, leading to loss of elasticity of the lungs and alveoli merging into bullae). The result is lungs with decreased compliance, less surface area (hence the decreased FVC), and lots of mucus that cannot be cleared. As a consequence, patients suffer chronically from poor gas exchange in their lungs and recurrent infections.

Notice that spirometry in COPD patients often shows both a reduced FER (forced expiratory ratio = FEV_1/FVC) due to obstructed airways and a reduced FVC (although the lungs are hyperinflated, their lack of elasticity means they shift a smaller volume of air as much remains trapped in the lungs). This is not the case in asthma, where usually only the FER is affected as it is the speed with which air can be moved in/out of the lungs (FEV_1) that is affected, rather than the actual volume (FVC). Notice also that the shortness of breath in COPD is persistent and largely irreversible. Again, this is not the case in asthma, where patients are not short of breath between attacks.

The management of COPD (as per the NICE 2010 guidelines) involves:

- **Smoking cessation.** This is the single most important factor in limiting the progression of the disease.
- **Inhaled therapy.** As in asthma, short- and long-acting β_2-agonists and/or antimuscarinics can be used to control symptoms and improve exercise tolerance in patients. Inhaled corticosteroids should be added to long-acting bronchodilators to decrease exacerbation frequency in patients with an FEV_1 ≤50% predicted who have had two or more exacerbations requiring treatment with antibiotics or oral corticosteroids in a 12-month period.
- **Pulmonary rehabilitation** (for all patients who are functionally limited by their COPD). This programme of physiotherapy, exercise, education, etc. increases exercise tolerance and quality of life.
- **Vaccination** (flu and pneumococcal) should be offered to all patients with COPD.
- **Non-invasive ventilation (NIV).** This is the treatment of choice when medical therapy fails to control persistent hypercapnic ventilatory failure during exacerbations.
- **Long-term oxygen.** Patients who are hypoxic with an arterial partial pressure of oxygen (P_aO_2) <7.3 kPa on air, or <8.0 kPa and pulmonary hypertension, should use long-term oxygen for 15 hours each day. This prevents progression to cor pulmonale (heart failure secondary to high pulmonary vessel pressures) but does not improve symptoms. Ambulatory oxygen can be given to those who desaturate when walking, while short-burst oxygen is for symptomatic relief only.
- **Manage exacerbations.** Appropriate use of inhaled steroids, bronchodilators, and vaccines should be used to reduce the incidence of exacerbations. The impact of exacerbations should be minimized by:
    - Giving self-management advice on responding promptly to the symptoms of an exacerbation
    - Starting appropriate treatment with oral corticosteroids and/or antibiotics
    - Use of NIV when indicated
    - Use of hospital-at-home or assisted-discharge schemes.

SHORT CASE

Mr Marley (from the previous case) is admitted to hospital 5 months after he is diagnosed with COPD by the respiratory physicians. He has become very short of breath, confused, and unable to complete full sentences. His daughter explains that he has been deteriorating gradually over the past week and was due to see the respiratory physicians again next week. He is immediately given high-flow 100% oxygen. An arterial blood gas (ABG) is performed and shows pO_2 = 6.2 kPa, pCO_2 = 7.3 kPa, pH = 7.28, bicarbonate = 33 mM, base excess = -1 (on 15 L of O_2). A chest radiograph shows no signs of consolidation (pneumonia) or pulmonary oedema. His ECG, FBC, and serum biochemistry are normal.

What is the problem? How would you proceed?

Mr Marley's ABG shows **type II respiratory failure** (Pao_2 <8 kPa and $Paco_2$ >6.5 kPa). With his history and ABG results (indicating a degree of metabolic compensation but with an acute acidosis), this is an acute-on-chronic picture.

Type II respiratory failure is **a medical emergency.** Untreated, the rising CO_2 will narcose the patient, who will fall into an irreversible coma and die. Treatment involves:

1. **Controlled oxygen therapy.** The high CO_2 that defines type II respiratory failure often means that patients no longer rely on CO_2 levels to stimulate breathing. If you give 100% oxygen, you risk causing a respiratory arrest so this must be stopped in Mr Marley's case. Instead, give controlled oxygen (24–35% using a special Venturi connector on the oxygen mask) aiming for oxygen saturations of 88–92%. Perform repeated blood gases, looking for a drop in $Paco_2$.

2. **Improve ventilation.** If the CO_2 does not drop with controlled oxygen therapy, ensure the airway is fully patent and involve the relevant physicians as the patient will need NIV (usually only available in select locations with appropriately trained nurses, not on every ward).

3. **Treat the underlying cause.** Assess for reversible causes of reduced gas exchange (e.g. pneumothorax—which is a contraindication to NIV, pneumonia, pulmonary oedema, PE) and reversible causes of reduced ventilation (e.g. airway obstruction due to reduced consciousness, opiate medication).

SHORT CASE

Miss Chanda is a 27-year-old factory worker from Zambia who has been referred to the medical admissions unit of her hospital because of severe shortness of breath, which has been present for the last few days. She finds she is always breathless but it is worse with even mild exertion such as walking. She has felt very weak for the last few days and has had a dry cough and fever. On hindsight, she thinks she has probably been losing weight for the past few months. Her past medical history is unremarkable and she takes no regular medications.

On examination, Miss Chanda has a temperature of 37.6°C and a respiratory rate of 25/min. Her JVP is not raised, there is no peripheral oedema, and both heart sounds are present without any added sounds. There are fine crackles heard over the entirety of both lung fields. The rest of the examination is entirely normal. Her oxygen saturations are 90% on air but the attending nurse comments that when Miss Chanda came back from walking to the toilet, her saturations had dropped to 82%. A chest radiograph shows diffuse interstitial shadowing throughout both lung fields.

What is the likely diagnosis? What tests will you arrange?

The clinical picture of dry cough, shortness of breath, low oxygen saturation/desaturation on exercise, and diffuse interstitial shadowing throughout the lungs on a chest radiograph in a young patient from Africa should always make you suspicious of **Pneumocystis jiroveci pneumonia** (previously known as *Pneumocystis carinii* pneumonia, or PCP). *Pneumocystis* is an opportunistic organism that rarely causes problems in healthy adults but commonly causes pneumonia in immunosuppressed patients. Indeed, PCP is a common complication of patients with AIDS. It is diagnosed by performing microscopy (+ silver staining) and culture on sputum and bronchoalveolar lavage samples.

If you suspect *Pneumocystis* pneumonia, you should arrange to test for two other infections:

- **HIV.** Offer Miss Chanda an HIV test. If this is positive, you will need to check her CD4+ lymphocyte levels and viral load, as these dictate the need for antiretroviral therapy.

- **Tuberculosis**, as this is a frequent cause of pulmonary pathology in HIV-positive patients. Testing is by microscopy (+ Ziehl–Neelsen staining) and culture of sputum and/or bronchoalveolar lavage samples.

SHORT CASE

Mrs Betts is a 48-year-old magistrate who attends your clinic complaining of persistent breathlessness that has been getting worse over the last year. It is worst when she takes her dog for a brisk walk, but is always present, even at rest. She denies any cough, weight loss, or night sweats. She smokes 'the odd cigarette' at social events, but never more than five cigarettes a month. A recent blood test ordered by her referring GP shows:

Haematology		Biochemistry			
Hb	115 g/L	Glucose	4.8 mM	HbA1c	5%
RBC	4.7×10^{12} cells/L	Cholesterol	4.3 mM	ESR	72 mm/h
WCC	8.0×10^{9} cells/L	LDL	2.2 mM		
		HDL	2.1 mM		

Her past medical history includes rheumatoid arthritis, for which she takes methotrexate.

On examination, you notice swelling of the metacarpophalangeal joints (MCPJs) and ulnar deviation of her fingers on both hands. Her pulse is 80 bpm and regular, her blood pressure is 120/80 mmHg, and she is apyrexial. There are no signs of peripheral or central cyanosis, anaemia, or lymphadenopathy. Her trachea is central and her apex beat undisplaced. Heart sounds I and II are present with no added sounds, and no carotid bruits. Her lungs expand symmetrically and show normal resonance to percussion. However, very fine crackles can be heard all over her lung fields. She has no peripheral oedema and her abdominal and neurological examinations are entirely normal.

Flow spirometry reveals FVC = 65% and FEV$_1$ = 88%. An ECG shows sinus rhythm with no abnormalities.

What is the most likely cause of Mrs Betts's shortness of breath? How would you confirm this?

Mrs Betts does not have any features that are strongly suggestive of the 'most likely' or 'must exclude' diagnoses listed in Figure 10.2. Her flow spirometry suggests a *restrictive lung pathology* as her expiratory rate is normal (FEV$_1$ >70%) but her lung capacity is reduced (FVC <70% predicted value)—in other words, the problem is not getting air out but how much air her lungs can hold. The fine crackles heard all over her lungs, combined with her flow spirometry and absence of another obvious diagnosis, suggest that Mrs Betts has **interstitial lung disease.** Interstitial lung disease can be caused by congenital diseases (e.g. neurofibromatosis, Gaucher disease), systemic inflammatory diseases (e.g. rheumatoid arthritis, ankylosing spondylitis, sarcoidosis), chemical irritation (e.g. silica, asbestos, coal dust, chlorine), drugs (e.g. methotrexate, amiodarone), allergic reactions (e.g. bird-fancier's lung), radiation, or the cause may not be known (e.g. usual interstitial pneumonitis).

The best way to confirm Mrs Betts's postulated diagnosis of interstitial lung disease is a high-resolution chest CT scan. Radiologists can diagnose interstitial lung disease with high sensitivity and specificity by looking for characteristic linear reticular opacities and a ground-glass appearance of the lung.

Mrs Betts should switch from methotrexate to another immunosuppresive agent in order to control her rheumatoid arthritis. Although this is unlikely to improve her condition significantly, it will at least prevent further deterioration, particularly if the fibrosis was mainly due to the methotrexate rather than the rheumatoid arthritis (which explains her elevated ESR).

SHORT CASE

Claire is a 15-year-old student who presents to her GP complaining of general fatigue and shortness of breath when she exercises. She has recently found herself feeling unusually tired towards the end of the day and complains that she is more breathless than usual during her netball training. She does not smoke, denies any cough, and is never woken at night feeling short of breath. She has never travelled further than Italy, and is otherwise fit and well. She has no family history of respiratory disease. When specifically asked, she reveals with some embarrassment that her periods are 'a bit heavy' but she denies her faeces ever being dark or bloody. Physical examination is unremarkable. Spirometry reveals an FVC = 90% and FER = 88%.

What tests should the GP arrange? What is the most likely diagnosis?

This patient complains of fatigue and admits to having menorrhagia (heavy menstrual periods), in the absence of any of the clinical features of respiratory or cardiac causes of breathlessness. It is therefore very likely that this patient is **anaemic**, as the most common cause for anaemia in menstruating women is menorrhagia. The GP should order an FBC (which will probably reveal a microcytic hypochromic anaemia, compatible with an iron-deficiency anaemia) and clotting studies (to rule out a clotting disorder that may be causing or exacerbating her menorrhagia). If a gynaecology referral does not reveal any abnormality causing the menorrhagia, the patient will probably benefit from pharmacological treatment. NICE guidelines recommend a levonorgestrel-releasing intrauterine device (LNG-IUD) or the combined oral contraceptive pill.

SHORT CASE

Mr Andreyov is a 42-year-old investment banker who presents to your clinic complaining of shortness of breath. He says the sensation of breathlessness is always present. He doesn't think it is connected, but mentions that he has found it increasingly difficult to type at his computer recently and he has noticed some twitching of his thighs that he initially put down to stress. He has no relevant past medical history and is not on any medication. He has never smoked and drinks approximately 10 units of wine a week with evening meals. He sleeps well and has not noticed any change in his appetite nor any bloody or dark faeces or urine. He is worried he may be developing heart problems because he admits his diet is not very healthy and he doesn't exercise enough.

Cardiovascular, respiratory, and abdominal examination is unremarkable. Neurological examination reveals that the first dorsal interossei on both hands are wasted. In addition, you note fasciculations over both his thighs, reduced power (4/5) on knee flexion, and an upgoing plantar reflex. Flow spirometry reveals FVC = 60% and FEV$_1$ = 58%.

What important diagnosis should you consider in this patient?

Mr Andreyov has presented with shortness of breath and a history suggestive of weakness/poor coordination in distal muscle groups of his upper limbs. He has wasting of his hand muscles (suggesting a lower motor neuron or muscular pathology). He also has fasciculations in his right leg (suggesting a lower motor neuron pathology) but an upgoing plantar reflex (suggesting an upper motor neuron pathology). The combination of upper and lower motor neuron pathology signs in any patient should always arouse the suspicion of **motor neuron disease** and warrants referral to a neurologist. The shortness of breath is likely to be due to diaphragmatic weakness, usually a late sign of this disease.

SHORT CASE

Mr O'Hara is a 27-year-old former paratrooper who presents to your clinic complaining of shortness of breath. He first noticed this a month ago when he was jogging, but says he now feels breathless with minimal exertion. He has not had a cough and has never smoked. He drinks a few pints of ale every weekend. His only past medical history is a fractured right tibia 2 years ago. He has not noticed any changes in his bowel habit or urine, but admits that he has probably lost weight over the past few months.

On examination, you can feel several enlarged lymph nodes in the right anterior cervical chain of his neck. His right lung shows decreased expansion and is dull to percussion in the bases. Vocal fremitus is markedly reduced on the right. His cardiovascular, abdominal, and neurological examinations are all normal.

What diagnosis should you consider for Mr O'Hara? What are your next steps?

Mr O'Hara gives a history of worsening shortness of breath and weight loss. His respiratory examination reveals lymphadenopathy of the neck and signs consistent with a right-sided **pleural effusion**. The combination of weight loss, lymphadenopathy, and pleural effusion should make you think of a **malignant pleural effusion** caused by infiltration of the pleural space by metastatic cancer cells.

Your next step should be to arrange a **chest radiograph**. If this confirms a right-sided pleural effusion, the effusion should be sampled (**thoracocentesis**) to determine if the fluid in the pleural space is due to changes in osmotic forces (*transudate*, with protein <25 g/L) or due to infiltration of the pleural space by metastatic cancer cells, infectious agents or inflammatory proteins (*exudate*, with protein >35 g/L). A finding of protein between 25 and 35 g/L is considered indeterminate and you should then use Light's criteria (see Chapter 8).

You should also arrange for a **lymph node fine needle aspiration (FNA)**, as Mr O'Hara's history of weight loss should alert you to the possibility of a malignancy.

Mr O'Hara's chest radiograph showed a massive pleural effusion in his right lung. Thoracocentesis showed it to be an exudate, with low glucose and abnormal-looking lymphocytes. A lymph node biopsy confirmed the presence of binucleated lymphocytes (Reed–Sternberg cells), which are diagnostic of Hodgkin's lymphoma.

Viva questions

The notes of a patient you are asked to see state that his past medical history is of 'asthma/COPD'. Is such a diagnosis possible?

It is obviously possible to have both COPD and asthma at the same time, but it is much more likely that a clear diagnosis has simply not been made. Asthma and COPD are very different diseases and should not be confused:

- Asthma is a *reversible* and *transient* obstruction of the airways caused by excessive mucus production, airway inflammation, and constriction of the bronchi. Flow spirometry shows only obstructive changes (i.e. drop in FEV_1 <70% but normal FVC, that is, a reduced rate of air flow but a normal lung capacity), although it may be normal when the patient is not symptomatic. The FEV_1 improves with bronchodilators, hence it is 'reversible'. It is usually accompanied by a cough and is often worse at night. It is often linked to triggers such as pollen, dust mites, or cold air and is common in patients who are atopic (i.e. who suffer from multiple diseases caused by excessive IgE-mediated hypersensitivity, such as eczema, hay fever, or urticaria).

- COPD is an *irreversible* and *progressive* obstruction of the airways. There is a history of chronic bronchitis and/or emphysema. Flow spirometry shows obstructive changes (i.e. drop in FEV_1 <70%) that are largely irreversible after bronchodilator therapy. There is often also a degree of restrictive change (i.e. FVC <70%). Patients are usually older and have a smoking history of >10 pack years.

Which different classes of inhaled drugs are used in obstructive airways disease (asthma and/or COPD)? What is the mechanism of action of each drug?

1 **Short-acting bronchodilators**
   - Salbutamol (UK: blue, Ventolin): selective β_2-agonist. Acts on a G-protein-coupled receptor, activating adenylate cyclase and increasing the formation of cAMP, leading to relaxation of the smooth muscle lining the airways.
   - Ipratropium (UK: white + green, Atrovent): antimuscarinic/cholinergic. Antagonizes muscarinic acetylcholine receptors in the airways, preventing parasympathetic-mediated smooth muscle contraction. Often used in COPD, but less often in asthma.
   - Salbutamol + ipratropium (UK: white + orange, Combivent).

2 **Inhaled steroids**
   - For example beclometasone, budesonide (UK: brown inhalers), fluticasone (UK: orange inhaler). Work by affecting intracellular transcription of various proteins to reduce inflammation in the airways. Used in asthma and COPD as second-line treatment.

3 **Long-acting bronchodilators**
   - Salmeterol, formoterol, vilanterol: long-acting β_2-agonist (LABA). Mechanism like the short-acting variant.
   - Tiotropium: long-acting muscarinic agents (LAMA). Mechanism like the short-acting variant. Used in COPD but not asthma.
   - Long-acting bronchodilators can also be combined with inhaled steroids, e.g. budesonide + formoterol (UK: red, Symbicort) or fluticasone + salmeterol (UK: purple, Seretide).

CONTINUED ➤

CONTINUED

4   **Oxygen.** Don't forget that this is a drug! It may be given acutely, e.g. in an ambulance or in hospital, or long-term, e.g. in severe COPD.

Oral drugs are also sometimes used, including oral steroids, xanthine derivatives (theophylline, aminophylline), leukotriene antagonists (montelukast), biologics (e.g. omalizumab, a monoclonal antibody targeted at IgE), and phosphodiesterase inhibitors (e.g. roflumilast).

What is the difference between bronchitis and pneumonia, and between broncho- and lobar pneumonia?

Both are lower respiratory tract illnesses, but bronchitis is a disease of the airways whereas pneumonia is a disease of the alveoli. In bronchitis, airways inflammation leads to excess mucus production and partial airway obstruction, thereby causing cough but not usually breathlessness. In pneumonia, pus accumulates in the alveoli impairing gas exchange and appearing as consolidation on a chest radiograph.

Pneumonia can be classified by the pattern of anatomical involvement. In bronchopneumonia, focal areas are affected in a patchy distribution that may involve one or more lobes. Lobar pneumonia, as the name suggests, involves most or all of a single lobe.

Why do we get short of breath at altitude? What is the pharmacological mechanism of action of the altitude sickness drug acetazolamide (Diamox)? How might this influence breathlessness at altitude?

At altitude, there is a lower partial pressure of oxygen in the environment. Thus there is a smaller concentration gradient driving oxygen from air in the alveoli into the blood. As a result there is a reduction in gas exchange, leading to hypoxia. This causes breathlessness and compensatory hyperventilation to correct the hypoxia. The hyperventilation causes a respiratory alkalosis, which makes one feel lightheaded. One either feels breathless (from hypoxia) or dizzy (from hyperventilation).

Acetazolamide inhibits carbonic anhydrase, an enzyme that catalyses the conversion of CO_2 and H_2O into HCO_3^- and H^+. There are two theories as to how this might alleviate breathlessness. The first suggests the inhibition of carbonic anhydrase leads to a build-up of CO_2, stimulating the respiratory centre and increasing the ventilatory drive. The other theory suggests that the inhibition of carbonic anhydrase in the kidneys leads to a bicarbonaturia (loss of bicarbonate in the urine) and hence a metabolic acidosis (loss of bicarbonate drives carbonic anhydrase to produce more of it to compensate, and as a consequence, more H^+), which offsets the respiratory alkalosis due to hyperventilation at altitude. The acidosis caused by acetazolamide enables one to hyperventilate at altitude (thus reducing hypoxia and shortness of breath) without becoming lightheaded from the alkalosis that would otherwise result from hyperventilating.

There has been a large decrease in the incidence of epiglottitis in the last 20 years, particularly in children. How can you explain this?

Historically, epiglottitis primarily affected children and was a severe, sometimes fatal, condition. It is nearly always due to bacterial infection by *Haemophilus influenzae* B (HiB). The development and introduction of a HiB vaccine into the UK vaccination schedule in the mid-1990s has led to a decrease in both meningitis (another condition often caused by HiB) and epiglottitis.

What is the difference between type I and type II respiratory failure? What are some of the causes?

Respiratory failure is defined as impairment of pulmonary gas exchange sufficient to result in hypoxaemia (Pao_2 <8 kPa or 60 mmHg) and/or hypercapnia ($Paco_2$ >6 kPa or 45 mmHg). It is divided into two types depending on whether CO_2 is expelled (and therefore normal or low) or retained (and therefore raised):

Type I respiratory failure

- Pathology: this is a problem with *one* gas (oxygen), i.e. **hypoxaemic respiratory failure.** It is caused by any disease pathology affecting how much oxygen can get into the pulmonary blood either because of problems with gas exchange at the alveolar membrane or because of ventilation of the lungs.
- Causes: any lung disease, e.g. asthma, COPD, pneumonia, pulmonary fibrosis, pulmonary oedema.

Type II respiratory failure

- Pathology: this is a problem with *two* gases (oxygen and carbon dioxide), i.e. **hypercapnic respiratory failure** (low Pao_2 and a raised $Paco_2$). This is caused by **ventilatory failure,** i.e. impairment of the respiratory 'bellows', resulting in alveolar hypoventilation. CO_2 is highly soluble, so problems affecting gas exchange across the alveolar membrane will usually affect oxygenation of blood but not CO_2 removal. If CO_2 builds up it implies that air isn't being shifted in/out of the lungs adequately i.e. there is a ventilation problem.
- Causes:
  - Decreased respiratory drive, e.g. opiates, central neurological damage (stroke, head trauma)
  - Impaired lung movements, e.g. reduced compliance and hyperinflated lungs with increased dead space (in COPD), chest wall deformity (e.g. kyphoscoliosis), increased chest wall load (obesity), neuromuscular impairment (e.g. motor neuron disease)

What is the difference between a 'pink puffer' and a 'blue bloater'?

Note that these terms are not synonymous with type I and type II respiratory failure! They are outdated terms but still sometimes used on the wards to describe two distinct clinical pictures that arise in chronic lung disease (e.g. COPD), although this is of course a simplification and every patient will be different:

- 'Pink puffers' respond to hypercapnia and hypoxaemia by increasing their respiratory rate, resulting in normal Pao_2 levels and a 'pink' appearance. As a result of the hard work to maintain their oxygenation, they often have a barrel-shaped, hyperinflated chest and may breathe through pursed lips. They nonetheless complain of shortness of breath on mild exertion. Broadly speaking, their prognosis is better than that of 'blue bloaters'.
- In 'blue bloaters' the presence of chronically high $Paco_2$ levels results in desensitization of the respiratory centre to $Paco_2$ and chronic cyanosis, giving them a 'blue' appearance. They are chronic CO_2 retainers, becoming reliant on their hypoxic (rather than hypercapnic) drive. They are often bloated because of widespread peripheral oedema caused by right heart failure secondary to the lung problems (cor pulmonale). In general, their prognosis is poor.

What is Eisenmenger's syndrome?

Eisenmenger's syndrome describes the situation where a left-to-right cardiac shunt becomes a right-to-left (or bidirectional) shunt. It follows a sequence of events beginning with a left-to-right cardiac shunt, due to, for example, a ventricular and/or atrial septal defect, or patent ductus arteriosus. Over time this causes progressive pulmonary hypertension as the delicate pulmonary vasculature is subjected to blood emerging from the left ventricle, via the shunt, at greater pressures than normal pulmonary pressures. Eventually the pulmonary hypertension provides enough resistance to reverse the direction of the shunt.

Ultimately it leads to heart failure and can only be cured by heart–lung transplant. Women of childbearing age must be warned about the increased mortality in pregnancy associated with Eisenmenger's syndrome (>50%) and strongly advised against it. This condition has become relatively rare in the UK due to early surgical correction of cardiac defects (indeed this is the rationale behind early correction of such defects).

Which muscles are responsible for inspiration and expiration: (a) at rest and (b) during exercise or respiratory distress? (see Table 10.1).

Table 10.1 **Muscles responsible for inspiration and expiration**

	Inspiration	Expiration
At rest	Diaphragm External intercostals	(Passive—natural elastic recoil of lung)
During exercise/ respiratory distress	Diaphragm External intercostals Scalene Sternocleidomastoids	Natural elastic recoil of lung PLUS: Internal intercostals Abdominal muscles (rectus and transversus abdominus, internal and external obliques)

What is the differential diagnosis for bibasal crepitations? Which features in the history and examination will help you to distinguish them? (see Table 10.2.)

Table 10.2 **Differential diagnosis for bibasal crepitations**

Cause of crepitations	Key clue
Pulmonary oedema	Displaced apex, raised JVP, ankle oedema, orthopnoea, old age, history of ischaemic heart disease
Interstitial lung disease	Reduced expansion, clubbing, crepitations that do not vary with cough
Bronchiectasis	Chronic productive cough, wheeze, and crepitations that vary with cough, clubbing
Pneumonia	Acute productive cough, fever, chest pain, bronchial breathing, dull percussion

What is your differential diagnosis for shortness of breath in a postoperative patient? What key clues will help you identify the most likely cause? How will you manage each cause? (Table 10.3)

Table 10.3 **Common causes of postoperative dyspnoea**

Cause	Key clue	Management
Pulmonary oedema	Displaced apex, raised JVP, ankle oedema, frothy sputum ± evidence of MI on ECG or biochemically (troponins)	Sit patient up, furosemide, oxygen, nitrates
PE	Tachycardia, signs of DVT in leg, pleuritic chest pain, fever. Onset typically 10 days after surgery	LMWH, start warfarin, TED (anti-embolism) stockings to prevent more DVTs
Atelectasis	Crepitations, mild fever, fruity and painful cough. Onset typically during first 48 h after surgery	Analgesia, oxygen, and chest physiotherapy
Pneumonia	Productive cough, fever, chest pain, bronchial breathing, dull percussion, increased vocal resonance, consolidation on chest radiograph	Antibiotics, oxygen (titrated to appropriate saturations) and IV fluids (titrated to appropriate heart rate and blood pressure)
Pneumothorax	Area of lung with decreased air entry, hyper-resonance and air in pleural space on chest radiograph	Chest drain (if meets appropriate British Thoracic Society criteria)

LMWH, low molecular weight heparin.

Once a patient has been diagnosed with chronic heart failure, there are several medications that can help reduce their mortality. What are the key trials demonstrating mortality benefit in chronic heart failure?

- **ACE inhibitors:** the **SAVE**[1] and **SOLVD**[2] trials both showed that ACE inhibitors can significantly reduce mortality from chronic heart failure, from 8–28% depending on how symptomatic the patient is (more symptomatic patients gain more benefit). In patients who cannot tolerate ACE inhibitors because of their side effects (e.g. cough), the **ELITE II**[3] study and **Valsartan Heart Failure Trial**[4] have shown that **ARBs** are as effective as ACE inhibitors in reducing mortality. However, a third trial (**RESOLVD**[5]) had to be stopped because of increased mortality in the group receiving the ARB.

- **β-Blockers:** Several trials[6] including **CIBIS-II**[7] and **MERIT-HF**[8] have shown that β-blockers reduce mortality from chronic heart failure by about 25%.

- **Spironolactone:** the **RALES**[9] trial found that the aldosterone receptor spironolactone reduced mortality from chronic heart failure by about 30%.

[1] Pfeffer MA, Braunwald E, Moye LA, Basta L, Brown EJJ, Cuddy TE, *et al*. Effect of captopril on mortality and morbidity in patients with left ventricular dysfunction after myocardial infarction. Results of the survival and ventricular enlargement trial. The SAVE Investigators. *New Engl J Med*, 1992;327: 669–677.

CONTINUED ➤

CONTINUED

2 SOLVD Investigators. Effect of enalapril on survival in patients with reduced left ventricular ejection fractions and congestive heart failure. The SOLVD Investigators. *New Engl J Med*, 1991;325: 293–302.

3 Pitt B, Poole-Wilson PA, Segal R, Martinez FA, Dickstein K, Camm AJ, *et al*. Effect of losartan compared with captopril on mortality in patients with symptomatic heart failure: randomised trial—the Losartan Heart Failure Survival Study ELITE II. *Lancet*, 2000;3551: 1582–1587.

4 Cohn JN, Tognoni G. A randomized trial of the angiotensin-receptor blocker valsartan in chronic heart failure. *New Engl J Med*, 2001;345: 1667–1675.

5 Tsuyuki RT, Yusuf S, Rouleau JL, Maggioni AP, McKelvie RS, Wiecek EM, *et al*. Combination neurohormonal blockade with ACE inhibitors, angiotensin II antagonists and beta-blockers in patients with congestive heart failure: design of the Randomized Evaluation of Strategies for Left Ventricular Dysfunction (RESOLVD) Pilot Study. *Can J Cardiol*, 1997;13: 1166–1174.

6 Doughty RN, Rodgers A, Sharpe N, MacMahon S. Effects of beta-blocker therapy on mortality in patients with heart failure. A systematic overview of randomized controlled trials. *Eur Heart J*, 1997;18: 560–565.

7 CIBIS-II Investigators. The Cardiac Insufficiency Bisoprolol Study II (CIBIS-II): a randomised trial. *Lancet*, 1999;353: 9–13.

8 Hjalmarson A, Goldstein S, Fagerberg B, Wedel H, Waagstein F, Kjekshus J, *et al*. Effects of controlled-release metoprolol on total mortality, hospitalizations, and well-being in patients with heart failure: the Metoprolol CR/XL Randomized Intervention Trial in Congestive Heart Failure (MERIT-HF). MERIT-HF Study Group. *JAMA*, 2000;283: 1295–1302.

9 Pitt B, Zannad F, Remme WJ, Cody R, Castaigne A, Perez A, *et al*. The effect of spironolactone on morbidity and mortality in patients with severe heart failure. Randomized Aldactone Evaluation Study Investigators. *New Engl J Med*, 1999;341: 709–717.

Single Best Answers

1. Which of the following statements about chronic obstructive pulmonary disease (COPD) is false?

a. COPD is caused by smoking
b. COPD can be caused by α-1 antitrypsin deficiency
c. COPD often responds to salbutamol inhalers

d. Patients with COPD should generally not be given 100% oxygen
e. COPD is a risk factor for pneumothorax

2. A patient with shortness of breath is diagnosed, after chest radiograph and CT scans, as having hypersensitivity pneumonitis. Which of their medications could be responsible?

a. Warfarin
b. Simvastatin
c. Atenolol

d. Amiodarone
e. Furosemide

3. A patient presenting to the Emergency Department with shortness of breath is diagnosed as having an infective exacerbation of their chronic obstructive pulmonary disease (COPD). Treatment should include which of the following?

a. Non-steroidal anti-inflammatory drugs (NSAIDs)
b. Steroids

c. Immunoglobulin
d. Gentamicin
e. Metronidazole

4. Which of the following is contraindicated in chronic heart failure?

a. Aspirin
b. Bisoprolol
c. Ramipril

d. Amlodipine
e. Diltiazem

5. Which of the following findings on spirometry would be consistent with a purely restrictive lung disease?

a. FEV_1 <80% predicted, FVC >80% predicted, FEV_1:FVC <70%
b. FEV_1 <80% predicted, FVC <80% predicted, FEV_1:FVC ~70%

c. FEV_1 >80% predicted, FVC >80% predicted, FEV_1:FVC >70%
d. FEV_1 >80% predicted, FVC <80% predicted, FEV_1:FVC >70%
e. None of the above

Breast lump

Core case

 Read through the sections in the case boxes, covering up the sections that follow so that you don't see the answer. At the end of each case box, try to answer the question before reading on.

CORE CASE

Miss Collins is a 28-year-old teacher who presents to her GP because she has noticed a lump in her breast.

What is your differential diagnosis for a breast lump?

Consider which diagnoses are more or less likely, and try to stratify your differential according to the age of the patient.

The four most common diagnoses for a breast lump are:

- Benign cystic change (also known as fibrocystic change, fibroadenosis, or benign breast change)
- Fibroadenoma
- Cyst
- Carcinoma

If we consider women of all ages, there are a number of other potential diagnoses:

- Fat necrosis
- Periductal mastitis
- Abscess
- Galactocele
- Phyllodes tumour
- Sarcoma
- Duct papilloma
- 'Non-breast' lumps, e.g. lipoma, sebaceous cyst, prominent costal cartilage/rib.

The age of the patient is one of the most useful pieces of information for narrowing the differential (see Figure 11.1). As an approximate guide, the most common diagnoses in the following age groups are:

- **<30 years:** physiologically normal lumpy breast; benign cystic change; fibroadenoma; abscess (if breast-feeding); galactocele (if breast-feeding)
- **30–45 years:** benign cystic change; cyst; abscess (especially smokers); carcinoma
- **45–60 years:** cyst; abscess (smokers); carcinoma
- **>60 years:** carcinoma

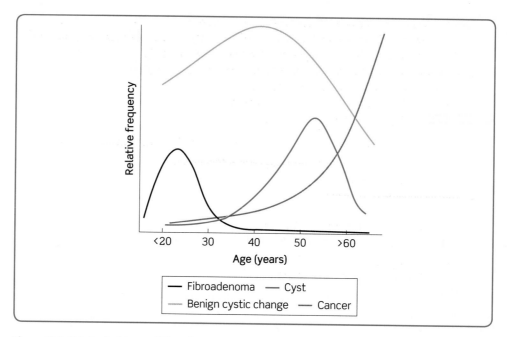

Figure 11.1 Relative incidence of fibroadenoma, benign cystic change, cyst, and carcinoma by age.

▲ Note: It is worth emphasizing that breast cancer is possible in all ages, is common, and is potentially very serious. Therefore you must exclude it in any presentation of breast lump, regardless of how benign it seems. Failure to diagnose breast cancer is one of the most common malpractice claims in the USA.

Are there any diagnoses that you would only encounter in breast-feeding women?

Galactoceles may occur during or shortly after the cessation of lactation. They may present as a firm mass (often subareolar) and are caused by the obstruction of a lactiferous duct. The duct gradually becomes more distended with milk and epithelial cells, and may rarely be complicated by a secondary infection leading to abscess formation. Clinically, a galactocele is very similar to a cyst on examination.

In addition, lactating women are predisposed to **mastitis** (whether or not they have a galactocele). The causative organisms are usually skin commensals such as *Staphylococcus aureus* or *Staphylococcus epidermidis*—this is in contrast to the periductal mastitis and abscess formation seen in older women, in whom anaerobic bacteria may also be implicated.

The vast majority of women who present with a breast lump will be concerned that they have breast cancer. As part of a thorough history-taking it is obviously important to enquire about risk factors.

What are the main risk factors for breast cancer?

Two of the greatest risk factors for breast cancer are being female and increasing age. Otherwise, the following are recognized as important factors:

- **Previous breast cancer**

- **Family history of breast cancer.**[†] Suspicions should be raised if:
  - Three close blood relatives (on the same side of the family) develop breast cancer at any age
  - Two close blood relatives develop breast cancer before the age of 60
  - One close blood relative develops breast cancer before the age of 40
  - One male close blood relative develops breast cancer
  - One close blood relative develops bilateral breast cancer
- **Previous ovarian, endometrial, or bowel cancer**
- **Irradiation to the chest wall** (such as mantle irradiation for Hodgkin's lymphoma)
- **Increased exposure to oestrogens,** especially cyclical stimulation:
  - Early menarche (<13 years)
  - Late menopause (>51 years)
  - Nulliparity
  - Having a first child after the age of about 30 years
  - Not breast-feeding
  - Hormone replacement therapy (HRT)[‡]
  - Use of combined oral contraceptive pill (COCP)
  - Obesity.

The first stage is to take a history from Miss Collins.

What are the relevant pieces of information to obtain from the history?

While addressing the history of the presenting complaint, you will need to establish:

- **How long has the lump been there? Why was it first noticed?** An abscess or cyst can appear very rapidly, whereas tumours such as fibroadenomas or carcinomas typically grow more slowly. Of course, it is perfectly possible for a mass such as a carcinoma to be present for a long time before it is noticed. It may be that a lump was noticed during routine self-examination, or by a partner, or because of associated skin changes, or perhaps due to pain.

- **Has there been any breast trauma?** Trauma, whether accidental (such as a seat-belt injury) or iatrogenic (e.g. aspiration of a cyst, recent breast surgery), predisposes to fat necrosis and infective sequelae such as an abscess.

- **Has the lump got bigger, smaller, or stayed the same size? Are changes related to the menses?** Just as an abscess or cyst can appear 'almost overnight', they can also undergo rapid increases in size. Lumps that undergo cyclical changes in size or character (for example, becoming more tender) are far more likely to represent benign cystic breast disease than a more sinister condition such as carcinoma.

---

† Remember that the vast majority of women presenting with a breast lump will be concerned that they have cancer—even if they do not voice these concerns explicitly. A frank but sensitive discussion of any familial cases of breast cancer serves to illustrate your familiarity with these concerns and expectations. Although many patients will consider that breast cancer in their 82-year-old grandmother constitutes a significant family history, this is not the case. While it is important to establish how many family members have been affected by breast cancer, it is also informative to ascertain how many women in the family have *not* had breast cancer. For example, a history of an aunt and a sister with breast cancer becomes less significant if the patient is one of 10 sisters and has 7 aunts.

‡ Not only does HRT usage increase the risk of breast carcinoma, but it also extends the normal age range of benign cystic disease and cysts—which are not normally seen in postmenopausal women. Combined HRT (oestrogen and a progestogen) increases the risk of breast cancer more than oestrogen-only HRT.

- **Is the lump painful?** Benign cystic change, acute mastitis, and abscesses classically cause breast pain and tenderness. Benign cystic change may, however, be painless. Simple cysts may or may not be tender. While it is perfectly possible for a carcinoma to be painful, it is more common for carcinoma to present as a non-tender lump. Indeed, breast pain (mastalgia) as an isolated symptom is rarely a presenting feature of breast carcinoma.

- **Has she noticed any skin changes on her breasts?** Warm erythematous skin should raise your suspicions of an infective or inflammatory process such as mastitis or an abscess, or perhaps an inflammatory breast carcinoma (rare). The patient may have noticed puckering of the overlying skin ('peau d'orange'), and this suggests carcinoma until proven otherwise.

- **Has she noticed any changes to her nipples?** Some women will naturally have inverted nipples, but any recent distortion of the nipple also hints at carcinoma.

- **Has she noticed any discharge from her nipples?** A nipple discharge in the context of a breast mass is suggestive of:
  - carcinoma (bloody discharge)
  - intraductal papilloma (serous or serosanguinous discharge)
  - periductal mastitis arising from duct ectasia (green, brown, or yellow discharge) or
  - a galactocele (milky discharge).

  → Unilateral nipple discharge is less likely to be physiological.

- **Is the patient otherwise fit and well?** The majority of patients presenting with a breast lump will have no other symptoms. Patients with mastitis or an abscess may be febrile. Breast carcinoma rarely presents with generalized systemic symptoms—such as weight loss, night sweats, and fevers—that are sometimes seen with other forms of malignancy. They may, however, present with signs of metastasis, such as back pain (spinal metastases). This is also relevant in assessing their fitness for any treatment (e.g. surgery, chemo- or radiotherapy), should they require it.

- **Does the patient have any of the risk factors mentioned earlier?**

Miss Collins reports that she noticed the lump in her right breast 2 days ago while she was showering. The lump has not changed in size or location since she first noticed it. It is non-tender. There is no reported history of breast trauma and she is otherwise fit and well. She is a non-smoker and is taking no medications. She started having periods when she was 13 years old, but has no children and has no significant gynaecological history. Her stepmother was diagnosed with ovarian cancer at the age of 52, and her paternal grandmother died of breast cancer aged 79.

You perform a breast examination.

What will you look for on *inspection* of the breasts?

The key features to look for are:

- **Asymmetry:** many women will have one breast that is larger than the other, but any new change is significant.

- **Contours:** any disruption to the normally smooth curvature of the breast is suspicious, although it could simply be due to fibrocystic change or naturally lumpy breasts.

- **Skin changes:** look for erythema, ulceration, dimpling, peau d'orange. Radiotherapy tattoos (small black/blue dots) may be visible in patients who have had previous treatment.

- **Nipple changes or discharge:** note any new inversion of the nipple, and the colour of any discharge.

Miss Collins' breasts appear normal on gross inspection. There is no asymmetry, skin abnormality, or nipple inversion. Having inspected Miss Collins' breasts, the GP moves on to palpation. Having palpated the normal breast, axillary tail, and axilla, she then asks Miss Collins to point to the lump in her right breast.

As with any lump, it is important to characterize the site, size, shape, surface, borders, and consistency.

Which of these features are most useful for distinguishing between a carcinoma, fibroadenoma, cyst, and benign cystic disease? What other information should the GP hope to gain from the examination?

The four most common presentations of a breast lump (across all age groups) classically differ, in the ways listed in Table 11.1.

Table 11.1 The four most common presentations of a breast lump

Lump	Surface	Borders	Consistency	Mobility	Fixity[a]	Lymphadenopathy
Solitary cyst	Smooth	Distinct	Firm to lax	No	No	No
Fibroadenoma	Smooth	Distinct	Rubbery	Yes	No	No
Benign cystic change	Irregular	Indistinct	Mixed	No	No	No
Carcinoma[b]	Irregular	Indistinct	Hard	No	Maybe	Maybe

[a] Fixity or tethering to skin or underlying muscle: It will not be possible to move intradermal masses such as sebaceous cysts independently of the overlying skin. If a deeper mass shows the same fixity to skin and/or underlying pectoralis muscle (assessed by asking the woman to push her hands into her hips, hence contracting the muscle) it is highly suggestive of a malignancy. Fixation to skin is almost diagnostic of cancer—the only conditions that may mimic this are fat necrosis or a pointing abscess.

[b] Please bear in mind that this is a classical presentation of breast carcinoma—but not all carcinoma has read the books. You must retain a high index of suspicion for any solid breast lump, particularly those presenting in older women.

Miss Collins has an oblong-shaped lump in the upper inner quadrant of her right breast. The lump is approximately 2 cm × 1 cm. It has a smooth surface, clearly defined margins, a rubbery consistency, and is highly mobile.

What diagnosis is most likely? What features of history and examination make other common diagnoses in a 28-year-old woman less likely?

It is most likely that Miss Collins has a **fibroadenoma**. Fibroadenomas are aberrations of normal breast development that contain both stromal and epithelial elements. As many as 7–13% of young women will have a fibroadenoma at some stage during their teens or twenties.

The most common breast lumps in women of Miss Collins' age are fibroadenomas, benign cystic change, normally lumpy breasts, and lactation-related abscesses. As Miss Collins is not lactating, and has no breast tenderness, warmth, or erythema, we can effectively rule out an abscess. The fact that her lump is very clearly delineated points us away from diffuse benign cystic disease, and the fact that she has recently noticed a new lump argues against this being part of normally lumpy breasts.

We should at least consider a cyst or carcinoma, even though they are rare in women of this age. The clearly defined borders of this lump are consistent with those of a cyst, but the rubbery nature of the lump is not cyst-like (cysts are either firm or lax, according to the pressure of fluid within them). Furthermore, cysts are not highly mobile lumps. Miss Collins has no risk factors for breast carcinoma (her family history is non-significant) and malignant breast lumps are typically hard with irregular margins—although it is often hard to differentiate the characteristics of a lump on clinical examination.

What should the GP do next?

All women with a palpable breast lump should be referred to a surgical breast clinic, even if you are fairly certain from your history and examination that the lump is benign—the risk of misdiagnosis is simply too high. The GP should aim to reassure Miss Collins that findings are consistent with this being a benign lump, but that she will be further assessed in a specialist 'one stop' breast clinic (where she will be seen by breast surgeons ± radiologists and pathologists). Most guidelines would suggest that as she is under 30, and the lump is neither enlarging nor fixed and hard, that she would not qualify as a 2-week wait referral.

How are all solid lumps investigated in the breast clinic?

Breast lumps undergo **triple assessment** (ideally on the same day, at the same clinic), the components of which are:

1 **Clinical examination.**
2 **Radiological examination:**
   - Ultrasound if <35 years old. The breast tissue in younger women is too dense to evaluate by radiography (mammography).
   - Two-view mammogram (± ultrasound) if >35 years old. Cancer is suggested by increased density, irregular margins, spiculation (like shards of glass), and accompanying clustered irregular microcalcifications.
3 **Fine needle aspiration** (FNA) or **core biopsy**. FNA will only provide information on the type of cells (and whether they are dysplastic or not) whereas core biopsy will additionally provide information on local architecture (e.g. invasion of surrounding structures).

Miss Collins was referred to the breast clinic. She underwent triple assessment at a 'one stop' clinic which confirmed that the lump was a fibroadenoma.

What treatment options are available to Miss Collins?

There are two treatment options. The majority of fibroadenomas will resolve over several years and pose no increased risk of malignancy. As such, it is often appropriate to adopt a conservative stance and **reassure** the patient that this is a benign lesion.

The second option is to remove the fibroadenoma by **excisional biopsy**. Indications for this include patient preference, a lump that is increasing in size (either clinically or as measured by ultrasound), or a lump that is causing discomfort.

Short cases

Mrs Sowerby is a 78-year-old woman who presents to her GP with a lump in her right breast. She reports that the lump has been there for some time, but that she didn't want to bother the doctor unnecessarily. She has had two breast cysts aspirated in the past—one in her early fifties and one in her early sixties. Her delay in presentation to the GP was because she thought that this was another cyst and, as she remembers being told that cysts are harmless, she wanted to see if it would go away of its own accord. However, this lump now feels different from her previous cysts and she is now keen for the doctor to take a look.

The lump has gradually got bigger over the past few months, but she reports that it is not painful. She is not aware of any trauma to her breast. When specifically asked about any changes to her nipples, or any nipple discharge, she says that the right nipple is now quite flat whereas it used to be prominent. She has not, however, noticed any discharge.

Mrs Sowerby has one daughter, aged 55, whom she breast-fed. She started having periods 'at the same time as everyone else', and underwent the menopause aged 50. She did not use HRT. She wears a ring pessary for vaginal prolapse but has no other significant gynaecological history.

When asked about any family history of breast cancer, she says that her daughter was told she had a 'breast mouse' when she was younger, but she is unaware of any other breast disease in the family. Her husband died of prostate cancer aged 81.

She is otherwise fit and well. She takes a thiazide and angiotensin-converting enzyme (ACE) inhibitor for hypertension.

On examination, Mrs Sowerby has an obvious lump in the upper outer quadrant of her right breast. The lump extends towards her nipple, which is observed to be inverted. There is skin tethering over the superior portion of the lump. Palpation of the mass reveals a hard irregular lump approximately 5 cm × 4 cm. The edges are irregular and poorly defined. The mass is non-mobile and appears fixed to the overlying skin. Several lymph nodes are palpable in the right axilla. The left breast and axilla appear normal.

What is the most likely diagnosis? What is the next step for Mrs Sowerby?

The long history of a progressively enlarging non-tender lump, together with skin and nipple changes, and examination findings of an irregular, hard, fixed mass with local lymphadenopathy are highly suggestive of breast **carcinoma**.

Mrs Sowerby should be **urgently referred** to the breast surgeons for triple assessment. Note that the term 'breast mouse' is sometimes used colloquially to describe fibroadenomas because of their small and highly mobile nature, so this is likely what the patient was referring to in her daughter.

Mrs Sowerby was seen by the surgeons within a fortnight. She underwent triple assessment. Core biopsy revealed a poorly differentiated ductal carcinoma.

Where are the most likely sites of metastasis and how should these potential sites be investigated if there is any suggestion of metastasis?

Breast carcinoma most commonly metastasizes to lungs, liver, bone, and brain. NICE guidelines recommend that all patients with suspected metastatic breast cancer undergo investigation for possible bone and liver metastases. Chest and brain metastases are often investigated only if clinically suspected.

- **Liver:** All patients with suspected metastatic breast cancer should have either CT abdomen, MRI abdomen or contrast-enhanced ultrasound.
- **Bone:** All patients with suspected metastatic breast cancer should have imaging of axial skeleton (bone scintigraphy or CT or MRI) *plus* imaging of long bones (bone scintigraphy or plain radiographs). Blood tests such as serum calcium, phosphate and ALP can be a useful adjunct.
- **Chest:** CT usually only if symptoms or signs suggest chest pathology.
- **Brain:** CT usually only if there are symptoms or signs suggestive of brain metastases, such as fitting or early morning headache and nausea.
- Some hospitals will advocate staging patients with whole body CT ± PET.

SHORT CASE

Mrs Sowerby underwent a bone scintigraphy scan and a CT of her abdomen which revealed no bony nor liver metastases.

In broad terms, what treatment options are available to her?

Treatment options include:

- Local treatments: surgery, radiotherapy
- Systemic treatments: chemotherapy, hormonal therapy, monoclonal antibodies (e.g. herceptin)

The precise treatment will depend on size, stage, and grade of the tumour, nodal status, receptor status, suitability for surgery, and other comorbidities.

Hormonal therapy is usually given to all women who have tumours expressing oestrogen receptors ('ER positive') and/or progesterone receptors ('PR positive'). Such therapy decreases oestrogen synthesis (aromatase inhibitors) or selectively blocks oestrogen receptors (e.g. tamoxifen).

SHORT CASE

Mrs Regan is a 55-year-old woman who presents to her GP with a lump in her left breast. She first noticed the lump as a painful swelling above her nipple 2 days ago. The lump has increased in size slightly during that time. She says that the overlying skin is quite red and tender, but that there have been no nipple changes. She has felt a bit feverish for the past day or so but is otherwise well.

She underwent the menarche aged 13 and the menopause aged 52. She has four children, all of whom are in their thirties, and all of whom were breast-fed. She has been taking HRT for the last 3 years. She is not aware of any previous breast disease and has had no gynaecological operations. There is no family history of breast cancer.

She smokes cigarettes and has a 21-pack-year history. She drinks 12–15 units of white wine per week. She reports that she is otherwise fit and well, and only occasionally takes sumatriptan for migraines.

On examination, there is periareolar erythema of the left breast. The reddened skin is warm to the touch. An irregular firm mass, approximately 1.5 cm in diameter is palpable medial to the nipple, within the boundaries of the erythema. There is skin tethering. Two lymph nodes are palpable in the left axilla. The right breast and axilla appear normal. Mrs Regan is febrile.

What is the likely diagnosis? How should Mrs Regan be managed?

The sudden appearance of a painful lump in the breast of a middle-aged smoker, combined with examination findings of fever, skin erythema, and tethering, make it highly likely that this is a **breast abscess**.

Mrs Regan should be started on appropriate antibiotics that give anaerobic cover. She will also need referring to the surgeons to either have the abscess drained surgically or aspirated. Any residual solid mass that remains after drainage and antibiotic treatment will need triple assessment.

She should be encouraged to stop smoking as smokers have a significantly higher risk of non-lactational mastitis and abscess formation.

SHORT CASE

Mrs Dean is a 42-year-old woman who presents to her GP because she noticed a tender lump in her right breast 2 days previously. She first noticed the lump while examining her breasts in the bathroom mirror (she does this each month). She says that she has not had any previous breast lumps. She feels well.

She started having periods aged 13, and is premenopausal. She has no children. She uses the combined oral contraceptive pill. There is no family history of breast cancer. She does not smoke or drink alcohol, and takes no regular medications.

Her breasts appear normal on gross inspection. Palpation of the right breast reveals a well-circumscribed tender mass in the lower inner quadrant. The lump is approximately 2 cm in diameter, has a smooth surface, and is firm to the touch. It is non-mobile and is not fixed or tethered to the overlying skin. Both axillae and the left breast appear normal.

The GP refers Mrs Dean for triple assessment. Ultrasound reveals a well-defined hypoechoic mass in the left lower inner quadrant.

What is the most likely diagnosis? How should Mrs Dean be managed?

The history and examination findings are most consistent with a **cyst**. The well-circumscribed nature of the lump, combined with the smooth surface and firm texture, could possibly be confused for a fibroadenoma, but fibroadenomas are not typically painful and would be unusual in a woman of this age. Furthermore, the ultrasound scan indicates a cystic mass (a solid mass will be hyperechoic on ultrasound, whereas a fluid-filled cyst will be hypoechoic).

The diagnosis can be confirmed by aspirating the cyst. Most cysts contain fluid that is a shade of green (ranging to almost black), brown, or yellow. If the aspirate is bloodstained it should be sent for cytology. The breast should be re-examined after the cyst has been aspirated to dryness. If there is not complete resolution of the lump it will require triple assessment as carcinoma may occur within a cyst.

SHORT CASE

Miss Pennyweather is a 34-year-old woman who presents to her GP because her left breast is 'lumpy' and tender. She says that she first noticed that her breast felt tender 3 months ago. She has not noticed any skin or nipple changes and has not had any nipple discharge. When asked directly about any relationship to menstrual cycle, Miss Pennyweather describes how her left breast is more tender in the build-up to her period. Her breast also feels more 'lumpy' during this time, but the lumpiness appears to fade once her period has begun.

She started having periods when she was 13 years old, and has no children. She uses the combined oral contraceptive pill. She was referred to the breast clinic with a lump in her left breast when she was 21 years old. This was diagnosed as a fibroadenoma and was managed conservatively. Her mother was diagnosed with breast cancer aged 61 and had a mastectomy.

She has no significant past medical or gynaecological history, and takes no medications. She enjoys the odd social cigarette, but does not drink alcohol.

On examination, Miss Pennyweather's breasts appear normal on gross inspection. Palpation reveals an indistinct area of tender nodularity in the upper outer quadrant of the left breast. The nodularity spans an area of approximately 10 cm in diameter. Discernible lumps within the nodularity have a rubbery texture. The right breast and both axillae appear normal.

What is the most likely diagnosis and how should Miss Pennyweather be managed?

This diffuse nodularity, which shows cyclical variation in both prominence and tenderness, is most likely **benign cystic change** (fibrocystic change, fibroadenosis, or benign breast change). As there are areas of discrete nodularity within the breast these will require triple assessment, and reassurance if no abnormality is detected.

SHORT CASE

Mr John is a 50-year-old wine merchant. He presents to his GP because he is concerned that he is developing what he refers to as 'moobs'. He has recently started playing rugby for a local veterans team and says that he has become the butt of incessant jokes about his prominent breasts. He says that he has had prominent breast tissue for a few years but would now like to know what is causing it and whether anything can be done about it.

Mr John is not aware of any recent change in the size of his breasts, but he says that they are occasionally tender. There is no family history of breast cancer.

Mr John had a cholecystectomy when he was 43 years old. He takes allopurinol for gout, and a thiazide and ACE inhibitor for hypertension. He smokes a dozen cigars each week, and is not quite sure how much alcohol he actually drinks each week, but estimates that it is approximately three bottles of wine.

On inspection, Mr John has a feminine contour to both breasts, with bilateral areolar prominence. There are no skin changes. The swelling is tender to palpation, but is of uniform consistency. There are no areas of nodularity and both axillae are normal.

What is the most likely diagnosis? What can cause this condition?

This generalized enlargement of the male breasts is almost certainly **gynaecomastia**. Although 1% of breast cancer does occur in men, this would be a very unusual presentation as male breast cancer is typically unilateral, non-tender, with an irregular surface, indistinct margins, and a hard consistency (just as in women).

Palpable breast tissue is present in almost a third of adult men and two-thirds of pubertal boys, but is more prominent in some men than others. The majority (two-thirds) of gynaecomastia is 'physiological', and occurs at times of hormonal fluctuation, such as during the neonatal period, puberty, and old age. Pathological causes include:

- Liver disease

- Drugs (e.g. cimetidine, spironolactone, phenothiazines, finasteride, anabolic steroids)

- Primary testicular failure (e.g. anorchia, bilateral cryptorchidism)
- Acquired testicular failure (e.g. mumps orchitis)
- Secondary testicular failure (e.g. panhypopituitarism)
- Endocrine tumours (e.g. testicle, adrenal, pituitary)
- Non-endocrine tumours (e.g. bronchial carcinoma)

Viva questions

What factors determine the prognosis with breast carcinoma?

The principal determinants of prognosis are:

- tumour stage (which reflects the spread of the cancer and therefore incorporates tumour size, nodal status, and presence of metastasis)
- tumour grade (which reflects the loss of differentiation of the cancerous cells and therefore incorporates their histopathological appearance)
- hormone receptor status (oestrogen, progestogen, and human epidermal growth factor receptor 2 (HER2))
- tumour type (such as lobular or ductal)
- patient age, and
- treatment type.

There are various scoring systems, such as the Nottingham Prognostic Index, which incorporate some or all of these factors to produce an estimate of survival.

What is peau d'orange and what causes it?

Peau d'orange ('orange peel') refers to the skin changes that may occur with an infiltrating carcinoma of the breast. The skin has a dimpled appearance—much like the skin of an orange. Blockage of the dermal lymphatics by a tumour, surgery, or radiotherapy results in cutaneous oedema. Sweat ducts and hair follicles tether the skin, thus resulting in dimples within the oedematous areas.

What is the difference between skin fixity and skin tethering?

If a lesion is fixed to the skin, it cannot be moved independently of the overlying skin. A lesion that is tethered to the skin can be moved independently of the skin to some extent. However, if you imagine that the lesion is tethered to the skin as if by a length of string, it will only move independently of the skin within the limits of the length of string. If you try to move the lesion beyond those limits it will distort and dimple the overlying skin.

Contrast the roles of adjuvant and neo-adjuvant chemotherapy.

Adjuvant chemotherapy is used after surgery and thus the main aim is to treat any micrometastases which remain following surgical excision of the primary. By contrast, neo-adjuvant chemotherapy is delivered before surgery and aims to shrink the primary tumour (thus making it operable, or more amenable to surgical removal) as well as minimizing the metastatic tumour burden. The main advantage of neo-adjuvant chemotherapy is that tumour size can be assessed for response to therapy (which is obviously not possible after surgical resection), and non-response can lead to second-line treatments. Patients selected for neo-adjuvant chemotherapy are typically those at highest risk of micrometastases—young patients, those with large tumours, and those with palpable lymph nodes.

When is mastectomy preferred over breast-conserving surgery?

Breast-conserving surgery by wide local excision (WLE) followed by radiotherapy has been shown to produce equal long-term survival to mastectomy, with only a slight increase in the rates of local recurrence. However, not all patients will have cancer that is suitable for WLE. Mastectomy may be necessary to achieve tumour clearance if the tumour is of a large size relative to the breast (i.e. a large tumour, small breast, or both), a tumour that occupies a central position within the breast, multifocal tumours, recurrent tumours, or if the patient prefers this to a WLE. Mastectomy is also indicated for the treatment of male breast cancer.

Although WLE has the theoretical advantage that it may produce better cosmesis, the patient will need to be counselled about the requirement for adjuvant radiotherapy, and perhaps further surgery if there are positive surgical margins or local recurrence. By contrast, mastectomy may obviate the need for further surgery or radiotherapy. Mastectomy may also produce an acceptable cosmetic result if combined with reconstructive procedures (such as free or pedicled flaps, and/or breast prostheses), either as a simultaneous or delayed procedure.

What are the advantages and disadvantages of FNA over core biopsy?

FNA:
- Advantages:
  - Quick
  - Minimally invasive
  - Low risk of bruising or local complications
  - Adequate for assessing the hormone receptor status of the cancerous cells.

- Disadvantages:
  - May have poor sensitivity (inadequate specimens)
  - *In situ* and invasive disease cannot be differentiated as local architecture is lost during the aspiration (you end up with a solution of floating cells).

Core biopsy:
- Advantages:

  - *In situ* and invasive disease can be differentiated as local architecture is preserved during the biopsy.

- Disadvantages:
  - Higher risk of local complications and bruising than FNA
  - Results are not immediate (compared with FNA)
  - Requires local anaesthesia
  - More invasive and time consuming than FNA.

What methods exist for axillary staging of breast cancer?

There are three main techniques for axillary staging of breast cancer:

1. **Axillary clearance:** removal of all local lymph nodes. Three levels of clearance (I, II, and III) refer to removal of increasing numbers of lymph nodes lateral, posterior, and medial to pectoralis minor.

2. **Axillary sampling:** a minimal dissection of the axilla is undertaken and a selection of at least four nodes is removed from the low axilla for histological analysis.

CONTINUED ➤

CONTINUED

3 **Sentinel lymph node biopsy:** aims to identify the first node which drains the breast (and is thus the most likely site of metastasis). Blue dye and/or radio-isotope is injected into the periareolar tissue in the same breast quadrant as the cancerous tissue. The sentinel node will take up this dye and/or radio-isotope and is identified intraoperatively as 'hot', 'blue', or 'hot and blue'. This single sentinel node can then be removed and sent for histology. The sentinel node is located in the low axilla in >90% of cases. The main advantage of the technique is a considerable increase in sensitivity of lymph node analysis, and avoidance of the high morbidity (such as lymphoedema, long thoracic nerve injury, axillary vein thrombosis, etc.) associated with axillary clearance.

A woman is discussed during a multidisciplinary team (MDT) meeting as having a P4R4C4B5 breast lump. What does this mean?

There are two components to this scoring system. The letters refer to triple assessment:

P = physical examination
R = radiological examination
C = cytology (FNA)
B = biopsy (core)

Each aspect of the triple assessment is then given a score out of 5:

1 = normal (in the context of examination, radiology, biopsy) or inadequate sample (cytology)
2 = benign
3 = probably benign
4 = probably malignant
5 = malignant

Hence a P4R4C4B5 lump had a high probability of being malignant that has been confirmed by biopsy. The overall sensitivity of triple assessment in most UK units is >99.5%.

What is ANDI?

ANDI refers to 'aberrations of normal development and involution'. These aberrations include fibroadenomas, benign cystic changes (fibroadenosis), intraductal papillomas, duct ectasia, and cysts.

A 40-year-old woman comes to see you, her GP, because she is concerned that two of her younger sisters have developed breast cancer in their thirties. She has not had any genetic testing but has heard about *BRCA* genes on the news. She is convinced that she must be *BRCA*-positive and would like to be referred to a breast surgeon for a prophylactic bilateral mastectomy. How would you approach such a consultation?

It is of course perfectly understandable that this patient is anxious about her chances of developing breast cancer, and it is vital that her concerns are addressed in a sensitive manner. The notion of 'risk' is open to a huge amount of personal interpretation, and part of the challenge in such a consultation

CONTINUED

CONTINUED

is to establish the patient's frame of reference. While it may be all too easy for medics to talk about absolute and relative risk as definable entities, such values will be skewed by socioeconomic and cultural factors and by the patient's personal experience. It is also of paramount importance to use language that the patient understands—some patients may be very familiar with terms such as heritability and dominant traits, whereas for other patients it may be more appropriate to talk about familial or inherited conditions.

A consultation such as the one described here will obviously be directed to a large part by the patient's questions. However, as the GP you may wish to address the following points—if the patient wishes to hear them:

- What does she know about breast cancer, its risk factors, and potential genetic predisposition?

- What is her frame of reference? What were the circumstances surrounding the diagnosis in her two sisters? What was the outcome for her sisters?

- What constitutes a significant family history of breast cancer? (See earlier in this chapter.)

- What proportion of breast cancer is familial? It is important to explain that only a minority (~5%) of breast cancer is familial. This patient, however, is likely to be in that minority as she has two sisters who have been diagnosed before the age of 40.

- What would genetic counselling and genetic testing involve? Many patients are under the false impression that testing will give an immediate result, and are unaware that affected relatives will need to give blood and that test results may take weeks.

- If testing reveals that she is positive for *BRCA1* or *BRCA2*, does this imply that she will definitely develop breast cancer? Does it have implications for the risk of developing other cancers such as ovarian cancer, malignant melanoma, or prostate cancer (in male relatives)? What does a positive result imply for any other of the patient's siblings or children?[†]

- She has mentioned prophylactic bilateral mastectomy, but is she aware of any other options? What about annual mammogram screening? Is she aware that bilateral mastectomy does not entirely eliminate breast cancer risk? Is she aware that some women will also request prophylactic oophorectomy as this reduces risks of both breast and ovarian carcinoma?

- Has she considered any potential effect that genetic testing may have on insurance premiums?— this may sound rather callous, but is a real concern for some patients.

- Is she aware of patient support websites such as <http://www.breastcancercare.org.uk/> or <http://www.breastcancergenetics.co.uk/>?

[†] There are three main genes (*BRCA1*, *BRCA2*, and *TP53*) that are known to carry an increased risk of breast cancer. Possession of one of these mutations significantly increases the risk of developing breast cancer, but does not imply that breast cancer is inevitable. It is, however, important to remember that the *BRCA* mutations also predispose to other cancers. *BRCA1* is associated with an increased risk of ovarian and bowel cancer, while *BRCA2* is associated with an increased risk of ovarian and prostate cancer, male breast cancer, and malignant melanoma.

Single Best Answers

1. **A patient with a breast lump is assessed and diagnosed as having fat necrosis. What is the most likely cause?**

   a. Smoking
   b. Trauma
   c. Ductal carcinoma in situ (DCIS)

   d. Fibrocystic changes
   e. Breast-feeding

2. **A patient is diagnosed as having breast cancer. Which of the following is the most likely risk factor?**

   a. Smoking
   b. Previous fibrocystic disease
   c. Exposure to hydrocarbon compounds

   d. Human papillomavirus
   e. Mother had breast cancer

3. **In patients with breast cancer, which feature(s) suggest worse prognosis?**

   a. Current smoker
   b. Positive family history
   c. HER2 receptor positive

   d. Axillary lymph node metastases
   e. ER receptor positive

4. **A patient is found to have a 4 cm calcified lesion on mammography, confirmed as a malignant lesion on fine needle aspiration (FNA). A biopsy shows it to be non-invasive, and oestrogen receptor and HER2 negative. It is removed by wide local excision with clear margins. At the same time sentinel node biopsy is performed and found to be negative. What is the most likely outcome?**

   a. Response to axillary radiotherapy
   b. Response to tamoxifen
   c. No further therapy and no recurrence

   d. Development of Paget's disease of the nipple
   e. Axillary node clearance with no recurrence subsequently

5. **A man goes to his GP complaining of swollen, tender breasts of several months duration. You review his medications: which could have caused this?**

   a. Aspirin
   b. Atorvastatin
   c. Lisinopril

   d. Metformin
   e. Digoxin

Core case

Read through the sections in the case boxes, covering up the sections that follow so that you don't see the answer. At the end of each case box, try to answer the question before reading on.

Mr Simpson is a 40-year-old man who presents to the Emergency Department with acute epigastric pain.

What is your differential diagnosis for acute epigastric pain?

Try to also identify those conditions that you must attempt to exclude at the earliest possible opportunity because they require urgent treatment (surgical or medical).

We have arranged the differential diagnosis in order of likelihood in a man of this age with more likely diagnoses in larger font and less likely diagnoses in smaller font in Figure 12.1. Pathologies that should be excluded at the earliest possible opportunity are shown in **bold**. Bear in mind that this differential

Acute pancreatitis
Perforated peptic ulcer
Gastritis/duodenitis
Peptic ulcer disease (gastric or duodenal)
Biliary colic
Acute cholecystitis
Ascending cholangitis
Myocardial infarction
Ruptured abdominal aortic aneurysm (AAA)
Mesenteric ischaemia
Basal pneumonia
Oesophagitis (due to gastro-oesophageal reflux disease, GORD)
Non-ulcer dyspepsia (NUD, also called idiopathic dyspepsia)[†]
Chronic pancreatitis
Incomplete bowel obstruction
Boerhaave's perforation
Gastric cancer
Pancreatic cancer (although cancer in the head of the pancreas is normally painless)
Acute hepatitis (although this is usually painless unless there is hepatomegaly and stretch of the liver capsule)

[†] *Also known as functional dyspepsia; this is a diagnosis of exclusion, made in approximately 30% of patients who are investigated for dyspepsia whose endoscopy is negative. Patients typically complain of discomfort rather than pain and it is unusual for this to present acutely to hospital.*

Figure 12.1 Differential diagnosis for acute epigastric pain in adults. Diagnoses that require exclusion due to their need for immediate management are shown in **bold**.

diagnosis refers to epigastric pain as a presentation of 'acute abdomen' and thus differs markedly from epigastric pain presenting as outpatient dyspepsia.

Note that although we have adopted a standard approach of history, examination, and investigations over the course of the following pages, you should use clinical judgement to deviate from this path if one of the 'must exclude' diagnoses is suspected, or if there is a need for urgent resuscitation. For example, if a 69-year-old male diabetic patient with known unstable angina presents with exercise-induced epigastric pain, you would be wise to perform an electrocardiogram (ECG) and obtain baseline observations at the earliest opportunity.

> The first step when taking the history is to characterize the pain using a system such as SOCRATES.
>
> **What key features of the pain would point you to some of the diagnoses in Figure 12.1?**

Various characteristics of the pain will help to narrow our differential diagnosis of epigastric pain:

Site:

- Pain that has spread from the epigastrium to involve the rest of the abdomen may suggest peritonitis from a perforated GI tract (e.g. perforated gastric ulcer, which causes epigastric pain because the stomach is embryologically a foregut structure).
- Pain that has spread from the epigastrium to involve the chest may be cardiac.
- Biliary disease, although anatomically located in the right upper quadrant, may present with purely epigastric symptoms.

Onset:

- Pain that is of very sudden onset suggests perforation of a viscus (e.g. a perforated duodenal ulcer or Boerhaave's perforation) or myocardial infarction.
- Pain from acute pancreatitis and biliary colic develops maximal intensity over 10–20 minutes.
- Inflammatory processes such as acute cholecystitis or pneumonia typically take hours to reach their peak.

Character:

- 'Crushing' or 'tightness' qualities are typical of cardiac pathology.
- Sharp, 'burning' pain is typical of peptic ulcers, gastritis, and duodenitis.
- Deep, 'boring' pain is typical of pancreatitis.

Radiation:

- Back pain is classically associated with pancreatitis, leaking abdominal aortic aneurysms, and some-times seen with peptic ulcers.
- Shoulder-tip pain due to irritation of the phrenic nerve suggests diaphragmatic involvement (for example by a basal pneumonia or subphrenic abscess).
- Jaw, neck, or arm pain suggests cardiac pathology.
- Retrosternal chest pain suggests oesophagitis or myocardial ischaemia.

Attenuating factors:

- Patients with acute pancreatitis may find that sitting forwards relieves their pain.
- Surgical dogma suggests that eating makes the pain of gastric ulcers worse but relieves the pain from duodenal ulcers, but these are unreliable features for distinguishing the two in clinical practice.

Timing:

- Biliary colic, uncomplicated peptic ulcer disease, gastritis, duodenitis and non-ulcer dyspepsia are likely to be self-limiting over timescales of less than 6–8 hours (although in many cases there will be recurrent episodes).
- Bear in mind that biliary colic does *not* produce truly colicky pain (where the pain waxes and wanes during a single episode), but rather the pain is relatively constant for the duration of the attack.
- Epigastric pain made worse by exercise must make you consider cardiac pathology.

Exacerbating factors:

- Movement worsens severe pain of intra-abdominal origin and peritonitis.
- Deep breathing (pleuritic pain) can worsen epigastric pain when it is due to basal pneumonia, pulmonary embolus, pneumothorax, pericarditis or any cause of pleural inflammation.
- The triggering of self-limiting pain by fatty meals is highly suggestive of biliary colic.

Severity:

- Uncomplicated peptic ulcer disease, gastritis, duodenitis, and non-ulcer dyspepsia are usually not severe (and many patients will not present to hospital).
- Severe pancreatitis, perforated peptic ulcers, and myocardial infarction are typically very painful.

Once you have characterized the pain, which other symptoms should you ask about?

- **Nausea and/or vomiting?** Small bowel obstruction can present as colicky epigastric pain associated with nausea and vomiting. An inferior MI can also cause vomiting by irritation of the diaphragm. Boerhaave's perforation is precipitated by forceful vomiting. Be clear about whether the vomiting immediately preceded the pain or immediately followed it.
- **Fever?** Could suggest an infection (e.g. viral hepatitis, pneumonia) or widespread inflammation in the peritoneum (i.e. peritonitis).
- **Dyspepsia and/or waterbrash?** Patients who describe the constellation of symptoms including heartburn, retrosternal discomfort, and a bitter taste in the mouth are very likely to be suffering from gastro-oesophageal reflux disease (GORD), or sequelae such as oesophagitis.
- **Have they noticed any change in their stool recently?** Pale stools indicate that bile is not reaching the bowel. Foul-smelling, floating stools (steatorrhoea) indicate poor digestion of fat, usually due to pancreatic exocrine insufficiency or long-standing biliary disease (as it implies chronic obstruction).
- **Cough?** In the absence of abdominal symptoms other than epigastric pain, an acute cough and/or productive sputum raises the likelihood of basal pneumonia. A more chronic cough with epigastric pain suggests GORD, where the refluxed stomach acid irritates the vocal cords.

What is the particular relevance of the past medical/surgical history?

There are four diseases or groups of diseases that you should pay particular attention to. However, patients may not have a proven diagnosis and may not have related previous symptoms to a particular disease process. For example, while many patients are adept at recognizing angina, few may recognize the symptoms of biliary colic. Clinical judgement may thus be required to tease out such conditions from the history of the presenting complaint and past medical history.

- **Biliary disease:** patients with a known history of gallstone disease are prone both to recurrence of the biliary disease and to complications such as acute pancreatitis, acute cholecystitis or ascending cholangitis. Note that even patients who have had a previous cholecystectomy can suffer the effects of gallstones retained in the common bile duct.

- **Peptic ulcer disease:** a wise maxim is to regard all patients with known peptic ulcer disease, presenting with sudden-onset severe epigastric pain, as having a perforated ulcer until proven otherwise.

- **GORD:** has a high rate of recurrence.

- **Vascular disease:** patients with widespread arterial disease are at increased risk of both myocardial infarction and mesenteric ischaemia. Mesenteric ischaemia may occur as an acute presentation, or as chronic 'mesenteric angina'. The latter can be regarded in a similar way to cardiac ischaemia in that it may be preceded by work-related pain which, in the case of the gut, is manifested as colicky postprandial abdominal pain. Risk factors for *chronic* mesenteric ischaemia include smoking, hypertension, diabetes mellitus, hypercholesterolaemia, and a family history of cardiovascular disease. Risk factors for *acute* mesenteria ischaemia reflect potential sources of emboli, and thus include atrial fibrillation, recent myocardial infarction, and cardiac valvular disease.

When asking about drug history, are there any particular medications that would predispose to conditions in our differential diagnosis?

Both peptic ulcer disease and acute pancreatitis can be drug induced, although the link is far stronger for the former. Drugs to consider include:

- **Peptic ulcer disease:** non-steroidal anti-inflammatory drugs (NSAIDs), steroids, bisphosphonates, salicylates (e.g. aspirin). Bear in mind that steroids not only predispose to peptic ulcer disease, but they can also dampen the inflammatory response to any subsequent ulcer perforation and hence partially mask signs of peritonism.

- **Acute pancreatitis:** while many drugs have been linked to acute pancreatitis by way of sporadic case reports, some of the more robust links to be aware of include sodium valproate, steroids, thiazides, and azathioprine.

Does family history have any relevance to the presentation of acute epigastric pain?

The most compelling reason to ask about family history in the context of epigastric pain is to establish cardiovascular disease risk. However, there are also some very rare hereditary causes of acute pancreatitis (such as mutations in *PRSS1*, *SPINK1*, and *CFTR*) that may be significant if there is a strong family history.

Why is Mr Simpson's social history of particular relevance?

While you should always ask about smoking and alcohol intake, it is particularly important that you spend some time establishing alcohol intake when faced with a patient complaining of epigastric pain.

Acute pancreatitis can be caused both by chronic alcohol consumption (developing in about 10% of chronic alcohol abusers) and by binge drinking. Smoking is a risk factor for both peptic ulcer disease and vascular causes of epigastric pain (e.g. myocardial infarction, mesenteric ischaemia).

Mr Simpson describes his pain as severe and constant. He says it came on suddenly while he was preparing lunch about 5 hours ago. The pain gradually increased in intensity over the first 15 minutes or so. He rates it as 9/10 and says that it radiates to his back. He has been sick several times, including twice since he arrived at the hospital half an hour ago. He says that he is no longer bringing very much up, but feels very nauseated and is retching. He has had no cough, fever, or dyspepsia, and denies any change to his stool. He has lost his appetite.

He has a history of episodes of right upper quadrant pain; most recently a couple of years ago. Mr Simpson did not seek medical help during any of these episodes as he was able to control the pain with paracetamol and the pain resolved within a few hours. He is not aware of any particular triggers for these episodes, but direct questioning reveals that they may have followed meals. He has taken paracetamol today but it has not helped to relieve his pain. He has no other significant medical history, takes no medications, and has no allergies. There is no significant family history. He does not smoke, and states that he drinks perhaps two or three glasses of red wine with meals each week.

What signs should you look for on examination?

First you should check Mr Simpson's need for resuscitation (airway, breathing, circulation—ABC). If his condition is severe, he may have a fever, tachycardia, hypotension, tachypnoea, and low oxygen saturations, and may require transfer to intensive care.

When examining Mr Simpson, particularly focus on:

- **Position:** patients with peritonitis lie completely still and rigid; any movement (e.g. the car ride to the hospital) is exquisitely painful. The pain of pancreatitis is said to be positional, improving when patients sit forwards or lie in the recovery position (on their side, facing slightly down into the bed). Patients with severe pancreatitis may, however, lie completely still.

- **Jaundice:** this may be seen with posthepatic causes of biliary obstruction such as ascending cholangitis and gallstone-induced acute pancreatitis, or with acute hepatitis (although this rarely causes pain). Acute pancreatitis can also cause jaundice in the absence of gallstones, because oedema of the head of the pancreas compresses the common bile duct (usually 2–3 days after symptom onset).

- **Cullen's or Grey Turner's signs:** discoloration due to extravasated blood in the retroperitoneum, around the umbilicus, and flank respectively. These may be seen in acute haemorrhagic pancreatitis but are rare, non-specific, and late (>48 hours) signs. Figure 12.2 shows Grey Turner's sign in a patient with severe pancreatitis.

- **Signs of small bowel obstruction:** a distended abdomen (which may be hard to appreciate in a patient with a high body mass index (BMI)) and absent or tinkling bowel sounds.

- **Tenderness and guarding:** there may be localized tenderness, as in the case of acute cholecystitis (Murphy's sign), or mild pancreatitis. Acute mild pancreatitis may produce a degree of local peritonism. If the tenderness is more severe, generalized, and seen in combination with guarding and board-like rigidity, this is likely to be peritonitis.

- **Masses:** check for the presence of a central, laterally expansile, pulsatile mass (AAA). Don't forget to check the inguinal folds and femoral canal for hernias which may be causing bowel obstruction (although epigastric pain would be an unusual presentation of such an obstruction).

Figure 12.2 Grey Turner's sign (flank discoloration due to severe pancreatitis).

- **Respiratory examination:** never forget that pathology of the lung bases may on rare occasions masquerade as upper abdominal pain. Check for signs of consolidation including decreased expansion, dullness to percussion, decreased breath sounds, and increased vocal resonance.

Looking at Mr Simpson, you note that he is sitting forwards in bed—a position he says he finds more comfortable. On palpation there is mild epigastric tenderness, but no rebound tenderness or guarding. There are no palpable masses, obvious abdominal distension, or discoloration. A digital rectal examination (DRE) is unremarkable. The lung bases are clear.

His observations are as follows: temperature of 38.6 °C, heart rate 111 bpm, blood pressure 106/79 mmHg, respiratory rate 17/min, oxygen saturations 97% on room air.

Which investigations should you request for Mr Simpson?

Bloods

- **Full blood count (FBC):** look for signs of infection or inflammation (elevated white cell count), or blood loss (low haemoglobin), for example due to a bleeding peptic ulcer. Neutrophilia is a prognostic indicator in pancreatitis.

- **C-reactive protein (CRP):** elevated in the case of inflammation or infection, but non-specific as to the cause. Establishing a baseline enables you to monitor progression.

- **Pancreatic amylase or lipase:** slight increases (200 to 600 U/L) in amylase levels are most commonly caused by pancreatitis, but such concentrations are relatively non-specific (see Viva questions for other causes). However, very high amylase levels (>1000 U/L) or elevated lipase levels (>300 U/L) are usually regarded as diagnostic of acute pancreatitis, as they are released following autodigestion of the pancreas (exact cut-offs will depend on your local laboratory protocols). There are a number of points to note regarding the interpretation of pancreatic enzymes. Firstly, if the amylase is not raised you cannot exclude acute pancreatitis. Values should be interpreted in the context of time elapsed since the onset of abdominal pain. Amylase levels usually rise within hours of onset of pancreatitis, but fall back to normal within 3–5 days. Lipase has a longer half-life and thus may be a more suitable marker if the patient presents late (urinary amylase also takes longer to fall than serum amylase). As many as 30% of patients presenting with acute pancreatitis will have a normal amylase level—either because of a late presentation, very severe pancreatitis, or acute-on-chronic pancreatitis (as there is little active pancreas left).

- **Liver enzymes:** look for hepatic pathology. Elevated levels of aspartate aminotransferase (AST) and alanine aminotransferase (ALT) suggest pathology *within the liver* as these are released by damaged hepatocytes. A raised alkaline phosphatase (ALP), bilirubin, and gamma-glutamyl transferase (GGT) suggests pathology *in the biliary tree*, or extrinsic compression of the biliary tree (such as by pancreatic oedema). A rise in ALP in the absence of a raised GGT suggests a source other than the liver (e.g. bone or placenta). An isolated rise in GGT is more likely to reflect alcohol excess (but *not* necessarily alcoholism).

- **Albumin:** this is useful as a prognostic factor if the patient has pancreatitis.

- **Urea and electrolytes (U&Es) and creatinine:** as a baseline prior to fluid resuscitation. Also these may be deranged due to renal hypoperfusion if the patient is in shock, or if the patient has been vomiting.

- **Calcium:** Hypercalcaemia can cause pancreatitis (the mechanism is unclear) and established pancreatitis can cause hypocalcaemia (the calcium binds to the digested lipids from the pancreas to form soap in a process known as saponification of the pancreas), hence a low calcium is a prognostic indicator of severity in pancreatitis.

- **Glucose:** a capillary glucose (BM) will suffice. [†] Hyperglycaemia is a marker of severity of pancreatitis as it reflects lack of insulin production from the damaged pancreas.

- **Arterial blood gas (ABG):** should be obtained if the patient is hypoxic (oxygen saturations <94%), as acute respiratory distress syndrome (ARDS) is a complication of acute pancreatitis. Low Pao_2 is also a poor prognostic indicator in pancreatitis. In the absence of hypoxia, a **venous blood gas (VBG)** is adequate and will give you the pH and lactate, both elevated in conditions causing severe inflammatory responses (e.g. acute pancreatitis, peritonitis) as the vasodilation leads to hypoperfusion of tissues with a subsequent increase in anaerobic respiration and lactic acid production.

- **Troponin:** although myocardial infarction does not usually present with epigastric pain, you will not want to miss it. Troponin levels are usually taken on admission and at 3–12 hours (depending on local test and protocol) from the onset of pain, although some higher sensitivity assays can be checked sooner. Use clinical judgement as to whether this test is indicated.

ECG

While Mr Simpson's history is atypical, and he has no known risk factors for cardiovascular disease, you should still exclude cardiac ischaemia. In higher-risk patients you should perform an ECG at the earliest possible opportunity.

[†] You may be interested to know that BM stands for *Boehringer-Mannheim*, a company that made some of the first glucose strips used in the UK.

Imaging

- **Erect chest radiograph:**
  - Air under the diaphragm may suggest a perforated peptic ulcer but is not always visible and usually requires the patient to have been sitting upright for 10 minutes.
  - Lower lobe consolidation suggests a basal pneumonia.
  - A pleural effusion is not uncommon in pancreatitis or with a Boerhaave's perforation.
- **Abdominal radiograph:**
  - Abdominal radiographs are requested far too often in patients with abdominal pain by junior doctors (who are unaware that they don't alter clinical management in 90% of cases even when requested for the right reasons). They are only helpful to look for bowel dilatation (in suspected bowel obstruction or possible toxic megacolon), or to look for foreign bodies. While one can occasionally see calcification of the head of the pancreas (in some cases chronic pancreatitis), loss of a psoas muscle shadow (in rare cases of AAA rupture), gallstones (but only 10% are radio-opaque), pneumoperitoneum (in some patients with a perforated viscus) or small segments of dilated loops (called 'sentinel loops' and possible in almost any cause of intra-abdominal pathology), the reality is that plain abdominal radiography has been superseded by ultrasound and CT scans for most patients with abdominal pain who need imaging, as they are more sensitive and specific.

> Mr Simpson's wife has arrived. She says she has read in a newspaper about ultrasounds and CT scans, and she wonders if her husband needs one of these to help diagnose the problem. Does Mr Simpson need an abdominal ultrasound at this stage?

An ultrasound performed by an experienced ultrasonographer can help visualize many intra-abdominal organs but is unhelpful in establishing the actual diagnosis in most cases of acute epigastric pain. An exception to this is when a leaking (or ruptured) **abdominal aortic aneurysm is suspected**, but this is **not** the case for Mr Simpson based on his age, history and examination. If an AAA is seen on ultrasound (>3 cm in diameter) and the patient has abdominal pain, a leak or rupture of the aneurysm will still need ruling out either by CT aortogram (if the patient is stable) or surgically (if the patient is unstable). The reason for this is that abdominal aortic aneurysms bleed into the retroperitoneum and this is much harder to visualize on ultrasound than fluid in the peritoneal cavity.

If a diagnosis of acute pancreatitis is made, an ultrasound is helpful to look for **gallstones** as a cause. If no stones are viewed by ultrasound, the patient should either be rescanned several days later (as dilated loops of bowel may mask the view in the acute setting) or sent for magnetic resonance cholangiopancreatography (MRCP). Ultrasound can also help **exclude biliary dilation** (>6 mm common bile duct diameter) and/or thickened walls of the biliary tree secondary to obstruction or inflammation.

> Should patients presenting with epigastric pain have a CT scan?

In the acute setting, CT is only useful if the clinical, biochemical, and other radiological findings are inconclusive, if **mesenteric infarction is suspected** clinically or if an **AAA is suspected** clinically or radiographically. In the context of acute pancreatitis, contrast-enhanced CT may be indicated if there is persisting organ failure, signs of sepsis, or a deterioration in clinical status 6–10 days after admission (note that pancreatic necrosis is not visible until 4 days after symptom onset). CT may be diagnostic of acute pancreatitis in situations where clinical and biochemical findings are inconclusive.

You request bloods and an erect chest radiograph. The chest radiograph is normal. The blood results are:

Haematology		Biochemistry	
Hb	137 g/L	CRP	46 mg/L
WCC	15.3 × 10⁹ cells/L	Total bilirubin	16 µM
Platelets	276 × 10⁹ cells/L	ALT	97 U/L
		AST	41 U/L
Venous blood gas		ALP	158 U/L
pH	7.37	GGT	20 U/L
Lactate	1.4 mM	Serum amylase	1264 U/L
Bicarbonate	25 mM	Ca (corrected)	2.32 mM
		Na	137 mM
		K	3.9 mM
		Urea	9.1 mM
		Creatinine	132 µM
		Glucose	4 mM

Given the history, examination, and investigations, what is the most likely diagnosis?

The most likely diagnosis is **acute pancreatitis**, an inflammatory condition of the pancreas in which activated pancreatic enzymes are released and begin to autodigest the gland. Mr Simpson has sudden-onset epigastric pain, which radiates to the back and is relieved by sitting forwards. He has a past medical history suggestive of biliary colic, but minimal alcohol intake—hence making a gallstone aetiology for the pancreatitis most likely. He has minimal abdominal signs (a common finding in mild pancreatitis). His amylase is significantly raised and there are no other obvious causes for such a high level given his history and examination findings.

What are the causes of acute pancreatitis? How will you start investigating the aetiology?

The causes can be remembered with the mnemonic I GET SMASHED:

Idiopathic† (10-20%)

Gallstones

Ethanol

Trauma

Steroids

Mumps/HIV/Coxsackie infection

Autoimmune

Scorpion bites—vanishingly rare, so do not mention this until you have covered common causes first!

---

† You should be reluctant to label pancreatitis as 'idiopathic' until you have performed a vigorous search for gallstones. Modern use of endoscopic ultrasound and MRCP has shown that many cases of pancreatitis that would have previously been labelled as 'idiopathic' are actually due to microlithiasis (gallstones <3 mm in diameter) or sludge (crystals) in the biliary tree.

Hyperlipidaemia/hypercalcaemia/hypothermia

Endoscopic retrograde cholangiopancreatography (ERCP)

Drugs (e.g. sodium valproate, steroids, thiazides, and azathioprine)

Given that by far the most common causes are gallstones and ethanol, these should be the first you investigate. The exact contribution varies according to geography—for example, gallstones are the most common cause in the UK but alcohol is more common in the USA.

An ultrasound is requested and indeed reveals gallstones in the gallbladder and no dilation of the biliary tree. In Mr Simpson's case, his probable pre-existing gallstone disease is likely to be the underlying cause, with a stone having damaged and/or temporarily blocked the pancreatic duct causing a release of digestive pancreatic enzymes into the surrounding tissues.

Do you know of a scoring mechanism used clinically for assessing severity and prognosis of pancreatitis? Using the results given earlier, what is Mr Simpson's score?

There are two scoring scales commonly used in clinical practice—the Ranson scale, developed and more commonly used in the USA, and the Glasgow (or Imrie) scale, developed and more commonly used in the UK. Both include criteria predictive for outcome. They are fairly similar, but the Glasgow scale is a little simpler, using 8 rather than 11 criteria. Both have been validated, although Ranson's was validated in a sample of predominantly alcohol-induced pancreatitis whereas the Glasgow scale has been validated in patients with both alcohol- and gallstone-induced pancreatitis.

The Glasgow scale can be remembered using the mnemonic PANCREAS (it should be based on results within 48 hours of admission)[*]

Pao$_2$ <8 kPa or <60 mmHg

Age >55 years

Neutrophilia >15 × 10^9 cells/L (WCC)

Calcium <2.0 mM

Renal function: urea >16 mM

Enzymes: lactate dehydrogenase (LDH) >600 U/L or AST >200 U/L

Albumin <32 g/L

Sugar >10 mM (in non-diabetics)

Each criterion scores a single point, totalling 8. A score of 3 or more is considered severe pancreatitis, requiring more intensive management in an intensive therapy unit (ITU)/high-dependency unit (HDU) setting. Note that pancreatic amylase and lipase levels are *not* prognostic indicators.

Mr Simpson scores 2/8 on the Glasgow scale (elevated white cells, and age >55; we can assume his Pao$_2$ >8 kPa given that his oxygen saturations are ≥94%). He therefore has **mild pancreatitis** and will require regular observations to intervene promptly if he deteriorates (e.g. rapid development of shock needing fluid resuscitation). Remember that these scoring systems are only a guide and should not be a substitute for regularly checking the patient's clinical condition.

How should Mr Simpson be managed?

* Reproduced from Moore EM, 'A useful mnemonic for severity stratification in acute pancreatitis', *Annals of the Royal College of Surgeons of England*, **82**,1, pp. 16–17, copyright 2000, with permission from the Royal College of Surgeons of England.

First, as always, you must have initially checked Mr Simpson's need for resuscitation (ABC). Even patients with mild pancreatitis can decompensate rapidly so you must continually reassess:

- Airway.
- Breathing—severe cases may develop ARDS, so you must monitor oxygen saturations and work of breathing closely (whether the patient is getting exhausted from breathing).
- Circulation—patients with severe pancreatitis can become hypotensive due to the so-called 'third space' fluid loss that follows the severe inflammatory response. Decreased intravascular volume may be due to a combination of increased capillary permeability, ascites, and ileus. Fluid leaking through the vasculature into an unusual location such as the peritoneum is referred to as 'third space' fluid loss; the first space is vascular, the second space is the natural reservoirs like the bladder. You must monitor fluid balance very closely. All patients will require large-bore intravenous (IV) access. A urinary catheter will aid monitoring of fluid balance if Mr Simpson's condition deteriorates. **Be prepared for a transfer to ITU/HDU** if his condition suddenly deteriorates.

Having ensured that Mr Simpson is stable, you can begin treating the symptoms and the relevant underlying factors—in this case, gallstones. In the acute setting, Mr Simpson will primarily need supportive care. This includes:

- IV fluids, titrated to total output and clinical parameters such as heart rate, blood pressure and respiratory effort to avoid overloading the patient with fluid.
- Oxygen.
- Analgesia. Patients with pancreatitis often have high analgesic requirements, so don't forget to prescribe regular and 'as required' analgesia. Patients with high analgesic requirements often benefit from patient-controlled analgesia (PCA), a special syringe pump which allows the patient to self-administer opiates (e.g. morphine) in a safe and regulated way.
- Antiemetics.
- Deep vein thrombosis (DVT) prophylaxis.
- Low-fat diet if tolerated. If the patient is unable to tolerate food (e.g. due to abdominal pain), nasojejunal feeding may be indicated as it is important to maintain his calorie intake when he is acutely unwell. Enteral (i.e. via the gut) nutrition is far preferable to parenteral (i.e. IV) nutrition as the latter requires dedicated central venous lines and daily blood tests, and can cause significant problems to patients.

How will you prevent a recurrence of this condition in Mr Simpson?

Most patients will recover without further therapy within a week. If complications develop (see Viva questions), for example sepsis, these should be treated as appropriate. There is, however, no specific treatment for severe pancreatitis per se.

Unless the underlying gallstone aetiology is dealt with, Mr Simpson is liable to suffer another attack of acute pancreatitis. In the case of *mild* pancreatitis, gallstones are usually identified by biliary ultrasound and a **laparoscopic cholecystectomy** is done within the same hospital admission or within 2 weeks of discharge. In the case of patients with *severe* pancreatitis, the patient should have **ERCP** within 72 hours of the onset of the pain if biliary obstruction, biliary sepsis, or persistent organ dysfunction are present. ERCP is accompanied by sphincterotomy, and is followed by delayed cholecystectomy once the patient is fit enough to undergo surgery.

In patients who have alcohol-induced pancreatitis, prevention of recurrence is focused on cessation of drinking.

Short cases

Mr Bickerstaff is a 38-year-old accountant who presents to his GP with a 2-week history of epigastric pain. The pain can come on at any time, he says, but typically follows meals. It is a burning pain and does not radiate anywhere. He has not suffered from waterbrash and has not vomited. The symptoms are no worse at night or when Mr Bickerstaff bends forwards. He has tried over-the-counter antacids with no success. He does not take any regular medications, but smokes 20 cigarettes a day, and drinks 25–30 units of alcohol a week.

On examination, Mr Bickerstaff is obese. There are no obvious stigmata of gastrointestinal disease on inspection. He complains a little of tenderness in the epigastric region on deep palpation, but his abdomen is otherwise soft and non-tender, with no masses or organomegaly. Bowel sounds are present and normal.

What is the most likely diagnosis? How should the patient be managed?

It is most likely that Mr Bickerstaff is suffering from **peptic ulcer disease, gastritis,** or **non-ulcer dyspepsia (NUD, also called idiopathic dyspepsia)**. It is possible that he has **GORD,** but the episodic nature of the pain, inability to recreate the discomfort with a positional change (touching his toes), and lack of history of an acid taste in the mouth make it less likely. His risk factors for peptic ulcer disease include smoking and alcohol. The ineffectiveness of antacids in treating his pain is not unusual; severe dyspepsia often requires stronger medications, such as histamine H_2 receptor antagonists or proton pump inhibitors (PPIs).

Mr Bickerstaff should initially be given lifestyle advice. In the short term he may derive symptomatic benefit from reducing or eliminating his intake of alcohol, caffeine, chocolate, and fatty foods, and stopping smoking. Weight loss will also help him in the longer term.

If conservative management fails to resolve Mr Bickerstaff's symptoms he should be given a trial of either **full-dose PPIs** for 1 month, or should be offered **'test and treat'** therapy for *Helicobacter pylori,* the most common cause of peptic ulcers. If present (as detected by a ^{13}C-urea breath test, anti-*Helicobacter* blood serology or an *H. pylori*-positive endoscopic biopsy), eradicating it with triple therapy should allow the ulcers to heal. There are numerous variations so local guidelines should be checked; NICE guidelines suggest a 7-day, twice-daily course of a full-dose PPI with either metronidazole 400 mg and clarithromycin 250 mg, or amoxicillin 1 g and clarithromycin 500 mg.

There are specific recommendations regarding which patients with dyspepsia should be referred for endoscopy (see Viva questions).

Mr Singh is a 58-year-old man with epigastric pain who has reluctantly been brought to the Emergency Department by his wife. He insists that he only has 'indigestion', as he ate a large meal a couple of hours earlier—around the time that the pain started. His wife confirms that he does suffer from indigestion at times, but is concerned that the pain has not yet subsided and that the over-the-counter antacids she gave him haven't worked. You also discover that her father was recently diagnosed with gastric cancer, which may be a factor in her anxiety.

Mr Singh describes his pain as a burning pain and points to just below the xiphisternum. He says it hasn't radiated or changed in character, and is 8/10 in severity. He has felt nauseated but has not vomited, and has experienced no other symptoms. He has diabetes, for which he takes metformin. He has had no recent health complaints or GP visits, and no previous hospital admissions. He has no risk factors for hepatitis infection or peptic ulcer disease.

On examination, he appears uncomfortable but is haemodynamically stable with a pulse of 87 bpm and blood pressure of 137/88 mmHg.

At this stage, the team managing Mr Singh feel that he is suffering from dyspepsia ('heartburn'). They nonetheless request an ECG and blood tests. His ECG is unremarkable. His blood tests on admission include a haemoglobin of 14.3 mg/dL, white cell count of 6.3×10^9 cells/litre, urea of 5 mg/dL, creatinine of 80 μM, and high-sensitivity troponin T of 56 ng/litre (normal range <14 ng/litre).

What is the most likely diagnosis and why?

Mr Singh has almost certainly had a (partial thickness) **non-ST elevation myocardial infarction** (NSTEMI), based on his elevated troponin. He is in some ways lucky—had his troponin on admission been normal and his symptoms improved, he might have been discharged without waiting for a repeat troponin level (and with a normal ECG).

Mistaking myocardial infarction for 'heartburn' or 'indigestion' is common—cases of a missed diagnosis of myocardial infarction account for the most dollars recovered in medical malpractice suits in the USA. An estimated 6% of patients with myocardial infarction are thought to be misdiagnosed in the UK. Prompt treatment is crucial in the prognosis after myocardial infarction, thus the delay caused by a missed diagnosis is very serious. You must therefore keep myocardial infarction in mind in a patient presenting with epigastric pain—if you don't think about it, you won't diagnose it.

SHORT CASE

Mrs Lloyd is a 54-year-old advertising sales manager who was brought into hospital by ambulance with severe epigastric pain. The pain came on spontaneously while she was in a meeting 3 hours ago, and is described as a constant stabbing pain. The pain has not radiated and has not been relieved by ibuprofen. She has felt nauseated but has not vomited or had any other symptoms. She rates the pain as 10/10 in severity. She last opened her bowels first thing in the morning (8 hours ago) and has noticed no recent change in her stool. In her past medical history she suffers from chronic back pain, for which she takes regular over-the-counter NSAIDs (ibuprofen). She has not been diagnosed with gallstone disease nor recalls suffering from right upper quadrant pain. She has never smoked but drinks 'maybe 20 units' a week at social events with clients.

Her initial observations are: heart rate 104 bpm regular; blood pressure 126/81 mmHg; respiratory rate 17/min; saturations of 100% on room air; temperature 36.6 °C.

As you are examining her, she complains of worsening pain. She is lying motionless on the bed. There is widespread guarding and percussion tenderness. Bowel sounds are absent. The lung bases are clear.

The results of routine bloods requested on admission come back:

Haematology		Biochemistry	
Hb	118 g/L	AST	28 U/L
WCC	13.3×10^9 cells/L	ALT	31 U/L
Platelets	243×10^9 cells/L	ALP	23 U/L
MCV	102 fL	Urea	7 mM
		Creatinine	77 μM
		Ca (corrected)	2.43 mM
		Amylase	387 U/L
		Troponin	<0.2 ng/mL

Her erect chest radiograph is shown in Figure 12.3.

Figure 12.3 Mrs Lloyd's erect chest radiograph.

What is the most likely cause of her presenting symptoms? What happened while she was in hospital to make her symptoms worse?

The most likely diagnosis is **peptic ulcer perforation**. This is consistent with severe epigastric pain, and in her history she has two risk factors for duodenal ulcers: long-term NSAID use and significant alcohol consumption. She also describes suffering from occasional heartburn. Of the blood results, the amylase is significant: it is not as elevated as is typical in acute pancreatitis (>1000 U/L), but is sufficiently elevated to be consistent with a perforated peptic ulcer, bowel obstruction, mesenteric ischaemia, mumps, pancreatic carcinoma, or opiate medications. Notice that the erect chest radiograph shows air under the diaphragm (bilaterally, in this case). Air under the diaphragm (pneumoperitoneum) is diagnostic of a perforated gastrointestinal tract, unless the patient has had recent abdominal surgery to explain this presence of air in the peritoneal cavity.

While in hospital she has developed **peritonitis**. This is identified by the triad of a motionless patient, tenderness and guarding on abdominal palpation, and absent bowel sounds.

Her case is a surgical emergency and she should be referred immediately to the surgeons. In the meantime, she should be given adequate **analgesia, IV fluid resuscitation** and **IV antibiotics, oxygen** as required, be made **nil by mouth**, have a **nasogastric tube** passed (so that gastric contents can come up the NG tube rather than out of her perforated ulcer) and have her **urine output monitored** (which may require a urinary catheter).

Miss O'Riley is a 31-year-old woman referred to your gastrointestinal outpatients clinic for review of her epigastric pain. She has had epigastric pain for the last 12 months, for which she has seen the GP three times and gone to the Emergency Department once. The Emergency Department admission was followed by an outpatient biliary ultrasound, which was reported as normal. There are no obvious precipitants to painful episodes. It is a moderately severe (5/10), burning pain that does not radiate. It is not alleviated by food or defecation. She adds that she often feels bloated and uncomfortable after meals. Miss O'Riley has had no other symptoms. She tells you that, so far, no one has been able to find a cause, much to her distress.

She is taking an antidepressant (citalopram), having recently suffered a traumatic relationship breakup, but no other medications. She has no smoking history and drinks modestly, less than 5 units a week.

An abdominal examination is unremarkable. Her GP's letter adds that he has requested an FBC, CRP, U&Es, creatinine, calcium, and liver function tests, and that all were within the normal ranges. The GP says a therapeutic trial of a PPI for 6 weeks was also unsuccessful in alleviating her symptoms.

You arrange for an oesophagogastroduodenoscopy (OGD) to be performed as an outpatient. Nothing remarkable is seen, and you meet with her for a further consultation.

What is the most likely diagnosis? What will you tell Miss O'Riley?

No organic cause can be found for Miss O'Riley's chronic epigastric pain, as evidenced by normal blood tests, a normal OGD, and normal biliary ultrasound, so the most likely diagnosis is **NUD**. This is a diagnosis of exclusion, albeit a common one, accounting for about 30% of cases of investigated dyspepsia.

As with other functional disorders, the doctor–patient relationship is key to management. You must be sensitive to her concerns in your consultation, particularly as she sees you as something of a last resort and you will not want her to feel alienated by the health service. Each individual case should be treated differently, but in your discussion you may wish to:

- Acknowledge that her symptoms are real. Remember that not being able to find an organic cause does not make her symptoms any less real.

- Reassure her that the good news is that the tests have shown no signs of any of the worrying causes of epigastric pain. You may wish to add that her condition is very common.

- Managing her expectations:
  - Take care not to overly investigate her. Excessive investigation (e.g. MRI) is not only costly, but runs the risk of identifying asymptomatic 'incidentalomas' which may require invasive and risky testing.
  - Be honest about the limitations of medical treatment. She is likely to be worried about prognosis and so you should address it. Prokinetic agents, H_2-receptor antagonists, and PPIs have been shown to have some beneficial effect in some patients and may all be considered (although a PPI has not worked in this case).
  - You should also be honest about her prognosis. Idiopathic dyspepsia is typically a relapsing condition (60–90% of patients have symptoms 2–3 years after diagnosis). However, diagnosis and the lifestyle and medical therapies available make most patients feel better.

- Suggest that she starts with simple measures such as dietary and lifestyle modification. Some patients benefit from avoiding fatty foods and eating smaller, more frequent meals. It is also sensible to avoid drugs that irritate the lining of the gastrointestinal tract (e.g. NSAIDs), and to stop smoking for the same reason.

- She may be interested in the cause. If she is, you should explain that the causes are poorly understood at present. You can direct her to sources of more information if she is interested.
- Keep the door open. This is partly in case any organic disease manifests itself, but also to protect her relationship with health professionals.

Viva questions

What are the indications for endoscopic investigation of dyspepsia?

According to the 2007 NICE guidelines, urgent (within 2 weeks) endoscopic investigation is indicated if any of the following 'red flag' signs are present:

- persistent vomiting
- chronic gastrointestinal bleeding
- weight loss
- progressive dysphagia
- iron deficiency anaemia
- epigastric mass
- suspicious barium meal
- age ≥55 with unexplained and persistent, recent-onset dyspepsia.

How does the breath test for *H. pylori* work?

The carbon urea breath test works as follows: the patient is given a drink of ^{14}C- or ^{13}C-labelled urea. This is metabolized by the bacteria, if present, into labelled CO_2. A breath test is conducted 15 minutes later, and will detect the labelled CO_2 if *H. pylori* is present.

What are the complications of peptic ulcers?

The five main complications of peptic ulcers are:

- **Haemorrhage.** This is associated with high morbidity, and can be particularly severe in patients on anticoagulant therapy. Cardinal symptoms include haematemesis and/or melaena.
- **Perforation.** Patients taking NSAIDs are most at risk. Perforation usually leads to peritonitis.
- **Penetration.** This refers to penetration of the ulcer through the bowel wall without leakage into the peritoneum (as in perforation). This may occur into the pancreas, omentum, biliary tract, colon, and vasculature. Patients typically have a chronic history of peptic ulcer disease. They will report a change in symptoms, such that there is no relationship between pain and mealtimes, and it is no longer relieved by antacids. Weight loss and diarrhoea may also be seen.
- **Scarring.** If sufficiently severe, this can cause gastric outlet obstruction. The patient experiences early satiety, bloating, and/or vomiting of partially digested food.
- **Malignancy.** Chronic gastric ulcers are a risk factor for adenocarcinoma of the stomach.

What are the complications of pancreatitis?

The complications of pancreatitis can be divided into local and systemic:

Local

- Pancreatic
  - Necrosis of the pancreas
  - Abscess formation
  - Pseudocyst (accumulation of fluid in the lesser peritoneal sac)
- Other
  - Paralytic ileus
  - Duodenal stress ulceration
  - Fistula formation to colon
  - Obstructive jaundice due to choledocholithiasis or pancreatic oedema

Systemic

- Sepsis
- Shock, due to release of inflammatory mediators and loss of fluid to the peritoneum ('third space loss') or haemorrhage through the pancreas
- Acute renal failure, secondary to hypoperfusion
- Respiratory compromise, due to release of inflammatory mediators and increased permeability of the alveoli. This ranges from mild atelectasis to pleural effusion to ARDS
- Disseminated intravascular coagulation (DIC), triggered by the strong prothombotic stimulus provided by the pancreatic inflammation
- Metabolic
  - Hypocalcaemia due to saponification of fats in the retroperitoneum
  - Hyperglycaemia due to massive release of glucagon (also insulin but this is more than offset by glucagon release)/due to the inability to produce insulin
- Pancreatic encephalopathy, due to cerebral hypoperfusion, ranging from confusion to coma.

What is the role of stool elastase in chronic pancreatitis management? Why?

Stool elastase is a very good marker of pancreatic function as it is:

- Only synthesized in and excreted by the pancreas
- Stable in transit through the gastrointestinal tract, thus there is a direct correlation between elastase in the stool and in pancreatic fluid

A low stool elastase has a high sensitivity for pancreatic compromise (100% for severe and 77% for moderate disease), with a specificity of about 93%. The specificity of stool elastase levels is compromised in patients with diseases of the small bowel such as coeliac disease, Crohn's, and short gut syndrome.

What are Cushing's and Curling's ulcers?

Cushing's and Curling's ulcers are peptic ulcers distinguished by aetiology. Cushing's ulcers arise after brain injury (remember that Harvey Cushing was a neurosurgeon). Curling's ulcers occur after burns.

What is the differential diagnosis of a raised serum amylase level?

An elevated serum amylase level may be due to:

- Pancreatic pathology
  - Pancreatitis
  - Pancreatic trauma
  - Pancreatic carcinoma
- Other intra-abdominal pathology
  - Perforated peptic ulcer
  - Acute appendicitis
  - Acute cholecystitis
  - Ectopic pregnancy
  - Pelvic inflammatory disease
  - Mesenteric ischaemia
  - Leaking AAA
- Decreased amylase clearance
  - Renal failure (amylase is renally excreted)
  - Macroamylasaemia (amylase is bound to immunoglobulin and cannot be renally excreted)
- Miscellaneous conditions
  - Diabetic ketoacidosis
  - Head injury

Single Best Answers

1. A patient presents with severe epigastric pain and a markedly raised amylase. Which of the following biochemical abnormalities might you also see?

a. Hypercholesteraemia
b. Hypertriglyceridaemia
c. Hypokalaemia

d. Hyponatraemia
e. Positive sweat test

2. A young man presents with a history of several months of upper abdominal pain and a 2 week history of nausea. Examination is normal, but a faecal occult blood test (FOBt) is positive. Oesophagogastroduodenoscopy (OGD) is performed and a solitary 1.5 cm diameter shallow, sharply demarcated ulceration is noted in the stomach. Which of the following is most likely to be true?

a. The lesion is probably malignant
b. Because the lesion is small, a biopsy is not necessary

c. A pancreatic gastrinoma is probably present
d. This patient is probably an alcoholic
e. The lesion is probably located in the antrum

3. You request an oesophagogastroduodenoscopy for a patient with a history of chronic epigastric pain. The report comments on areas of erythematous mucosa extending 3–4 cm proximally from the gastro-oesophageal junction. Which of the following statements is true?

a. This patient has a high alcohol consumption
b. This patient has an increased risk of squamous cell carcinoma

c. This patient is likely to develop a hiatus hernia
d. This patient has iron deficiency anaemia
e. This patient has chronic gastro-oesophageal reflux disease (GORD)

4. Which of the following is not a prognostic indicator in acute pancreatitis?

a. Amylase
b. Calcium
c. Pao_2

d. Urea
e. Age

Core case

Read through the sections in the case boxes, covering up the sections that follow so that you don't see the answer. At the end of each case box, try to answer the question before reading on.

Mr Price is a 47-year-old electrician who presents to his local Emergency Department complaining of nausea and vomiting.

Nausea and vomiting has a very wide differential. Broadly speaking, what can cause nausea and vomiting?

The **vomiting centre** (mainly histamine and acetylcholine receptors) in the medulla oblongata can be activated by four main input systems shown in Figure 13.1: the **vestibular system**, the **central nervous system**, the **chemoreceptor trigger zone** (in the fourth ventricle of the brain), and **cranial nerves IX and X**.

With these four inputs in mind, it becomes easier to understand some of the pathologies that can activate the vomiting centre and cause nausea and vomiting, as is shown in Figure 13.2.

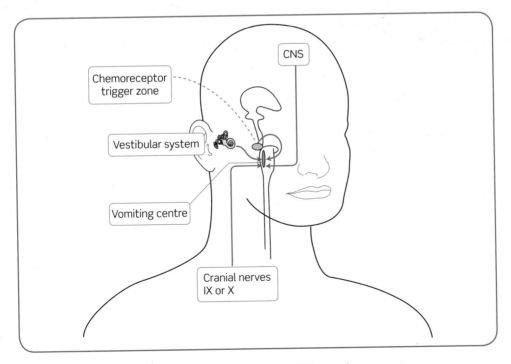

Figure 13.1 The four inputs that activate the vomiting centre. CNS, central nervous system.

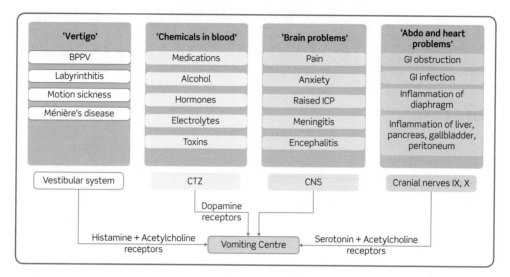

Figure 13.2 Causes of nausea and vomiting. BPPV, benign paroxysmal positional vertigo; CNS, central nervous system; CTZ, chemoreceptor trigger zone; GI, gastrointestinal; ICP, intracranial pressure.

What initial questions will help you narrow down your differential?

Details of the vomit:

- **Contents**
  - **Undigested:** oesophageal disorders, e.g. achalasia, pharyngeal pouch
  - **Partially digested:** gastric outlet obstruction, gastroparesis (delayed stomach emptying, e.g. seen in diabetes mellitus)
  - **Bile (green):** small bowel obstruction (distal to the ampulla of Vater)
  - **Faeculent:** distal intestinal or colonic obstruction. Note: the only time you will see faecal (i.e. true faeces), as opposed to faeculent (i.e. foul looking), vomiting is in patients with a gastrocolonic fistula... or coprophagia
  - **Blood/coffee-ground:** haematemesis (see Chapter 5)
  - **Large volume:** less likely to be functional.

- **Timing**
  - **Early morning:** classically in pregnancy and raised intracranial pressure.
  - **Duration:** this is useful in identifying the severity (patients with severe nausea and vomiting present early) and a longer time course makes acute pathologies such as bowel obstruction less likely, as untreated this will either deteriorate or resolve.

- **Association with eating?**
  - Vomiting within an hour of eating suggests an obstruction high in the gastrointestinal (GI) tract proximal to the gastric outlet. If this is the case, you should ask about peptic ulcer disease (or a history of dyspepsia) as this can cause scarring and pyloric stenosis.

- Vomiting after a longer postprandial delay is consistent with an obstruction lower in the GI tract, usually in the small bowel.
- Early satiety, postprandial bloating, and abdominal discomfort together suggest gastroparesis or outlet obstruction.

Details of any pain:

- Use the **SOCRATES** mnemonic to characterize the pain (see Chapter 12).
- The site is indicative of certain pathologies (e.g. right upper quadrant suggests a hepatobiliary cause, epigastric suggests a pancreatic or gastroduodenal cause). However, localization of pain is far from accurate in abdominal pathology due to the neural wiring and embryology, and also anatomical variations.
- Relief after vomiting is consistent with obstruction.

Other symptoms?

- **Fever?** Any infectious or inflammatory cause: gastroenteritis, appendicitis, cholecystitis, cholangitis, pancreatitis, hepatitis, urinary tract infection (UTI), meningoencephalitis.
- **Headache? Visual disturbance? Any other neurological symptoms? (e.g. cranial nerve palsies, limb weakness, paraesthesia)** Meningitis, encephalitis, migraine, raised intracranial pressure.
- **Vertigo ('the room is spinning')? Difficulty standing/walking (as a consequence of vertigo)?** Labyrinthitis, Ménière's, benign paroxysmal positional vertigo (BPPV).

Bowel movements?

You should always ask when a patient's bowels were last open. This includes passing both faeces and flatus.

- **Delay/absolute constipation:** a long delay could suggest bowel obstruction (either mechanical or functional, i.e. ileus). Constipation may simply be a feature of eating less and vomiting, but *absolute* constipation of faeces and flatus is a serious sign, suggesting bowel obstruction. Constipation is also important as patients with extensive faecal loading may well become nauseated and vomit.
- **Diarrhoea?** Diarrhoea and vomiting suggests infectious gastroenteritis.

Exposure to infectious bowel pathogens?

- **Close contacts also suffering nausea and vomiting?** Suggests contagious aetiology such as rotavirus, adenovirus, norovirus, etc. or sharing contaminated food (e.g. buffet food infected with *Staphylococcus aureus* enterotoxin).
- **Living in close quarters?** Hospitals, army barracks, boarding schools, and cruise ships are all notorious for outbreaks of infectious GI pathogens.
- **Recent foreign travel?** Differing hygiene standards and local pathogens make travelling abroad a high risk for GI infections.
- **Unusual meals recently?** A recent barbeque, wedding buffet, late-night kebab, restaurant meal, etc. may all suggest exposure to an infectious GI pathogen.

Exposure to potential drugs and toxins?

- **Medications?** Opiates, chemotherapy, anticonvulsants, antibiotics, and many other drugs can cause nausea and vomiting.
- **Industrial chemicals?** Arsenic and organophosphate fertilizers, for example, can cause vomiting.
- **Alcohol? Illicit drugs?**

History of previous abdominal surgery?

Previous surgery predisposes to adhesions between the peritoneum and the bowel, which can cause bowel obstruction.

The principal components of this approach are summarized in the flowchart in Figure 13.3, along with some examples of the pathologies they could indicate.

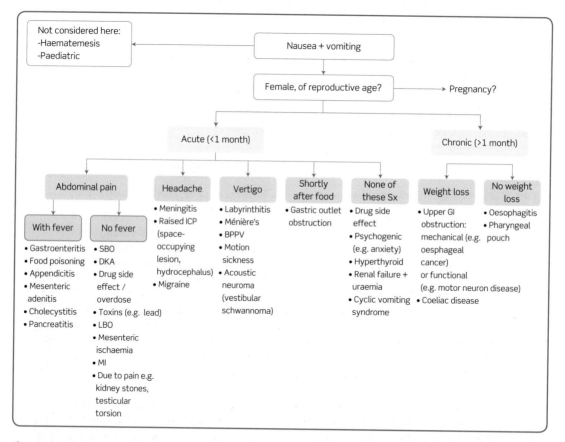

Figure 13.3 Flowchart for investigating nausea and vomiting. BPPV, benign paroxysmal positional vertigo; DKA, diabetic ketoacidosis; GI, gastrointestinal; ICP, intracranial pressure; LBO, large bowel obstruction; MI, myocardial infarction; SBO, small bowel obstruction; Sx, symptoms.

As mentioned earlier, the differential diagnosis for nausea and vomiting is very broad, including some potentially serious causes.

What signs and/or symptoms will help alert you to these?

First and foremost you will be concerned about any patient who requires resuscitation on a primary survey of their airway, breathing, and circulation (ABC). In particular, persistent large-volume vomiting can result in dehydration, which may be severe enough to decrease the patient's consciousness.

Specific worrying symptoms and signs are shown in Table 13.1.

You should also be worried about a drug overdose; the signs and symptoms of overdose will depend on the drug taken.

Table 13.1 Worrying signs and symptoms in nausea and vomiting

Features	Serious condition suggested
Motionless patient, rigid abdomen, absent bowel sounds	?Peritonitis (any cause)
Bilious or faeculent vomiting, distended abdomen, absolute constipation, abdominal pain	?Bowel obstruction
Very high fever (>38.5 °C)	?Infection
Early morning vomiting, headache worse when lying down, nerve VI palsy	?Raised intracranial pressure
Central, crushing chest pain	?Myocardial infarction
Meningism (stiff neck, photophobia, headache)	?Meningitis
Reduced consciousness	?Diabetic ketoacidosis ?Meningitis ?Raised intracranial pressure
Haematemesis	?Bleeding peptic ulcer ?Oesophageal varices

Mr Price tells you that he started vomiting a couple of hours after eating dinner the night before last. The vomit was 'normal vomit', by which he means digested food, and is not obviously associated with meals although he has barely eaten during the past 36 hours. The pain has been 'cramping' and is vaguely umbilical but not well localized. He gets mild relief from vomiting, and says the pain is severe (8/10). He has felt generally unwell but has not taken his temperature. He has, however, had no night sweats. None of his close contacts have reported any vomiting. He last opened his bowels yesterday morning and he cannot recall passing any flatus today. About 20 years ago he had an appendicectomy, but has had no other surgery.

Mr Price tells you he takes sumatriptan for occasional migraines, when he needs to. He also uses some herbal remedies and aromatherapy. He takes no regular medications. He has no allergies and is a non-smoker who drinks about a bottle of wine a week at most. He denies taking any recreational drugs.

What signs would you specifically look for on examination?

You should of course conduct a full examination. However, specific signs you would look for in Mr Price's case include:

On inspection

- **Hydration status:** e.g. dry mucous membranes. It is useful to ask the patient if they feel thirsty, as this is a reasonable indicator of patients being dehydrated
- **Abdominal distension:** suggestive of obstruction—but remember this can be caused by six Fs: faeces, flatus, fluid, fetus (not in Mr Price's case!), fat, filthy great tumour
- **Scars:** from previous abdominal surgery, which could be associated with adhesions
- **Hernias:** (particularly irreducible hernias) that could contain trapped bowel and cause the obstruction or which could appear due to obstruction and raised intra-abdominal pressure
- **Jaundice:** consistent with a hepatobiliary cause

On palpation

- **Tender abdomen:** suggesting inflammation somewhere in the peritoneal cavity
- **Signs of dehydration:** cold peripheries, delayed capillary refill time
- **Masses:** could be causing an obstruction
- **Guarding and rigidity:** suggests peritonitis

On auscultation

- **Bowel sounds:** absent in ileus (e.g. due to peritonitis) and high-pitched or 'tinkling' in mechanical obstruction

You examine Mr Price. He is lying in bed but in some discomfort from the 'stomach cramps'. He is not jaundiced but has an appendicectomy scar and mild distension of his abdomen. There are no other peripheral stigmata of disease. His abdomen is soft with mild discomfort but no focal tenderness or peritonism, and no palpable masses or organomegaly. You hear high-pitched bowel sounds on auscultation.

His observations are as follows: temperature 36.5 °C, heart rate 66 bpm, blood pressure 128/69 mmHg, respiratory rate 12/min, oxygen saturations 99% on room air.

In light of the history and examination, which investigations would you request?

You should request the follow investigations:

Bloods

- **Full blood count (FBC)** and **C-reactive protein (CRP):** raised inflammatory markers (white cell count (WCC), CRP) would indicate infection or inflammation.
- **Urea and electrolytes (U&Es):** in protracted or severe vomiting there may be an electrolyte imbalance. The urea may be raised due to dehydration with subsequent renal hypoperfusion. A baseline is also needed if the patient may go to surgery.
- **Venous blood gas (VBG):** The pH and lactate will give you an idea of how sick this patient is (a metabolic acidosis with a raised lactate implying the patient is critically ill). VBGs are also a quick way

of obtaining results for Na$^+$, K$^+$ and in some machines a creatinine (when working in the Emergency Department, where blood gas analysers are readily available).

- **Liver enzymes:** hepatobiliary pathologies will lead to deranged liver enzymes, e.g. biliary disease causes a cholestatic picture (raised alkaline phosphatase (ALP) and gamma glutamyl transferase (GGT)), whereas hepatitis causes a transaminitis (raised alanine aminotransferase (ALT) and aspartate aminotransferase (AST)).

- **Amylase:** to help confirm or exclude pancreatitis. Note this may be normal in pancreatitis, particularly in chronic pancreatitis when it is thought that the chronicity of the insult causes necrosis and depletes the store of amylase.

- **Group and save:** As Mr Price may need surgery on this admission it would be wise to 'group and save' his blood group, so that blood is available if he proceeds to theatre.

Imaging

- **Supine abdominal radiograph:** you must request this to look for signs of intestinal obstruction. Indeed, looking for signs of bowel obstruction on abdominal radiograph is one of the few indications for requesting this investigation nowadays (a foreign body and toxic megacolon being the others).

- **Erect chest radiograph:** this is used to look for air under the diaphragm, which may be seen if the bowel has perforated and is a serious sign. The patient needs to be able to sit up for ~ 10 min before the radiograph is obtained, to allow air to migrate up towards the diaphragm.

Other potential investigations:

You would not initially order these for Mr Price but might consider them in patients with a different history and examination:

- **Pregnancy test:** you must consider (and test for) pregnancy in any woman of potentially childbearing age. You should enquire if they are sexually active, and explain that you need to perform a pregnancy test if only to exclude pregnancy. It is worth noting that no contraceptive method is failsafe (e.g. the combined oral contraceptive pill, properly taken, still has a failure rate of 1 in every 100 women per year). It is interesting to note that in some studies β-human chorionic gonadotropin (β-HCG) is associated with the nausea and vomiting seen in pregnancy, and that the hyperemesis (exaggerated nausea and vomiting) seen with multiple pregnancies and molar pregnancies may reflect the greater production of β-HCG in these states.

- **Toxicology screen:** if there is suspicion of accidental or deliberate overdose of specific medications (e.g. paracetamol, aspirin) then it would be worthwhile to screen for these drugs. Remember there is no such thing as a generic 'tox screen' that tests for everything!

- **Contrast studies:** e.g. small bowel follow-through, looking for obstruction if this was not evident on abdominal radiography.

- **Abdominal CT:** looking for intraperitoneal pathology.

- **Head CT:** looking for intracranial pathology such as dilated ventricles or mass lesions (if the history suggests raised intracranial pressure).

Older textbooks may refer to the 'saline load test', which was used to distinguish gastric outlet obstruction from gastroparesis (delayed gastric emptying). The advent of endoscopy has made it redundant.

Stool gazing yields pitifully little information and is therefore (thankfully!) a dying art.

Mr Price's blood tests come back and show:

Haematology		Biochemistry			
WCC	7.8×10^9 cells/L	Na	138 mM	AST	28 U/L
		K	3.8 mM	ALT	26 U/L
		Urea	4.3 mM	ALP	30 U/L
		Creatinine	90 µM	Amylase	154 U/dL
		CRP	22 mg/L		

His chest radiograph is normal and his abdominal radiograph is shown in Figure 13.4.

Figure 13.4 Mr Price's abdominal radiograph taken on admission.

What does the abdominal radiograph show? Based on all the information you have, what is the most likely diagnosis? What is a possible aetiology in Mr Price?

The abdominal radiograph shows centrally located loops of distended (>3 cm diameter) small bowel with valvulae conniventes.

The most likely diagnosis is **small bowel obstruction**. A possible aetiology is entanglement of a loop of bowel in **postoperative adhesions** from his previous appendicectomy. Postsurgical inflammatory response leads, over time, to the formation of fibrous 'adhesions' between the bowel and the parietal peritoneum. Obstruction may occur shortly after the operation or, as in the case of Mr Price, many years later if a loop of bowel gets twisted in a pre-existing adhesion.

Small bowel obstruction accounts for 20% of acute surgical admissions.

The patient is referred for admission under the care of the surgeons.

While you await a surgical bed and review, how should you manage Mr Price?

As always, you should have checked Mr Price's need for resuscitation (ABC) on admission (and on an ongoing basis as necessary).

You should also start the following:

- **Nil by mouth** (NBM), in case Mr Price needs to go to theatre (an empty stomach reduces the risk of aspiration on induction of anaesthesia) and to 'rest the bowel'.

- **'Drip and suck'**, i.e. IV fluids and aspiration of gastric contents via a nasogastric (NG) tube. He will need the fluids as he may be dehydrated from vomiting and is NBM, plus you may need to correct any electrolyte imbalance. Aspirating the gastric contents will decompress the stomach, making the patient feel considerably better in most cases, and will reduce the risk of aspiration following vomiting.

- **Analgesia.** You must not forget this—patients will be very grateful! However don't forget that opiates can cause nausea and constipation, and NSAIDs are nephrotoxic so should be avoided in dehydrated individuals or those with acute kidney injury.

- **Antiemetics.** Caution must be exercised with the use of antiemetics: metoclopramide is a prokinetic and can make things worse if obstruction is present. Cyclizine or ondansetron are better alternatives in this situation.

Mr Price goes to the surgical unit for review.

How are the surgeons likely to manage Mr Price?

A sensible approach would be:

1 **A trial of conservative management**, i.e. fluids and NG aspiration ('drip and suck'), to see if the obstruction resolves of its own accord. He should be reviewed regularly to ensure he does not deteriorate (e.g. bowel strangulation).

2 **CT scan**: To clearly demonstrate the exact level of obstruction (looking for a transition point), and establish whether there is a closed loop obstruction (which will not decompress of its own accord), ischaemic bowel, or a cause for obstruction other than adhesions (such as intussusception or a mass lesion).

If the patient has a virgin abdomen it is likely that the surgical team will request a CT at an early stage. If the patient has undergone previous surgery, and thus is at risk of adhesional obstruction, the surgical team may choose to wait ~24 hours to see if the obstruction settles prior to requesting a scan (unless there are worrying features on abdominal radiograph).

3 **Surgery**, if:
   - there are signs of strangulation or peritonism
   - after ~48 hours the obstruction has not resolved; or
   - there is no history of abdominal surgery, making adhesions less likely and more sinister causes more likely.

In Mr Price's case, the surgeons attempted conservative management, but 48 hours later he was still in pain and had not been able to keep anything down. A CT scan revealed a single transition point in the small bowel with no masses or suggestion of ischaemia. The surgeons then performed a laparotomy and divided postoperative adhesions.

About a quarter of patients with small bowel obstruction will undergo surgery, to divide postoperative adhesions or repair hernias, with or without small bowel resection.

Short cases

Mrs O'Connor is a 31-year-old woman who is 34 weeks pregnant and is referred to her local maternity unit by her GP with a 48 hour history of nausea and vomiting. The vomit looks like digested food, and she has been unable to keep anything down other than a bit of water and some soup. She has had diarrhoea and abdominal pain, which she still complains of. She is multiparous, with four previous children and says she never had any morning sickness (or any other problems) during those pregnancies. Two of her children have also been unwell with vomiting and diarrhoea over the past week.

On examination, her pulse is 88 bpm, blood pressure 110/66 mmHg (her pregnancy notes show a previous baseline blood pressure in pregnancy of 105/60 mmHg), temperature 37.7 °C, respiratory rate 12/min, and oxygen saturations of 98% on room air. Her abdomen is soft and non-tender, and the fetal heart rate is present and normal on cardiotocography (CTG) at admission. Her blood tests on the day are:

Haematology		Biochemistry			
Hb	123 g/L	Na	136 mM	Bilirubin	11 μM
WCC	11.5×10^9 cells/L	K	3.8 mM	AST	10 U/L
		Urea	4.5 mM	Uric acid	2.8 mg/dL
		Creatinine	81 μM	(baseline 43 μM at the start of pregnancy)	

Urinalysis shows ketonuria 1+ but no proteinuria, haematuria, glycosuria, pyuria or nitrites.

What is the most likely diagnosis?

Mrs O'Connor has a 2-day history of vomiting with probable affected contacts (her children) and diarrhoea as well as vomiting. Vomiting alone could potentially represent an atypical presentation of pre-eclampsia, but this is unlikely as her BP is not raised, her liver enzymes and uric acid are normal, and she has no proteinuria. A UTI is unlikely as her urinalysis has no pyuria nor nitrites. The most likely diagnosis is **gastroenteritis** (i.e. infection of the bowel), particularly given the combination of diarrhoea and vomiting. It is unlikely to be 'morning sickness' as this is most common in the first trimester and she has no history of it in previous pregnancies; moreover this would not explain the diarrhoea. It is also unlikely to be 'food poisoning', i.e. due to a toxin in the food (which may be a bacterial or environmental toxin) rather than infection, as toxins do not usually persist for more than 24 hours, whereas infections often do.

It may be tempting to discharge Mrs O'Connor home as gastroenteritis is a benign, common, self-limiting, usually harmless condition in almost all patients. However, she has ketonuria suggesting she in a state of metabolic starvation (due to not eating because of the vomiting), which is less than ideal in a pregnant woman whose caloric and metabolic requirements will be slightly above those of a non-pregnant woman. More worryingly, while her creatinine falls within normal limits for a non-pregnant woman, 80 mM/L is the top end of the normal range for pregnancy and, worse yet, is double her previous baseline level during pregnancy. This doubling implies that she has **acute kidney injury** (AKI).

AKI is a medical emergency as it is associated with increased morbidity and mortality in all patient groups. Despite this, a recent National Confidential Enquiry into Patient Outcome and Death (NCEPOD) revealed that only 50% of patients with AKI get good care. This patient needs admission for intravenous fluids (some of which will need to include dextrose given her state of metabolic starvation), a fluid in/out chart, daily weight chart, monitoring of electrolytes and renal function, and discussion with a senior renal physician (if nothing else to arrange follow-up for her AKI). Discharge will require resolution of her symptoms and demonstration that her renal function has returned to baseline or is improving.

SHORT CASE

A 16-year-old girl is brought into the Emergency Department after several episodes of vomiting. She is also becoming drowsy and difficult to rouse. She had a history of thirst and polyuria in the previous days, and had abdominal pain with her nausea and vomiting. Her parents say she has vomited her last meals but there has been no bile or blood in the vomitus.

On examination, her pulse is 103 bpm, blood pressure 111/63 mmHg, temperature 36.2 °C, respiratory rate 25/min, and oxygen saturations of 100% on room air. She has dry mucous membranes but the rest of the physical examination was unremarkable.

Her capillary glucose is 24.7 mM. Her capillary ketones are 7 mM. Urinalysis revealed ++ glucose, +++ ketones and a negative pregnancy test. A VBG and formal bloods are performed and show:

Venous blood gas		Haematology		Biochemistry	
pH	7.25	Hb	123 g/L	Na	128 mM
Lactate	2.8 mM	RCC	4.1×10^{12} cells/L	K	4.9 mM
Glucose	25.2	WCC	6.6×10^9 cells/L	Urea	8.3 mM
Cl	101 mM			Creatinine	168 µM
HCO_3	7.2 mM				

What is the most likely diagnosis? How would you interpret the VBG in the context of your diagnosis? What is the anion gap?

This girl has **diabetic ketoacidosis**, based on her symptoms, urinalysis, and the results of her initial tests which demonstrate *diabetes mellitus* (raised glucose), *ketosis*, and *acidaemia*. Diabetic ketoacidosis can present with vomiting, abdominal pain, polydipsia, polyuria, headache, and, in more extreme cases, decreased consciousness and Kussmaul breathing. The urinalysis shows ketone production, which is a common finding in starved patients (who have low insulin levels and a normal glucose maintained by glycogen breakdown and gluconeogenesis), but is very abnormal in the presence of high glucose, as high glucose should result in the production of raised insulin levels which block the production of ketone bodies. There is also glucosuria, also consistent with insufficient insulin production and sustained hyperglycaemia. Her serum glucose is elevated (>11 mM). Her creatinine is also high, probably due to her dehydration (supported by the clinical finding of dry mucous membranes). Her sodium is low, probably artificially so ('pseudohyponatraemia') due to the high glucose in the serum that is distorting the readings made by the laboratory machine (blood gas machines are not prone to this artefact).

Her VBG shows an acidosis (pH <7.35). The low bicarbonate (<22 mM) indicates that this is a **metabolic acidosis**. The anion gap is calculated as $[K^+] + [Na^+] - [Cl^-] - [HCO_3^-]$. In this case, it is raised (>16 mM) at 24.7 mM. Put simplistically, a raised anion gap suggests the presence of extra acid groups in the blood (e.g. ketone bodies, lactate, aspirin) rather than the loss of alkali (e.g. bicarbonate in diarrhoea).

The chronic management of type 1 diabetes mellitus is discussed in other textbooks. In the acute setting, diabetic ketoacidosis may seem daunting but there are step-by-step guidelines that can be followed (such as those from <http://www.diabetes.org.uk[†]>). Essentially, this involves giving IV fluids to rehydrate the patient and IV insulin as an infusion (not a bolus) to suppress ketosis, until the ketones have disappeared from repeat blood tests. In fact, these patients need intensive monitoring: of their fluid balance, capillary glucose, ketones, and serum potassium (in case of a drop in potassium while on IV insulin; which will invariably need replacing). Potassium therapy is often called for (indeed most guidelines call for 20 mmol of potassium to be added in each 500 ml of fluid given), but bicarbonate is rarely given to correct the acidosis. Patients should be transferred to subcutaneous insulin once capillary ketones are <0.3 mM and pH is >7.3.

SHORT CASE

Miss Agar is a 15-year-old schoolgirl who presents to the hospital (she is worried her GP is overly friendly with her parents) with a history of several days early morning nausea and vomiting. The vomit consists of her last meal and sometimes 'some bile', which she describes as a slight yellowing (true bile, however, is green). She has had no abdominal pain, no fever, headache, visual disturbance, vertigo, or other symptoms except for feeling a bit tired. You ask her if she could be pregnant; she tells you she has had sex four times in the last month using the withdrawal method. Her last period was around 4 or 5 weeks ago, she cannot quite remember but says she is late.

Her pulse is 63 bpm, blood pressure 108/61 mmHg, temperature 36.1 °C, respiratory rate 10/min, and she has oxygen saturations of 100% on room air. Her abdomen is soft and non-tender with no organomegaly, and the rest of her examination is unremarkable. No abnormalities are noted on urinalysis.

What is the most likely diagnosis and how would you confirm this? What medications could you use to treat Miss Agar?

The most likely diagnosis is **pregnancy**, and you must perform a pregnancy test. 70–85% of pregnant women suffer with nausea or vomiting and 50% have both, especially in the first trimester.

Before jumping in with medications, you should consider conservative measures such as lifestyle advice. Eating smaller meals more slowly can reduce symptoms in pregnancy, and some women may find that dietary adjustments (e.g. avoiding spicy/fatty/acidic foods) also help.

If non-pharmacological measures are unsuccessful, you should consider antiemetic drugs. You need to be very careful about the drugs and doses you give in pregnancy. In large part this is because trials are rarely conducted on pregnant women and so the effects of many drugs in pregnancy are not known. Antihistamines (e.g. meclizine or promethazine), electrolyte replacement, and thiamine supplementation are recommended for morning sickness. In severe cases (hyperemesis gravidarum) prochlorperazine, chlorpromazine, metoclopramide, ondansetron, or, if symptoms are refractory to antiemetics, corticosteroids can be used.

[†] The Diabetes UK Guideline on Management of Diabetic Ketoacidosis in Adults can be found online at <http://tinyurl.com/cerg9zl>.

SHORT CASE

Mrs Bray is a 74-year-old woman brought in to her GP by her daughter who says she has been vomiting regularly over the last few days. This has happened mainly in the mornings, and she has also had a headache that is worst in the mornings. Mrs Bray has noticed no change in her vision but it is a little blurry in any case as she is developing cataracts. On questioning she tells you the vomit is small amounts of food, and is not accompanied with abdominal pain or fever. She can think of no recent head trauma and has no other symptoms. She is a diabetic for which she is on metformin, and also takes ramipril and simvastatin. She has been taking paracetamol for the headaches but it hasn't worked. She does not drink or smoke, but smoked 10 cigarettes a day until her husband died of a heart attack 25 years ago (a total of 30 years, or 15 pack years).

Her vital signs are pulse 86 bpm, blood pressure 138/63 mmHg, temperature 36.7 °C, respiratory rate 12/min, and oxygen saturations of 99% on room air. On examination, her abdomen is soft and non-tender with no organomegaly. Her chest is clear, and her heart sounds are present with no added sounds. She has no focal neurological signs on examination of her limbs. Cranial nerve examination reveals double vision on extreme right gaze and failure of the right eye to abduct. The rest of her cranial nerve examination is normal.

What is the most likely cause of her vomiting? What bedside examination would help you confirm this?

You must suspect **raised intracranial pressure** as the cause of Mrs Bray's nausea and vomiting because she has two key features of this:

- Headaches that are worse on lying down
- Early morning nausea and vomiting. This is thought to be because during sleep we tend to hypoventilate, causing a rise in pCO_2. The cerebral vasculature dilates slightly in response to the rising CO_2, with the increased blood flow resulting in a further increase in ICP and more pronounced symptoms on waking.

Mrs Bray also has signs suggestive of a cranial nerve VI palsy. This is the commonest focal neurological deficit in raised intracranial pressure because of the long intracranial course of nerve VI, which increases the points at which it can be compressed. The most likely underlying cause is metastatic spread of a cancer to the brain, although it could also be a primary brain tumour or another space-occupying lesion (such as a large subdural haematoma).

At the bedside you should perform **fundoscopy**, to look for papilloedema. This is not always present but when it is, is a good sign of raised intracranial pressure. Mrs Bray will need imaging (CT and/or MRI) of her head looking for a space-occupying lesion.

SHORT CASE

Mr Pitman is an electrical engineer in his mid-20s who comes into hospital suffering with severe abdominal pain and vomiting. He says it began 2 or 3 days ago but has been getting progressively worse. You ask about the pain and he tells you it was like a diffuse ache which he thought would pass, but is now much sharper and points to his right iliac fossa. It is uncomfortable whatever position he is in and has not been alleviated by eating, fasting, vomiting, or the large doses of paracetamol and ibuprofen he says he has tried. You ask about the journey to the hospital and he tells you it was very painful. He tells you he has vomited four times and brings up partially digested food, but there has been less of this in the past 24 hours as he has lost his appetite and not eaten. He adds that he has been feverish, although he did not actually take his temperature. He last opened his bowels the previous evening but has passed flatus since then. There is no history of affected contacts. He is usually fit and well, with no current diagnoses or surgical history. Other than the painkillers, he takes no medications.

His pulse is 124 bpm, blood pressure 113/65 mmHg, temperature 38.3 °C, respiratory rate 14/min, and oxygen saturations of 99% on room air. He is lying very still when you examine him and his abdomen is rigid and tender to light palpation throughout, with rebound tenderness also present. Bowel sounds are decreased. The rest of your examination is unremarkable.

Blood tests include:

Haematology		Biochemistry	
Hb	147 g/L	Na	142 mM
WCC	14.2×10^9 cells/L	K	3.9 mM
		Urea	8.6 mM
		Creatinine	81 µM

What is the most likely diagnosis?

Mr Pitman gives a good history for **appendicitis**, reinforced by the clinical signs and investigations. Key symptoms include a pain that was poorly localized but now localizes to the site of the appendix, anorexia, fever, and vomiting. Clinically he is febrile and has signs of peritonism (he is motionless with a rigid, very tender abdomen), suggesting a **perforated appendix**. This is a surgical emergency as the patient is at very high risk of deteriorating into septic shock from the gut contents spilling into this peritoneal cavity.

Mr Pitman will require resuscitation with IV fluid boluses (titrated to response in his heart rate), broad spectrum IV antibiotics, analgesia, antiemetics and to be kept nil by mouth in preparation for surgery. He then requires an urgent referral to a senior surgeon for consideration of emergency surgery (an appendicectomy and washout of any contamination from the perforated appendix).

Viva questions

If a dehydrated patient is able to tolerate oral fluids, what is the best fluid to use and why?

The best fluid is oral rehydration solution. This contains sodium, glucose, and water in the correct proportions to make optimal use of the sodium–glucose cotransporter in the gut wall that drives fluid absorption. The best way to give it is to encourage patients to take it *'little and often'* as they will find this easier than trying to gulp down large volumes in one go when they are unwell.

What is the basis of the pregnancy test available over the counter?

The pregnancy test measures β-HCG. This is produced by the placenta after implantation of the fertilized ovum and can be detected around 12 days after fertilization.

A patient with terminal lung cancer presents with nausea and vomiting. They have widespread metastatic disease and are receiving palliative chemotherapy. What mechanisms could be mediating their nausea and vomiting? (Hint: there are lots!)

There are a variety of mechanisms:

- Metabolic: hypercalcaemia (bone involvement), uraemia
- Intracranial: raised intracranial pressure due to brain metastases
- GI: constipation, bowel obstruction or ileus, hepatomegaly (pressing on the stomach)
- Psychogenic: anxiety
- Chemotherapy (particularly platinum-based) or opiate analgesia

---

Name the common surgical scars on the schematic diagram in Figure 13.5, and give an example of the operations each approach might be used for.

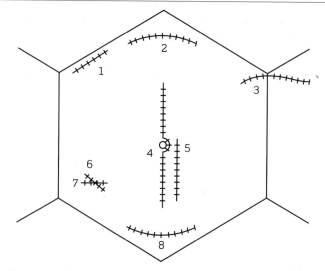

Figure 13.5 Common surgical scars. See text for key.

CONTINUED ➤

CONTINUED

1 Kocher's (or subcostal) incision: cholecystectomy

2 Rooftop incision: Whipple's surgery, gastric surgery

3 Transverse abdominal incision for nephrectomy

4 Midline incision: laparotomy, e.g. exploratory, bowel obstruction, gynaecological

5 Paramedian incision: as for midline incision

6 Gridiron or McBurney's incision: appendicectomy

7 Lanz incision: appendicectomy

8 Pfannensteil incision: Caesarean section, gynaecological operation.

Don't forget to look for porthole scars (including one in the umbilicus) for laparoscopic surgery.

What are the mechanisms of action of the following antiemetics: cyclizine; metoclopramide; ondansetron; haloperidol? Based on this, give an example of a condition where each might be indicated.

- **Cyclizine** is an antihistamine and antimuscarinic that blocks acetylcholine receptors in vestibular and vomiting centres. It is useful in postoperative nausea, bowel obstruction nausea (as it is antikinetic), motion sickness and other labyrinthine aetiologies, and also in conditions causing raised intracranial pressure.

- **Metoclopramide** has agonist properties at $5\text{-}HT_4$ (serotonin) receptors and antagonist properties at dopamine (D_2) receptors such as those found in the chemoreceptor trigger zone and myenteric plexus of the GI tract. It is prokinetic, particularly in the stomach, and therefore indicated in causes of delayed stomach emptying, e.g. as a side effect of opiates, gastroparesis. Because it is a prokinetic, it is *contraindicated* in bowel obstruction. Its antidopaminergic mechanism means that it should also be used with caution in patients with Parkinson's disease.

- **Ondansetron** is a $5\text{-}HT_3$ (serotonin) receptor antagonist that acts on receptors in the gut and the chemoreceptor trigger zone. It is useful for chemotherapy-induced and postoperative vomiting.

- **Haloperidol** is an antagonist of dopamine (D_2) receptors such as those found in the chemoreceptor trigger zone and myenteric plexus of the GI tract. At low doses (rather than the higher doses used in psychosis), it acts both centrally and on the GI tract to remove inhibition to normal motility. It is useful in treating drug-induced and metabolic causes of nausea and vomiting, and also vomiting due to raised intracranial pressure.

What are the potential complications of vomiting?

Vomiting can cause:

- Dehydration and renal impairment
- Electrolyte imbalance, particularly hypokalaemia and hypochloraemia
- Metabolic alkalosis
- Aspiration and aspiration pneumonia
- Mallory–Weiss tear in the mucosa of the upper oesophagus, leading to bleeding
- Boerhaave's syndrome—rupture of the oesophagus
- Loss of tooth enamel in chronic vomiting (e.g. bulimia nervosa) leading to dental caries.

Nausea and vomiting is common in postoperative patients. What factors might be contributing to this?

There are a number of reasons why patients might be expected to suffer from postoperative nausea and vomiting (PONV):

- Preoperative factors
    - Patient factors, e.g. obesity, female, non-smokers
    - Prolonged preoperative fasting
    - Anxiety
    - Previous postoperative nausea and vomiting
- Intraoperative factors
    - Opioid use
    - Inhalation (volatile) anaesthetics
    - Drugs such as teicoplanin, syntocinon and ergometrine.
    - Site of surgery: ENT surgery, gynaecological and abdominal surgery
- Postoperative factors
    - Pain
    - Postoperative opioid analgesia
    - Early postoperative intake of food
    - 'Dizziness'/light-headedness due to dehydration, hypotension
    - Ileus

Single Best Answers

1. **A patient presents complaining of a 1 week history of constant vertigo and nausea. They say the vertigo persists regardless of their position or movement. Their hearing is intact. Which of the following is the most likely cause?**

   a. Benign paroxysmal positional vertigo (BPPV)
   b. Labyrinthitis
   c. Motion sickness
   d. Orthostatic hypotension
   e. Ménière's disease

2. **There is an outbreak of vomiting and watery, non-bloody diarrhoea in an old people's home. Which of the following is the most likely causative agent?**

   a. Rotavirus
   b. Norovirus
   c. Giardia
   d. Shigella
   e. *E. coli* O157

3. **A young patient with acute onset abdominal pain and vomiting is operated on for suspected appendicitis. The pathologist examines the resected appendix and finds the inflammation is limited to the serosa. Which should they suspect?**

   a. Normal appendix
   b. Mild early acute appendicitis
   c. Chronic appendicitis
   d. Peritonitis
   e. Polyarteritis nodosa

4. **A previously healthy 4-week-old boy with no apparent congenital anomalies is brought to hospital with projectile vomiting after each meal. He is afebrile and has not had any diarrhoea, although is dehydrated. Which of the following is the most probable cause?**

   a. Hirschsprung disease
   b. Tracheo-oesophageal fistula
   c. Congenital duodenal atresia
   d. Pyloric stenosis
   e. Gastroenteritis

5. **An elderly man has died after 6 months of anorexia, vomiting, abdominal pain, and 15 kg weight loss. His autopsy reports a shrunken stomach with a thickened gastric wall and extensive overlying mucosal erosions. The liver is characterized by several tan mass lesions. Which of the following most likely preceded his terminal illness?**

   a. Chronic alcohol abuse
   b. NSAID use
   c. Diabetes mellitus
   d. Pernicious anaemia
   e. HIV infection

Jaundice

Core case

Read through the sections in the case boxes, covering up the sections that follow so that you don't see the answer. At the end of each case box, try to answer the question before reading on.

Miss Watroba is a 28-year-old woman from Poland who has recently moved to the UK. She has attended her GP because she has developed 'yellow eyes'. As soon as she walks into your office, you can see she is jaundiced. Jaundice is due to the excessive accumulation of bilirubin in tissues.

What is the normal metabolism of bilirubin?

The metabolism of bilirubin in humans is summarized in Figure 14.1 and can be divided into three sequential steps:

1 **Production of unconjugated bilirubin.** Red blood cells are broken down by macrophages (mainly in the spleen), which degrade haemoglobin into iron and unconjugated (water insoluble) bilirubin (point 2 in Figure 14.1). The iron is stored inside transferrin proteins. Unconjugated bilirubin travels to the liver bound to albumin. In disease, unconjugated bilirubin can be produced by haemolysis of red cells intravascularly, rather than in the spleen (point 1 in Figure 14.1).

2 **Conjugation of bilirubin.** Liver hepatocytes uptake unconjugated bilirubin (point 3 in Figure 14.1) and conjugate it to glucuronate, thus making water soluble, conjugated bilirubin (point 4 in Figure 14.1).

3 **Excretion of bilirubin.** Once conjugated, bilirubin is secreted into the bile canaliculi (point 5 in Figure 14.1). Conjugated bilirubin flows with bile down the bile ducts and into the duodenum (point 6 in Figure 14.1). Inside the bowel, conjugated bilirubin is metabolized by bacteria into colourless products (urobilinogen, stercobilinogen). Some of these can be reabsorbed by the gut and excreted via the kidneys, but the vast majority are oxidized in the gut into coloured pigments (urobilin, stercobilin) which give faeces their brown colour. Consequently, if there is *complete* obstruction of the bile ducts there will be no flow of conjugated bilirubin into the gut, no conversion into urobilinogen, and therefore not even a trace of urobilinogen in the urine.

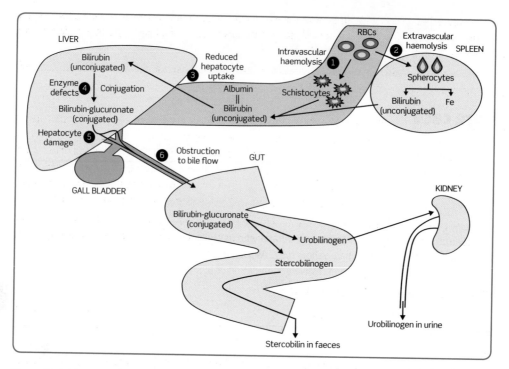

Figure 14.1 The metabolism of bilirubin in humans. The numbers 1 to 6 indicate points in the pathway that can lead to the accumulation of bilirubin and jaundice.

Clinicians often talk about jaundice being prehepatic, hepatic, or posthepatic in origin; obstructive; cholestatic; and conjugated or unconjugated.

What does all this terminology mean?

The terminology is confusing because different people mean different things. If you are going to use this terminology, make sure that you and your colleagues agree on the definitions. Nonetheless, this is what people usually mean:

- **Prehepatic jaundice:** this refers to jaundice caused by an excessive production of bilirubin. Remember that bilirubin is produced by the breakdown of haemoglobin in the blood vessels or the spleen, hence the term prehepatic (points 1 and 2 in Figure 14.1).

- **Hepatic jaundice:** for some people, this means any jaundice due to pathology in the liver (anatomically), such as points 3, 4, and 5 in Figure 14.1, and can thus include problems with hepatocytes (e.g. hepatitis) or with the bile canaliculi (e.g. primary sclerosing cholangitis, PSC). For other people, hepatic jaundice refers strictly to pathology affecting hepatocytes but not the bile canaliculi, which they consider part of the posthepatic system.

- **Posthepatic jaundice:** everyone agrees that posthepatic jaundice refers to a problem with biliary flow (point 6 in Figure 14.1). However, some people only talk of posthepatic jaundice when the flow is obstructed outside the liver (e.g. common bile duct obstruction) whereas others would include obstruction inside the liver (e.g. PSC). Confusing!

- **Obstructive jaundice:** this refers to jaundice caused by the lack of bile flow into the gut (point 6 in Figure 14.1), which manifests as pale faeces (lack of urobilin/stercobilin) and dark urine (conjugated bilirubin). Strictly speaking, the obstruction can be anywhere in the biliary system and therefore can be in the liver (bile canaliculi) or after the liver (common bile duct). However, some authors use the term 'obstructive jaundice' to refer only to obstructions affecting the biliary system outside the liver. Again … confusing!

- **Cholestatic jaundice:** this refers to jaundice caused by bilirubin not flowing out via the common bile duct (again, point 6 in Figure 14.1). This could be due to obstruction (e.g. a gallstone) or due to paralysis (ileus) of the common bile duct peristalsis (e.g. drug induced).
- **Unconjugated jaundice:** this refers to jaundice caused by the accumulation of unconjugated bilirubin (which is water insoluble, cannot dissolve in urine, and is thus sometimes called 'acholuric jaundice'). This can be due to excessive production of unconjugated bilirubin (increased breakdown of red blood cells, points 1 and 2 in Figure 14.1) or due to decreased capacity to conjugate bilirubin (hepatocyte pathology, points 3 and 4 in Figure 14.1). Thus, by definition, all prehepatic jaundice is unconjugated. Hepatic jaundice may be conjugated or unconjugated, depending on your definition of 'hepatic'.
- **Conjugated jaundice:** this refers to the accumulation of conjugated bilirubin. Thus, posthepatic jaundice is always conjugated but hepatic jaundice can be conjugated or unconjugated depending, again, on your definition of 'hepatic'.

What is your differential diagnosis for jaundice?

It is helpful to divide your list into problems that affect either bilirubin production, bilirubin conjugation, or bilirubin excretion.

The following list of differential diagnoses is not comprehensive but includes the most common causes of jaundice:

Increased production of bilirubin

Increased breakdown of red blood cells (haemolysis) can lead to excessive amounts of bilirubin in the circulation that the normal liver is unable to cope with. This can be due to:

- **Intravascular haemolysis** (point 1 in Figure 14.1): if the increased haemolysis is taking place in the circulation, one might find *black urine* due to free haemoglobin being degraded via an alternative pathway into haemosiderin (which is very dark but water soluble), and *schistocytes* on a blood film (fragments of red blood cells).
    - **Congenital causes:** for example, glucose-6-phosphate dehydrogenase (G6PDH) deficiency, pyruvate kinase (PK) deficiency, sickle cell disease, thalassaemia, etc.
    - **Acquired causes:** for example artificial heart valves, blood group mismatch, disseminated intravascular coagulopathy (DIC), malaria (hence the old-fashioned name 'blackwater fever'), HELLP syndrome in pregnant women, medications, etc.
- **Extravascular haemolysis** (point 2 in Figure 14.1): if the increased haemolysis is taking place in the spleen, one might find *splenomegaly* on examination and *spherocytes* on a blood film (due to the red blood cells being 'nibbled' at by splenic and liver macrophages into spherocytes):
    - **Congenital causes:** hereditary spherocytosis
    - **Acquired causes:** autoimmune haemolysis

Decreased conjugation of bilirubin

This is either because not enough unconjugated bilirubin is getting into the hepatocytes for conjugation (*reduced hepatocyte uptake*) or because the hepatocytes aren't conjugating bilirubin adequately (*enzymatic problems*). The excess bilirubin will be *unconjugated*. Decreased conjugation is rarely due to hepatocyte damage, because hepatocytes need to be *very damaged* before they stop conjugating bilirubin—so damaged that jaundice would be the least of one's problems.

- **Reduced hepatocyte uptake** (point 3 in Figure 14.1): cholecystographic contrast agents, portosystemic shunts to bypass a cirrhotic liver
- **Congenital enzymatic problems** (point 4 in Figure 14.1): Gilbert's syndrome (common), Crigler-Najjar syndrome (rare)

Decreased excretion of bilirubin

In this case, normal amounts of bilirubin are being produced, and the liver can cope adequately with conjugating the bilirubin, but the conjugated bilirubin either cannot make it out of damaged hepatocytes (because the active exporter of bilirubin is very sensitive to damage, point 5 in Figure 14.1) or cannot make it into the bowel (due to obstruction, point 6 in Figure 14.1). The consequence is that faeces may become pale (due to lack of stercobilin), foul smelling, and floating (steatorrhoea, due to lack of bile salts which normally solubilize fat in food) and the urine may become dark (due to conjugated bilirubin, which is water soluble, being excreted by the kidneys). The excess bilirubin is *conjugated*. There are many causes that can lead to reduced excretion of bilirubin from hepatocytes and into the duodenum. Congenital causes such as Dubin–Johnson syndrome are very rare. Acquired causes are much more common and different people have different ways of remembering them. Here, we offer a 'surgical sieve' using the acronym INVITED MD—although, as you can see, surgical sieves don't always work:

Infection: viral hepatitis, bacterial hepatitis (e.g. leptospirosis or Weil's disease), ascending cholangitis, liver abscess, *Echinococcus* (tapeworm) infection (causing hydatid cysts)

Neoplasia: metastatic liver cancer, hepatocellular carcinoma, pancreatic cancer, cholangiocarcinoma (cancer of the bile duct)

Vascular: Budd–Chiari syndrome (thrombosis in the hepatic vein)

Inflammation: primary biliary cirrhosis (PBC), PSC, autoimmune hepatitis, pancreatitis

Trauma: gallstones, stricture (e.g. after an endoscopic retrograde cholangiopan creatography (ERCP) or cholecystectomy)

Endocrine: intrahepatic cholestasis of pregnancy (although the exact mechanism is unclear, hormone changes in pregnancy appear to play a role)

Degenerative: likewise, there aren't really any degenerative causes

Metabolic: Wilson's disease, haemochromatosis

Drugs: some drugs affect the ability of hepatocytes to excrete bilirubin (e.g. alcohol abuse, paracetamol overdose, valproate, rifampicin) while others can induce a paralysis (ileus) of the biliary system (e.g. co-amoxiclav, nitrofurantoin, oral contraceptive pill).

Having formulated a broad differential diagnosis for jaundice, you proceed to take a history from Miss Watroba. Your history will contain the usual elements of personal information, presenting complaint, past medical history, medications and allergies, family history, social history, and patient concerns.

Can you think of key clues in each of these sections that might suggest certain diagnoses?

Personal information

- **Ethnic background:** sickle cell disease affects mainly West African and Afro-Caribbean patients, whereas thalassaemias and G6PDH deficiency mainly affect Mediterranean, east Asian, and African patients.

Presenting complaint

- Is this an **acute** or **chronic** illness?
- Is this patient **pregnant**? If so, consider whether the patient could have intrahepatic cholestasis of pregnancy, pre-eclampsia with HELLP syndrome or acute fatty liver of pregnancy.

  Ask about potential associated symptoms:

- **Right upper quadrant discomfort, nausea, vomiting**, and **pruritus** (itch) are all features of hepatitis of any cause (virus, autoimmune, drugs, alcohol).
- **Fever** or **diarrhoea** may additionally be present if the liver is infected (e.g. viral hepatitis, abscess).
- **Steatorrhoea** (pale, floating, foul-smelling faeces), **dark urine**, and **pruritus** are seen in obstruction to biliary flow.
- **Weight loss, fever**, and **night sweats** could indicate a malignancy of the liver, bile duct, or pancreas.
- **Bronzed skin** and **signs of diabetes mellitus** (polyuria, weight loss, infections) are suggestive of haemochromatosis. This condition is hereditary so check for family history.
- **Exposure to outdoor water/sewage** (which may be contaminated by rat urine and faeces) is a risk factor for leptospirosis.

Past medical history

- **Gallstones?** Consider obstructive jaundice due to gallstones or ascending cholangitis blocking the common bile duct.
- **Liver disease?** Alcoholic liver disease, non-alcoholic fatty liver disease (NAFLD or 'fatty liver' due to dyslipidaemia), hepatitis B and C, haemochromatosis, Wilson's disease, α_1-antitrypsin deficiency, PBC, and PSC are all causes of jaundice per se and also significant risk factors for liver cirrhosis.
- **Haemophilia?** Such patients may have received blood products contaminated with hepatitis C, a scenario which was tragically the case up until the 1980s.
- **Recent blood transfusion or surgery?** This may suggest a blood group incompatibility, although this is thankfully rare in hospitals today.
- **Ulcerative colitis?** This makes PSC more likely, as there is a strong association between these conditions.
- **Diabetes mellitus?** As mentioned earlier, this is seen in haemochromatosis.
- **Emphysema?** Suggests α_1-antitrypsin deficiency.
- **Psychosis?** May suggest Wilson's disease (rare!).

Medications

Medications can cause haemolysis by four mechanisms:

- **Intravascular haemolysis** (e.g. sulphonamides, aspirin in G6PDH-deficient patients).
- **Autoimmune, extravascular haemolysis** (e.g. methyldopa).
- **Hepatitis** (e.g. paracetamol overdose).
- **Cholestasis** (e.g. co-amoxiclav).

Family history

There are various familial conditions which can cause jaundice, such as Gilbert's disease, haemochromatosis, Wilson's disease, sickle cell disease, thalassaemia, hereditary spherocytosis, G6PDH deficiency (although the latter is unlikely to affect Miss Watroba as it is X-linked).

Social history

- **Excessive alcohol consumption?** Quantify exactly how many units a week the patient consumes and remember that recommended levels are <14 units/week for females and <21 units/week for males. Levels above 35 units/week for females or 50 units/week for males are very dangerous.
- **Intravenous drug use?**
- **Unprotected sex** or **multiple partners?**
- **Foreign travel?** You must consider the possibility of malaria, hepatitis A, and hepatitis E (particularly if they have been to east Asia, although hepatitis E can be acquired in the UK, possibly through undercooked pork or venison).
- **Tattoos?** The unsterile conditions under which some tattoos are created, particularly those acquired abroad, increases the risk of blood-borne transmission (e.g. viral hepatitis).

Concerns

First, patient concerns can provide important clues that can alter clinical management: a patient who is very worried that their jaundice is due to IV drug use or unprotected sex may need advice on the need to screen for a variety of pathogens such as hepatitis B, hepatitis C, HIV, *Chlamydia*, gonorrhoea, syphilis, etc.

Secondly, if you don't address a patient's concerns you are failing in your duty as a doctor. A patient whose jaundice is due to hepatitis A contracted abroad from contaminated food but who fears they have liver cancer needs reassurance.

Miss Watroba was born in Poznan, Poland. She has lived in Frankfurt for the past 4 years, and only moved to the UK 2 months ago. She has been well until 4 days ago when she began feeling nauseated and vomited a couple of times. She was initially worried that she might be pregnant, but then developed diarrhoea and mild discomfort in the right upper quadrant of her abdomen. She relaxed, assuming this meant she was suffering from an upset stomach. However, yesterday morning her flatmates noticed that her eyes were a bit yellow. The diarrhoea resolved, but by the evening, her eyes were more noticeably yellow and she decided to seek medical help. She has not lost any weight in the last few months, her faeces are brown, and she denies any urinary symptoms.

Her past medical history is remarkable only for chest infections as an infant. She has never had any surgery or transfusions of blood products. She takes paracetamol for occasional headaches but hasn't taken any in the past week. She is not allergic to any medications.

Her family are all from Poland. Her father and grandfather had heart problems and required coronary artery bypass surgery, and she has a younger brother with Down's syndrome. She does not recall anyone in her family ever being jaundiced or having hepatitis.

She shares a flat with three other Polish girls. She has smoked 10 cigarettes a day since she was 16 but says she never drinks more than 10 units of alcohol a week and she has never taken any recreational drugs. She does not have a boyfriend and appears reluctant to discuss her sexual history. You explain this information is important and that everything discussed is confidential. She hesitantly tells you that she has slept with three men in the last few months, and that some of the sexual encounters have involved unprotected intercourse. She does not undertake any regular exercise and has no history suggesting she is at risk of leptospirosis.

She is worried that she is pregnant or that she may have a sexually transmitted illness.

You examine Miss Watroba. Is there anything in particular that you will be looking out for?

Basic observations

- **Signs of dehydration:** tachycardia, a narrow pulse pressure, and hypotension (a late sign)
- **Fever**

On inspection

- Confirm the patient is **icteric** (yellow eyes) and **jaundiced** (yellow skin)
- Does the patient look **cachectic?** If so, consider malignancy
- Does the patient have **scratch marks,** suggesting pruritus (itch)?
- Does the patient have **needle marks,** suggesting intravenous drug use?
- Does the patient have **spider naevi, palmar erythema, clubbing, bruising** or **gynaecomastia** (if they are male) that might suggest chronic liver disease?
- Does the patient have a **bronzed tan,** suggesting haemochromatosis?
- Does the patient have **Kayser–Fleischer** (green) **rings** in the iris, suggesting Wilson's disease?

On palpation

- Does the patient have any **hepatomegaly, splenomegaly,** or an **epigastric mass?** If so consider malignancy (liver or pancreatic respectively), extravascular haemolysis (splenomegaly) or acute hepatitis (hepatomegaly)
- Does the patient have **right upper quadrant tenderness?** Consider acute hepatitis or gallbladder disease (e.g. cholecystitis or cholangitis)
- Does the patient have **ascites?** Consider chronic liver disease
- Does the patient have **palpable lymphadenopathy?** Consider malignancy.

On examination, Miss Watroba is jaundiced but has no other signs. Her basic observations show a regular heart rate of 75 bpm, a respiratory rate of 15/min, a blood pressure of 125/85 mmHg and a temperature of 36.8 °C.

What investigations will you perform to help narrow your differential diagnosis?

The history makes particular diagnoses unlikely (blood mismatch, alcoholic liver disease, drug-induced hepatitis, abnormal red blood cells, malaria, and G6PDH deficiency). The examination has been unhelpful in further narrowing your differential diagnoses, but the following investigations can help (key investigations for a jaundiced patient are summarized in Figure 14.2).

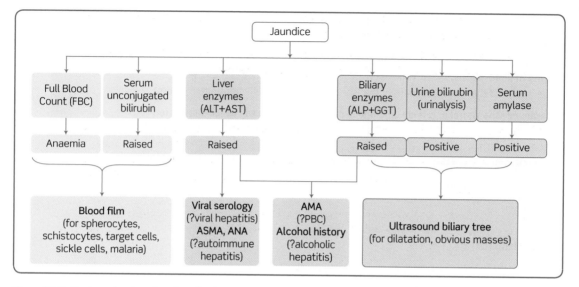

Figure 14.2 Key investigations for a jaundiced patient: ALP, alkaline phosphatase; ALT, alanine aminotransferase; AMA, antimitochondrial antibodies; ANA, antinuclear antibodies; ASMA, antismooth muscle antibodies; AST, aspartate aminotransferase; GGT, gamma-glutamyl transferase; PBC, primary biliary cirrhosis.

Initial screen

Bloods

- **Full blood count (FBC) and reticulocyte levels.** A low red blood cell (RBC) count with a high (>2%) reticulocyte count suggests increased RBC turnover consistent with haemolysis or a recent bleed. Remember that reticulocytes are precursors to RBCs and if the bone marrow is struggling to keep up with RBC destruction, it will end up throwing reticulocytes out into the circulation. A low RBC volume (microcytosis) would be consistent with thalassaemia (or iron deficiency anaemia).

- **Serum bilirubin levels.** This will confirm that the jaundice is due to hyperbilirubinaemia. If the proportion of conjugated bilirubin is >20% of the total bilirubin, it suggests that the problem is obstruction to bile flow (as the liver can cope with conjugating all the bilirubin that reaches it). In Gilbert's disease, total bilirubin levels will not be >100 μM. You may have to specifically ask the lab to report the conjugated and unconjugated fractions.

- **Liver enzymes.** Alanine aminotransferase (ALT) and aspartate aminotransferase (AST) are raised if there is damage to hepatocytes, and are very high in acute viral hepatitis. In general, elevation of AST > ALT suggests excessive alcohol intake whereas elevation of ALT > AST suggests viral hepatitis. However most hospitals only routinely report one of the two. Levels of ALT/AST in the thousands are typically only seen in viral hepatitis, paracetamol overdoses and ischaemic hepatitis.

- **Alkaline phosphatase (ALP) and gamma-glutamyl transferase (GGT).** ALP and GGT are useful tests if bile flow obstruction is suspected. ALP is released from damaged biliary epithelial cells, bones with high turnover, and/or a placenta (remember that she might be pregnant!). GGT is expressed almost exclusively by biliary epithelial cells. Consequently, a raised ALP and raised GGT suggest bile duct pathology (e.g. obstruction), whereas a raised ALP but normal GGT suggests increased bone turnover (e.g. malignant bone metastases, primary hyperparathyroidism) or pregnancy. Hepatitis is often associated with an element of intrahepatic obstruction and a rise in GGT and ALP. A raised GGT in isolation is seen after recent alcohol consumption.

- **Serum amylase or lipase.** Elevated levels of either of these pancreatic enzymes is highly suggestive (although not 100% specific) of pancreatic pathology (e.g. pancreatitis).

Urine

- **Urinalysis.** Bilirubin in the urine (which may be visible to the naked eye as brown urine) is always pathological and indicates posthepatic obstruction. Urobilinogen is sometimes found in the urine of healthy adults and is the result of bilirubin being metabolized by gut bacteria and then reabsorbed in the gut. Thus in posthepatic obstruction, bilirubin cannot reach the gut and therefore no urobilinogen appears in the urine.

- **Pregnancy test.** A number of causes of jaundice are specific to pregnancy, such as intrahepatic cholestasis of pregnancy, pre-eclampsia with HELLP syndrome (seen only in pregnancies > 20 weeks) and acute fatty liver of pregnancy.

Second-line investigations

Bloods

- **Haemolysis screen.** If the initial screen suggests that the jaundice is due to haemolysis (anaemia, elevated unconjugated bilirubin), consider checking:
  - **haptoglobins** (a protein that binds haemoglobin released by haemolysed RBCs, becoming depleted in haemolysis)
  - **lactate dehydrogenase** (LDH) released by haemolysed RBCs
  - a **direct antiglobulin test** (DAT, or Coombs) for autoimmune haemolysis, and
  - a **blood film**, which will allow you to directly assess whether there are schistocytes, sickle cells, target cells (thalassaemia), spherocytes, or malaria.

- **Viral screen.** If the initial screen reveals elevated liver enzymes, it is worth checking serology for hepatitis A, hepatitis B, and hepatitis C in anyone with jaundice of unclear aetiology. Epstein–Barr virus (EBV, causing glandular fever) and cytomegalovirus (CMV) are also relatively common in the younger population and would be worth checking in a patient like Miss Watroba. Given the patient's unprotected intercourse with multiple partners, you should check HIV status. Note that 2008 British HIV Association (BHIVA) guidelines advise that in areas of high prevalence (>2:1000), all new medical admissions should be tested routinely. This includes nearly every borough in London.

- **Autoimmune screen.** Check antinuclear antibodies (ANA), antismooth muscle antibodies (ASMA), and antimitochondrial antibodies (AMA). These should be checked if the initial screen reveals elevated liver enzymes, i.e. hepatocyte damage. ASMA are positive in (type I) autoimmune hepatitis. AMA is elevated in 95% of patients with PBC and in some patients with autoimmune hepatitis.

- **Congenital screen.** Check for haemochromatosis (high ferritin, high transferrin saturation), α_1-antitrypsin deficiency (low α_1-antitrypsin levels) and Wilson's disease (high Cu, low caeruloplasmin).

Imaging

- **Ultrasound of abdomen.** A useful, safe, non-invasive imaging modality that will show, for example, liver cirrhosis or liver carcinoma. If the history, examination, and blood results suggest problems with biliary outflow (pale faeces, dark urine, high ALP + GGT), an ultrasound of the common bile duct may show dilatation, suggesting mechanical obstruction (e.g. cholangiocarcinoma, or a choledochal cyst). The cause may be obvious (e.g. gallstone) but if not, further imaging (e.g. magnetic resonance chol-angiopancreatography (MRCP), endoscopic ultrasound, CT scan of the abdomen) will be necessary. If the common bile duct is not dilated, but you think the problem is biliary outflow, you should think of other causes of cholestasis: drugs, PBC or PSC.

Further investigations

- **Clotting studies** and **albumin.** Along with bilirubin, these are measures of liver synthetic function and form the basis of prognostic scoring systems in cirrhosis (e.g. Child–Pugh and Model for End-stage Liver Disease (MELD) scores). They should be measured if liver pathology is suspected. Deranged PT is one of the earliest markers of compromised liver function. Albumin takes about 20 days to fall and may be due to either reduced synthesis (e.g. liver damage, severe malnutrition) or increased albumin loss (e.g. nephrotic syndrome).

- **Liver biopsy.** This invasive procedure may be necessary to establish the diagnosis in liver disease, particularly if blood tests and imaging prove inconclusive.

Blood and urine samples are taken and sent off to labs. Initial results show:

Haematology		Biochemistry			
Hb	126 g/L	Na	132 mM	Bilirubin	95 µM
WCC	14.0 × 10⁹ cells/L	K	4.2 mM	ALT	1650 U/L
Platelets	280 × 10⁹ cells/L	Urea	12.3 mM	AST	1200 U/L
MCV	92 fL	Creatinine	103 µM	ALP	60 U/L
				GGT	20 U/L
Clotting				Albumin	36 g/L
PT	12 seconds			Amylase	36 U/L
APTT	35 seconds				

Urinalysis is positive for bilirubin. All other results are pending.

How would you interpret these results? What is the likely diagnosis? What is your next step?

The presence of bilirubin in the urine is always pathological and suggests problems in conjugated bilirubin getting out of hepatocytes into bile and down to the duodenum. The high WCC suggests infection. The elevated ALT and AST suggest damage to hepatocytes. Thus, there appears to be an infection that is damaging hepatocytes and compromising the ability of conjugated bilirubin to reach the duodenum. Several infections could do this but the *very* high ALT and AST levels (>1000 U/L) are strongly suggestive of a **viral hepatitis**. If you haven't already, you should send for **viral serology**, a **liver autoimmune profile** and request a **liver ultrasound** (to check for vascular causes of acute liver failure).

Viral serology is requested and shows:

Anti-HepA IgM/IgG	Negative
Hepatitis C Virus RNA	Undetectable
HBsAg (HepB surface antigen)	Positive
Anti-HBcAg IgM (HepB core antigen IgM)	Positive
Anti-HBsAg IgG	Negative
AMA	Undetectable
ASMA	Undetectable
ANA	Undetectable

What is the diagnosis and prognosis for this condition?

Miss Watroba is suffering **acute viral hepatitis B**. The prognosis for acute viral hepatitis B is:

- **'Full recovery'.** In the majority of cases, hepatitis B is a self-limiting condition with full *clinical* recovery, although evidence suggests that the virus is rarely cleared completely but kept in check by cytotoxic T-cells. Thus, immunosuppression at any stage in later life can lead to reactivation of the virus. However, if patients recover from acute hepatitis B and have undetectable levels of virus (HBsAg), the long-term sequelae are negligible.

- **Carrier status.** About 10% will become asymptomatic carriers (no symptoms but virus still detectable in the blood). In such patients, the long-term prognosis is good with most studies suggesting that the risk of long-term complications is <1%.

- **Chronic hepatitis B.** About 5–10% will develop chronic (symptomatic) hepatitis B. Rates are 90% if the infection was acquired at birth from the mother. Of the patients who develop chronic infection, about 20% will develop cirrhosis and 6% will develop hepatocellular carcinoma.

- **Fulminant hepatitis.** About 0.5% of patients with acute hepatitis B will develop fulminant hepatitis B, which has a mortality rate of 80%.

How should Miss Watroba be managed?

Miss Watroba needs referral to a specialist hepatologist. Management of the acute phase is supportive and largely involves:

- Practising 'safe sex' with barrier protection until she becomes non-infectious or her partner has been vaccinated
- Minimizing alcohol consumption to <10 units/week during the acute phase
- Avoid sharing any toothbrushes or razors
- Contact tracing
- Vaccination of current sexual partners and children, who are at risk of exposure via cuts and scratches

Miss Watroba probably contracted hepatitis B during her unprotected sexual encounters. She should therefore be advised to attend a genitourinary medicine (GUM) clinic to screen for other sexually transmitted diseases and for advice on precautions during future sexual encounters.

If she progresses to chronic hepatitis B infection, whether or not she is treated with antivirals will depend on levels of HBV DNA, ongoing hepatocyte damage (as indicated by elevations in ALT and AST), and fibrosis on liver biopsy or ultrasound (transient elastography) scan. This algorithm is complicated and changing, hence the need for referral to a specialist liver centre.

Short cases

Ms Jones is a 21-year-old woman who attends her GP complaining of 'yellow eyes'. For the past few days she has been feeling unwell with a cough and fever, but she is most distressed about the unusual colour of her eyes. She has never received blood or coagulation factors, denies any intravenous drug use, and she denies any sexual intercourse in the last 6 months. Blood tests taken by the GP reveal:

Hb	137 g/L
RBC	6.1×10^{12} cells/L
WCC	13×10^9 cells/L
Platelets	180×10^9 cells/L
Total bilirubin	60 µM
Conjugated bilirubin	2 µM

Markers for viral hepatitis are negative. Liver enzymes and reticulocyte count are within the normal range. A blood film is reported as unremarkable. A urine dipstick and pregnancy test normal.

What is the likely diagnosis? How should it be managed?

The most likely diagnosis is **Gilbert's syndrome**, a diagnosis of exclusion. Thus you need to demonstrate normal liver enzymes, normal haemoglobin levels, a serum bilirubin <100 µM and no bilirubin on a urine dipstick. This is an autosomal recessive condition affecting approximately 3–8% of Caucasian people that results in the liver not being able to conjugate bilirubin at an adequate rate in times of physiological stress (e.g. acute infection, excessive alcohol, pregnancy, starvation). There is no need for management for Gilbert's syndrome as it is asymptomatic except for the occasional episode of icterus. Patients should be reassured there is nothing they can do beyond leading as healthy a life as possible.

Mrs Gupta is a 43-year-old marketing director who attends her local Emergency Department complaining of yellow eyes, nausea, and pain in her abdomen. It all started a few days ago after dinner, when she developed a stabbing pain in the right upper quadrant. The pain 'comes and goes' several times a day, with each wave of pain lasting about 40 minutes. She has developed smelly, loose stools that are slightly pale and her urine is dark.

Her past medical history is unremarkable. She takes no medications and does not smoke or drink. On examination, she is afebrile but jaundiced. She is tachycardic and has tenderness on deep palpation of her right upper quadrant. The rest of her examination is normal.

Initial blood results show:

Haematology		Biochemistry	
Hb	134 g/L	Bilirubin	134 µM
WCC	11.8×10^9/L	ALT	98 U/L
Plt	320×10^9/L	AST	92 U/L
INR	1.2	ALP	410 U/L
		GGT	231 U/L

(INR, international normalized ratio)

> An abdominal ultrasound reveals a common bile duct that is dilated proximal to an echogenic mass in the lumen of the duct, but no other pathology.
>
> What is the diagnosis? What related surgical emergencies must you rule out?

Mrs Gupta has presented with jaundice, steatorrhoea, and dark urine. This suggests that the jaundice is due to reduced excretion of conjugated bilirubin via the normal route. The elevated ALP and GGT together suggest damage to biliary epithelia, and the raised ALT and AST suggest damage to hepatocytes. Put together, this suggests that the jaundice is due to obstruction in the biliary system (**obstructive jaundice**). Several aetiologies are possible, but the history of waves of right upper quadrant pain and nausea are suggestive of biliary colic due to a **gallstone**. The ultrasound confirms an echogenic mass in the common bile duct which is almost certainly a gallstone. If the ultrasound had been inconclusive, one could request MRCP to visualize the biliary tree and pancreas. Most gallstones pass by themselves, but if they cause obstructive jaundice they need removing via **ERCP**.

In anyone presenting acutely with gallstone pathology you have to rule out two related conditions that are surgical emergencies:

* **Cholecystitis:** the patient will usually present with constant, unresolving (>6 hours) fever, a tender abdomen (Murphy's sign positive) that is often distended, nausea, and possibly vomiting. Cholecystitis is an emergency that requires prompt antibiotics, analgesia, nil by mouth, and intravenous (IV) fluids, plus a cholecystectomy. Mrs Gupta does not have cholecystitis (yet) as her symptoms are intermittent and she is afebrile.

* **Ascending cholangitis:** such patients often present with Charcot's triad of febrile rigors, jaundice, and right upper quadrant pain. This is also an emergency and requires blood cultures, careful monitoring, broad-spectrum antibiotics, and an ERCP (or percutaneous transhepatic cholangiography (PTC)) to drain the common bile duct of pus. Mrs Gupta does not have ascending cholangitis: she is afebrile and far too well.

SHORT CASE

Mrs Gonzalez is a 48-year-old woman presenting with jaundice. She has become increasingly lethargic over the past month. For the past month she has felt exhausted and had yellow, itchy skin and pale, offensive stools. Her past medical history is unremarkable and she takes no medications. She does not smoke and drinks less than 10 units of alcohol a week.

On inspection, she is jaundiced and looks unwell. Several spider naevi are evident on her chest and a number of bruises are noticeable on her limbs. Her liver is tender to palpation. The rest of her examination is unremarkable.

Her urine dipstick is positive for bilirubin, despite her urine not being dark to the naked eye. An abdominal ultrasound does not reveal any abdominal masses, gallstones, or dilated common bile duct. Her blood results are:

Haematology		Biochemistry		Immunology	
Hb	123 g/L	Bilirubin	120 µM	AMA	60 IU/L
WCC	11 × 10⁹/L	Albumin	41 g/L	ASMA	Negative
Plt	220 × 10⁹/L	ALT	100 U/L	ANA	Negative
INR	1.7	AST	85 U/L	Anti-HepA IgM/IgG	Undetectable
		ALP	320 U/L	Anti-HBsAg	Positive
		GGT	210 U/L	Anti-HBcAg	Negative
		Total cholesterol	4.1 mM	HCV RNA	Undetectable

What is the diagnosis? How should this patient be managed?

Mrs Gonzalez is jaundiced. The elevated ESR and a borderline high WCC suggest an inflammatory process. Her INR is elevated, suggesting poor liver synthetic function or decreased absorption of fat-soluble vitamin K. Her ALT and AST are elevated, suggesting active liver damage. Viral serology is negative (the positive anti-HBsAg but negative anti-HBcAg result indicates past vaccination), making viral hepatitis unlikely. ALP and GGT are elevated, suggesting damage to the biliary epithelial cells. She has bilirubin in her urine and steatorrhoea suggesting obstruction to the biliary tree.

There are multiple causes of posthepatic (obstructive) jaundice but her positive AMA suggests this is a case of **PBC**. This is an autoimmune disorder characterized by T-cell-mediated destruction of the biliary ducts (the autoantibodies form as a secondary consequence of this damage). As the biliary ducts are destroyed (hence the high ALP and GGT), outflow of bile contents (including bilirubin) from the liver is obstructed. This explains the pale faeces (lack of urobilin and stercobilin), smelly faeces (undissolved fat due to lack of bile salts), itch (due to accumulation of bile salt in the skin), and jaundice.

Management of PBC involves:

- **Referral to hepatologist,** for ongoing care
- **Confirming diagnosis,** via MRCP and liver biopsy
- **Immunosuppression** (as this is an autoimmune condition), using agents such as corticosteroids, methotrexate, or ciclosporin
- **Bile salt replacement,** using agents such as ursodeoxycholic acid
- **Fat-soluble vitamin replacement:** supplement the fat-soluble vitamins A, D, E, and K
- **Pruritus (itch) management,** using agents such as cholestyramine (which sequesters bile salts in the gut lumen to prevent their reabsorption) and antihistamines
- **Liver transplantation,** to be considered once the patient becomes cirrhotic.

SHORT CASE

Mr Al-Iqbal is a 38-year-old mathematics teacher with ulcerative colitis. His wife has noticed he is icteric and he has been referred to the gastroenterology clinic by his GP. Mr Al-Iqbal denies feeling unwell. He has never received any blood transfusions or clotting factors and never drinks any alcohol. He has not noticed any change in his bowel motions or urine. Bloods sent by the GP show:

Haematology		Biochemistry		Immunology	
Hb	132 g/L	Bilirubin	70 µM	AMA	Negative
WCC	5.4 × 10⁹/L	ALT	60 U/L	ASMA	Negative
Plt	189 × 10⁹/L	AST	32 U/L	ANA	Negative
INR	1.1	ALP	200 U/L	Anti-HepA IgM/IgG	Undetectable
		GGT	80 U/L	Anti-HBsAg	Negative
				Anti-HBcAg	Negative
				HCV RNA	Undetectable

The mildly elevated ALT, ALP, and GGT suggest a posthepatic (obstructive) cause to Mr Al-Iqbal's jaundice. Worried about potential gallstones, but concerned about an alternative diagnosis, the gastroenterology registrar requests an MRCP study of his liver, bile duct, and pancreas. The MRCP shows that the bile ducts are dilated in some areas but have strictures in others, all along their course from inside the liver down to midway along the cystic duct.

Why did the gastroenterology registrar opt to perform an MRCP rather than an ultrasound? What is the likely diagnosis?

Mr Al-Iqbal appears to have jaundice caused by cholestasis due to pathology in the biliary system (hence his elevated ALP and GGT). The best way to determine the cause of the obstruction is to use some form of imaging. This usually involves ultrasound, which is good at showing masses (e.g. gallstones, tumours) but less good at showing the fine detail of the biliary tree. The gastroenterology registrar knew that patients with ulcerative colitis are at increased risk of PSC, a disease which affects the biliary tree—hence the decision to go for an MRCP, which will show any masses compressing the biliary tree but also any strictures within the bile ducts.

The MRCP did not show any masses, but instead multiple areas of biliary strictures that had led to dilatation upstream. This is highly suggestive of **PSC**. This is also a T-cell-mediated autoimmune destruction of biliary epithelial cells, leading to multifocal scarring of the biliary ducts. Approximately 90% of patients with PSC have underlying **ulcerative colitis** (although only 5% of patients with ulcerative colitis develop PSC). Patients with PSC also have elevated perinuclear antineutrophil cytoplasmic autoantibodies (pANCA) in 60–80% of cases.

Management of PSC is broadly the same as for PBC (described earlier).

SHORT CASE

Mr MacDonald is a 72-year-old man referred to the surgical admissions unit by his GP. He is jaundiced and has noticed his trousers becoming looser over the past few months. He initially attributed his jaundice to excessive alcohol consumption, as he drinks 2 pints of Guinness every day before going to bed. He says that he is otherwise well and denies any abdominal pain, but on inspection you notice that he is severely cachectic, with the skin around his ribs and abdomen looking too big for him. Lymph nodes are palpable in his left supraclavicular fossa, and on deep palpation of his abdomen a mass is noted in his epigastrium.

What is the likely diagnosis? What initial investigations will you perform?

Few people successfully lose *significant* weight on purpose (despite many people dieting) and so weight loss should always alert you to the possibility of a catabolic (energy-consuming) process such as cancer. The combination of significant weight loss, an epigastric mass, Virchow's lymphadenopathy, and painless jaundice should make you suspicious of **pancreatic carcinoma**.

Initial investigations should include:

- **FBC:** cancer patients are often anaemic
- **Serum amylase:** this may be raised in any form of pancreatic disease
- **Liver enzymes:** to see if there is liver pathology secondary to the obstruction
- **Imaging:** CT scans of the abdomen are the first-line imaging modality as they offer a greater sensitivity than transabdominal ultrasound. Endoscopic ultrasound appears to be as good as CT scans but requires specialist staff and equipment (not always available) and is more invasive than CT for the patient.

A CT abdomen of the patient revealed a mass in the head of the pancreas compressing the common bile duct, which was later found to be a **pancreatic adenocarcinoma**. Pancreatic cancer has a very bad prognosis, despite heroic surgical attempts to remove it (known as a Whipple's procedure). Five-year mortality is around 97% without surgery and 80% (at best) with surgery. He will require formal staging and discussion in the upper gastrointestinal cancer MDT as a matter of priority.

SHORT CASE

Miss Hoeder is a 26-year-old journalist who presents to her GP complaining of increasing fatigue. She claims that she is usually a highly active individual who runs 10 km twice a week and is always 'up for a party'. Over the past month, she has become unusually tired. At first, she put this down to 'flu or something' but her fatigue and lethargy have remained, and she is worried because she gets short of breath when she goes for even a gentle run. Her periods have not been unusual in any way but she has noticed that her eyes are yellow and she thinks her skin might be slightly yellow, too. Her family history is unremarkable.

On examination, Miss Hoeder is indeed icteric and jaundiced. Her spleen is palpable just below her left costal margin. The rest of the examination is unremarkable.

The GP sends off some blood for analysis. It reveals:

Haematology		Biochemistry	
Hb	92 g/L	Total bilirubin	72 µM
MCV	95 fL	Conjugated bilirubin	7 µM
WCC	4.5×10^9/L		
Plt	210×10^9/L		
Reticulocytes	6%		
INR	1.0		
Blood film	Spherocytes and reticulocytes evident		

What is the likely diagnosis? What is the next step?

Miss Hoeder has a normocytic anaemia with a reticulocytosis, spherocytosis, and jaundice. This suggests a **haemolytic anaemia**.

The next step is to diagnose the cause for her haemolytic anaemia by referring her to a haematologist. The combination of spherocytes and elevated bilirubin in Miss Hoeder suggests that she is suffering from extravascular haemolysis. This is either due to hereditary spherocytosis or due to an autoimmune haemolytic anaemia (including drug-induced). The lack of family history makes hereditary spherocytosis unlikely. Thus, autoimmune haemolytic anaemia is the most likely diagnosis, and hence tests to detect antierythrocyte antibodies (e.g. DAT or Coomb's test) should be performed.

Viva questions

A medical student is asked to take urgent bloods for cross-matching from an IV drug user and alcohol-dependent patient who has presented to the Emergency Department with bleeding oesophageal varices. Having successfully obtained the blood, the student cannot see a sharps disposal bin within easy access. Ignoring all previous health and safety advice, the student tries to re-sheath the used needle into its cap, and in doing so sustains a needlestick injury. What infections is the student most at risk of catching?

Most people worry about HIV transmission from needlestick injuries. This concern is understandable, because despite great advances in the management of HIV infection, there is still no cure. However, HIV is a rather fragile virus (it won't last more than a few hours at room temperature) and the risk of infection from a single needlestick injury is estimated to be 0.3%.

Hepatitis C has an infection risk following needlestick injury of 3%. Hepatitis B virus, by contrast, is a robust virus that will survive for up to a week at 44 °C. Risk of infection after a needlestick injury is 30%. These statistics assume that the injury occurred from a patient who is a carrier for the virus, rather than the population as a whole. Either way, contaminated needlestick injuries are a medical emergency and the student needs seeing urgently either in the Emergency Department (where he currently is) or in Occupational Health so that postexposure prophylaxis (for HIV) can be started as soon as possible if required, as the efficacy of antiretrovirals at preventing seroconversion of HIV drops with time over the first 72 hours after exposure. His hepatitis B immunity status will also need checking as he may require a booster within the first 48 hours after exposure.

If a patient is clinically jaundiced, how high will his bilirubin levels be at a minimum?

Jaundice is due to the accumulation of bilirubin above its normal range of 3–17 μM (of which at least 10% will be conjugated bilirubin). For jaundice to be visible to the naked eye, serum bilirubin levels must be >40 μM.

A medical student is asked to provide proof of his hepatitis B immunization status. As he has lost his relevant paperwork, Occupational Health take a blood sample for serological studies. These reveal that the student has

HBsAg	Positive
IgG anti-HBs	Positive
IgG anti-HBc	Positive
IgM anti-HBc	Negative

What do these results mean?

Like any virus, hepatitis B virus contains multiple proteins. The surface antigen (HBsAg or HBs) is present on the surface of the virus and is used, in isolation, for immunization. The core antigen (HBcAg) is buried deep inside the virus and is absent from the vaccine preparation, as is the e antigen (HBeAg).

He has positive IgG anti-HBs which could be due to vaccination or infection. However, he also has high levels of HBsAg suggesting either the presence of the virus or a *very recent* vaccination. Most importantly, he has positive IgG anti-HBc, suggesting infection with the hepatitis B virus (as HBc is *not* a part of the vaccine). The lack of IgM anti-HBc (remember that IgM is an acute antibody) suggests this is **chronic hepatitis B**. This has potential implications for his medical career, so he should seek advice from both a hepatologist and from Occupational Health, and practise safe sex at all times.

Which tumours could cause obstructive jaundice?

The most common tumours causing obstructive jaundice are carcinoma of the head of the pancreas and malignant lymph nodes at the porta hepatis. Liver metastases or a carcinoma at the ampulla of Vater are less common, while cholangiocarcinoma (cancer of the biliary tree) is rare. For interest, a Klatskin tumour is a cholangiocarcinoma at the confluence of right and left hepatic ducts.

Why does obstruction of the common bile duct result in steatorrhoea?

Steatorrhoea is stool with a high fat content—it is typically foul-smelling, greasy, pale, and floats in water. Bile salts provide stool with its colour and normally emulsify (solubilize) fats in the intestine, which facilitates absorption through the enterocyte brush border. If bile is not reaching the intestine then less fat will be absorbed and more will be excreted with the faeces. As a consequence, the patient will have steatorrhoea but may also develop deficiency of fat-soluble vitamins (A, D, E, K).

Single Best Answers

1. Which of the following is a cause of intravascular haemolytic anaemia?

a. Thalassaemia
b. Iron deficiency
c. Alcohol

d. Hypothyroidism
e. Pyruvate kinase deficiency

2. A patient presents with jaundice. Initial blood tests reveal raised conjugated bilirubin and liver enzymes, and a normal haemoglobin. You suspect primary biliary cirrhosis (PBC). Which of the following investigations would be most useful in confirming your diagnosis?

a. Antimitochondrial antibodies (AMA)
b. Antismooth muscle antibodies (ASMA)
c. Antinuclear antibodies (ANA)

d. Antineutrophil cytoplasmic antibodies (ANCA)
e. Antihepatitis B surface antigen (anti-HBsAg)

3. A patient presents with fatigue and jaundice. His past medical history is notable for a previous episode of jaundice about 15 years ago that self-resolved. He has otherwise been healthy. Blood tests include reduced albumin, raised ALT and AST, a mildly elevated conjugated bilirubin, and a normal haemoglobin. A liver biopsy shows focal ballooning degeneration of hepatocytes and inflammation in the triads extending into the lobules. Which of the following findings would be most characteristic of this disease?

a. Low serum caeruloplasmin
b. High serum ferritin
c. Positive hepatitis B surface antigen (HBsAg)

d. Negative antihepatitis B surface antigen (anti-HBsAg) antibody
e. Positive antismooth muscle antibodies (ASMA)

4. A patient presents with a 2 month history of fatigue and jaundice. Their past medical history is notable for a total colectomy performed several years ago. ERCP reveals widespread loss of intrahepatic bile ducts. A liver biopsy is reported as showing periductal 'onion skin' fibrosis with a lymphocytic infiltrate, loss of intrahepatic bile ducts but no focal areas of necrosis. Which underlying disease is this patient most likely to have?

a. Systemic lupus erythematosus (SLE)
b. Microscopic polyangitis (MPA)
c. Hepatitis B

d. Ulcerative colitis (UC)
e. Primary biliary cirrhosis (PBC)

5. An elderly man presents with a 2 month history of nausea, jaundice and 5 kg weight loss. There is no abdominal tenderness. Blood tests include a normal haemoglobin, albumin, AST, and ALT but a raised ALP and raised conjugated bilirubin. Which of the following is most likely?

a. Chronic hepatitis

b. Primary biliary cirrhosis

c. Haemolytic anaemia

d. Gilbert's disease

e. Pancreatic adenocarcinoma

Right upper quadrant pain

Core case

Read through the sections in the case boxes, covering up the sections that follow so that you don't see the answer. At the end of each case box, try to answer the question before reading on.

Mrs Cole is an overweight 38-year-old Caucasian woman who presents to the Emergency Department at 11 p.m. complaining of severe pain in the right upper quadrant (RUQ) of her abdomen, together with nausea and vomiting.

What is your differential diagnosis for this patient's current presentation?

Think anatomically of which structures might give you pain in the RUQ of the abdomen. Try to arrange your list of possible diagnoses in order of likelihood given this patient's sex, age, and presentation.

Figure 15.1 shows the differential diagnosis arranged in order of likelihood in a woman of this age.

Biliary colic
Cholecystitis
Duodenal ulcer
Pancreatitis
Basal pneumonia (irritating the right hemidiaphragm)
Ascending cholangitis
Gastric ulcer
Small bowel obstruction
Appendicitis
Hepatitis (autoimmune, infective, or drug-induced)
Pyelonephritis
Fitz-Hugh-Curtis syndrome (formation of adhesions around the liver capsule due to *N. gonorrhoeae* or *Chlamydia*).

Figure 15.1 List of the main differential diagnoses for right upper quadrant abdominal pain in a young woman. Bigger font sizes indicate more likely diagnoses and **bold** fonts imply diagnoses that need to be ruled out due to their high morbidity and/or mortality.

Suppose that Mrs Cole was 68 years old, rather than 38 years old.

Would your differential diagnosis list change?

Yes, the likelihood of certain diseases would change considerably. In older patients, certain pathologies are relatively more common, such as pneumonia, cancer (e.g. hepatocellular carcinoma), or vascular disease (aortic dissection, abdominal aortic aneurysm, inferior myocardial infarction). Of course, the differential would still include those diseases seen in a 38-year-old Mrs Cole.

What questions should you ask in a history to narrow your differential diagnoses?

Characterize the pain. One useful way is to follow the mnemonic SOCRATES:

Site of pain, and has it moved since it began?

Onset of pain—was it sudden or gradual, and did something trigger it?

Character of pain—stabbing, dull, deep, superficial, gripping, tearing, burning?

Radiation of pain—does the patient have pain elsewhere?

Attenuating factors—does anything make the pain better (position? medications?)

Timing of pain—how long has it gone on for, has it been constant or coming and going?

Exacerbating factors—does anything make the pain worse (moving? breathing?)

Severity—on a scale of 0-10, where 10 is the worst pain ever (e.g. childbirth).

Once you have characterized the pain, you should ask:

- **Has the patient had any symptoms other than pain?** (e.g. fever, weight loss). The reason is that certain other symptoms will help you refine your diagnosis. Thus, fever suggests an infective process and makes a myocardial infarction less likely. Significant weight loss over the preceding months may be due to a cancer, which is a catabolic process (breakdown of tissues for energy).

- **When did they last open their bowels or pass any flatus (wind)?** A patient who hasn't opened their bowels may be constipated, but a patient who isn't even managing to pass wind ('absolute constipation') may be obstructed—a surgical emergency.

- **Have they noticed any change in their stool recently?** (e.g. colour, floating, smelly). If the common bile duct is obstructed, bilirubin and fat-dissolving bile salts won't reach the bowel and thus stools will be pale, floating, and smelly (steatorrhoea). If blood is entering the bowel lumen via a bleeding ulcer, the iron (haemoglobin) in the blood will be oxidized, making stools appear very dark, black, tarry, and smelly (melaena).

- **If the patient is female, is she pregnant?** If the patient is a woman of fertile age, you must exclude pregnancy, even if the patient insists she is not pregnant or sexually active. This is partly because radiography of a pregnant woman needs careful consideration, partly because certain causes of RUQ pain are exclusive to pregnancy (e.g. pre-eclampsia, cholestasis of pregnancy) and partly because potentially fatal ectopic pregnancies are a major source of abdominal pain—even if pain in the RUQ would be an unusual presentation.

Mrs Cole's pain is in the RUQ of her abdomen. It came on gradually 16 hours ago when she went to bed. It is deep, sharp, constant, and 8/10 in severity. She also gets the occasional sharp stabbing sensation on her back and she points to her right scapula very specifically (this is known as Boas's sign). She has not found anything that makes it better or worse. She last opened her bowels before she went to bed but has been passing flatus this morning. She reports no significant weight change recently.

In the history, she also reveals that every couple of months, usually after a heavy, fatty meal, she develops a sharp, stabbing pain in the same area of her abdomen and which usually gets better after a few hours. Her past medical history includes heartburn (dyspepsia), which is well controlled with omeprazole (a proton pump inhibitor, PPI). However, the pain this time 'feels different' and she feels 'very sick'.

Just from this history, particular diagnoses become very likely. The next steps will be to examine the patient and arrange first-line investigations with the aim of confirming your suspected diagnosis and ruling out those diseases that would require urgent management (those emphasized in **bold** in Figure 15.1).

What key features on examination would you look out for?

- **Jaundice:** most easily seen in the whites of the eyes (sclera); it is typical of diseases that block the common bile duct such as choledocholithiasis (gallstones in the common bile duct), ascending cholangitis, acute pancreatitis, pancreatic cancer, or cholangiocarcinoma.

- **Bruising and discoloration around the umbilicus and flank** (Cullen's sign or Grey Turner's sign, respectively). Sometimes seen in severe pancreatitis, as shown in Figure 12.2.

- **A pulsatile and laterally expansile central mass.** This indicates an abdominal aortic aneurysm, but remember that not feeling one clinically doesn't mean it isn't there.

- **Murphy's sign:** palpate the abdomen just below the tip of the right ninth costal cartilage, apply pressure, and ask the patient to take a deep breath. This will cause the liver and hence gallbladder to descend and press against your fingers. If the gallbladder is tender it will cause the patient to arrest inspiration as the gallbladder strikes your fingers. This is strongly suggestive of an inflamed gallbladder (cholecystitis).

- **Peritonitis:** the patient will lie very still, have a rigid and exquisitely tender abdomen, and exhibit guarding when you try to palpate lightly. There may be no bowel sounds. In the case of Mrs Cole, this would suggest perforation of a peptic ulcer or the gallbladder.

- **Signs of small bowel obstruction:** a distended abdomen (which may be hard to appreciate in a patient with a high body mass index (BMI)) and absent or tinkling bowel sounds. If the bowel becomes strangulated, signs of peritonitis would predominate.

On examination, Mrs Cole is febrile (38.3 °C) and tachycardic (108 bpm). Her cardiovascular and respiratory systems are otherwise unremarkable. She is not jaundiced, has no hernias, and no palpable abdominal masses. Her abdominal aorta is palpable but does not feel laterally expansile. Her RUQ is tender to light palpation with a positive Murphy's sign. A digital rectal examination (in the presence of a female nurse) reveals soft faeces in the rectum but no signs of blood.

Her history and physical examination are very typical of a particular diagnosis. The next step is to arrange first-line investigations that will confirm this diagnosis and help rule out other diagnoses that you should exclude because of their need for urgent management.

What investigations will you request?

Blood tests

- **Full blood count:** the patient may be anaemic from a chronically bleeding gastric or duodenal ulcer. Her white cell count will be elevated if she has any inflammatory condition (e.g. cholecystitis, ascending cholangitis, or basal pneumonia).

- **Serum amylase (or lipase) levels:** slight increases (200–600 U/L) in amylase levels are most commonly caused by pancreatitis, but also by various other pathologies such as bowel obstruction, mesenteric ischaemia, a posteriorly perforated duodenal ulcer, mumps, pancreatic carcinoma, or opiate medications. However, very high amylase levels (>1000 U/L) or elevated lipase levels (>300 U/L) are almost exclusively found in pancreatitis. (The exact cut offs will depend on your local laboratory protocols.)

- **Liver enzymes:** elevated levels of aspartate aminotransferase (AST) and alanine aminotransferase (ALT), sometimes called a 'transaminitis', suggest damage to hepatocytes owing to inflammation in the liver. This could be due to viral hepatitis, autoimmune hepatitis, or obstruction of the common bile duct because of a gallstone, infection of the duct, tumour of the duct, inflammation of the pancreas or tumour of the pancreas. A raised alkaline phosphatase (ALP) level by itself can be due to increased bone breakdown (e.g. metastatic bone disease, Paget's disease). However, a raised ALP level that is more elevated than AST/ALT levels and/or accompanied by a raised gamma-glutamyl transferase (GGT) level suggests obstruction of the common bile duct (a 'cholestatic' picture).

- **Bilirubin:** elevated levels of *unconjugated* bilirubin suggest that the liver cannot conjugate it fast enough, either because there is too much breakdown of haemoglobin into bilirubin (e.g. haemolytic anaemia) or because of a hereditary deficiency of conjugating enzyme (e.g. Gilbert's syndrome). Elevated levels of *conjugated* bilirubin suggest the liver is working (conjugating) but that there is obstruction of bile flow either in the liver (e.g. primary biliary cirrhosis with intrahepatic scarring affecting flow through the bile canaliculi to the bile ducts) or outside the liver (e.g. gallstones blocking the common bile duct).

Imaging

- **Erect chest radiograph:** air under the diaphragm strongly suggests a perforated viscus such as a gastric or duodenal ulcer (but can also be a sign of recent abdominal surgery). Bear in mind that if this patient had suffered a perforated peptic ulcer we would have found signs of peritonism during the abdominal examination. A wide mediastinum and/or heart shadow can suggest aortic dissection. Don't forget to do a pregnancy test before any radiography on a woman of fertile age—this not only rules out certain gynaecological pathologies (e.g. ectopic pregnancies) but is important from a patient safety and medico-legal point of view.

- **Ultrasound of pancreas, common bile duct, and gallbladder:** Pay particular attention to the thickness of the gallbladder wall (a thickened, inflamed wall suggests cholecystitis), presence or absence of gallstones or biliary sludge, and presence of intra- or extrahepatic duct dilatation (the 'normal' diameter of the common bile duct is age-related, but >6–7 mm is usually abnormal).

- **Abdominal radiograph:** Plain abdominal films would not be first-line investigations for the majority of RUQ pain presentations. Remember that only ~10% of gallstones are radio-opaque. However, if there is a clinical suspicion of bowel obstruction or perforation (look for Rigler's sign), then plain abdominal films are indicated.

Mrs Cole's blood tests, and chest radiograph are normal. The abdominal ultrasound reveals a common bile duct (CBD) of normal diameter with no wall thickening, no masses in the pancreas but a thick-walled gallbladder containing multiple calculi.

In light of the history, examination, and first-line investigations, what is the most likely diagnosis? How does this explain her symptoms?

This is a classical clinical picture for someone with **cholecystitis**: a middle-aged, Caucasian woman with RUQ pain, positive Murphy's sign, fever, and a previous history of pains in this area after heavy, fatty meals. The normal serum amylase levels rule out pancreatitis. The lack of jaundice or raised serum bilirubin, and normal CBD diameter with no wall thickening on ultrasound, suggest that there is no obstruction of the common bile duct. There were no signs on examination suggestive of bowel obstruction or peritonism, and the chest radiograph was normal, so a perforated peptic ulcer is unlikely. The ultrasound did not reveal any pancreatic or CBD masses, suggesting that there is no pancreatic cancer nor cholangiocarcinoma, but it showed a thick gallbladder wall, suggesting it is inflamed.

Cholecystitis (*chole* = bile, *cyst* = bladder, *-itis* = inflammation) is inflammation of the gallbladder, caused in 95% of cases by a stone in the gallbladder. The gallbladder suffers a chemical inflammation and this often leads to subsequent infection affecting the surrounding tissue. The inflamed gallbladder irritates the parietal peritoneum, causing a *constant* pain. Irritation of the visceral peritoneum in the initial stages produces a poorly localized, dull, midline epigastric pain. As the irritation spreads outwards to the parietal peritoneum, the pain becomes sharply localized to the RUQ. The inflamed gallbladder can also irritate the liver capsule, which in turn can irritate the diaphragm above it. The diaphragm is supplied by nerve roots C3, C4, and C5 ('*3, 4, 5 keep the diaphragm alive*') which also supply sensation to the shoulder. The referred pain in the right scapula is believed to be because the central nervous system (probably the dorsal spinal cord, but perhaps the sensory cortex in the brain) confuses the incoming signals from the right shoulder and the right hemidiaphragm.

How will the team manage Mrs Cole's cholecystitis?

When asked about management in exams, remember that you must start from the beginning and not dive into drugs or surgery. Thus, having assessed her need for resuscitation (airway, breathing, and circulation, ABC), taken a full history, examined the patient, carried out first-line investigations, and suggested a diagnosis of cholecystitis, Mrs Cole's therapeutic management can be divided into operative and non-operative:

- **Non-operative:**
  - **Clear fluids.** Mrs Cole should avoid all food and be restricted to clear fluids if her nausea and vomiting permit oral intake. This is partly to avoid food in the duodenum triggering gallbladder contractions and partly to prepare her if there is a need for surgery.
  - **Intravenous (IV) fluids.** To avoid and/or treat dehydration (remember that she has been vomiting at home and thus is likely to be partially fluid depleted, and may not be able to meet her requirements orally).
  - **Analgesia.** Regular multimodal analgesia with paracetamol and opioids may be necessary in the initial stages. Orally administered analgesics should be avoided if the patient is vomiting.
  - **Antibiotics.** Choice will be dictated by local hospital guidelines but will need to provide cover against the likely Gram-negative pathogens such as *E.coli* and *Enterococcus*. This will start to combat the infection if surgery is delayed and will reduce the risk of systemic or peritoneal infection as a consequence of the surgery.

- **Operative:** Mrs Cole should undergo a **laparoscopic cholecystectomy** to remove her inflamed gall-bladder. Controversy exists over whether the best strategy is urgent laparoscopic cholecystectomy within the first 72 hours or treating the acute episode and then returning the patient for an elective cholecystectomy 6–12 weeks later. The arguments in favour of the latter are that conversion rates from laparoscopic to open surgery are reduced. However, waiting for an elective procedure may mean that patients have repeat admissions in the interim—and this entails increased morbidity, expense, and lost time (for the patient).

Short cases

Mrs Cole (the patient from the core case) was admitted on to a surgical ward. While awaiting her laparoscopic cholecystectomy, Mrs Cole's RUQ abdominal pain becomes worse. She also becomes jaundiced, her temperature rises to 40.1 °C, and she starts to shake uncontrollably with rigors.

What are the complications of cholecystitis, and what has happened to Mrs Cole? How must she be managed?

Complications of cholecystitis include empyema (a collection of pus in the gallbladder that will need draining), formation of a cholecystoduodenal fistula (a connecting fistula between the gallbladder and small bowel, which allows bowel air into the gallbladder—seen on radiography—but also allows gallstones to travel into the small bowel, eventually getting stuck in the terminal ileum and causing 'gallstone ileus'), or even gallbladder carcinoma. However, Mrs Cole has more likely developed **ascending cholangitis**, which is characterized by *Charcot's triad* of signs:

- RUQ pain
- Jaundice
- Fever with rigors.

Ascending cholangitis (*chole* = *bile*, angio = vessel, *-itis* = inflammation) is inflammation of the CBD because of an infected stone in the CBD or due to spread from an infected gallbladder (cholecystitis). Inflammation in the CBD leads to it becoming obstructed, so that conjugated bilirubin can no longer drain through it, its build-up causing **jaundice**. Unlike cholecystitis, where the infection is confined to the gallbladder, in cholangitis the infection can easily spread up the CBD, into the liver, and thence into the systemic circulation—this is why it is called *ascending* cholangitis. The presence of proinflammatory molecules in the systemic circulation leads to the swinging fever and rigors.

Management of ascending cholangitis: ascending cholangitis is a surgical emergency that carries a high mortality (~10–30%) if intervention is not started early, because of the high risk of the infection spreading upwards to the liver and ultimately entering the circulation (sepsis). Management should include:

- **Blood cultures,** in an attempt to establish the identity and antibiotic sensitivities of the infective bacteria.
- **Antibiotics.** The patient may need broader-spectrum antibiotics until the exact antibiotic sensitivities of the bacteria are known—always check your local guidelines as these are determined by local patterns of resistance. Mrs Cole's case should be discussed with the microbiologists as she has deteriorated despite early antibiotic therapy.
- **Endoscopic retrograde cholangiopancreatography (ERCP) drainage.** The patient must have their blocked CBD physically drained via ERCP. An endoscope is passed via the oesophagus from the patient's mouth into the duodenum. From here, a fine catheter is passed via the sphincter of Oddi and into the CBD, where the pus is drained and sent for culturing to determine the identity and antibiotic sensitivities of the infective bacteria. At the time of ERCP a small basket can be 'trawled' through the CBD to remove obstructing calculi or sludge, and a sphincterotomy is usually performed to aid the passage of any further calculi or sludge out of the CBD into the dudodenum. If, for some reason,

an ERCP fails, the patient may require percutaneous transhepatic cholangiography (PTC), a surgical procedure that allows biliary drainage.

- **Monitoring.** Once the CBD has been drained, the patient is kept in hospital on antibiotics, nil by mouth, fluids (IV), and analgesia and the patient's vital signs are monitored carefully for any signs of systemic infection (sepsis).

- **Definitive management.** ERCP is usually only a temporizing measure in patients who are fit enough for surgery. Remember that Mrs Cole will still need an elective cholecystectomy to prevent further attacks of cholecystitis and associated syndromes.

SHORT CASE

Mrs Cole mentioned in her initial history that she often suffered from a sharp, stabbing pain in her RUQ, typically a few hours after a fatty meal. The pain came and went over a period of several hours but always self-resolved within half a day.

What pathological process was Mrs Cole most likely describing?

Mrs Cole was probably suffering from bouts of **biliary colic** due to **cholelithiasis** (*chole* = bile, *lithiasis* = stone formation). About 20% of the population have small stones in their gallbladder, but in 90% of cases these cause no problems at all. In some people, however, the stones can irritate Hartmann's pouch (where the gallbladder meets the cystic duct) or the CBD, causing a sharp, stabbing pain which, despite being called 'biliary colic', is rarely a true colic (i.e. waxing and waning pain), as the pain is usually fairly constant. In most patients the gallstone eventually passes into the small bowel but in some the gallstone requires removal via ERCP.

SHORT CASE

Mr Goldstone is a 52-year-old restaurant manager who presents to his hospital with severe RUQ pain. The pain started a few hours after lunch and has been present since. He says that for the last month he has been suffering from a burning pain in his upper abdomen, often after meals. This time, the pain is stabbing in nature and much worse in severity. He has not opened his bowels since the pain started, about 4 hours ago. He has a past medical history of osteoarthrosis of his right hip, for which he takes regular NSAIDs (diclofenac) while he awaits his hip replacement. Examination reveals heart rate 90 bpm, blood pressure 137/84 mmHg, respiration 18/min, temperature 37.1 °C, and a mildly tender RUQ. Rectal examination shows dark, black, tarry stool. His erect chest radiograph is normal, with no air under the diaphragm.

What diagnosis is likely in this patient? How would he be investigated?

Mr Goldstone gives a history of upper abdominal burning pain for the last month, which is highly suggestive of a peptic ulcer (you cannot tell if it is gastric or duodenal from associations with meals and times of the day, contrary to myth). He has melaena (dark, tarry stool caused by digestion of blood from an upper GI source) and this combined with his more severe, stabbing pain suggests that Mr Goldstone may have developed a **bleeding peptic ulcer**.

The next step would be to visualize the gut wall for sources of blood using **endoscopy**. An oesophago-gastroduodenoscopy (OGD) will look at the oesophagus, stomach, and duodenum. If endoscopy doesn't reveal the source of bleeding, one can consider looking for a bleed in the jejunum and ileum using either an abdominal **CT angiogram** (which will only pick up relatively large bleeds), **video capsule endoscopy**, or a **red cell scan**.

Mr Goldstone was admitted to hospital and underwent an OGD. This showed a duodenal ulcer just distal to the pylorus with stigmata of recent bleeding. Biopsies of the ulcer were positive for *Helicobacter pylori* but showed no signs of malignancy. Mr Goldstone had his NSAID stopped and went on to receive triple eradication therapy for his ulcer: a PPI (e.g. omeprazole) and two antibiotics (e.g. amoxicillin and clarithromycin) for 1 week.

Viva questions

Explain the difference between biliary colic, cholecystitis, and ascending cholangitis.

Biliary colic occurs when the gallbladder attempts to contract against an obstruction—usually a gall-stone at Hartmann's pouch. At this stage the gallbladder is not inflamed or infected. Pain only lasts until the stone falls back into the gallbladder or is passed along the cystic duct and then CBD—but this can be anything from minutes to hours.

Cholecystitis: a significant proportion of patients presenting with biliary colic go on to develop acute cholecystitis—at which point the gallbladder is inflamed (*chole* = bile, *cyst* = bladder, *-itis* = inflammation). If a stone impacts in Hartmann's pouch or the cystic duct, the gallbladder may be full of bile that cannot escape. As water is absorbed by the gallbladder, the bile becomes very concentrated and irritates the gallbladder causing a sterile, chemical cholecystitis. As the bile and gallstone cannot drain, they often become infected causing an infective cholecystitis. Hence, both biliary colic and cholecystitis can be regarded as consequences of stones in the gallbladder (*cholelithiasis; chole* = bile, *lithiasis* = stone formation). Bowel rest (nil by mouth), antibiotics, and analgesia are sufficient in 90% of cases of cholecystitis, although many surgeons will opt for either urgent cholecystectomy or elective cholecystectomy at a later date to avoid repeated attacks.

Ascending cholangitis is usually a complication of *choledocholithiasis* (*chole* = bile, *docho* = duct, *lithiasis* = stone formation)—stone(s) in the CBD. These stones block the CBD causing jaundice, but they can also become infected by gut bacteria and the infection can spread via the liver into the circulation, causing high fever and rigors. This is the most serious presentation of gallstone disease and carries a mortality of about 15%. Ascending cholangitis may also occur if the CBD is blocked by a stricture (due to recent surgery) or a tumour, or if gut bacteria have been pushed up into the CBD by a doctor during an ERCP. Charcot's triad of fever, RUQ pain, and jaundice is present. The patient needs urgent drainage of the CBD, broad-spectrum antibiotics, and careful monitoring in hospital for signs of deterioration.

What is bile? How are bile salts conserved by the body?

Bile is made up of four main components:

- **Water:** although much of this is reabsorbed while bile is stored in the gallbladder
- **Fat:** mainly cholesterol and some phospholipids
- **Bile salts:** which serve to solubilize the fats in bile but also fats and fat-soluble vitamins (A, D, E, K) found in food
- **Conjugated bilirubin:** digested by gut bacteria into a brown pigment (stercobilin) which gives faeces its colour.

Bile salts are absorbed from the terminal ileum and then travel back to the liver via the enterohepatic circulation. Bile salts may be recycled up to 10 times each day.

Both liver disease or a blocked CBD (obstructive jaundice) can cause patients
to have prolonged blood clotting times, but administering parenteral (not oral)
vitamin K will only correct the problem in one of the cases: which one, and why?

Remember that the extrinsic arm of the clotting cascade, as measured by the prothrombin time (PT),
relies upon the liver making clotting factors II, VII, IX, and X. This process depends on vitamin K which
is fat soluble and therefore absorbed thanks to bile salts. Liver disease may result in an increased PT
due to impaired synthesis of these clotting factors within the liver. By contrast, if the patient is suffering from a blocked CBD (obstructive jaundice) then there will be little or no bile salts reaching the
gut and emulsifying fats. Thus there will be severely impaired vitamin K absorption from the terminal
ileum, and this in turn impairs clotting factor synthesis.

   An increased PT due to liver disease will not be corrected by the parenteral administration of vitamin K
as the problem is not a lack of vitamin K but that the liver has lost its synthetic function. Conversely, parenteral vitamin K will correct a prolonged PT that is due to obstructive jaundice (because clotting factor synthesis is only being hindered by a lack of raw material—vitamin K—rather than impaired synthetic ability).

What sorts of gallstones are there? Which groups of patients are prone
to particular sorts of gallstones?

There are three main types of gallstones: approximately 5% are bile pigment stones, 20% are cholesterol, and 75% are mixed composition. Note that only about 10% of gallstones are radio-opaque and
thus the vast majority will not show on plain abdominal radiographs (which is why we look for them
on ultrasound, not abdominal radiographs). Contrast this with renal/ureteric stones, about 90% of
which are radio-opaque.

   Certain patients are predisposed to particular gallstones:

- **Bile pigment stones:** bile pigments are haemoglobin breakdown products and thus patients with
  haemolytic anaemias (such as hereditary spherocystosis, sickle cell disease, or G6PD deficiency)
  are predisposed to these sorts of stones. Long-term total parenteral nutrition (TPN) is also associated with pigment gallstone disease.

- **Cholesterol stones:** it is said that the classic cholesterol gallstone patient is a fair, fat, fertile
  female of forty (the five Fs). Some add 'flatulent' as a further alliterative compliment to the
  unfortunate patient. The use of oral contraceptive therapy further increases the risk of cholesterol
  stones. Patients with Crohn's disease may suffer higher rates of cholesterol stones because the
  terminal ileum pathology impairs reabsorption and enterohepatic circulation of bile salts, thus
  making bile-based stones less likely.

What are the potential consequences of gallstones?

Remember that gallstones usually cause no pathology—they may uneventfully pass down the biliary
tree and then into the duodenum. Otherwise think anatomically. Stones may remain in the gallbladder and cause biliary colic, acute or chronic cholecystitis, a mucocoele (mucus-filled gallbladder),
empyema (pus-filled gallbladder), or (in the long term, presumably as a result of chronic inflammation) cancer of the gallbladder or CBD (cholangiocarcinoma). Stones may pass into the CBD and block
it (obstructive jaundice) or get infected (ascending cholangitis). If the stone travels down the CBD it
may become lodged at the ampulla of Vater and thus cause acute pancreatitis. Lastly, the stone may
cause gallstone ileus. This latter pathology causes some confusion and is worth elaborating on. When

CONTINUED ➤

CONTINUED

the gallbladder becomes inflamed, its neighbouring structures, namely duodenum, transverse colon, and omentum, may wrap around the gallbladder to 'wall off' the inflammation. This raises the possibility of fistula formation. A stone that travels through a cholecystocolic fistula (to the large bowel) is unlikely to cause any problems, and will most likely be passed from the body with the next stool. However, if a stone passes through a cholecystoduodenal fistula (to the small bowel) it is liable to get stuck at the narrowest part of the intestinal tract—the terminal ileum. This represents a mechanical obstruction and the term 'gallstone ileus' is thus rather a misnomer as ileus usually refers to functional obstruction of the gut. Gallstone ileus can be diagnosed on a plain abdominal radiograph by looking for signs of small bowel obstruction, air in the biliary tree, and perhaps a stone at the terminal ileum (remembering that radio-opaque gallstones are rare).

Explain why the consumption of fatty foods can exacerbate the pain of biliary colic and chronic cholecystitis.

Cholecystokinin (CCK) is released from the duodenum in response to fatty foods. CCK stimulates the secretion of digestive enzymes from pancreatic acinar cells, and also stimulates contraction of the gallbladder and relaxation of the sphincter of Oddi. These last two actions would release bile into the duodenum to aid with fat digestion and absorption. However, CCK-induced gallbladder contraction can exacerbate the pain of biliary colic and chronic cholecystitis. It would also accentuate the pain of acute cholecystitis, but you are unlikely to be eating if you have this disease!

During cholecystectomy the surgeon will look for Calot's triangle—what is it?

Calot's triangle (see Figure 15.2) is an anatomical zone used to define the usual path of the cystic artery, the cystic duct, and the common hepatic duct. It is essential to visualize and dissect this triangle during a

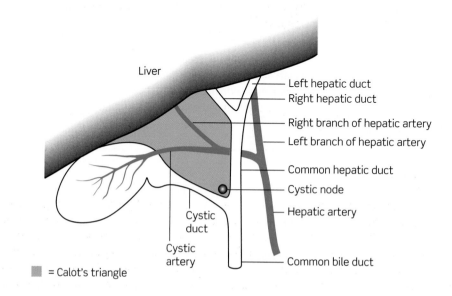

Liver

Left hepatic duct
Right hepatic duct

Right branch of hepatic artery
Left branch of hepatic artery

Common hepatic duct
Cystic node

Hepatic artery

Cystic duct

Cystic artery

Common bile duct

■ = Calot's triangle

Figure 15.2 Anatomy of Calot's triangle.

CONTINUED ➤

cholecystectomy so that one can be sure that one is ligating and cutting the cystic artery and cystic duct, and not the right hepatic artery, hepatic duct, or CBD. The superior border of the triangle is the liver, the inferior border is the cystic duct, and the medial border is the common hepatic duct. The cystic artery is a branch of the right hepatic artery, which usually passes behind the common hepatic duct. However, in about 25% of patients, the right hepatic artery passes in front of the common hepatic duct.

Where would a gallstone need to be in order to cause obstructive jaundice?

Typically the stone would need to be in the CBD or the ampulla of Vater. However, it is worth remembering that a stone in Hartmann's pouch (see Figure 15.3) may also press extrinsically on the CBD (Mirizzi's syndrome).

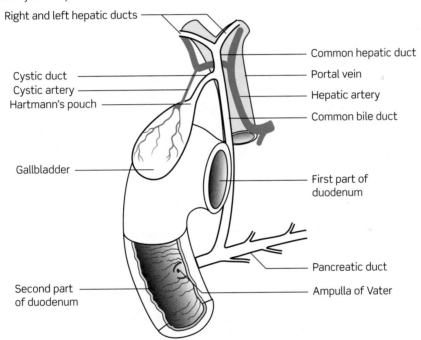

Figure 15.3 Anatomy of the biliary tree.

Reproduced from MacKinnon PCB and Morris JF, *Oxford Textbook of Functional Anatomy, Vol. 2 Thorax and Abdomen*, 2nd edition, 2005, Figure 6.6.4, page 162, with permission from Oxford University Press.

What is Courvoisier's law?

This 'law' states that if the gallbladder is palpable in the presence of jaundice then the jaundice is unlikely to be due to stones. The rationale is as follows: if the obstruction is caused by a stone in the CBD then the gallbladder is likely to be thickened and fibrotic (as the gallbladder is the source of the stone) and thus not distended and palpable, but rather shrivelled up. By contrast, if the CBD is obstructed for some other reason, such as a tumour, then the gallbladder is likely to be normal and it will dilate due to back-pressure. Note the phrasing of Courvoisier's law—it does *not* state that if the

CONTINUED ➤

CONTINUED

gallbladder is not palpable then the jaundice is due to a stone. This is because it is perfectly possible for the gallbladder to be dilated (perhaps due to a distal tumour causing back-pressure of bile) but not palpable because it is obscured by the liver or layers of fat in the abdominal wall.

What is an ERCP? What is the advantage of ERCP over MRCP? What are the complications of ERCP?

ERCP is endoscopic retrograde cholangiopancreatography. A side-viewing endoscope is passed via the mouth, past the oesophagogastric junction and pylorus, and down to the second part of the duodenum. At this point a fine catheter emerges from the endoscope and is passed through the duodenal papilla and into the ampulla of Vater. It is possible to inject contrast medium directly into the biliary tree, which is then visualized radiographically.

MRCP is magnetic resonance cholangiopancreatography. It enables detailed visualization of the biliary tree, but is purely a diagnostic procedure. ERCP has a therapeutic role as it is possible to both remove stones (using a Dormia basket) and perform endoscopic sphincterotomy (cutting the sphincter of Oddi with a fine diathermy wire in order to facilitate the passage of any stones within the CBD).

Aside from being a rather unpleasant procedure to undergo, the **risks of ERCP** include bleeding, perforation of the biliary tree, cholangitis, and pancreatitis. There is about a 1–3% risk of pancreatitis and, for reasons that are not entirely clear, this pancreatitis carries a 20% mortality risk (which is higher than normal for pancreatitis).

Single Best Answers

1. **A patient presents with right upper quadrant pain. The examining doctor palpates over the tip of the right 9th costal cartilage and asks the patient to take a deep breath. The patient winces and arrests inspiration. What is the name of this clinical sign?**

   a. Grey Turner's sign
   b. Murphy's sign
   c. Cullen's sign
   d. Prehn's sign
   e. Boas's sign

2. **Which of the following investigations is not relevant to biliary disease?**

   a. MRCP
   b. Ultrasound
   c. HIDA
   d. MIBG
   e. ERCP

3. **Into which part of the duodenum does the common bile duct drain?**

   a. D1
   b. D2
   c. D3
   d. D4
   e. D5

4. **In the majority of cases, the cystic artery (which supplies the gallbladder) arises from which artery?**

   a. Hepatic artery
   b. Common hepatic artery
   c. Left hepatic artery
   d. Right hepatic artery
   e. Gastroduodenal artery

5. **Which of the following biochemical markers is the most specific indicator of hepatocyte damage?**

   a. Amylase
   b. ALP
   c. AST
   d. ALT
   e. Bilirubin

Right iliac fossa pain

Core case

Read through the sections in the case boxes, covering up the sections that follow so that you don't see the answer. At the end of each case box, try to answer the question before reading on.

> Mr Beck is a 28-year-old builder who presents to the Emergency Department on Sunday evening with a 3-hour history of right iliac fossa (RIF) pain. He is nauseated and has vomited once.
>
> **What is your differential diagnosis? Try to prioritize into those conditions that are most likely (or most common), those that you must exclude, and the remainder.**

The differential diagnosis for acute RIF pain is shown in Figure 16.1.

Appendicitis
Gastroenteritis
Ureteric colic
Inguinal hernia (especially **if encarcerated or strangulated**)

Epididymitis and/or orchitis
Mesenteric adenitis
Acute pancreatitis
Testicular torsion
Meckel's diverticulitis
Cholecystitis
Pyelonephritis
Psoas abscess
Small bowel obstruction
Diabetic ketoacidosis
Urinary tract infection
Constipation
Acute onset ileitis (bacterial or Crohn's)
Caecal volvulus
Perforated peptic ulcer
Caecal diverticulitis
Shingles
Rectus sheath haematoma
Femoral hernia (especially **if encarcerated or strangulated**)

Figure 16.1 Differential diagnoses for acute right iliac fossa pain in an adult male. Diagnoses shown in **bold** are all surgical emergencies that you must exclude as you clerk the patient. The most common diagnoses are in large font at the top.

Note that certain diagnoses are going to be more likely in different patient groups. Children and elderly people are more likely to have a longer differential as symptoms are often less pronounced and non-specific. Intussusception is almost exclusively seen in children, and the vast majority of cases of mesenteric adenitis are also seen in children. By contrast, caecal pathology (tumours, volvulus, or a solitary mesenteric diverticulum) is usually associated with advancing age. An abdominal aortic aneurysm would be extraordinarily rare in a young adult but should be considered in anyone >50 years of age.

What other diagnoses must you consider in a female patient?

You must of course consider gynaecological pathology, such as ectopic pregnancy, pelvic inflammatory disease/salpingitis, torsion/haemorrhage/rupture of an ovarian tumour or cyst, mittelschmerz (mid-cycle pain corresponding to a ruptured ovarian follicle), threatened abortion, fibroid degeneration, or uterine dehiscence.

In any woman of reproductive age you *must* perform a pregnancy test—this is not only to exclude particular diagnoses such as ectopic pregnancy, but is also essential to help weigh up the risk of radiation to the fetus against the diagnostic usefulness of the test.

On further questioning we establish that Mr Beck had a milder, poorly localized, central abdominal pain for about 12 hours before the onset of the RIF pain. The pain worsened about 3 hours ago, at which time he felt that it had shifted to the right. The pain has been constant ever since. He says that the pain doesn't radiate anywhere else, but struggles to give much more of a description when asked to characterize it—'pain is pain'. He hasn't taken anything for the pain but states that he'd rate it as 8 out of 10. He is not aware of anything that makes the pain worse, but is reluctant to lie flat on the bed, and you notice that he keeps his right hip slightly flexed. He had his customary Saturday night curry yesterday. He ordered the hottest dish on the menu, but says that he always does this and never suffers any ill effects. None of his friends from the meal have had similar symptoms. He has completely lost his appetite today and has not opened his bowels either. He has felt otherwise well over the preceding week. Mr Beck's face appears flushed and, as already noted, he is reluctant to lie flat.

With this history in mind, you need to examine Mr Beck to try and narrow your differential. In particular, you need to establish the site and extent of abdominal tenderness. How will you do this?

Note that *tenderness is a sign whereas pain is a symptom.*

It is very useful to have an idea of the degree of abdominal tenderness before you even lay a hand on the patient. Remember that you will win no prizes (either in exams or with patients themselves) if you actually cause a patient pain. So, start by asking the patient to suck their tummy in as far as possible and then puff it out again (this is particularly useful in children). A patient with board-like abdominal rigidity secondary to generalized peritonism will only make very minor movements. Now ask the patient to cough: patients with inflammation of the parietal peritoneum will be reluctant to cough deeply and may well place their hands over the area of tenderness.

Whether you palpate the abdomen in quadrants or nine zones, be sure to start in the opposite area to that which the patient states is most painful. Start by palpating gently and keep looking at the patient's face for a reaction. Patients are likely to demonstrate guarding (involuntary muscular rigidity in tender areas of the abdomen). Percussion tenderness, when percussion over an area causes the patient pain, is a sensitive means of demonstrating parietal peritoneum irritation and is far kinder to the patient than assessing rebound tenderness.

What else will you be looking for on examination?

- **Is he ill?** As a first line you should establish whether Mr Beck is febrile and/or tachycardic, hypotensive, or tachypnoeic. If he looks ill, make sure you flag the patient as soon as possible to your seniors so they are aware that you are dealing with an unwell patient who may need their involvement at short notice.

- **Scars:** scars in particular anatomical sites can be particularly informative—for example, has this patient still got an appendix? Remember that any previous abdominal surgery will also make small bowel obstruction more likely as postsurgical adhesions predispose to obstruction.

- **Abdominal distension:** in a thin patient you may be able to observe these signs of small bowel obstruction.

- **Cervical lymphadenopathy:** particularly important for trying to rule out mesenteric adenitis, which is inflammation and enlargement of the mesenteric lymph nodes. It often follows an upper respiratory tract viral infection (hence cervical lymphadenopathy may be present) and is one of the most difficult conditions to differentiate from appendicitis in young patients.

- **Masses:** the greater omentum can wrap around inflamed organs, hence creating a localized mass (such as an appendix mass). Other palpable masses may be due to a tumour or a rectus sheath haematoma. The history in Mr Beck's case is rather short, but in someone with a longer history of constipation you may be able to palpate faecal loading in the sigmoid and colon.

- **Bowel sounds:** these will be absent if there is functional bowel obstruction (ileus) or perhaps 'tinkling' if there is small bowel obstruction.

- **Hernias:** a particularly important cause of small bowel obstruction.

- **Rectal exam:** A rectal examination can sometimes provide useful clues such as constipation (and whether it is caused by a rectal mass) or blood (suggestive of inflammatory bowel disease, a bleeding Meckel's or caecal diverticulum) but most patients with RIF pain will be able to tell you if they are constipated or having rectal bleeding, and in them, a rectal examination is unlikely to aid your diagnosis.

- **External genitalia:** you *must* examine the testicles for signs of torsion—particularly in young men. Torsion, epididymitis and orchitis can present with referred pain to the abdomen via T10 sympathetic innervation. The window of opportunity for surgical rescue of torted testes is only about 6 hours since onset.

Mr Beck is febrile (37.8 °C), tachycardic (102 bpm), and normotensive (134/78 mmHg) with a respiratory rate of 20/min. He is asked to cough and finds this incredibly painful—clutching his hands over his right side. There is guarding in the RIF. In addition, palpation in the left iliac fossa results in greater pain in the RIF than the left (Rovsing's sign positive). There are no palpable cervical lymph nodes and no abdominal masses. No obvious organomegaly is palpable. His abdominal aorta is pulsatile but not expansile. Percussion tenderness is maximal over a point approximately two-thirds of the distance from the umbilicus laterally towards the anterior superior iliac spine (McBurney's point). Bowel sounds are normal. Examination of the hernial orifices is normal. A chaperone is present during examination of the external genitalia which feel normal to palpation and are not tender. Mr Beck denies constipation or blood in his faeces so a rectal examination is not performed.

Although Mr Beck's history and examination are highly suggestive of a particular diagnosis, there are still a number of other contenders to rule out. What investigations would you like to request to refine your differential diagnosis?

Blood tests

- **Full blood count (FBC):** the white cell count may be elevated in response to any inflammatory condition (e.g. appendicitis, cholecystitis, or basal pneumonia).

- **C-reactive protein (CRP):** elevated inflammatory markers point towards an inflammatory picture although, as with the white cell count, they are non-specific regarding the cause. An entirely normal neutrophil count and CRP make an inflammatory process unlikely (but not impossible).

- **Venous blood gas:** A raised lactate and/or a metabolic acidosis (pH <7.35, low/normal pCO_2 and BE (base excess) <−2) are signs of ischaemia or severe sepsis. If either of these signs is present, alert your seniors as this suggests the patient is unwell.

- **Urea and electrolytes (U&Es):** useful for establishing the baseline electrolyte status of the patient (remembering that a number of the diagnoses on our differential will require intravenous (IV) fluids and/or surgery). Urea is also used as a prognostic indicator for pancreatitis as part of the modified Glasgow criteria (see p. 220).

- **Serum amylase (or lipase) levels:** high amylase (or lipase) levels are strongly suggestive of pancreatitis, although they are non-specific and thus must be viewed in the context of the clinical picture. Slight increases (200–600 U/L) in amylase levels are most commonly caused by pancreatitis, but also by various other pathologies such as bowel obstruction, mesenteric ischaemia, a posteriorly perforated duodenal ulcer, mumps, pancreatic carcinoma, or opiate medications. However, very high amylase levels (>1000 U/L) or elevated lipase levels (>300 U/L) are almost exclusively found in pancreatitis. (The exact cutoffs will depend on your local laboratory protocols.) If you have any clinical suspicion of pancreatitis you should also request markers used in the modified Glasgow score for pancreatitis severity (FBC, calcium, urea, liver enzymes, lactate dehydrogenase (LDH), albumin, glucose, arterial blood gas).

- **Glucose:** remember that diabetic ketoacidosis can present with an acute abdomen and that infection is likely to cause disturbed glycaemic control in diabetic patients. Glucose levels are also part of the Glasgow pancreatitis criteria.

- **Liver enzymes:** within the context of a raised amylase, these provide useful prognostic information for pancreatitis (which can result in elevated aspartate aminotransferase (AST) and low albumin). Liver enzymes are also essential if there is any clinical suspicion of biliary pathology.

Urine

- **Urinalysis:** in the context of the acute abdomen, haematuria may result from infection, renal/ureteric calculi, or rarely an inflamed pelvic appendix that is irritating the bladder or retrocaecal appendix irritating the ureter. Glucose and ketones are indicative of diabetic ketoacidosis. A combination of positive leucocyte esterase and nitrites is highly suggestive of a urinary tract infection. Both urinary tract infection and appendiceal irritation of the bladder can result in proteinuria but these could be distinguished by performing urine microscopy looking for bacteria, which would confirm the urinary tract infection.

Imaging

- **Abdominal ultrasound:** this can be a very useful test if there is an atypical history such that renal or biliary pathology are likely differentials. Appendicitis can be suggested by a positive ultrasound scan, but not ruled out by a negative one. Ultrasound is also a useful test for detecting free fluid in the abdomen. Ultrasound (both transabdominal and transvaginal) may be particularly useful in female patients, where the differential diagnosis is broadened by gynaecological pathology.

Other investigations to consider are:

- **Erect chest radiograph:** request if there is any clinical suspicion of a perforated viscus. Air under the diaphragm could result from a perforated peptic ulcer, Meckel's diverticulum, caecal diverticulum, or appendix.
- **Abdominal CT:** CT scans involve a considerable dose of radiation, and the delay in obtaining a scan may be unacceptable for some diagnoses such as acute appendicitis. However, CT is useful for equivocal cases or for determining the extent of intra-abdominal collections and masses.
- **ECG:** Useful if the patient is tachycardic (and especially if general anaesthesia is likely) to confirm they have a standard sinus tachycardia.
- **Abdominal radiograph?** This is useful only:
  - if one suspects bowel obstruction (to look for dilated loops of bowel)
  - in the context of known inflammatory bowel disease (IBD) to rule out toxic megacolon
  - or to look for a foreign body.
  - As the patient is not vomiting (bowel obstruction unlikely), is not known to have IBD, and we don't suspect a foreign body, there is *no reason* to request an abdominal radiograph at this point. Patients with acute abdominal pain often have plain abdominal radiographs requested by inexperienced junior doctors, but in the overwhelming majority of cases there is no medico-legal justification for this radiation exposure.

Blood tests are taken:

Haematology		Biochemistry		Venous gas	
WCC	13.2×10^9 cells/L	CRP	32 mg/L	pH	7.37
Neutrophils	10.5×10^9 cells/L	Amylase	200 U/L	Lactate	0.5
				Glucose	4.7 mM

All other blood tests are unremarkable.
Urine dipstick is negative for protein, blood, leucocyte esterase, nitrites, glucose, and ketones.

In light of the history, examination and first-line investigations, what is the most likely diagnosis?

This is a classical clinical picture for **acute appendicitis**: low-grade central abdominal pain that gradually migrates to the RIF over 12–24 hours and becomes more intense. Anorexia is a reliable feature. The patient is flushed, febrile, tachycardic, and is lying still. Examination reveals guarding and percussion tenderness in the RIF—perhaps over McBurney's point. Digital rectal examination may also show right-sided tenderness. Rovsing's sign may be positive but is an unreliable sign. Bear in mind that this classical presentation is only seen in about 50% of patients. The appendix can lie in various positions relative to the caecum and thus produces various different examination findings when inflamed. Furthermore, there is no single test that is diagnostic for appendicitis.

What features of the history, clinical examination, and investigations help you rule out other diagnoses?

We can go through the differential diagnosis given initially and try to rule out alternatives to appendicitis:

- **Mesenteric adenitis?** Typically follows an upper respiratory tract infection or sore throat, thus cervical lymphadenopathy may be present. It is most common in children less than 15 years old. In truth, it is very difficult to distinguish between appendicitis and mesenteric adenitis, with the final diagnosis being made intraoperatively in many cases. The pain with mesenteric adenitis is often more diffuse than that of appendicitis, and signs of peritonitis are often absent. Mesenteric adenitis doesn't result in rectal tenderness, but appendicitis rarely results in this sign in any case. Fever is said to be slightly higher in mesenteric adenitis (>38.5 °C), but this too is unreliable. Mesenteric adenitis often settles quickly.

- **Meckel's diverticulitis?** As with mesenteric adenitis, it is almost impossible to definitively exclude an inflamed/ruptured Meckel's diverticulum preoperatively. Signs and symptoms are classically indistinguishable from appendicitis.

- **Constipation?** This would not cause a migration of pain to the RIF. There is almost invariably a history of infrequent and/or difficult bowel motions. Constipation virtually never results in fever or tachycardia.

- **Acute-onset Crohn's disease?** Although the acute signs and symptoms can mimic appendicitis, there is often a history of diarrhoea and weight loss for weeks/months leading up to the acute presentation.

- **Gastroenteritis?** Vomiting and diarrhoea predominate. The shifting nature of pain, and localized abdominal tenderness are not typical. In addition, you may expect to see similar symptoms in other family members or close contacts.

- **Renal/ureteric colic?** The patient would typically be writhing in pain (rather than lying still). Pain would not migrate from the central abdomen. Urine dipstick would usually (but not always) show haematuria.

- **Pancreatitis?** The migration of the pain to the RIF would be atypical for pancreatitis. Furthermore, if there is RIF pain we'd also expect there to be epigastric pain. Although the serum amylase is very slightly raised, it is not high enough to raise suspicions of pancreatitis (typically >1000 U/L, but levels may be normal even in severe pancreatitis). It is worth remembering that other intestinal pathology such as appendicitis, intestinal infarction, and perforated duodenal ulcer can also cause raised amylase levels, as can head injury, diabetic ketoacidosis, and drugs such as opioids. If Mr Beck did have pancreatitis it would be mild according to the prognostic Glasgow score (zero in his case; see Chapter 12).

- **Testicular pathology:** there are no signs of testicular tenderness or any palpable abnormality (see Chapter 25).

How would you manage Mr Beck?

Mr Beck has a slight tachycardia, so you should give him IV fluid boluses aiming to settle this. He should also be given adequate **analgesia**, which in itself is likely to help the tachycardia as the pain settles. The first-line treatment for appendicitis is **appendicectomy**, either open or laparoscopic. Patients should be **nil by mouth** for solids and non-clear fluids for 6 hours prior to surgery and clear fluids 2 hours prior to surgery, although most appendicitis patients have usually lost their appetite anyway. Intraoperative mortality in the UK is <0.2%, but rises to about 5% in very young or elderly patients as the difficulty of diagnosis in these patient groups means that they are more likely to present with perforation. Perioperative **broad-spectrum antibiotics** should be used in all appendicectomies as they reduce wound infection and abscess formation. The patient should also be prescribed some form of **deep vein thrombosis (DVT) prophylaxis** such as a daily injection of low molecular weight heparin and elastic compression stockings for the calves.

Mr Beck is taken to theatre for a diagnostic laparoscopy which confirms a friable, gangrenous appendix. Removal of the appendix is challenging. He remains well for the first 24 hours after the operation but you are then called at 2 a.m. by one of the ward nurses who is concerned that something is wrong. Mr Beck was initially comfortable but is now complaining of generalized abdominal pain and has vomited twice. You attend the ward and find that Mr Beck is clammy and pale. He is taking shallow, fast breaths and has a fast radial pulse. His chest sounds clear. He is tender and guarding throughout his abdomen and retches into a sick bowl while you are there. He tells you he has been feeling increasingly unwell since dinnertime and he confirms that he has passed wind several times since surgery, but not yet opened his bowels. His observation chart, including the most recent observations, is shown in Figure 16.2.

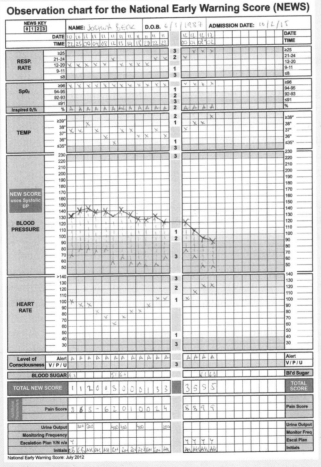

Figure 16.2 Observation chart for Mr Beck.

Reproduced from: Royal College of Physicians. *National Early Warning Score (NEWS): Standardising the assessment of acute illness severity in the NHS.* Report of a working party. London: RCP, 2012. Copyright © 2012 Royal College of Physicians. Reproduced with permission.

How will you manage Mr Beck? What is the likely diagnosis?

Mr Beck is acutely unwell. His airway is patent but he is breathing fast (30/min). He is tachycardic (125 bpm) and hypotensive (90/50 mmHg). He has a fever (39.5 °C). This patient is in **septic shock** and this is an emergency. First, **call for help**, even if this involves waking up your seniors. Then, manage his septic shock using the Sepsis Six interventions of the Surviving Sepsis campaign (Box 16.1). You have examined the patient and found that he is febrile and has a tender abdomen after gastrointestinal surgery. Although it is possible that he has postoperative ileus causing nausea and vomiting, he has only vomited twice (not enough to explain the hyptension), has passed wind (making ileus unlikely), and is febrile with a tender abdomen, so you should be suspecting that he has an intra-abdominal collection and subsequent development of generalized peritonitis. Septic shock kills even young patients if left untreated, so act promptly and give the patient broad-spectrum IV antibiotics.

Ultimately, this patient may need to return to theatre for a washout. In the meantime, the priority is to ensure that he is adequately resuscitated and has an urgent senior review to guide further management (whether that is CT with or without percutaneous drainage, and/or returning to the operating theatre).

Box 16.1 The Sepsis Six

1 **Administer high-flow oxygen.** You need to maximize oxygen delivery to his tissues so you should aim for oxygen saturations of ≥96%. Start with 15 L/min of oxygen via a reservoir bag mask and then titrate down if able.

2 **Take blood cultures.** These will help guide antimicrobial therapy in the subsequent days and if they are not taken now, they are likely to be forgotten.

3 **Give broad-spectrum antibiotics**, as soon as possible and certainly within 1 hour of recognizing the problem.

4 **Give IV fluid challenges.** This patient has a heart rate that is greater than his systolic blood pressure, suggesting he is shocked and will not be able to perfuse his organs adequately. Young patients don't drop their blood pressure until they are very unwell, so this is particularly worrying in Mr Beck's case. Ensure that he has large-bore IV access, and use IV fluids rationally and with regular reviews to see if they are working: give fluid boluses (e.g. 250 mL of a crystalloid solution) aiming to increase his blood pressure and reduce his heart rate to more normal values.

5 **Measure serum lactate and haemoglobin.** The quickest way to do this is by obtaining a venous blood gas, which will also give you the pH, electrolytes, glucose and (in some cases) creatinine. A raised lactate is an indicator of tissue ischaemia and severity of sepsis. A low haemoglobin is unlikely in Mr Beck, but useful in elderly patients or patients with cancer, in whom an Hb <70 g/L will exacerbate tissue ischaemia and worsen their prognosis.

6 **Measure accurate hourly urine output.** A decreasing urine output is one of earliest signs of impending acute kidney injury. If monitoring cannot be done using disposable urinary bottles, the patient will need a urinary catheter with a urometer.

© The UK Sepsis Trust/Dr Ron Daniel <http://survivesepsis.org/the-sepsis-six>

Short cases

Mr Briggs is a 46-year-old solicitor admitted to the surgical unit at the same time as Mr Beck. He describes a similar history of central abdominal pain that migrated to the RIF. However, he has waited 3 days before seeking help. He has been taking paracetamol 1 gram q.d.s. (four times a day) at home, but this has not controlled his pain. He has not eaten a proper meal for 3 days, and has only passed minimal amounts of stool. On examination, he is flushed, tachycardic, and febrile. There is marked halitosis. There is muscular rigidity in the RIF, and a tender mass is palpable in the RIF. The rest of the abdomen is soft and non-tender. Per rectum, genital, and hernial orifice examinations are all unremarkable.

What has happened to Mr Briggs?

It is likely that Mr Briggs has also had acute appendicitis but that he has suffered a complication and has now developed an **appendix mass**. The greater omentum, caecum, and/or adherent loops of small bowel wrap themselves around the inflamed or perforated appendix to form a localized mass. CT or ultrasound scan may clinch the diagnosis. The fact that Mr Briggs has waited 3 days before presenting to hospital does not necessarily mean that he is any more stoical or able to tolerate more pain than our previous patient. Rather, patients who develop an appendix mass are usually those who have had a less intense pain resulting from 'milder' inflammation of the appendix.

Initial conservative therapy is usually indicated for an appendix mass. This involves keeping patients nil by mouth, ensuring adequate IV fluids, antibiotic cover, analgesia, and DVT prophylaxis, and then marking out the size of the mass on the abdominal wall. Surgery is indicated if the mass increases in size, if the patient becomes more septic, or if the patient develops small bowel obstruction due to the adhesions.

If early surgery is not indicated and the mass resolves with conservative treatment, it is usual to perform an elective appendicectomy 6–8 weeks after resolution of the mass, although elective removal of the appendix following resolution of the mass remains controversial.

It is worth emphasizing the difference between an appendix mass and appendix abscess. The former is a phlegmon (an inflammatory mass) whereas an abscess contains pus, and it is often possible to distinguish between the two with appropriate imaging (CT or ultrasound). Hence a conservative approach can be adopted for an appendix mass but an abscess must be drained—either as an open procedure or percutaneously. Furthermore, once patients have recovered from the initial inflammatory episode they will often be booked for a colonoscopy or barium enema to exclude other causes of ileocaecal perforation such as a carcinoma (particularly for older patients).

Mr Fuhr is a 16-year-old student who presents to the surgical emergency unit with a 3-hour history of RIF pain. He has vomited once. He was specifically asked whether he had any central abdominal pain prior to the RIF pain but he is unsure. He was playing rugby earlier in the day and, as he doesn't like to play with a full stomach, says that it is usual for him to have some rumbling stomach pains before a big match. He has otherwise been fit and well. On examination, his temperature is 37.4 °C and pulse is 134 bpm, regular. He is in obvious discomfort. However, abdominal examination is unremarkable—there are no local areas of tenderness; no palpable masses; bowel sounds are present. Urine dipstick is negative. Bloods are sent for analysis.

Which critical examination has not yet been performed? Which diagnosis must we consider?

Mr Fuhr is exactly the right sort of age to present with **testicular torsion**. It is absolutely critical that all boys/young men have their testes examined when presenting with an acute abdomen. A thorough gastrointestinal examination of patients of any age should feature inspection of external genitalia and hernial orifices, and a digital rectal examination if appropriate.

Signs of testicular torsion include an exquisitely tender testicle and scrotal erythema. The abdominal pain is referred via the T10 sympathetic supply and reflects the embryological origin of the testes. Nausea and vomiting are commonplace. The affected testis will lie higher in the scrotum than a normal testis. A testis that lies horizontally is more likely to tort, so examine the other testis as well. Prehn's sign is said to help distinguish between epididymitis and testicular torsion: elevating the affected scrotum relieves the pain of epididymitis (positive Prehn's), but will not relieve the pain of torsion. However, although you may hear Prehn's sign being mentioned on the wards, it is not a reliable sign. More information would be gleaned by attempting to elicit the cremasteric reflex (downwards stroking of the superomedial aspect of the thigh should result in elevation of the ipsilateral scrotum/testicle). Although the absence of the cremasteric reflex does not diagnose torsion (as it is very frequently absent), it has a negative predictive value of 96%—in other words, its *presence* is strongly suggestive of another pathology.

Although the majority of testicular torsions appear to happen spontaneously (often at night), they may follow minor trauma. Doppler ultrasound of the testes may aid diagnosis, but if there is any suspicion of torsion it is safest to send the patient to theatre as time really does matter (90% chance of rescuing testis at 6 hours, 5% at 24 hours). If there is a delay in reaching theatre it may be appropriate to attempt manual de-rotation of the testis. It is important to warn patients and parents prior to theatre that both testicles will need fixing to avoid future torsions, and that the affected testicle may need to be removed if it appears necrotic.

SHORT CASE

Miss Norton is a 12-year-old girl who presents to her GP with RIF pain. It is difficult to establish much of a pain history, but it seems as though she has had this pain for about a day. The GP notes that one of his colleagues saw Miss Norton last week and diagnosed a suspected viral pharyngitis. Upon examination today, her abdomen is soft and there is only slight periumbilical and RIF tenderness to light palpation, but no guarding or rebound. The GP decides that it would not be appropriate to perform a digital rectal examination. He does, however, ask her to provide a urine sample. There are no signs of urinary tract infection or pregnancy on urine dipstick testing. Miss Norton has a fever of 38.6 °C and pulse 121 bpm, regular. The rest of the examination is unremarkable, except for a palpable right-sided submandibular lymph node. The GP decides to refer Miss Norton to the local hospital. He rings the admissions unit to warn of her arrival.

What is he likely to mention as the differential diagnoses?

Given that we can rule out ectopic pregnancy or threatened miscarriage, our most likely diagnoses would be **appendicitis** or **mesenteric adenitis**. The slightly higher fever, lack of guarding, and history of upper respiratory tract infection perhaps swing the pendulum in favour of mesenteric adenitis, but Miss Norton will need to be admitted for observation in case this is appendicitis. Miss Norton may proceed to surgery (laparoscopy) if her condition worsens enough to warrant it (so that appendicitis can be ruled out). It is, however, rare to need surgery in cases of mesenteric adenitis and patients remain well on observation.

SHORT CASE

Mrs Riley is a 36-year-old woman who presents with a 7-hour history of RIF pain that she rates as 7 out of 10. She also describes a 5-month history of painless loose stools that she has self-diagnosed as irritable bowel syndrome and is treating with probiotic yoghurts and peppermint tea (with minor benefit). She is nauseated and has vomited twice since the onset of the pain. She is not aware of any radiation of the current pain. There are no particular alleviating or aggravating factors.

On examination she is febrile (37.8 °C) and tachycardic (103 bpm regular). There are no peripheral stigmata of gastrointestinal disease. Abdominal examination reveals guarding and percussion tenderness in the RIF, but no palpable masses. The abdominal aorta is pulsatile but not expansile. Rectal examination is performed and is unremarkable. There are no hernias.

Blood tests show:

Haematology		Biochemistry	
WCC	12.3×10^9 cells/L	Urea	11.3 mM
		Creatinine	87 µM
		Na	129 mM
		K	3.3 mM
		CRP	45 mg/L

Other blood results are within normal ranges.

Urine analysis shows nothing abnormal. A pregnancy test is negative. Stool samples are sent for culture. The surgical team decide to perform laparoscopy. The appendix appears normal, but the terminal ileum is inflamed and mesenteric fat is seen to wrap around the ileum. The pattern of inflammation is discontinuous, and there are also isolated patches of inflammation in the proximal colon.

In light of the laparoscopy findings and clinical history, what is the most likely diagnosis?

It is most likely that Mrs Riley is suffering from an acute presentation of **Crohn's disease**. While only about 5% of Crohn's patients present in this way, it is important to consider the diagnosis when you have patients with a chronic history of disturbed bowel habit. Further tests such as barium meal and follow-through, and ileocolonoscopy with biopsy, would be required to confirm the diagnosis. Mrs Riley's low sodium, low potassium, and slightly raised urea with normal creatinine are most likely due to her diarrhoea and dehydration and will need monitoring to ensure they resolve (and correcting if not).

SHORT CASE

Miss Jackson is a 23-year-old company secretary who calls her GP, requesting a home visit because she has abdominal pain. On further questioning, she describes how the pain started quite suddenly, and has now been present for about 2 hours. The pain is focused in her RIF, and has not radiated. It is not influenced by her body position. When asked to rate the pain out of 10, she gives it a 4. She says that she feels slightly embarrassed calling the GP for a pain that is only 4/10, but explains that she has had similar pain a couple of times over the last few months and that she wanted the doctor to see her during one of these painful episodes in order to make sure that nothing sinister was going on. The last time that she had similar pain was about a month ago—it was also in her RIF, lasted about 4 hours, and was relieved by ibuprofen that she bought from the chemist. Prior to that, she remembers a similar unprovoked episode of abdominal pain about 2 months ago, but mentions that this pain was on the left side of her abdomen.

When specifically asked whether she could be pregnant, Miss Jackson says that this is impossible as she has not been sexually active since her last period. She has regular 28-day menstrual cycles and had her last period 2 weeks ago.

The GP explains that he feels that Miss Jackson is probably well enough to visit the surgery, rather than requiring a home visit, but that he will gladly see her if she is able to come in. While waiting for her to arrive, he looks through her medical record and establishes that she has no significant medical history and takes no regular medications. When Miss Jackson arrives at the surgery she looks well. She is, however, still complaining of abdominal pain and the GP therefore examines her. An abdominal examination is performed and nothing abnormal is noted. A urine dipstick and pregnancy test are negative.

What is the most likely diagnosis given the history and examination findings?

The most likely diagnosis is that Miss Jackson is suffering from **mittelschmerz** (German for 'middle pain'). This is a relatively common condition, affecting as many as one in five menstruating women. The key points in the history are that the pain is relatively mild, short-lived, and cyclical in nature—she has regular periods and reports how the pain appears around the time of ovulation (day 14 in a 28-day cycle). The fact that previous painful episodes have been on both the right and left sides is entirely consistent with mittelschmerz. Although some women experience a generalized lower abdominal pain mid-cycle, other women are able to perceive which of their ovaries has provided the egg in any given month. Whether the right or left ovary provides the egg each month is unpredictable and variable. The absence of any findings on abdominal examination is also consistent with mittelschmerz.

Viva questions

What are the main causes of appendicitis?

The main cause is thought to be obstruction by a faecolith or foreign body in the lumen of the appendix. Other important causes are lymphoid hyperplasia of Peyer's patches, or fibrous strictures at the base of the appendix following previous inflammation. A rare cause is a carcinoid tumour: such tumours are rare, but when they do occur, it is most often in the appendix. This is why all appendices removed at the time of surgery are sent for histological analysis.

What is the neuroanatomical basis of the shifting location of the pain in appendicitis?

The key to understanding the shift in location is to think about the distinction between visceral and somatic pain. There are two pain sensation systems in the abdomen—the splanchnic system, which only senses stretch and spasm, and the cerebrospinal pathway that can sense the same array of painful stimuli as skin. The embryonic gut arises as a midline organ and its splanchnic innervation is bilateral, thus visceral pain is felt in the midline. The splanchnic nerves carrying this information synapse on neurons which also receive inputs from the anterior abdominal wall—the brain misinterprets this visceral signal as arising from the anterior abdomen. The appendix, being an embryological midgut organ, is innervated by the lesser splanchnic nerve (T10–T11) and thus initial pain is felt around the umbilicus. There is no somatic innervation of the visceral peritoneum, but as the appendix progressively distends and the inflammatory process extends to involve the parietal peritoneum the pain signals are carried in somatic nerves and inflammation can be localized to the actual site of the appendix—usually in the RIF. This shift in pain location usually occurs in less than 24 hours.

What is the difference between SIRS (systemic inflammatory response syndrome), sepsis, severe sepsis, septic shock and multiorgan failure?

- **SIRS** is the body's response to a wide range of proinflammatory processes (not just infection but also e.g. pancreatitis, anaphylaxis, pulmonary embolus) and is defined as two or more of the following criteria:
  - Temperature >38 °C or < 36 °C
  - Heart rate >90 bpm
  - Respiratory rate >20/min or pCO_2 <4.3 kPa
  - White cell count > 12×10^9 cells/L or < 4×10^9 cells/L or >10% immature forms.
- **Sepsis** is SIRS caused by a suspected or proven infection.
- **Severe sepsis** is sepsis causing hypotension (systolic blood pressure <90 mmHg or ≥40 mmHg drop compared to normal for that patient) and end organ hypoperfusion (lactic acidosis on a venous blood gas).
- **Septic shock** is severe sepsis that is refractory to fluid resuscitation (and therefore in need of vasopressors).
- **Multiorgan dysfunction syndrome (MODS) or multiorgan failure:** evidence of two or more organs failing (e.g. confusion due to cerebral hypoperfusion, renal failure, respiratory failure, liver failure).

Which two incisions are commonly used for an open appendicectomy?

The classic approach was the gridiron incision, which is made perpendicular to the imaginary line between the umbilicus and anterior superior iliac spine (ASIS), and centred over McBurney's point. This is rarely used now. More commonly you will see a Lanz incision—this is placed slightly lower in the RIF, starting about 2 cm medial to the ASIS, and follows a more horizontal course than the gridiron. The Lanz produces better cosmesis as it sits in a natural skin crease. The laparoscopic approach is becoming more commonplace.

At the time of the operation, in the presence of a normal appendix, the surgeon also inspects the distal 60 cm (2 feet) of the terminal ileum—why?

Remember that one of the differential diagnoses of appendicitis is an inflamed/ruptured Meckel's diverticulum. This remnant of the vitelline duct is often said to follow the 'rule of 2s'—it occurs in 2% of the population, may contain two types of ectopic cells (pancreatic and gastric), is typically situated within 60 cm (2 feet) of the ileocaecal valve, is about 5 cm (2 inches) long, and is usually symptomatic by 2 years. Cynics would also add that the rule is only true 2% of the time! Surgeons are only likely to look for an inflamed Meckel's or evidence of Crohn's ileitis if the appendix is not inflamed at the time of operation (a non-inflamed appendix is said to look 'lily white').

If the appendix does not look inflamed at the time of open operation why would the surgeon remove it anyway?

It is possible for an appendix that is inflamed due to a faecolith to spontaneously resolve without surgical intervention. However, even a non-inflamed appendix is usually removed if the patient proceeds to theatre. This is to help future surgeons as it would be all too easy to assume that a patient no longer had an appendix if a gridiron or Lanz scar is visible.

What is an interval appendicectomy?

Some surgeons advocate electively removing the appendix at some time after the successful conservative treatment of an appendix mass or abscess. The rationale is that this prevents recurrence, but the approach is controversial as only 10–35% of patients suffer further attacks.

Are you aware of any relationship between appendicectomy and IBD?

Epidemiological studies indicate that appendicectomy appears to protect against the development of **ulcerative colitis**. Patients who do develop ulcerative colitis post-appendicectomy are less likely to develop recurrent symptoms and less likely to require colectomy.

The risk of **Crohn's disease** appears to be increased during the first few years after appendicectomy, although this is probably because many patients with Crohn's disease initially present with a clinical picture that strongly resembles appendicitis but is in fact their first presentation of Crohn's disease.

Single Best Answers

1. **A patient presents with suspected appendicitis. Palpation in the patient's left iliac fossa produces pain in the right iliac fossa. What is the name of this clinical sign?**

   a. McBurney's sign
   b. Obturator sign
   c. Psoas sign

   d. Dunphy's sign
   e. Rovsing's sign

2. **Which of the following structures is not crossed when performing an open appendicectomy?**

   a. Camper's fascia
   b. Scarpa's fascia
   c. External oblique

   d. Rectus sheath
   e. Internal oblique

3. **Which of the following causes of right iliac fossa (RIF) pain is most likely to occur in older rather than young patients?**

   a. Mesenteric adenitis
   b. Acute appendicitis
   c. Meckel's diverticulitis

   d. Caecal carcinoma
   e. Intussusception

4. **What is the most common anatomical location of the appendix?**

   a. Retrocaecal
   b. Retroileal
   c. Preileal

   d. Subcaecal
   e. Pelvic

5. **Which of the following scoring systems may play a role in diagnosing acute appendicitis?**

   a. Ranson
   b. Apache
   c. Alvarado

   d. Helsinki
   e. Glasgow

Core case

Read through the sections in the case boxes, covering up the sections that follow so that you don't see the answer. At the end of each case box, try to answer the question before reading on.

> Mrs Hamilton is a 76-year-old woman who presents at her local Emergency Department with left iliac fossa (LIF) pain.
>
> **What is your differential diagnosis for LIF pain?**
>
> As we have done for previous presentations, try to think anatomically of what structures might give you pain in the LIF. Try to prioritize into those conditions that are most likely (or most common), those that you must exclude, and the remainder.

In Figure 17.1 the differential diagnosis is arranged in order of likelihood in a woman of this age, with more likely diagnoses in larger font and less likely diagnoses in smaller font. Pathologies that should be excluded at the earliest possible opportunity are shown in **bold**.

Acute diverticulitis†
Constipation
Inflammatory bowel disease (IBD)
Ischaemic colitis
Pseudomembranous colitis‡
Leaking abdominal aortic aneurysm (AAA)
Locally perforated sigmoid carcinoma
Urinary tract infection
Ureteric colic
Pyelonephritis
Irritable bowel syndrome (IBS)
Shingles
Rectus sheath haematoma
Diabetic ketoacidosis

Figure 17.1 Differential diagnoses for left iliac fossa pain in a postmenopausal woman. Diagnoses that need excluding due to a high acute morbidity or mortality are shown in **bold**.

† *Diverticulosis* refers to the presence of diverticula in the bowel (which may be asymptomatic). *Diverticular disease* is symptomatic diverticulosis, which can manifest as painless bleeding, altered bowel habit, or painful inflammation (*acute diverticulitis*).

‡ *Pseudomembranous colitis* is an acute inflammatory condition of the bowel that is usually, but not always, caused by *Clostridium difficile*.

> **If Mrs Hamilton had been premenopausal would there have been any other diagnoses to consider?**

There are a number of gynaecological pathologies that can cause acute LIF pain. Some, such as ectopic pregnancy, mittelschmerz (mid-cycle pain), or haemorrhage into a functional ovarian cyst, can only occur in menstruating women. Others, such as pelvic inflammatory disease or torsion/rupture of an ovarian cyst, are far more likely to be seen in women younger than Mrs Hamilton, but can be kept in mind as rare differentials for someone of her age.

> **Is there any pathology peculiar to males that may cause LIF pain?**

Testicular torsion can cause referred pain to either the left or right iliac fossa and tends to occur in boys and young men. Haemorrhage into a testicular tumour can also cause left or right iliac fossa pain. Thus, don't forget to examine the testes.

> **What questions would you like to ask Mrs Hamilton about the pain in order to help narrow your differential diagnosis?**

You should ask the standard array of questions about the pain—remember the mnemonic SOCRATES:

Site: Where is the pain, and has it always been there? Pain that is initially poorly localized, midline, and colicky but which then migrates to the LIF and becomes constant is highly suggestive of acute diverticulitis (akin to left-sided appendicitis). Pain that migrates down the left flank and iliac fossa is more consistent with the migration of a ureteric stone.

Onset: Gradual or sudden? Sudden onset of pain is suggestive of perforation of a viscus, or of acute haemorrhage (e.g. into an ovarian cyst or from a ruptured AAA) or torsion (of an ovary or testis).

Character: Is the pain colicky or constant? Is it sharp or dull? Acute diverticulitis is often preceded by colicky midline pain. Ureteric calculi may result in colicky pain. Established diverticulitis, and the other differential diagnoses from our list would all produce constant abdominal pain. Sharp pain is most suggestive of haemorrhage, perforation, or torsion.

Radiation: Does the pain radiate to the groin (typical of ureteric pain)?

Alleviating factors: Does anything make the pain better? Discomfort due to irritable bowel syndrome (IBS) may be relieved by defecation. Peritonitic patients will be most comfortable when lying still.

Timing: How long has the pain been present? Have there been any previous similar episodes? Patients with IBS may have suffered from abdominal discomfort for many months or years. Patients with acute diverticulitis often give a history of 2–3 days of LIF pain, and may have had a previous episode.

Exacerbating factors: Does anything make the pain worse? Patients with peritonitis (e.g. due to colonic perforation) are very sensitive to motion and may mention that the car journey to the hospital was painful (i.e. every time they hit a bump).

Severity: How severe is the pain (e.g. on a scale of 1–10)? Ureteric colic is excruciatingly painful, as is colonic perforation secondary to diverticulitis or a sigmoid carcinoma.

Mrs Hamilton's pain started about 24 hours ago. She woke in the morning with 'vague stomach cramps'. By mid-morning she was suffering from constant pain in her LIF. She took some paracetamol at home, but this did not relieve the pain, which she reports as dull but 7/10 intensity. The pain does not radiate.

Having characterized the pain, what other symptoms should you enquire about?

- **Nausea and vomiting?** Nausea and, to a lesser extent, vomiting, are seen with acute diverticulitis. They may also accompany pelvic inflammatory disease.
- **Fever?** Indicating an underlying infective or inflammatory disease such as acute diverticulitis.
- **Change of bowel habit?** A relatively non-specific symptom of most of the colonic diseases in our differential. IBS, diverticular disease, inflammatory bowel disease (IBD), and colorectal carcinoma may all result in prolonged changes in bowel habit.
- **Rectal bleeding?** Overt rectal bleeding may be seen with acute diverticulitis, but is more likely to be seen in the context of bloody diarrhoea with ulcerative colitis, pseudomembranous colitis, ischaemic colitis, or colorectal carcinoma.
- **Bloating?** This is a characteristic feature of IBS.
- **Weight loss?** Although acute pain is an atypical presentation of colorectal carcinoma, a history of unintentional weight loss may raise your suspicions.
- **Gynaecological symptoms?** New vaginal discharge and/or pain during sex (dyspareunia) are consistent with pelvic inflammatory disease. In women who are menstruating, ask about the timing of the last menstrual period, regularity of periods, painful periods, and whether there is any possibility that the woman could be pregnant.

Are there any particular medicines to look out for in the drug history?

The most important class of drugs to be aware of is **steroids**, as these can dampen the inflammatory response, thus masking signs and symptoms. Bear in mind that patients taking steroids may be more ill than they appear by clinical examination.

Recent use of **antibiotics** (or proton pump inhibitors) may raise your suspicions of pseudomembranous colitis (*Clostridium difficile* colitis) in patients presenting with LIF pain and diarrhoea.

On further questioning, Mrs Hamilton explains that she has felt nauseated since this morning, but has not actually vomited. She feels feverish. She has not had any diarrhoea or felt constipated, and has not passed any blood per rectum. There are no gynaecological symptoms to note. She says that she is otherwise fit and well, and that her weight has not changed recently. She takes no medications, does not smoke, and enjoys an occasional glass of wine.

Mrs Hamilton reports that she suffered from a similar pain last year, and that her GP had then advised her to drink lots of clear fluids and had prescribed her antibiotics and painkillers. However, Mrs Hamilton feels worse on this occasion, and thought that she should go to hospital instead of her GP.

What in particular will you look for when examining Mrs Hamilton?

General examination

- **How unwell** is Mrs Hamilton? Check her basic observations: heart rate, blood pressure, temperature, respiration and sats.

- Does she appear to have **generalized peritonitis**? Is she lying very still, taking shallow breaths, and looking pale?
- Is the patient **writhing in pain**, unable to keep still? This is typical for ureteric colic.
- Are there signs of gastrointestinal malignancy? Is she cachectic or jaundiced (e.g. liver metastases from a colon cancer)?

Abdominal examination

- You should examine the abdomen for any **focal tenderness**. Typically, uncomplicated acute diverticulitis presents with local tenderness and/or guarding.
- Does the patient have **generalized peritonitis** (tender, rigid abdomen with absent bowel sounds)? If so, you should suspect perforation of a colonic diverticulum, sigmoid carcinoma, or AAA.
- Are there any **masses**? A mass may be palpable in the LIF in patients with acute diverticulitis, even in the absence of a local abscess. A sigmoid carcinoma may also be palpable. A central, laterally pulsatile mass is an AAA until proven otherwise.
- Does she have left supraclavicular lymphadenopathy (Troisier's sign) suggesting gastrointestinal malignancy?

Rectal examination

- It may be possible to detect a pelvic abscess in patients with acute diverticulitis, and may also be possible to palpate a rectal malignancy.

Vaginal examination

- This is not indicated in Mrs Hamilton, but would be required in women presenting with LIF pain and new vaginal discharge, as cervical motion tenderness would lend weight to a diagnosis of pelvic inflammatory disease.

Mrs Hamilton is febrile (38.2 °C) and tachycardic (113 bpm regular), and looks flushed. Her blood pressure is 135/72 and her respiratory rate is 21/min. She does not appear to have generalized peritonitis. Her LIF is tender to palpation, but the rest of the abdomen is soft and non-tender. There is no guarding or percussion tenderness. No masses are palpable, there is no organomegaly, and no palpable AAA. Bowel sounds are present. A digital rectal examination is unremarkable. A urine dipstick (including pregnancy test) is normal.

Which blood tests would you like to request?

There are very few blood tests that are actually informative or necessary given this history:

- **Venous blood gas (VBG)**: a high lactate and/or a metabolic acidaemia should raise your suspicion that the patient is very unwell or has ischaemic bowel. A normal glucose will reassure you this is not diabetic ketoacidosis, although it would be extremely rare for someone this age to present in DKA. With some modern blood gas analysers you will get Na, K, and creatinine so you won't even need to wait for laboratory urea and electrolytes (U&E) results (see below).
- **Full blood count (FBC)**: the white cell count may be elevated in response to any inflammatory condition (e.g. acute diverticulitis, pseudomembranous colitis).

- **U&Es**: useful for establishing the baseline electrolyte status of the patient (remembering that a number of the diagnoses on our differential will require intravenous (IV) fluids and/or surgery) and checking she has not developed acute kidney injury (quite possible if she is unable to tolerate oral intake, has had vomiting and/or diarrhoea, and is septic, causing vasodilation and reduced renal perfusion). The presence of impaired renal function may influence any decision to give radiological contrast.

- **C-reactive protein (CRP):** This is useful in the context of ulcerative colitis and *C. difficile* colitis specifically, where it predicts outcomes.

Blood tests are done. The VBG shows a normal pH, lactate, and glucose. The white cell count (WCC) is 14.1×10^9 cells/L (neutrophils 11.2×10^9 cells/L), and U&Es are unremarkable. A CRP level has not been requested.

In light of the history, examination, and first-line investigations, what is the most likely diagnosis?

It is most likely that Mrs Hamilton has **acute diverticulitis**. She is an elderly patient with constant LIF pain, preceded by vague midline colicky pain, which is associated with nausea and fever. Examination confirms the LIF tenderness and shows no evidence of peritonism or an abscess. The leucocytosis confirms the underlying inflammatory response. Furthermore, there is a suggestion from the history that Mrs Hamilton has suffered from a previous episode of acute diverticulitis that was treated in the community.

Which imaging studies may be requested in the acute phase?

Mrs Hamilton appears clinically to have relatively mild diverticulitis, and there are some surgeons who would start empirical medical therapy without requesting any further imaging in the acute phase. However, a radiologically confirmed diagnosis is useful for determining whether surgery is indicated (discussed later in this case), and is also invaluable in more severely unwell patients, in those refractory to treatment, or those with a different history:

- **Abdominal CT with contrast**: this is the imaging modality of choice for diagnosing acute diverticulitis and planning future elective surgery. If there is a suspicion of an abscess complicating acute diverticulitis, or if the patient is seriously ill, clinically deteriorates, or the diagnosis is unclear, then abdominal CT is also invaluable.

- **Erect chest radiograph (CXR)**: request this if there is any clinical suspicion of a perforated viscus, looking for air under the diaphragm.

- **Abdominal radiograph (AXR)**: Although the AXR is abnormal in 30–50% of patients with diverticulitis (a common but non-specific finding being small and/or large bowel dilatation or ileus), it is only really useful for ruling out bowel obstruction if this is clinically suspected and the patient isn't going to have a CT abdomen, which is not the case here.

- Mrs Hamilton had a CT abdomen which confirmed **diverticulitis**.

If Mrs Hamilton had been premenopausal are there any other imaging modalities that you would request to investigate her LIF pain?

Transabdominal ± transvaginal ultrasound are particularly useful investigations in young female patients, where the differential diagnosis is broadened by gynaecological pathology.

> **Could Mrs Hamilton have had a colonoscopy or double-contrast barium enema to confirm the diagnosis in the acute phase of her illness?**

Mrs Hamilton **should not** have had either investigation in the acute phase. Colonoscopy and double-contrast barium enema are **contraindicated** in the acute setting as there is a risk of perforating the acutely inflamed colon. Furthermore, double-contrast barium enemas have been superseded by CT scans.

> **How should Mrs Hamilton be managed in the acute phase?**

Mrs Hamilton should be treated as follows:

- **Analgesia**
- **Bowel rest**: by clear fluids only
- **IV fluids**: if Mrs Hamilton is unable to maintain a sufficient oral intake
- **Antibiotics**: to cover Gram-negative bacteria and anaerobes (e.g. co-amoxiclav ± metronidazole, but consult local guidelines)
- **Venous thromboembolism prophylaxis**
- **Monitor**: if symptoms do not improve within 48–72 hours, further investigation is required to establish whether an abscess is present, or whether the initial diagnosis was flawed.

> **How will Mrs Hamilton be followed up? Is there any advice that she should be given?**

Given that the diagnosis of acute diverticulitis has been made on clinical and radiological grounds, Mrs Hamilton will be offered a **colonoscopy (or barium enema) 2–6 weeks after resolution of this episode** to directly visualize the colonic lumen and confirm the diagnosis. This assesses the extent of diverticulosis and the degree of stricturing secondary to inflammation, and can exclude other potential diagnoses such as colitis or carcinoma. CT colonography is being investigated as a potential alternative to conventional colonoscopy.

Mrs Hamilton should be advised to maintain a high intake of dietary fibre as this may reduce the chance of future episodes of diverticular disease.

> **Should Mrs Hamilton be offered an elective colonic resection?**

Following the successful conservative treatment of an episode of acute diverticulitis, about a third of patients will remain asymptomatic, a third will develop occasional abdominal cramps, and a third will suffer a further attack of acute diverticulitis. Further attacks of acute diverticulitis are less likely to respond to conservative treatment than the first episode. Various authorities have therefore recommended that patients with two *proven* episodes of acute diverticulitis requiring hospital admission, or with associated obstructive symptoms, or with contrast leak during CT abdomen should be offered elective resection of the affected portion of bowel if no emergency surgery has already been performed and if the benefits of surgery outweigh the risks for that individual. Mrs Hamilton did not have *proven* diverticulitis last year, and thus is not yet a candidate for elective surgery. Mrs Hamilton was admitted to hospital and received IV fluids, analgesia and antibiotics. She made an uneventful recovery and was discharged from hospital after 4 days. An outpatient colonoscopy 5 weeks later confirmed extensive diverticulosis of the sigmoid colon.

Short cases

Mr Arnold is a 67-year-old retired lecturer who presents to the Emergency Department with severe LIF pain. He reports that he has been in pain for the last 2 days, but that the pain suddenly increased in severity 1 hour ago. The pain is now sharp, does not radiate, and appears to be worsened by any degree of movement. Mr Arnold rates it as the worst pain he has ever experienced. For the past couple of days he has felt nauseated and feverish, but has not vomited. He has had slight diarrhoea, but has not noticed any blood in his stool. He reports no recent weight loss.

His past medical history is remarkable for two previous episodes of LIF pain. The first episode was 5 years ago and the second was 1 year ago. Mr Arnold reports that on both occasions the pain was very similar to that which he has had for the preceding 2 days—but was nowhere near as severe as the pain that he has experienced for the last hour. The episode 5 years ago was managed by his GP 'with antibiotics and paracetamol', and the second episode resulted in a 3-day hospital admission but no surgery.

Mr Arnold has no other significant medical history and takes no regular medications. He is a smoker with a 15-pack-year history, and is teetotal. He has no allergies.

On examination, Mr Arnold looks pale and clammy. He lies still on the examination couch and is taking shallow breaths. He is reluctant to cough as this causes him considerable pain. His basic observations are: heart rate 107 bpm regular, blood pressure 92/53 mmHg, temperature 38.3 °C, respiratory rate 19/min, and oxygen saturation 96% on room air. Examination reveals widespread guarding and absent bowel sounds.

What is the most likely diagnosis? How should Mr Arnold be managed?

Mr Arnold is **peritonitic**—he is shocked, lying still, displaying generalized guarding, and has absent bowel sounds. The sudden increase in pain and worsening of his symptoms suggests that Mr Arnold has probably perforated a viscus. More precisely, the combination of his past medical history and pain over the previous 2 days suggests that he has probably developed **perforated diverticulitis**.

Appropriate management differs considerably from the uncomplicated acute diverticulitis of the previous case. Mr Arnold will need to be treated as follows:

- **Fluid resuscitation** (titrated to response in BP, HR and urinary output), **oxygen** (if required to keep saturations >94%) and **urinary output monitoring** (which may require catheterization).
- **Blood tests**: VBG, FBC, U&E, and cross-match
- **Analgesia**
- **Antibiotics**
- **CT**: provided that imaging is readily available and doesn't delay transfer to theatre
- **Emergency laparotomy**.

The advantage of preoperative scanning is that a more precise diagnosis may be reached, hence the surgeon is better informed and the patient may be fully consented (for example, for a stoma). Preoperative knowledge aids the surgeon in planning incisions, choosing stoma sites etc.

There are two most common surgical options for the emergency treatment of perforated diverticulitis. Most patients have a Hartmann's procedure (see Chapter 21). In some patients it is safe to perform a primary anastomosis. To protect the primary anastomosis, the surgeon can also form a proximal loop ('defunctioning') ileostomy, which diverts bowel contents before they pass via the primary anastomosis.

SHORT CASES

Miss Sellers is a 31-year-old sales assistant who presents to her GP with LIF pain. She has suffered from the pain intermittently for over 6 months, and rates it as of moderate intensity. In addition, she often also has vague cramping abdominal pains. The pain does not radiate anywhere. The pain often follows meals, and may be relieved by defecation. She also reports feeling bloated. She has not felt nauseated or feverish. Her bowel habits are rather irregular—sometimes she has diarrhoea while at other times she tends towards constipation and finds herself straining to open her bowels. She has not noticed any rectal bleeding. Her weight has been stable. She reports no unusual vaginal discharge or itch, no intermenstrual bleeding, and no postcoital bleeding or pain. Her last menstrual period was 2 weeks ago.

She suffers from asthma, for which she uses fluticasone and salbutamol inhalers. She is otherwise well. She also takes the combined oral contraceptive pill and has no allergies. She does not drink alcohol or smoke. She has no family history of bowel cancer in anyone <50 years of age.

Examination is unremarkable. Miss Sellers is afebrile, normotensive, and has a pulse of 71 bpm regular. Her abdomen is soft and non-tender. Bowel sounds are audible. A rectal examination is unremarkable (in line with NICE guidance; a gynaecological examination is not performed at this stage as the GP does not feel it is indicated).

Given the history and examination findings, which diagnosis do you feel is most likely? What investigations would you like to request to confirm the diagnosis?

Miss Sellers has a history of chronic abdominal pain, with cramping, bloating, and altered bowel habit. She is otherwise well and has no signs on examination. It is most likely that Miss Sellers is suffering from **IBS**, but **IBD** should also be considered (in an older patient diverticular disease could lead to a similar presentation). The LIF pain is not a universal feature of IBS, but is consistent with the diagnosis. The fact that Miss Sellers is otherwise well, has lost no weight, and has passed no blood per rectum, favours IBS over IBD.

Before diagnosing Miss Sellers with IBS it is necessary to exclude other causes of chronic abdominal pain and altered bowel habit. Thus, as a first line, it would be appropriate to request the following investigations in a patient of Miss Sellers' age, explaining to her that you expect all the blood tests to be entirely normal:

- **Bloods**:
    - **FBC**: any signs of infection, inflammation, or anaemia of chronic disease?
    - **CRP**: any underlying chronic inflammation?
    - **Anti-endomysial antibodies** or **tissue transglutaminase (TTG)**: a positive result has a sensitivity and specificity of over 90% for coeliac disease. (Antigliadin antibodies have been used to test for coeliac disease but are less sensitive and specific.) You must always check **IgA levels** too, because IgA deficiency (found in 10% of the population) can cause a false negative result.

In Miss Seller's case, if these blood tests are normal, no further test should be necessary as she meets the NICE criteria for a clinical diagnosis of IBS: more than 6 months of abdominal pain associated with bloating and altered bowel habit. If the diagnosis was less clear, you might also wish to consider:

- **Stool culture**: does she have a chronic infection such as *Giardia*, which may account for her abdominal pain and altered bowel habit?
- **Flexible sigmoidoscopy**: any structural disease of the sigmoid, such as IBD?

SHORT CASE

Mrs Martinez is a 27-year-old woman who presents to the Emergency Department with acute LIF pain. She woke at 5 a.m. that morning with moderate dull pain in the LIF. The pain did not radiate, and was not relieved by simple analgesia. The pain has been constant for the past 4 hours. Mrs Martinez has not felt nauseated, and has not experienced any change in bowel habit. She last opened her bowels last night. She does not feel feverish.

Her last menstrual period was 35 days ago, and her usual menstrual cycle is 3–4/28 (bleeding for 3–4 days of a 28-day cycle). On direct questioning, she mentions that she has passed blood vaginally this morning, but that this is lighter than her usual period. She does not use any form of contraception with her husband. She reports no other gynaecological symptoms.

She had a laparoscopic appendicectomy 2 years ago, but has no other significant past medical history. She takes no regular medications, and has no allergies. She does not smoke, and drinks about 10 units of wine each week.

Mrs Martinez's observations are unremarkable, and she appears able to move with minimal discomfort. Her abdomen is tender to palpation in the LIF, but is otherwise soft and non-tender. There is no percussion tenderness or guarding, and bowel sounds are present. A rectal examination is not performed.

What single investigation must you request? How would you proceed with the results of this test?

Mrs Martinez is a sexually active young woman who presents with lower abdominal pain, vaginal bleeding, and amenorrhoea (her period is late). While it is possible that this morning's vaginal bleed represents the start of her period, the fact that she has pain should ring alarm bells that this is an **ectopic pregnancy**. Thus you must request an urgent **urine pregnancy test** to exclude this diagnosis. The fact that Mrs Martinez shows no signs of shock and has stable observations is reassuring as there is no current evidence that she has developed a perforated ectopic (a surgical emergency).

Mrs Martinez's pregnancy test was positive and thus she should be referred to the gynaecologists to confirm on ultrasound whether the pregnancy is intrauterine or ectopic.

SHORT CASE

Miss Efran is a 29-year-old salsa instructor who presents to her GP with LIF pain. She has had the pain for 3 days, and says that she decided to seek help as the pain has gradually become more uncomfortable for her. The pain is a dull ache that does not radiate. She can think of nothing that alleviates or exacerbates the pain. She has not taken any analgesia at home.

Miss Efran has vomited three times today. She says that she feels feverish, and that she has also been shaking/shivering. On direct questioning, she mentions that she has had some yellow vaginal discharge for the past 2 days, but has not passed any blood. She is sure that she cannot be pregnant because she is using the combined oral contraceptive pill with her new boyfriend. She reports no urinary symptoms and no change of bowel habit.

Miss Efran is otherwise fit and well. She has no significant past medical history, takes no regular medications other than the contraceptive pill, and has no allergies. She smokes about 10 cigarettes each day and drinks about 20 units of alcohol each week.

On examination, Miss Efran appears flushed, and is febrile (38.5 °C). Her heart rate is 103 bpm regular and her blood pressure is 123/71 mmHg. Her respiratory rate is 15/min. Her abdomen is soft, but tender to palpation in the LIF. There is no percussion tenderness. No organomegaly is detected. A digital rectal examination is not performed, but Miss Efran is consented for a bimanual pelvic examination that reveals marked adnexal tenderness.

A urinary pregnancy test is negative, and urinalysis reveals nil leucocytes, nitrites, protein, or blood.

In light of history and examination, what is the most likely diagnosis? How would you manage this?

It is most likely that Miss Efran has **acute pelvic inflammatory disease**—she is a sexually active woman (with a new partner), who has acute lower abdominal pain, new vaginal discharge, vomiting, and fever, combined with adnexal tenderness on vaginal examination. Her pregnancy test is negative.

The most likely causes of acute pelvic inflammatory disease are sexually transmitted bacterial infections such as *Chlamydia* or gonorrhoea. Appropriate further management of Miss Efran may involve the following steps:

- **Vaginal, urethral, and endocervical swabs**: to identify the pathogen
- **Empirical antibiotics**: to cover likely pathogens until culprit identified
- **Referral to a genitourinary medicine (GUM) clinic**
- **Avoidance of sexual intercourse while being treated**
- **Partner notification**: sexual partners from the preceding 6 months should be traced and offered testing in a GUM clinic; if they test positive they too should avoid sexual intercourse until they have completed their treatment
- **Consider alternative contraception:** condoms offer protection against sexually transmitted infections

Viva questions

How common is diverticulosis? Are there any known risk factors?

It is difficult to assess the true prevalence of diverticulosis as most patients are asymptomatic, but some data are available from autopsy series. Many patients are diagnosed incidentally. The prevalence is age dependent, such that about 5% of 40-year-olds, about 30% of 60-year-olds, and about 65% of 85-year-olds have colonic diverticula (mostly asymptomatic). There is a huge difference in prevalence between developed and developing countries: diverticulosis appears to be rare in developing countries. Much of this difference in prevalence is said to be due to variation in fibre intake—diets in the developed world are relatively fibre-depleted and this leads to high intraluminal colonic pressures that favour the development of pulsion diverticula.

What is the natural history of diverticulosis?

There are a number of possible outcomes for patients with diverticulosis:

- 70% remain asymptomatic
- 15–25% develop acute diverticulitis, 75% of which is 'uncomplicated' (as in Mrs Hamilton's initial presentation) and 25% of which is 'complicated' (as in Mr Arnold's initial presentation)
- 5–10% develop rectal bleeding (see Chapter 21).

What are the main complications of diverticulitis?

The main complications of diverticulitis are as follows:

- Perforation
  - May be localized/contained/walled-off as an abscess
  - May lead to generalized peritonitis
- Abscess formation
- Fistulation into adjacent structures (e.g. bladder)
- Chronic inflammatory strictures resulting in bowel obstruction
- Haemorrhage

Colovesical fistulas are the most common type of fistula caused by diverticulitis. Are they more common in men or women? Why?

A fistula can form between adjacent areas of inflammation. Colovesical fistulas are more common in men. This is thought to be because the uterus sits between the sigmoid and the bladder, forming a barrier to colovesical fistula formation.

Acute diverticulitis is sometimes nicknamed 'left-sided appendicitis'. Both are typically preceded by colicky midline abdominal pain. Would you expect this initial pain to be periumbilical for both presentations?

This question relates to the embryological anatomy of the gut. Remember that the initial midline colicky pain caused by inflammation of the gut is mediated by autonomic innervation. This pain is approximately referred to the epigastrium, umbilicus, or hypogastrium according to whether the inflamed structure is within the embryological foregut, midgut, or hindgut. As the appendix is a mid-gut structure you would expect the initial colicky pain to be periumbilical, whereas acute diverticulitis would cause referred colicky pain in the suprapubic area. In practice, it may be difficult to differentiate these sites from the patient's account of the history of the pain. In addition, diverticulitis may yield right-sided pain if the sigmoid loop is long and extends to the right iliac fossa.

What are the risk factors for ectopic pregnancy?

The main risk factors include:

- Previous ectopic pregnancy
- Pelvic inflammatory disease
- Tubular procedures, e.g. sterilization (some women may still become pregnant)
- Endometriosis
- Pelvic surgery
- *In vitro* fertilization (IVF)
- Intrauterine contraceptive device

The underlying mechanism for several of these risk factors is an alteration to the normal anatomy of the fallopian tubes. Inflammation or surgical manipulation of the tubes can lead to strictures or kinks that disrupt the normal passage of the egg.

What is Hinchey's classification[†]?

This classification represents an assessment of peritoneal contamination at the time of surgery in the context of acute diverticulitis. As such, it may be used as a guide to the suitability for primary anastomosis following resection. Four classes are recognized:

I   Pericolic or mesenteric abscess

II   Walled-off pelvic abscess

III Generalized purulent peritonitis (~5% mortality)

IV   Generalized faecal peritonitis (~35% mortality)

† This information was published in *Advances in Surgery*, **12**, 1, Hinchey EJ et al., 'Treatment of perforated diverticular disease of the colon', pp. 85-109, Copyright Elsevier 1978.

Single Best Answers

1. **In which of the following locations are diverticula least likely to occur?**

   a. Ascending colon
   b. Transverse colon
   c. Descending colon
   d. Sigmoid colon
   e. Rectum

2. **Which of the following complications of diverticular disease is not an indication for emergency surgery?**

   a. Generalized peritonitis
   b. Localized peritonitis unresponsive to medical treatment
   c. Paracolic abscess
   d. Bowel obstruction
   e. Unresolving haemorrhage

3. **Which of the following investigations are contraindicated in the context of acute diverticulitis?**

   a. Supine plain abdominal radiograph
   b. Erect chest radiograph
   c. CT abdomen with contrast
   d. CT colon
   e. Colonoscopy

4. **A patient with left iliac fossa pain is diagnosed with pseudomembranous colitis due to *Clostridium difficile* infection. Which of the following may be used to treat this infection?**

   a. IV vancomycin
   b. Oral vancomycin
   c. Oral cefuroxime
   d. Oral amoxicillin
   e. Oral ciprofloxacin

5. **Which of the following criteria can be used to make a diagnosis of irritable bowel syndrome?**

   a. Elevated ESR
   b. Positive antiendomysial antibody
   c. Low serum albumin
   d. Microcytic hypochromic anaemia
   e. None of the above

Flank pain

Core case

Read through the sections in the case boxes, covering up the sections that follow so that you don't see the answer. At the end of each case box, try to answer the question before reading on.

> Mr Kirk is a 61-year-old pilot who comes to the Emergency Department complaining of severe flank pain just below his ribs. The triage nurse has asked you to prescribe him analgesia and see him next. He has no known allergies so you prescribe paracetamol and codeine to start with.
>
> **What is your differential diagnosis for acute flank pain? Are any of your diagnoses surgical emergencies?**

Muscular sprain
Nephrolithiasis/ureteric colic
Spinal pathology (fractures, metastases, disc prolapse)
Leaking/ruptured abdominal aortic aneurysm (AAA)
Testicular torsion (very unusual in an elderly person)
Pyelonephritis (unusual in a man)
Perforated peptic ulcer
Renal cancer
Abscess (perinephric, renal)
Basal pneumonia

Figure 18.1 Differential diagnosis of flank pain in an adult male.

The diagnoses shown in **bold** in Figure 18.1 are all surgical emergencies that you must exclude as you clerk the patient.

In women, you should consider gynaecological causes, e.g. ectopic pregnancy, ovarian torsion (you can of course narrow these down depending on whether the woman is of childbearing age or not). Also, bear in mind that other abdominal pathology can occasionally present as flank pain (e.g. pancreatitis, diverticulitis, appendicitis).

> **What questions will you ask about the presenting complaint (i.e. flank pain) to help you narrow your diagnosis?**

You should ask the standard array of questions about the pain—remember the mnemonic SOCRATES:

Site: Where is the pain, and has it always been there? Is it unilateral or bilateral? Kidney stones are almost always unilateral, but the location of the pain may radiate from loin to groin. Often they start with a vague discomfort that is ignored until it becomes a severe pain.

Onset: Any trauma or other trigger, or spontaneous? Gradual or sudden? Trauma may lead to musculoskeletal pain or internal bleeding.

Character: Is the pain colicky or constant? Is it sharp or dull? Ureteric stones give a colicky (waxing and waning) pain because of periodic spasms of the ureteric smooth muscle walls trying to dislodge the blockage. A constant pain is more consistent with a stone lodged in the kidney, which does not periodically contract ('vermiculate') like the ureters, or an inflammatory cause. Musculoskeletal pain is more typically an ache, while nerve impingement causes shooting pains.

Radiation: Does the pain radiate to the groin (typical of ureteric pain)? Does it radiate down the leg (typical of lumbar nerve root pain)?

Alleviating factors: Does anything make the pain better, e.g. a given posture, eating/drinking, any medications, etc.?

Timing: How long has the pain been present? Musculoskeletal back pain can last many weeks, whereas a leaking abdominal aortic aneurysm (AAA) is unlikely to persist for more than a day without resolution, one way or another.

Exacerbating factors: Does anything make the pain worse? Patients with peritonitis (e.g. due to a perforated peptic ulcer) are very sensitive to movement.

Severity: How severe is the pain (e.g. on a scale of 1–10)? Kidney stones are said to be excruciatingly painful, comparable to childbirth.

> Mr Kirk's pain is unilateral. It is localized to his right flank, and has not moved. He says it came on spontaneously while he was watching television. At first it was just a dull constant ache, but a couple of hours ago it became colicky and started radiating from his flank into his groin. There is nothing he can do to make it better or worse.
>
> **Having characterized his pain, what further questions should you ask in the history?**

History of presenting complaint

- **Fever, rigors, night sweats?** A markedly raised fever indicates an inflammatory process such as pyelonephritis (or any other form of sepsis, such as a psoas abscess) or, less commonly, a malignancy (e.g. renal cell carcinoma).

- **Dehydration?** Persistent dehydration predisposes to concentrated urine and therefore to kidney stones.

- **Nausea and vomiting?** This is more typical of visceral organ pathology (e.g. ureteric stones, biliary colic, appendicitis) but rare in other causes of pain (e.g. musculoskeletal pain, nerve root compression, shingles).

- **Haematuria?** Although 70–90% of patients with kidney/ureteric stones are reported to have haematuria, this is usually microscopic (i.e. not visible to the naked eye) and of course means that 10–30% of patients with a renal tract stone won't even have microscopic haematuria. Nonetheless, it is worth asking whether they have had any macroscopic haematuria, as this can occur.

- **Lower urinary tract symptoms?** Urinary frequency, urgency, and dysuria are common in urinary tract infection. Hesitancy, reduced flow, dribbling, and incomplete voiding are more typical of ureteric obstruction (e.g. due to an enlarged prostate in men, or more unusually stones or tumours).

- **Cloudy or offensive-smelling urine?** Another sign of infection.

- **Leg weakness?** This could suggest spinal pathology.

Past medical history

- **Previous kidney stones?** Nephrolithiasis is associated with an ~50% 10 year recurrence rate.
- **Recurrent cystitis?** Recurrent episodes of urinary tract infection predispose to stones of the struvite type.
- **Atherosclerotic disease (e.g. angina, myocardial infarction, stroke, claudication)?** A strong risk factor for AAA.
- **Longstanding back pain?** This is usually due to pathology affecting the muscles, ligaments, and bones.
- **Kidney disease?** Polycystic kidney disease predisposes to pyelonephritis. If the patient only has one kidney, you need to know as obstruction of the only functional ureter is a medical emergency.

Drug history

- Aciclovir and indinavir may crystallize in the urine, whereas acetazolamide causes diuresis and potentially dehydration, predisposing to kidney stone formation.

Family history

- **Family history of kidney stones?** This may indicate a (rare) inherited condition such as cystinuria.

Mr Kirk says he has been feeling sick, although he has not actually vomited. He adds that he has never had anything like this before. He has type 2 diabetes mellitus which is well controlled by diet and daily metformin. His family history is unremarkable. He concedes that he probably doesn't drink enough fluids, but doesn't feel especially dehydrated.

You proceed to examine Mr Kirk.

What signs are you looking for on examination?

- **Position?** Whether your patient is restless or still can be very informative. Those with ureteric colic are unable to sit still and tend to writhe in pain. Those with peritonitis (e.g. from a ruptured AAA) are rigid and motionless, as any movement causes pain.
- **Tenderness?** Individuals with renal or ureteric stones may have flank or loin tenderness (particularly in the costovertebral angles), but tend not to have any other abdominal signs. Abdominal tenderness suggests a peritoneal cavity problem (e.g. appendicitis, pancreatitis).
- **Masses?** You should look specifically for a central, laterally expansile mass which could be a leaking AAA. This must be suspected in anyone >55 years of age. It is possible for the pain from an AAA to be misdiagnosed as ureteric colic. Note that physical examination does *not* exclude an AAA; if it is suspected, the patient should undergo imaging.
- **Spine?** You must also exclude spinal pathology by testing range of movement (e.g. straight leg raise) and feeling for tenderness along the vertebrae.
- **Lower limbs?** If spinal pathology is suspected from the history and examination so far (e.g. a prolapsed intervertebral disc), conduct a neurological exam of the lower limbs. If an AAA is suspected, conduct a vascular examination of the lower limbs, as an AAA can compromise blood supply to the lower limbs. If you can easily feel the popliteal pulse, you should suspect a popliteal aneurysm and remember that about 50% of patients with popliteal aneurysms also have AAAs.
- **Temperature?** Indicates whether an inflammatory process, potentially pyelonephritis, is ongoing.

Mr Kirk is restless, consistent with the description of his pain. His flanks are not particularly tender. His abdomen is soft and non-tender with no masses. Bowel sounds are present and normal. He is apyrexial. Examination of his lower limbs is unremarkable. Judging from the way Mr Kirk is writhing on the bed, he has a full range of motion in his back, and although you are not able to assess his spine formally, you establish there is no tenderness to palpation over bony landmarks.

What diagnosis do the history and examination suggest so far? What investigations will you arrange?

Mr Kirk has presented with a history of spontaneous, sudden-onset, 'loin to groin', colicky, severe pain that is highly suggestive of **renal or ureteric colic**. The lack of fever, and abdominal tenderness makes other diagnoses far less likely. Therefore, the following investigations would be appropriate in this patient:

Urine

- **Urinalysis:** you should note the presence of haematuria, white blood cells (pyuria), leucocyte esterase, and nitrites. You may also want to note the urine pH, as patients with urate stones usually have acidic urine; an alkali pH suggests the presence of urease-producing bacteria (e.g. *Proteus, Pseudomonas, Klebsiella*) that can predispose to stone formation.

- **Urine microscopy, culture, and sensitivity (MC&S):** performed only if the urinalysis is abnormal and shows either blood, leucocytes or nitrites. Look for red cells, evidence of infection (white cells, bacteria), and crystals. Identifying the type of crystal helps particularly in understanding the aetiology and secondary prevention of future stones. The presence of red cell casts or white cell casts indicates that the red or white cells are coming from the kidney (where, simplistically, cells are squeezed through the tiny nephrons into sausage shaped clumps of cells), rather than the ureters or bladder. Thus red cell casts indicate glomerular damage and white cell casts suggest pyelonephritis (although these are rarely found).

Bloods

- **Full blood count (FBC) and C-reactive protein (CRP):** look for a raised white cell count (WCC) and CRP, indicating infection or sepsis.

- **Urea, creatinine, and electrolytes:** assess renal function, as obstruction by a renal stone can precipitate renal damage. Renal failure is a medical emergency!

- **Serum calcium, phosphate, and urate:** these provide valuable clues as to the aetiology of kidney stones and should be requested in anyone with a proven stone.

Imaging

- **Bedside ultrasound:** It is increasingly common for registrars and new consultants in Emergency Departments to be competent in bedside ultrasound that can be used to look for an AAA >3 cm. Ultrasound will not tell you if an aneurysm is bleeding (as it will bleed into the retroperitoneal space, which is harder to visualize on ultrasound) so any patient with flank/back/abdominal pain and an AAA on ultrasound requires a contrast CT abdomen to look for a leak of their AAA (if haemodynamically stable enough). Equally, ultrasound of the abdominal aorta can be technically difficult to achieve in patients with a large body habitus or who are unfasted and have lots of air and peristalsis in their transverse colon.

- **Non-contrast CT-KUB (kidneys, ureters, and bladder):** this will show any stones in the kidney or ureter, but also any rare causes of ureter obstruction causing renal colic (e.g. a retroperitoneal tumour).

It is possibly the single most important test in anyone >55 years presenting with flank pain as it will also detect any AAAs. CT has a greater sensitivity and specificity than plain KUB radiographs for kidney stones, but KUB radiographs are still useful for following the progression of confirmed stones in a way that involves less exposure to ionizing radiation. A magnetic resonance urogram (MRU) can be used if the patient is pregnant and therefore unsuitable for any form of ionizing radiation. Although intravenous urography/pyelography (IVU or IVP) used to be the gold standard for detecting kidney stones, it has now been superseded by CT-KUB.

Remember! If pancreatitis is suspected, you should request a **serum amylase** or lipase level. If a perforated peptic ulcer is a concern, you should request an **erect chest radiograph** to look for air under the diaphragm.

You take Mr Kirk's basic observations. His heart rate is 98 bpm and regular, his blood pressure is 146/94 mmHg and his respiratory rate is 20/min with oxygen saturation of 99% on room air. He is afebrile.

Urinalysis shows microscopic haematuria, a urine pH of 6.0, and is weakly positive for white cells (+). His WCC is normal. Reassuringly, his urea and electrolytes (U&Es) are all within the normal ranges.

A CT-KUB scan is performed and a single slice is shown in Figure 18.2.

Figure 18.2 CT scan of kidneys, ureters, and bladder (CT-KUB) (single slice) for Mr Kirk.

What is the diagnosis?

Mr Kirk has renal colic caused by a **kidney stone** (aka *nephrolithiasis*, or *renal calculus*), lodged at the right pelviureteric junction (PUJ).

The CT-KUB report confirms a single 0.78 cm stone in the right PUJ. More importantly, it shows a normal-diameter abdominal aorta and no hydronephrosis due to the kidney stone.

How should Mr Kirk be managed during the acute episode? Does he require admission?

Having assessed his need for resuscitation (airway, breathing, circulation, ABC), you should decide whether or not to admit him. He should be admitted if:

- there is evidence of upper urinary tract infection (cloudy urine ± white cell casts, high WCC in blood, high CRP, fever,…). Infection proximal to an obstruction is a surgical emergency, requiring drainage
- there is evidence of renal impairment/failure (high creatinine, high urea, high K^+)
- there is refractory pain (despite analgesia)
- there are bilateral obstructing stones (or a single obstructing stone if only one kidney present)
- the patient is elderly, a child, or otherwise unwell (e.g. unable to tolerate oral fluids), for closer monitoring.

Your management of Mr Kirk acutely should include:

- **Regular multimodal analgesia** (e.g. regular paracetamol + non-steroidal anti-inflammatory drugs (NSAIDs)) as renal tract stones can be as painful as childbirth, and Mr Kirk won't be able to go home unless his pain is controlled. NSAIDs and paracetamol are preferred to opiates as studies show they provide equally adequate analgesia in the context of kidney stones (see Viva questions), may have some additional effect of decreasing ureteric smooth muscle tone, and lack some of the adverse effects of opiates, notably respiratory and central nervous system (CNS) depression, vomiting, and disorientation. Despite frequent patient concerns, long-term dependence of opiates is not an issue when they are used in the acute setting.
- You should also **encourage fluid intake**. If they cannot tolerate oral fluids, you should admit them and prescribe intravenous (IV) fluids.
- **Tamsulosin** (an α-blocker) or **nifedipine** (a calcium channel blocker)? Both relax the smooth muscle in ureters and both have been shown in meta-analyses to increase the chances of spontaneous passage of a renal tract stone, with tamsulosin being considerably superior to nifedipine. However, the results applied mainly to distal ureteric stones <10 mm. In Mr Kirk's case, where the stone is proximal (the PUJ of the kidney), the evidence for these medications is much less clear.
- **Active stone removal?** The major determinant of stone passage is size.
  - **Stones ≤5 mm** have a 50% chance of passing spontaneously. Patients with no reason for admission can be discharged and should be asked to strain their urine to recover the stone for analysis. **Follow-up** should be arranged for patients after 2–3 weeks. It is useful for patients to have a plain KUB radiograph before discharge which may also show the stone seen on CT-KUB. If it does, this allows the follow-up clinic to also perform a plain KUB radiograph and compare it directly to the KUB radiograph taken at original presentation, to see if the stone has moved. By comparing plain radiographs, one avoids the need for a repeat CT-KUB (which is a much higher dose of radiation) to monitor stone passage.
  - **Stones > 5 mm** are less likely to pass spontaneously, with those >7 mm in particular being very unlikely to pass. Stones that are >5 mm should therefore be discussed with the urologist on call for consideration of removal.

> Mr Kirk is given PR diclofenac (an NSAID) in addition to the paracetamol and codeine he was given at triage, and his pain subsides over the next hour. He now rates it as 1/10 in severity. As his stone is >5 mm, his case is discussed with the urologist on call.
>
> **How might Mr Kirk's 7.8 mm renal stone be removed?**

For renal tract stones > 5 mm (or smaller ones that haven't passed spontaneously after 4–6 weeks), various options are available to remove the stone:

- **Lithotripsy**, otherwise known as extracorporeal shock wave lithotripsy (ESWL) if small enough (renal stones <2 cm, ureteric stones <1 cm). This uses shock waves to break down the stone into smaller fragments that are then more likely to pass spontaneously.

- **Ureterorenoscopic removal** (using a fine telescope inserted via the urethra) with a dormia basket, holmium laser, mechanical lithotripsy, etc., if too large for ESWL. Note that this commonly requires a postoperative ureteric stent as it can cause ureteric stricture.

- **Percutaneous nephrolithotomy** (PCNL) is rarely used nowadays as it is invasive and thus there are risks of bleeding and damage to the collecting system and neighbouring structures.

- **Stenting** (using a JJ stent) or percutaneous nephrostomy may be performed in order to prevent hydro-nephrosis, if the obstruction cannot be resolved surgically.

- **Antibiotic cover** is given if an invasive procedure is employed. Of interest, certain occupations, nota-bly pilots, do not permit people to work even with an asymptomatic stone for fear of the unpredict-able onset of incapacitating pain while they are involved in a crucial task. Thus, patients such our Captain Kirk (who is a pilot) will require early definitive therapy rather than a more conservative approach.

In view of Mr Kirk's occupation and the fact that his renal tract stone is >7 mm and therefore very unlikely to pass spontaneously, the patient is admitted and the stone is removed by the urologists the following morning using a ureteroscope and dormia basket.

How should Mr Kirk be managed in the longer term? Are any further investigations or measures for secondary prevention appropriate?

All patients should be advised to increase their fluid intake.

In addition, it is appropriate to try to identify the underlying cause in those patients at greatest risk of recurrence, as there are some treatments available. Appropriate criteria for further testing could include:

- strong family history
- multiple stones at first diagnosis
- recurrent stone formation/passage

Mr Kirk has none of the above and so can be discharged without further investigation.

Short cases

Mr Kirk was discharged home after successful removal of his renal tract stone by the urologists. One month later he returns to hospital. He has a 2-day history of a dull ache in his right flank and is worried he has developed another kidney stone. However, this time he additionally has urinary frequency, dysuria, and a fever. He says he has vomited repeatedly. His heart rate is 124 bpm, blood pressure is 88/60 mmHg, respiratory rate 30/min, and temperature 40.2 °C. His urine dipstick reveals microscopic haematuria, pyuria (white cells +++), and nitrites (+++).

What is the most likely diagnosis? How should he be managed?

Mr Kirk has presented with a dull flank pain, high fever, and urinalysis suggestive of a urinary tract infection. He has most likely developed **acute pyelonephritis** secondary to obstruction from his previous kidney stone(s). The most common causal organism by far is *Escherichia coli*. Pyelonephritis requires rapid diagnosis and treatment as progression to septicaemia can be swift.

Management as always should begin with an assessment of Mr Kirk's need for resuscitation. This patient is hypotensive and needs to be resuscitated. Given that he is hypotensive, has an active infection, and has vomiting that precludes oral therapy, he will need admission.

You should then take a full history, conduct a thorough examination, request investigations, and instigate treatment for sepsis according to the Surviving Sepsis guidelines (see final section of long case in Chapter 16 for details):

- IV fluid boluses to restore his blood pressure to normal values, then orally if tolerated
- Oxygen, if required to maintain saturations > 94%
- Blood cultures
- Venous blood gas (to check lactate and Hb)
- Pyelonephritis should be treated with antibiotics for 2 weeks, initially on an empirical basis until the urine cultures return. Consult your local hospital guidelines for the appropriate antibiotic regimen.
- Monitor his renal function and urine output to assess his renal function. If his ureter is obstructed, he will need a percutaneous nephrostomy tube to give the urine an outlet and relieve pressure on the kidney.
- Don't forget the analgesia! (see Viva questions).
- During his admission, you should maintain a high index of suspicion for intrarenal or perinephric abscess. Watch out for a persistently high fever, bacteraemia (positive blood cultures), very high initial WCC, severe tenderness on examination, or failure to improve after appropriate therapy. If an abscess develops, it will require surgical drainage.

Mr McCoy is a 50-year-old truck driver with a high body mass index (BMI) who attends his GP complaining of right flank pain. The pain has been present for over a week, although he cannot remember a specific trigger. He describes it as an ache, worse in the morning or after a long day's drive. He has tried ibuprofen and this helps a little but he is unhappy as he sees it as only a temporary fix. Otherwise nothing relieves the pain.

He has no associated symptoms. In particular, he has not had any urinary or bowel symptoms, and has not noticed any weakness or changes in sensation in either leg. Examination is unremarkable except for limited flexion of the spine.

What is the most likely diagnosis? How should this patient be managed?

Mr McCoy is most likely suffering with **musculoskeletal back pain**. This will affect up to 80% of the population at some point. The majority will recover within 6 weeks, but 60% will have relapses in the future. Management should involve:

- **Maintaining activity and exercise.** It is better to avoid bed rest in patients with musculoskeletal lower back pain. Inactivity will make the problem worse. The key is to find mild, gentle exercise that they can tolerate on a regular basis. If the back pain becomes chronic there is also a proven role for cognitive behavioural therapy (CBT) to correct unhelpful negative beliefs regarding the back pain.

- **Regular multimodal analgesia.** Most over-the-counter analgesics (NSAIDs and paracetamol) work well for lower back pain but only if they are taken *regularly* and in *combination*. Back pain can take up to 6 weeks to recover, so opiates should be avoided if possible to avoid side effects (constipation), tolerance, and dependence.

- **Build up core muscles.** 'Core stability' muscle groups such as transversus abdominis, the internal and external obliques, and multifidus are crucial in maintaining the lower spine in a stable 'neutral position'. Weakness in these muscles predisposes to musculoskeletal back injury. Patients can be taught how to strengthen their core muscles at a gym or via a physiotherapy-directed programme such as an integrated back stability programme.

- **Weight loss.** Encourage patients to lose weight with the help of a dietitian if necessary.

- **General back care.** Most idiopathic back pain is the result of a combination of repeated bending (lumbar flexion) actions leading to accumulated strain on lumbar soft tissues. Recommend that a patient practices good back care—limit bending (bend the knees instead), and sit upright in a chair (don't slouch). When lifting or carrying, an object should be held close to the body to reduce leverage effects.

- **Avoid surgery.** For the overwhelming majority of patients, surgery is no better than conservative management involving exercise regimes, even when the lower back ache is due to clearly defined anatomical abnormalities such as herniated intervertebral discs or spondylolysis ± spondylolisthesis.

SHORT CASE

Mrs Chekov is a 76-year-old woman who presents to the Emergency Department with acute flank pain that came on suddenly and woke her at night. She has had back pain for many years, but this feels very different—it is sharper and more severe. Her initial observations are a heart rate of 116 bpm regular, blood pressure of 116/88 mmHg on lying, oxygen saturations of 98% on air and temperature of 36.4 °C.

She has been feeling fine recently, although she has a past medical history of lower back pain, angina, hypertension, and 'indigestion'. She takes regular aspirin, simvastatin, propranolol, diclofenac, co-codamol, and omeprazole. On examination, she is obese and has pitting oedema affecting both legs up to her knees. The oedema makes it impossible to palpate any pulses in her legs. Her body habitus makes it impossible to determine any masses on palpation of her abdomen or to visualize her abdominal aorta using a bedside ultrasound, but she does have mild epigastric tenderness. Her back is free of tenderness on palpation. Her spine has a very limited range of motion, but this is apparently longstanding. An urgent CT abdomen is done and is shown in Figure 18.3.

Figure 18.3 Abdominal CT scan for Mrs Chekov.

What is the diagnosis? How will you proceed?

Mrs Chekov is an elderly woman with a past medical history of ischaemic heart disease and hypertension who now presents with a sudden-onset, sharp flank pain. Her history and examination do not point to any clear diagnosis, but her age and risk factors suggest the possibility of either a **perforated duodenal ulcer** (indigestion, epigastric tenderness, use of NSAIDs) or a **leaking AAA** (age, atherosclerotic disease, hypertension). The fact that she is an elderly and female patient who is presenting with acute flank pain should raise alarm bells that this may be a leaking aneurysm and hence an urgent CT abdomen was done. This shows an enlarged abdominal aorta and blood that has leaked into the retroperitoneal cavity. Mrs Chekov thus has a **leaking AAA** which is a surgical emergency that carries a mortality rate of 50%.

The next step is to insert two large-bore IV access cannulae and **cross-match** 10 units of blood (= 5 L of blood or enough to replace the entire circulating volume), insert a **urinary catheter** (to monitor renal function), and **immediately notify** the vascular surgeon and anaesthetist on call.

Viva questions

What different types of kidney stones are there? How might you treat them?

In decreasing order of occurrence:

- **Calcium** (75–85%), which may be calcium oxalate, calcium phosphate, or mixed. These may be treated in different ways depending on the presence of an underlying metabolic imbalance. Patients with hypercalciuria should be investigated to exclude hyperparathyroidism. They then can be treated with thiazides (which decrease renal excretion of Ca^{2+}) and a low-calcium diet. Those with hyperuricosuria can be given allopurinol (which inhibits the production of uric acid during the breakdown of nucleic acids). Those with hypocitraturia can be given potassium citrate (citrate alkalinizes the urine and inhibits the formation of crystals).
- **Struvite** (10–20%), which is ammonium magnesium phosphate. These are most common in women and are secondary to infection with a urease-producing bacteria (e.g. *Proteus, Pseudomonas, Klebsiella*) which can break down urea into ammonium. Treatment of the underlying infection is indicated.
- **Urate** (5–10%). Urate crystals form in the presence of acid urine, so potassium citrate may be given to alkalinize the urine. Allopurinol can be used to lower urate production and subsequent excretion.
- **Cystine** (1%). These stones form secondary to cystinuria, a rare autosomal recessive disorder with increased cystine excretion. Patients should be advised to increase fluid intake as a means to diluting the urinary cystine concentration. As with urate stones, the solubility of cystine is pH dependent and so potassium citrate can also be given. Cystine-binding drugs may be given if all else fails, e.g. tiopronin.

A number of medical conditions can predispose to stone formation—can you name them?

- Metabolic:
  - Hypercalciuria
  - Hyperuricosuria
  - Hypocitraturia
  - Hyperoxaluria
  - Gout and other hyperuricaemic states e.g. malignancy, glucose-6-phosphate dehydrogenase (G6PDH) deficiency (urate stones)
  - Cystinuria
- Primary hyperparathyroidism
- Crohn's disease (often oxalate stones, although the exact mechanism for this remains unclear)
- Chronic urinary tract infection due to urease-producing bacteria (struvite stones)
- Medullary sponge or polycystic kidneys (resulting in static collections in which stones form)
- Renal tubular acidosis (stones result from hypercalciuria, alkalinization of the urine causing precipitation of calcium phosphate, and low urinary citrate)
- Sarcoidosis (causes a hypercalcaemia that can lead to stone formation)

What radiographic findings would you look for in a patient with suspected kidney stones? What are the 'soft-tissue rim' and 'tail' signs?

- The stones themselves
- Hydronephrosis and/or hydroureter (dilated ureters) due to obstruction
- Perinephric fluid

In the 'soft-tissue rim' sign stones may be surrounded by a rim of soft tissue, which can help differentiate stones in the ureter from a calcified pelvic vein (phlebolith).

The 'tail' sign is where a soft-tissue opacity extends away from the stone like a tail. This is consistent with a pelvic phlebolith (calcification of a previous thrombus in a vein) and is not a ureteric stone. Both the 'soft-tissue rim' and 'tail' sign refer to CT imaging.

What are the complications of kidney stones? How are they managed?

- **Ureteric stricture** from the passage of the stone (or ureteroscopic removal of a stone). If necessary a stent can be inserted.
- **Acute or chronic pyelonephritis**, potentially leading to sepsis. Managed as per the first short case.
- **Renal failure**, due to obstruction and back-pressure causing hydronephrosis and kidney damage. This requires stone removal and close medical management including monitoring of renal function and ensuring good renal perfusion.
- **Intrarenal or perinephric abscess**. Abscesses may occur as a complication of pyelonephritis, particularly if there are large 'staghorn' stones present blocking the ureters. As suggested by the name, a perinephric abscess forms when the pus discharges through the renal capsule into the perinephric fat. Patients present with systemic features and pyuria. Diagnosis is by finding a renal mass with a fluid level on ultrasound or radiology. Patients require drainage of the abscess.
- **Xanthogranulomatous pyelonephritis**. This is a type of chronic bacterial pyelonephritis characterized by the destruction of renal parenchyma and the presence of granulomas and abscesses. Patients are chronically ill with systemic symptoms. Nephrectomy is the standard treatment.
- **Urine extravasation** into the pelvic cavity. Although uncommon, this has severe consequences, as the combination of urine and the subsequent infection produces severe oedema, high fever, and dehydration. The extravasated urine must be drained and the urine flow diverted so that it does not continue to extravasate. The patient will also need fluids and antibiotics.

NSAIDs are now the first-line analgesic treatment for renal colic pain. What are the cautions and contraindications to NSAID use?

NSAIDs are contraindicated in:

- Asthma, unless the asthma is very mild or the patient has tried NSAIDs before without problem, in which case they can try them cautiously
- History of anaphylaxis with any NSAID
- Previous or active peptic ulcers

CONTINUED ➤

CONTINUED

- Severe heart failure
- COX-2 selective inhibitors (a subtype of NSAID) should not be used in ischaemic heart disease, cerebrovascular disease, or peripheral arterial disease as they are associated with an increased risk of thrombotic events

NSAIDs should be used with caution in:

- Coagulation defects: may be exacerbated due to antiplatelet effects.
- Renal, cardiac, or hepatic impairment: NSAIDs may impair renal function and cause fluid retention, leading to pulmonary oedema in patients with cardiac failure. This is more likely to occur if the patient has poor liver function (hepatic impairment) or pre-existing kidney disease (renal impairment).
- During pregnancy and breast-feeding: closure of the ductus arteriosus can occur in response to NSAIDs and this is a problem if it occurs *in utero*. There may also be delayed onset and increased duration of labour. NSAIDs are sometimes found in breast milk but there is little information on the risks presented. Nonetheless most manufacturers advise avoiding them if breast-feeding.
- Elderly patients as the risk of bleeding and renal failure is more common and is more likely to have a serious outcome.

Where along the renal tract are stones most likely to cause obstruction?

Stones are most likely to obstruct in the narrowest parts of the collecting system. These are:

- the pelvoureteric junction (PUJ)
- the pelvic brim
- the vesicoureteric junction (VUJ).

At what diameter is surgical intervention advisable for an unruptured AAA? What is the evidence for this?

Elective surgical repair of an AAA is a major operation that carries a 5% mortality rate. Left alone, AAAs with a diameter <5.5 cm have an annual risk of rupture <1%. However, AAAs with a diameter >6 cm have an annual risk of rupture of 25%(!). Thus the indications for surgery are:

- AAA diameter >5.5 cm
- AAA diameter growing >1 cm per year
- Symptomatic AAA

The evidence for this comes from the UK Small Aneurysm Trial[†] and the US Aneurysm Detection and Management Study.[‡] Both showed that aneurysms <5.5 cm are best managed non-operatively, finding no mortality benefit from surgery.

[†] UKSAT Investigators. Mortality results for randomised controlled trial of early elective surgery or ultrasonographic surveillance for small abdominal aortic aneurysms. The UK Small Aneurysm Trial Participants. *Lancet*, 1998;**352**: 1649-1655.

[‡] Lederle FA, Wilson SE, Johnson GR, Reinke DB, Littooy FN, Acher CW et al. Immediate repair compared with surveillance of small abdominal aortic aneurysms. *New Engl J Med*, 2002;**346**: 1437-1444.

What is the 'psoas sign' on abdominal radiographs?

You may occasionally hear reference to the 'psoas sign'. This is where one of the two psoas shadows on an abdominal radiograph is not visible. This can represent an AAA, as in the example in Figure 18.4. However, the psoas sign is also present in patients with other abdominal pathology (e.g. acute pancreatitis) and quite a few healthy individuals, too. It is thus an *unreliable* sign for AAA. Instead, AAAs are best assessed using either abdominal ultrasound (for simple detection and screening), plain abdominal CT or contrast abdominal CT (if a leaking AAA is suspected or surgery is planned).

Figure 18.4 (a) Plain abdominal radiograph of a patient with an abdominal aortic aneurysm (AAA) and absent psoas shadow on the patient's right side. (b) Three-dimensional reconstruction of a pre-operative abdominal CT scan of a patient with an AAA.

Part (a) Reproduced from John Reynard *et al.*, *Oxford Handbook of Urology*, 2006, Figure 3.4, page 49, with permission from Oxford University Press. Part (b) Reproduced from Gardiner MD and Borley NR, *Training in Surgery*, 2009, Figure 7.8, page 161, with permission from Oxford University Press.

A patient visits his GP complaining of ongoing lower back pain that is worse on the right side. What are the 'red flags' of back pain that warrant referral for further investigation (see Table 18.1)?

Table 18.1 Back pain: the 'red flags'

Red flags	Referral time
Sphincter problems	Immediate
Patient unable to self-care or walk	
Weight loss	Within 1 week
Fever	
Back tenderness to palpation	
Thoracic spinal pain	
Violent trauma (e.g. car accident)	
Age <20 years or >50 years	As soon as possible
Severe morning stiffness	
Structural deformity (e.g. scoliosis)	
Nerve root pain not resolving >6 weeks	

What medications would you prescribe for any patient in pain?

When prescribing analgesia, you should keep in mind the concept of using regular multimodal analgesia. The aim of this strategy is to target as many parts of the pain pathway as possible and to do so in a way that anticipates the pain, rather than simply reacting to it. One can broadly think of the pain pathway as having three components: the source of pain (often a site of inflammation), the pain nerves taking a signal from this site to the brain, and the brain itself. As a gross simplification, one can think of NSAIDs as decreasing inflammation at the site of pain, opioids as decreasing the transmission of pain signals along nerves to the brain, and paracetamol as reducing pain perception by the brain itself. Thus, the combination of regular paracetamol + NSAID (e.g. naproxen, ibuprofen) + weak opioid (e.g. codeine, tramadol) is more effective than these drugs taken alone and/or irregularly. The pain from ureteric colic is very severe and it is often tempting to prescribe strong opioids (e.g. morphine) for such patients. However, patients with opioid dependence occasionally present to hospital pretending to have ureteric colic in an attempt to obtain opioids and studies[†] have shown that NSAIDs are just as effective as opioids for the vast majority of patients with ureteric colic. It is thus good practice to start with paracetamol + NSAID ± weak opioid in such patients, adding a strong opioid (e.g. morphine) only if the pain is not controlled (as your priority is to relieve pain in all patients). There are circumstances in which NSAIDs will be contraindicated (see Viva question above) and when an opioid will be better.

† Holdgate A, Pollock T. Systematic review of the relative efficacy of non-steroidal anti-inflammatory drugs and opioids in the treatment of acute renal colic. *BMJ*, 2004;**328**: 1401.

Single Best Answers

1. What is the biochemical composition of struvite renal stones?

a. Calcium phosphate

b. Calcium oxalate

c. Cystine

d. Urate

e. Calcium magnesium ammonium phosphate

2. What is the approximate operative mortality for emergency surgical repair of a ruptured abdominal aortic aneurysm?

a. 10%

b. 25%

c. 40–50%

d. 75%

e. 90%

3. At which level of the spine does the abdominal aorta bifurcate?

a. L2

b. L3

c. L4

d. L5

e. S1

4. Which of the following is not a significant risk factor for the development of an abdominal aortic aneurysm?

a. Diabetes mellitus

b. Male sex

c. Family history

d. Tobacco smoking

e. Systemic hypertension

5. Elective abdominal aortic aneurysm repairs involve a trade-off between the risks of rupture versus the risks of surgery. There is no mortality benefit of elective surgery for aneurysms below which diameter?

a. 1.5 cm

b. 3.5 cm

c. 5.5 cm

d. 7.5 cm

e. 8.5 cm

Constipation

Core case

Mrs Crabbe is a 62-year-old retired secretary who has been referred by her GP to the gastroenterology department of her district general hospital, where you are one of the junior doctors. Her main complaint is constipation.

What does 'constipation' mean?

Constipation typically refers to stool that is passed infrequently and/or with difficulty. The most important thing to elucidate is what the patient means by 'constipation'. Therefore, writing 'constipation' in the notes is inadequate—you must say something about frequency, ease of passage, and volume.

Normal defecation requires that a person has adequate bowel peristalsis, relatively soft faeces, no obstruction to outflow, and the will and ability to push. With this in mind, it is possible to think of various mechanisms that might cause someone to be constipated.

What is your initial differential diagnosis for constipation in any patient?

Figure 19.1 shows the differential diagnosis for constipation.

Abnormal bowel peristalsis	Hard faeces	Bowel obstruction	Patient not pushing
• Irritable bowel syndrome	• Lack of dietary fibre	• Colorectal adenocarcinoma	• Haemorrhoids
• Medications (e.g. opiates, iron supplements, calcium-channel blockers)	• Dehydration	• Sigmoid volvulus	• Anal fissure
• Hypothyroidism		• Other pelvic masses (e.g. uterine fibroids, ovarian tumour)	• Pelvic floor dysfunction (e.g. after hysterectomy)
• Hypercalcaemia		• Colonic strictures (e.g. radiotherapy, Crohn's disease, diverticular disease)	
• Hypokalaemia			
• Multiple sclerosis			
• Parkinson's disease			
• Diabetic neuropathy			
• Idiopathic megacolon			
• Idiopathic slow transit			

Figure 19.1 Differential diagnosis for constipation.

Bear in mind that, in a hospital setting, one of the most common causes of constipation will not be due to any pathology per se but rather the embarrassment or discomfort of having to open one's bowels on a bed pan within earshot of others.

Equally, patients who are immobile for any reason (e.g. spinal pathology, old age) are prone to constipation, although the mechanism for this is unclear.

> Constipation is a very common symptom. It usually has a benign aetiology (lack of fibre, dehydration) and is successfully managed in primary care.
>
> **What 'red flags' would cause the GP to refer a patient with constipation for further investigation?**

There are a number of features from the history that should alert you to potentially sinister causes of constipation (especially colorectal cancer) and which warrant further investigation:

- Severe, persistent constipation that is unresponsive to treatment
- Absolute constipation, i.e. not passing either stool or flatus
- Rectal bleeding, tenesmus, or intermittent mucoid diarrhoea
- Significant weight loss, iron deficiency anaemia, and/or night sweats
- Past medical history of ulcerative colitis or colonic polyps
- Strong family history of colon cancer or colonic polyps, particularly if affected family members were <60 years old.

> The GP has referred Mrs Crabbe because of persistent constipation that has been refractory to primary care management with increased dietary fibre and two laxatives (macrogol and senna). You take a fresh history from Mrs Crabbe about her constipation.
>
> **What key clues will you look for in the history?**

About the constipation

- **Characterize what the patient means by 'constipation'.** Passing hard, lumpy stools suggests lack of fibre or dehydration, but not obstruction. No longer passing any faeces nor flatus ('absolute constipation') suggests complete bowel obstruction.

- **When did this start?** Recent change in bowel habit suggests pathology, whereas chronic constipation is usually benign.

Associated symptoms

- **Weight loss, night sweats, fevers?** May suggest malignancy.

- **Diarrhoea?** Intermittent diarrhoea and constipation can suggest irritable bowel syndrome (in younger patients), colorectal cancer (in patients >45 years, especially if the diarrhoea is mucoid), or diverticular disease (in patients >60 years, especially if they have had episodes of left iliac fossa pain).

- **Tenesmus?** Suggests a persistent mass in the rectum (e.g. tumour).

- **Blood on faeces, per rectum, or when wiping?** May suggest haemorrhoids, anal fissure, diverticular disease, or colorectal cancer (see Chapter 21).
- **Bloating?** A feature of irritable bowel syndrome.
- **Feeling cold, reduced appetite, gaining weight?** May suggest hypothyroidism.
- **Bone pains?** Could suggest bone metastases, which would lead to hypercalcaemia that can cause constipation.
- **Polyuria, thirst?** May suggest hypercalcaemia.

You should note any **abdominal pain** but it is unhelpful in narrowing the diagnosis as constipation itself can be a source of pain.

Risk factors for constipation

- **History of bowel disease, neurological disorders, back problems, or endocrine disease?**
- **Family history of bowel disorders?** In particular, look for a family history of bowel disorders that increase the risk of colorectal cancer such as colorectal cancer per se, familial adenomatous polyposis (FAP), hereditary non-polyposis colorectal cancer (HNPCC), or Peutz–Jegher's disease.
- **What medications are they on?** Check the British National Formulary (BNF) to see if the patient's medications can cause constipation as a side effect. Opiates, anticholinergics, tricyclic antidepressants, calcium channel blockers, and iron supplements are notorious for causing constipation.
- **Diet?** Do they eat a healthy, varied, fibre-rich diet? Do they keep adequately hydrated? Ask what colour their urine is (persistently yellow urine can suggest a degree of dehydration).

Mrs Crabbe tells you that she has always found it relatively hard to pass faeces, having had to strain and take her time on the toilet for most of her adult life. Despite this, she has always managed to pass faeces three or four times a week. However, for the past 2 months she has found it very difficult to pass any faeces at all, saying that she has only opened her bowels perhaps once a week. When she finally opens her bowels it is painless but only small amounts of 'surprisingly soft' faeces come out. She last opened her bowels 3 days ago but is still passing wind every day. Her faeces are not mucoid and she has not noticed any blood on her faeces or when she wipes.

Mrs Crabbe has not noticed any weight loss, fevers, or night sweats. She has not been unusually thirsty nor has she had any aches or pains. Her appetite has been reduced but she has not felt cold or lethargic. Her urine passes without difficulty and she thinks it is pale yellow in colour.

Mrs Crabbe has type 2 diabetes mellitus and hypertension. She had a kidney stone a few years ago but 'it passed' and no cause was ever found. She has two daughters, both of whom were delivered vaginally and weighed about 3.6 kg (8 lb), albeit requiring an episiotomy for the first. She takes metformin for her diabetes, amlodipine for her hypertension, and simvastatin for her cholesterol. She has never had any surgery.

Mrs Crabbe lost her husband 6 months ago quite suddenly and unexpectedly. She has since been living with her eldest daughter and her family. She describes her mood as having been low since her husband passed away, although the recent arrival of a granddaughter to the family has improved things. There is nil of note in her family history.

Mrs Crabbe smoked two packs of cigarettes a day from her teenage years until her father's death 20 years ago. She drinks a glass of sherry every evening and says her diet is 'very healthy' now that she is living with her daughter, who makes sure she eats plenty of 'greens'. She walks a couple of miles every day with her daughter and their dog.

Mrs Crabbe's main concern is that she will need some sort of surgery.

Can you narrow your initial differential diagnosis based on the information so far?

Based on her history, sex, and age, Mrs Crabbe's differential diagnosis can be narrowed down to that shown in Figure 19.2.

Dehydration
Colorectal cancer
Pelvic mass
Diabetic neuropathy
Hypothyroidism
Hypercalcaemia
Hypokalaemia

Figure 19.2 Differential diagnosis for Mrs Crabbe's constipation based on her history, sex, and age.

You move on to examination.

What clues should you look for on examination of someone with constipation?

General inspection

- **Cachexia?** Suggests malignancy.
- **Signs of hypothyroidism:** loss of hair (especially the outer third of eyebrows), brittle hair, dry skin, puffy eyes, malar flush?

Abdominal examination

- **Virchow's node** (left supraclavicular fossa)? Enlargement can suggest gastrointestinal (GI) malignancy.
- **Abdominal mass?** In the context of constipation, this could be impacted faeces, a colonic tumour, a Crohn's mass, or an ovarian mass.
- **Anal fissures or haemorrhoids?** This may explain the constipation—it can be too painful to push. However this is a little 'chicken and egg', in that it is hard to know whether the constipation or the fissure/haemorrhoid came first.
- **Mass on digital rectal examination?** This may suggest a rectal carcinoma or impacted faeces.

- **Lax anal tone?** This suggests neurological pathology, such as diabetic neuropathy or multiple sclerosis.

Neurological examination

- If the history is suggestive of diabetic neuropathy, multiple sclerosis, cord compression, or parkinsonism.

> There is nothing unusual on inspection of Mrs Crabbe. Her abdominal examination is remarkable only for what feels like a colon loaded with faeces down the left side of her abdomen on deep palpation. No other masses or organomegaly are present. There is no ascites, clubbing, or lymphadenopathy. You perform a rectal examination, with her consent, but it reveals no anal fissures or fistulae and an empty rectum.
>
> **What investigations will you arrange for Mrs Crabbe, and why?**

Ideally, no investigations will be necessary for the vast majority of patients with constipation, as the common diagnoses can be made clinically (diet, drugs, etc.). Moreover, there is no evidence to support the routine use of investigations in the diagnostic evaluation of patients with constipation. However, given that no obvious diagnosis can be made for Mrs Crabbe, a number of investigations may be useful:

- **Blood tests:**
    - **Full blood count:** a colonic mass can bleed and cause anaemia
    - **Electrolytes and calcium:** hypokalaemia and hypercalcaemia can cause constipation
    - **Thyroid function tests:** the history and examination do not suggest hypothyroidism as a cause of constipation, but it is easily excluded biochemically
    - **Glucose and HbA1c:** not routine examinations for constipation, but as Mrs Crabbe is a diabetic it would be helpful to investigate her diabetic control at present (glucose) and over the last few months (HbA1c).

The following investigations are not routinely requested when first investigating constipation but may be requested if the history and examination warrant them:

- **Faecal occult blood test (FOBT):** as she is nearly 65 years old, this would not be unreasonable. However remember that although this test is increasingly being used to screen for asymptomatic colon cancer, faecal blood can also be due to colonic angiodysplasia, colonic polyps, haemorrhoids, aspirin, or warfarin. Antiplatelets should be stopped 7 days before, if possible. The test has a low specificity and sensitivity for colon cancer, but a positive test warrants further investigation.
- **Carcinoembryonic antigen (CEA)/CA19-9/CA125:** these are all markers of colon cancer. However, they lack specificity (e.g. CA125 is more commonly elevated in ovarian malignancy) and sensitivity and therefore are *not* used to diagnose malignancy. They are, however, used to monitor response, relapse, and recurrence in patients with confirmed GI cancer.

The blood results and FOBT results for Mrs Crabbe are shown below:

Haematology		Biochemistry			
Hb	94 g/L ↓	Na	137 mM N	Ca (corrected)	2.2 mM little ↓
WCC	8.1×10^9 cells/L N	K	3.7 mM N	ALT	25 U/L N
Platelets	190×10^9 cells/L N	Urea	9.2 mM ↑	AST	22 U/L N
MCV	68 fL ↓ microcytic	Creatinine	122 µM ↑	ALP	98 U/L N
				GGT	18 U/L
		TSH	2.1 mU/L N		
		Free T_4	10 pmol/L N	Glucose	6.2 mM N
				HbA1c	5.9% N

Haematinics (requested after reviewing results above)

Ferritin	3 µg/L	↓
B$_{12}$	480 ng/L N	
Folate	6.8 ng/L N	

Fe def ↓ microcytic anaemia.

What is your next step?

Mrs Crabbe has iron deficiency anaemia in the context of a change in bowel habit (constipation). Given this and her age, your next step should be to request **imaging** of her upper and lower GI tract such as:

- **Proctoscopy.** A transparent dilator is used to visualize the anus and rectum. Can be done in the clinic or on the wards.

- **Rigid sigmoidoscopy.** Visualizes as far as the sigmoid colon. Can also be done in the clinic or on the wards.

- **Flexible sigmoidoscopy.** This involves a flexible sigmoidoscope, often with sedation (but not general anaesthetic) and limited bowel preparation (an enema may suffice). It can visualize as far as the splenic flexure (top of the descending colon), and be used to take biopsies and remove small polyps. It can be done as an outpatient and carries less morbidity than a complete colonoscopy. NICE guidelines (2011) advise that those with suspected colorectal cancer but without major comorbidity should be offered a colonoscopy instead, as flexible sigmoidoscopy will miss up to 40% of tumours that lie beyond the splenic flexure. If the patient has major comorbidities, they advise flexible sigmoidoscopy followed by a barium enema.

- **Colonoscopy.** Similar to a flexible sigmoidoscopy but involves more 'thorough' bowel preparation (which is less well tolerated), and can visualize as far as the ileocaecal valve.

- **CT colonography.** Also known as 'virtual colonoscopy' or 'CT pneumocolon'; this involves an abdominal CT scan after bowel preparation and insufflation (filling the colon with air). It shows the bowel lumen and surrounding structures (e.g. liver, ovaries). Usually done if patients are frail and unlikely to tolerate colonoscopy and/or sigmoidoscopy.

- **Double-contrast barium enema (DCBE).** As the name suggests, a barium enema is given to the patient and plain radiographs are taken at various times. Thus the lumen of the bowel can be visualized. This is very rarely used now there is better access to colonoscopy and with the advent of CT colonography for frail patients, both of which are more sensitive. Moreover, when asked, patients prefer colonoscopy (no doubt because sedation is used!).

- **Oesophagogastroduodenoscopy (OGD).** An endoscope is inserted via the mouth and used to visualize as far as the duodenum. An OGD should always be performed in the context of iron deficiency anaemia to exclude an upper GI source of blood loss.

You arrange for Mrs Crabbe to have a colonoscopy. The report is as follows:

Anal canal:	Internal, grade 1 haemorrhoids
Rectum:	Normal
Sigmoid colon:	Normal
Descending colon:	Large suspicious polypoid mass (see Figure 19.3). Biopsy taken
Spenic flexure:	Normal
Transverse colon:	Normal
Hepatic flexure:	Normal
Ascending colon:	Normal
Caecum:	Normal

Pathology report: Focalized adenocarcinoma, grade 2. The biopsy shows involvement of the mucosal lamina propria by neoplastic glands. The muscularis propria was clear of invasion in the biopsy specimen.

Figure 19.3 Colon mass at colonoscopy.
Reproduced from Gardiner MD and Borley NR, *Training in Surgery*, Figure 5.13, page 105, 2009, with permission from Oxford University Press.

What will you tell Mrs Crabbe? What is the next step?

Mrs Crabbe must be told that she has **colon cancer** but this must be done with care. Telling patients they have a serious condition (particularly cancer) can be devastating, so make sure you provide:

- **The right people.** Get an experienced and senior doctor (e.g. your consultant) to deliver the news. Involve the senior nurse, who will have more contact with the patient than doctors and can thus provide more support. Many hospitals will also have a colorectal clinical nurse specialist who can act as a single point of call for patients. Ideally, offer for family or friends to be present at the time so that they can offer support.

- **The right place.** Telling someone they have cancer on a rushed 'business' ward round and then leaving them to ponder the news is not good practice. Take patients into a quiet room.

- **The right time.** Make time to deliver bad news so that you don't have to rush off during the process (e.g. once your jobs are done, and don't be afraid to hand your bleep over to a colleague). Choose the right time for the patient, too: make sure the patient is able to understand, and await the arrival of family or friends.

- **The right message.** Make sure that Mrs Crabbe understands what she is being told. Many patients complain that doctors are euphemistic when talking about serious diseases such as cancer, which only confuses them. Find out how much she knows already. Explain to Mrs Crabbe that the colonoscopy found a mass in her bowel, on the left-hand side. The laboratories have confirmed it is a colon cancer. Explain that the spread of the cancer needs assessing, various treatment options are available, and the outcomes are nowadays good if colon cancer is caught before it spreads as the affected segment of bowel can be surgically removed. Unfortunately, you cannot say how far the cancer has spread from the pathology report, as the report reflects only a small biopsy. The next step is therefore to assess how far the cancer has spread.

Staging the cancer is important because it influences subsequent management and prognosis (see discussion later in the chapter). Staging needs to look at the main areas where the cancer might spread. In the case of colon cancer this is the liver and lungs, the ovaries in women, and the lymph nodes that drain the colon. Previously, staging was done by a combination of exploratory laparotomy (very invasive), liver ultrasound, and chest radiography. Nowadays this has been superseded by combined chest, abdomen, and pelvis CT scans with contrast, which offer a much better view in a quicker and less invasive way. No further imaging is necessary according to guidelines, but positron emission tomography (PET), which uses radiolabelled substrates taken up preferentially by highly metabolically active tumour cells, is being increasingly combined with CT scanning (PET-CT) to pick up even the smallest of metastases that are not seen by CT scans alone.

In the case of rectal tumours, MRI is additionally recommended for local staging, as there is evidence that it is superior to CT. If MRI is contraindicated, endorectal ultrasound is recommended.

All cases of colorectal cancer should be discussed at the colorectal MDT.

Mrs Crabbe has a chest, abdomen, and pelvis CT. It confirms a mass in the descending colon that does not appear to have invaded beyond the bowel wall. No obvious masses are apparent in any adjacent structures, the liver and lungs look normal, and there are no enlarged or suspicious lymph nodes. A small degree of prolapse is noted in her intervertebral disc at L4/L5 which is not impinging on either nerve root and is therefore likely to be an incidental finding. She is diagnosed with colorectal cancer that is provisionally staged as T2N0M0 (Dukes' A) and is referred to the colorectal surgeons. She receives a laparoscopic left hemicolectomy and is back home within a few days. Five years later, she remains free of recurrence.

Short cases

Mr Tanner is a 27-year-old lorry driver who has come to see his GP regarding long-standing constipation. He often fails to open his bowels for an entire week and this makes him irritable. The problem has been ongoing for many years, but he has finally come to see his GP to see if there is any medication that can help.

Mr Tanner has not had any pain or blood per rectum. His stools are often hard and his urine is always yellow in colour. He has not noticed any weight loss, change in appetite, heat intolerance, or lethargy. He occasionally uses a salbutamol inhaler for his asthma but his past medical and drug history is otherwise unremarkable. There is nil of note in his family history. He smokes a pack of cigarettes every day but drinks only the occasional pint of beer at weekends. On a typical day he eats white toast and jam with coffee for breakfast; a chocolate bar halfway through the morning; a sandwich (white bread) and packet of crisps for lunch; and meat with potatoes or chips for dinner. He rarely eats fruit or vegetables (other than potatoes). He drinks about six cups of coffee a day and rarely exercises.

On examination, Mr Tanner is overweight. His abdomen is soft and non-tender, with no masses or organomegaly. A digital rectal examination reveals a rectum loaded with hard faeces, normal anal tone, a normal feeling prostate, and no masses.

What are the most likely causes of Mr Tanner's constipation? How can it be managed?

The most likely cause of Mr Tanner's constipation is the most common aetiology: a combination of **lack of fibre** in the diet, **dehydration**, and a degree of **immobility**. Management can include the following options, introduced incrementally until the problem is solved:

- **Lifestyle changes:** this is likely to have the greatest long-term effect. Increase fluid intake and fibre intake. Explain the benefits of a high-fibre diet beyond improving constipation (it *may* reduce the risk of coronary heart disease and colon cancer). Exercise is also useful (e.g. he could start with brisk walk for 30 min every day).

- **Bulk producers:** fibre helps constipation by providing bulk (which activates stretch receptors in the bowel and triggers peristalsis) and by retaining water (which makes faeces softer). Simple dietary changes such as eating a fibre-rich cereal and changing from white to wholemeal bread could make a lot of difference to Mr Tanner. Various fibre supplements exist for patients who cannot achieve sufficient bulk by modifying their diet alone (e.g. methylcellulose tablets, ispaghula husk).

- **Stool softeners:** liquid paraffin and arachis oil enemas can be used to soften stool. They should only be used in the short term as they can lead to unpleasant side effects such as steatorrhoea and anal seepage.

- **Osmotic laxatives:** lactulose, macrogols/polyethylene glycols (e.g. Movicol), or magnesium salts act by retaining fluid in the bowel, thus causing a mild osmotic diarrhoea. Patients must therefore significantly increase their fluid intake for these to be effective. These should only ever be used as a short-term remedy as they can cause dehydration and tolerance without addressing the underlying cause. They should be used with caution in patients with renal impairment or who are being diuresed and/or fluid restricted for some other reason (e.g. heart failure).

- **Peristalsis stimulants:** glycerol suppositories, bisacodyl, or senna can all be used to stimulate peristalsis. Docusate probably acts as both a stimulant and stool softener, and as a result is a popular choice with geriatricians (for their patients, not themselves!).
- **Enemas:** these should be used as a last resort.

Note: A number of novel agents are emerging for constipation refractory to conventional treatments (e.g. the 5-HT$_4$ receptor agonist prucalopride). Consult your hospital pharmacy and/or seek gastroenterology advice should these become necessary.

SHORT CASE

Miss Pope is a 22-year-old woman complaining of a change in bowel habit. She is not sure how long it has been going on as it seems to have 'crept up on me gradually over many months'. With hindsight, she is sure that she used to open her bowels every day but now she only goes maybe once or twice a week. When she does go, she does not have to strain and there is no pain, blood, or tenesmus. She says her weight has been increasing despite the fact that she is eating less than before, although she no longer goes to the gym as she feels very tired all the time and her hands often hurt. When asked to expand on her hand symptoms, she explains she often gets a numbing, tingling feeling in her hands that she tries to shake off. She has not felt especially cold of late, although it is obvious she hasn't felt hot either to judge by the thick jumper she is wearing indoors. She does mention that her periods have been rather heavy lately, despite being on the combined oral contraceptive pill, which is the only medication she takes.

Miss Pope's past medical history and family history are unremarkable. She works in a call centre and lives with her boyfriend.

On examination, Miss Pope looks tired and has a heart rate of 55 bpm, regular. Phalen's test is performed and is positive, as is Tinel's test of the median nerve in both wrists. Examination of her cardiovascular, respiratory, and abdominal systems is unremarkable.

What is the likely diagnosis? What investigations would you order to confirm this? How is it managed?

Miss Pope describes reduced frequency of bowel motions along with lethargy, reduced appetite, weight gain, and features of carpal tunnel syndrome. There is also a suggestion of cold intolerance. On examination, her heart rate is on the low side for an adult who is not very athletic and provocation tests for carpal tunnel syndrome are positive. This is all highly suggestive of **hypothyroidism**. The most likely cause for hypothyroidism in a woman of this age is chronic autoimmune thyroiditis, also known as Hashimoto's hypothyroidism.

Hypothyroidism is easily confirmed by a blood test revealing a high TSH level, which is due to the lack of sufficient thyroxine to negatively feed back on its production. If this is Hashimoto's hypothyroidism, one will also find high antithyroid peroxidase antibodies.

Management is by daily oral levothyroxine and prognosis is very good (all symptoms should resolve), although patients have to remain on levothyroxine for life.

SHORT CASE

Mr Laporte is a 46-year-old retail manager suffering with constipation. He describes only opening his bowels twice a week for the past 2 months, although he previously opened his bowels almost daily. Defecation is not painful, but he has been getting aches and pains all over his body recently that he cannot explain. He has not noticed any blood in his faeces or on wiping. He has been passing a lot of urine lately but says this is probably because he has been drinking a lot of water. He feels very thirsty all the time, to the extent that he will wake up at least once every night and drink a pint glass of water. He has not noticed any change in his weight or appetite and does not feel unusually sensitive to heat or cold. His past medical history, drug history, and family history are unremarkable. He does not smoke or drink alcohol. He eats a healthy and varied diet that is rich in vegetables and fruit. He is an amateur triathlete who trains four times a week, although he admits he has not been keeping this up recently as he feels tired and low in mood after work. On examination, you find nothing remarkable. A quick capillary glucose measurement is done in the clinic to exclude diabetes mellitus, because of the polyuria and polydipsia, and it reads 5.1 mM.

What is the likely aetiology for Mr Laporte's symptoms based on his history? What tests will you arrange?

Mr Laporte describes constipation, but also polydipsia (excessive thirst), polyuria, aches and pains, and symptoms of depression (lethargy, low mood). This is all quite suggestive of **hypercalcaemia**, which produces a constellation of symptoms often described as 'moans, groans, bones, and stones' referring to the depression, aches and pains, and renal stones often found in this condition. Polydipsia and polyuria are also common, with the classic (but rarely seen) hypercalcaemia patient waking up at night to down a glass or two of water.

Hypercalcaemia is confirmed by checking serum calcium. The underlying cause can be ascertained by checking the blood results (Table 19.1).

Table 19.1 **Underlying causes of hypercalcaemia**

	Alkaline phosphatase (ALP)	Parathyroid hormone (PTH)	Phosphate
Bone metastases	High	Low	High
Myeloma	Normal	Low	High
Hyperparathyroidism (primary/ tertiary)	Normal/High	Normal/High	Low
Vitamin D overdose	Low	Low	High

- Bone metastases cause increased turnover of bones, hence the high ALP. This releases both calcium and phosphate from the bones.
- Myeloma causes a similar picture to bone metastases. However, in myeloma, osteoclasts are activated and osteoblasts are inhibited. As ALP comes from osteoblasts, it remains normal.
- In primary and tertiary hyperparathyroidism, PTH causes increased bone turnover; hence you also get high ALP (although this can be normal if the bone turnover is slow). Bone turnover releases both calcium and phosphate, but as PTH increases renal excretion of phosphate, this is low. Note that PTH levels are often in the 'normal range' but that this is actually abnormal as they should be low in the presence of high calcium (remember that PTH release is normally inhibited by high calcium levels).
- Vitamin D causes increased gut absorption of both calcium and phosphate. As there is no increased bone turnover, ALP is low, and because calcium levels are high, PTH is suppressed and also low.

Mr Laporte was found to have a serum calcium of 3.2 mM, phosphate 0.6 mM, ALP 309 U/L, and PTH 7.5 pM, suggesting primary hyperparathyroidism. This is usually caused by a solitary, benign para-thyroid adenoma, although parathyroid hyperplasia, parathyroid carcinoma, or PTH-secreting ectopic tumours also occur. Mr Laporte was referred to an experienced surgeon who ordered a ^{99}Tc-sestamibi scan to localize all parathyroid tissue and undertook a minimally invasive parathyroidectomy to remove the offending gland. The pathologist later confirmed that the removed tissue was indeed consistent with a benign parathyroid adenoma.

SHORT CASE

Mrs Doherty is a 78-year-old inpatient receiving palliative care for advanced metastatic breast cancer affecting her bones and liver. She has recently become constipated, having opened her bowels only once in the past 8 days. Despite having deep bone pains over her back and arms, she denies any abdominal pain or any new symptoms since her admission several weeks ago. The nurses say that when she did open her bowels, the faeces looked normal. For her breast cancer she takes pamidronate (to reduce bone turnover caused by the metastatic deposits), paracetamol and mor-phine sulphate (for the bone pain), and cyclizine (for the nausea caused by morphine). Her appetite has been low for some months, although she still manages at least one decent meal a day. Her fluid intake and urine output have both been adequate since her admission. Examination of Mrs Doherty reveals nothing other than some long-standing tenderness over a few ribs, caused by the metastatic bone disease. Her peripheral nervous system is normal and her abdomen is soft and non-tender with no masses or organomegaly. A digital rectal examination reveals normal anal tone and a rectum full of soft faeces.

There are many reasons for Mrs Doherty to be constipated—what are they?

Mrs Doherty's case is not unusual and constipation is commonly seen in such patients. Her constipa-tion is most likely multifactorial, with the following contributing factors:

- **Medications,** particularly opiates which reduce gut motility.
- **Hypercalcaemia** from bone metastases.
- **Immobility.** Mrs Doherty is elderly, unwell, and in hospital, and therefore likely to be fairly immobile.
- **Weakness.** Again, as she is elderly and unwell, she is likely to find it that much more difficult to strain.
- **Poor diet and dehydration.** Patients with cancer often lose their appetite and it is likely that her fibre intake is inadequate. Her fluid intake might also be low.
- **Megarectum.** Patients with chronic constipation can develop a dilated rectum that is susceptible to constipation.

Given Mrs Doherty's malignancy, one might also consider the possibility of the constipation being due to either spinal cord or cauda equina compression, although this is less likely to be the case given the normal peripheral neurological examination.

A reasonable first step would be to trial her on stimulant laxatives (to counteract the effect of the opiates) such as senna, with or without a faecal softener such as sodium docusate. This might then be fol-lowed by an osmotic laxative (e.g. macrogols (Movicol) or polyethylene glycol (Laxido)) or a bulking agent (e.g. ispaghula husk (Fybogel)) if she is able to increase her fluid intake. As she is being managed palliatively, co-danthramer may also be used: this is a combination of dantron, a stimulant, and poloxamer, a stool softener. Dantron is contraindicated in non-palliative patients due to adverse effects. Another alternative if standard laxatives do not work is the newer agent methylnaltrexone, which has been developed specifically for opioid-induced constipation. It acts as a peripheral opioid-receptor antagonist.

SHORT CASE

Mr Nikolaidis is a 68-year-old man who is referred to his local hospital by his GP because of his constipation. On arrival, he relates to the junior doctor that he often finds it hard to open his bowels, but that things are different this time: he has been unable to open his bowels for 2 days and he has developed severe, 'crampy' pains all over his lower abdomen which are worse after any food or cups of tea. He denies feeling sick, but admits he has probably not passed any wind for the last 48 hours either. His past medical history is remarkable for bilateral hip replacements and a right inguinal hernia, which was repaired 2 years ago. He is otherwise fit and well and does not take any regular medications.

On examination, Mr Nikolaidis has dry lips, a heart rate of 110 bpm (regular), a blood pressure of 115/78 mmHg, respiratory rate of 15/min, and temperature of 36.8 °C. His abdomen is distended, tympanic to percussion, and bowel sounds are present, albeit high pitched. No masses or organomegaly are palpable. A digital rectal examination reveals an empty rectum. His cardiovascular and respiratory examinations are unremarkable and his neurological system appears grossly intact.

The junior doctor arranges for an abdominal radiograph of Mr Nikolaidis, which is shown in Figure 19.4.

Figure 19.4 Abdominal radiograph for Mr Nikolaidis.

What is the most likely diagnosis? How will Mr Nikolaidis be managed?

Mr Nikolaidis has presented with most of the clinical features of bowel obstruction:

- Absolute constipation (no faeces or flatus passed)
- Colicky abdominal pain
- Distended abdomen
- Nausea and vomiting (this is mainly seen in *small* bowel obstruction).

The best way to confirm bowel obstruction is a plain abdominal radiograph. Small bowel loops with a diameter >3 cm, or large bowel loops with a diameter >6 cm, indicate bowel obstruction. Large bowel loops with a diameter >9 cm indicate risk of imminent perforation and the need for urgent surgery. Mr Nikolaidis's abdominal radiograph shows dilated loops of large bowel, confirming **large bowel obstruction**. This is usually due to mechanical obstruction by a colorectal tumour, sigmoid volvulus (twisting of the sigmoid colon), or inflamed diverticula (diverticulitis), but can be due to functional causes (e.g. hypothyroidism). Mr Nikolaidis's radiograph shows the 'coffee bean' sign (an enormous dilated loop of bowel, shaped like a coffee bean and extending from the pelvis up to the diaphragm), caused by the sigmoid portion of the bowel twisting on itself. Thus, Mr Nikolaidis has **sigmoid volvulus**.

Management of sigmoid volvulus involves:

- **'Drip and suck'.** The patient is placed nil by mouth, a nasogastric tube is inserted, and intravenous (IV) fluids are given, all in an effort to rest the bowel and replace the fluids and electrolytes that are building up in the obstructed bowel.

- **Removal of the obstruction.** In sigmoid volvulus, this is done using a sigmoidoscope with a long, soft flatus tube to untwist and decompress the bowel, or surgery if this is unsuccessful or the patient is peritonitic. In colorectal cancer, a metallic stent can be used to relieve the obstruction until the tumour is removed surgically. In diverticulitis, reduction of the inflammation with bowel rest and antibiotics may be enough to reduce the obstruction, although surgical resection is occasionally necessary.

Viva questions

What are the main advantages and disadvantages of the following methods for visualizing colon masses?

1. Rigid sigmoidoscopy
2. Flexible sigmoidoscopy
3. Colonoscopy
4. CT colon
5. CT colonography ('virtual colonoscopy' or 'CT pneumocolon')
6. DCBE

1. **Rigid sigmoidoscopy**
   - **Advantages:** quick, can be performed on the wards with minimal expertise, and allows both visualization of the rectum and biopsy taking.
   - **Disadvantages:** will only visualize the rectum, thus missing many masses.
2. **Flexible sigmoidoscopy**
   - **Advantages:** allows visualization and biopsy as far as the splenic flexure, which is not bad given that 60–75% of sporadic, non-familial colorectal cancers will be in the left colon. Only limited bowel preparation required.
   - **Disadvantages:** will obviously miss 25–40% of sporadic colorectal cancers and a greater proportion of familial ones. Invasive procedure so associated with a (very) small risk of bowel perforation.
3. **Colonoscopy**
   - **Advantages:** allows visualization and biopsy of the entire colon.
   - **Disadvantages:** uncomfortable as it requires the bowel to be filled with gas (gas insufflation) and has a risk of 1/500 for GI bleeding, 1/1000 for bowel perforation, and 1/10 000 for death. Requires 2 days of special diet ('bowel preparation') to empty the bowel of its contents, which may be poorly tolerated, especially in elderly, frail patients or those with major comorbidities. Limited visibility if bowel preparation is inadequate.
4. **CT colon**
   - **Advantages:** rapid and non-invasive visualization of the entire colon. Does not involve any bowel preparation and is thus suitable for frail patients.
   - **Disadvantages:** does not allow for biopsies and has a poorer sensitivity at detecting lesions than CT colonography because of the lack of bowel preparation (it can be hard to distinguish a malignant lesion from faeces).
5. **CT colonography** (aka virtual colonoscopy/CT pneumocolon)
   - **Advantages:** quick. Because it visualizes all the organs of the abdomen (rather than just the bowel lumen), it allows one to assess the degree of invasion of any bowel masses and look for masses in other organs, therefore allowing one not only to identify a cancer (e.g. colon, ovarian) but also assess how far it has spread (staging) all in one go.
   - **Disadvantages:** does not allow for biopsies. Also requires uncomfortable bowel preparation and gas insufflation. The radiation probably *contributes* to fatal cancer in about 1/2000 patient scans (0.05%). This may sound like a lot, but fatal cancer is so common (20%) that this would only increase the risk from 20% to 20.05%.
6. **DCBE**
   - Rarely used nowadays; included for historical reference and completeness.

Why is constipation very common after surgery?

The combination of anaesthesia, opiate analgesia, and (in abdominal surgery) bowel manipulation often sends the bowel into a state of paralysis called *ileus*. Electrolyte disturbances (e.g. hypokalae-mia, hypomagnesaemia) can further exacerbate this situation. On top of this, patients may find it difficult to pass faeces because of pain or the embarrassment of having to use a commode on the public wards.

Postoperative ileus is usually self-limiting, with normal peristalsis returning 24–72 hours after surgery.

The risk of postoperative ileus can be minimized by: using local/epidural anaesthesia where pos-sible; minimizing opiate analgesia (e.g. by using more local anaesthetics); minimizing bowel manipu-lation; and encouraging early mobilization of patients.

What staging classifications do you know for colon cancer?

Cancers are often staged using the international **TNM classification**[†] which, at its most basic, stands for:

Tumour size: scored from 1–4 depending on either size or local invasion.

Nodes: scored from 0 (none) to 3 (many and distant) depending on the lymph nodes affected by the cancer.

Metastasis: scored either 0 (none) or 1 (present) depending on spread of cancer in other organs.

Some cancers also have specific staging systems. For colon cancer, the older **Dukes classification**[*] is still often used:

Dukes A	No spread into muscularis propria
Dukes B	Tumour invading beyond muscularis propria
Dukes C	Tumour spread to lymph nodes
Dukes D	Tumour metastasized to other organs (although, curiously, there was no stage D in the original Dukes classification).

[†] Data from National Cancer Institute, USA. <http://www.cancer.gov/cancertopics/factsheet/detection/staging>

[*] Data from Dukes CE, 'The classification of cancer of the rectum', *Journal of Pathological Bacteriology*, 1932, **35**, p. 323

How is the Dukes staging system used for guiding management and prognosis?

Dukes A

- 90% survival at 5 years.

- Such patients are offered **surgical removal** of the tumour-affected portion of bowel, together with its enveloping blood vessels, adipose tissue, and lymph nodes (assuming they are fit enough). This was traditionally done via a laparotomy but is increasingly done laparascopically as studies have shown this is just as effective but has fewer complications in expert hands. Indeed, patients having a laparoscopic colectomy are often walking and eating with 24 hours

CONTINUED   ➤

CONTINUED

of surgery. Some studies suggest that the use of preoperative **radiotherapy** may further improve survival rates if the cancer is *rectal* but note that radiotherapy is not done if the tumour is proximal to the rectum as there is then a risk of damaging the highly radiosensitive small bowel.

Dukes B and C

- Approximately 65% and 30–45% survival at 5 years, respectively.
- Such patients will be offered **surgical removal** of the tumour plus multidrug adjuvant **chemotherapy.** Some patients with *rectal* tumours may also get preoperative **radiotherapy**. Multiple chemotherapy agents are needed because colon cancers are intrinsically very resistant to chemotherapy. This is a reflection of their adaptation to constant exposure to toxins in the diet (e.g. they naturally express multidrug efflux pumps such as P-glycoprotein).

Dukes D

- Approximately 5–10% survival at 5 years.
- Treatment in such patients is largely **palliative.** Patients may have surgical resection of the tumour and larger metastases (e.g. liver), chemotherapy (standard or experimental), stenting of the tumour if the patient is unfit for resection surgery, and/or palliative radiotherapy.

Patients often ask what can be done to reduce the risk of colon cancer when one of their family members has been diagnosed with this condition. Do you know of any key studies that have investigated modifiable risk factors for colorectal cancer?

- **Smoking: the Physicians Health Study**[1] and the **Women's Health Initiative**[2] study both found that smoking was an important, independent risk factor for colorectal cancer.
- **Exercise and obesity:** the observational, prospective **Nurses' Health Study**[3] found that people who exercise regularly (>4 hours a week) and are not obese were about 40% less likely to develop colorectal cancer than people who are sedentary (<1 hour of exercise a week) and obese. The link appears to be independent of healthy lifestyle factors often associated with people who regularly exercise and are not obese (e.g. they are less likely to smoke).
- **Fibre:** there remains a split on this topic in the literature, with some meta-analyses finding a reduced risk and others finding no difference.
- **Other dietary factors:** many studies have looked at the relationship between other details of dietary intake (e.g. red meat, saturated fats, fresh vegetables) and colorectal cancer. The short answer is that the data from these studies are contradictory. This probably reflects the fact that people's diets are complex and that the contribution of any one type of food to colorectal cancer may be too small to detect using an observational study. In lung cancer, the contribution of smoking is sufficiently large to avoid being confounded in observational studies. However, in colorectal cancer, the contribution of red meat or saturated fats may be small and therefore easily masked by other confounding factors (e.g. people who eat less red meat may eat more soya products, and both may increase the risk of colorectal cancer by a similarly small amount).
- **Aspirin.** The **BDAT** and **UKTIA** studies were randomized controlled trials investigating the role of *high-dose* daily aspirin in the prophylaxis of cerebrovascular thrombosis (TIAs and strokes). A meta-analysis of their data by Flossmann and Rothwell[4] incidentally found that patients on

CONTINUED ➤

CONTINUED

high-dose aspirin were about 50% less likely to develop colorectal cancer. However, the massive **Women's Health Study**[5] and **Physicians Health Study**[6] failed to find any association between *low-dose* aspirin and colorectal cancer.

[1] Sturmer, T, Glynn RJ, Lee IM, Christen WG, Hennekens CH. Lifetime cigarette smoking and colorectal cancer incidence in the Physicians Health Study I. *J Natl Cancer Inst*, 2000;**92**: 1178–1181.

[2] Paskett ED, Reeves KW, Rohan TE, Allison MA, Williams CD, Messina CR, et al. Association between cigarette smoking and colorectal cancer in the Women's Health Initiative. *J Natl Cancer Inst*, 2007;**99**: 1729–1735.

[3] Wolin KY, Lee IM, Colditz GA, Glynn RJ, Fuchs C, Giovannucci E. Leisure-time physical activity patterns and risk of colon cancer in women. *Int J Cancer*, 2007;**121**: 2776–2781.

[4] Flossmann E, Rothwell PM. Effect of aspirin on long-term risk of colorectal cancer: consistent evidence from randomised and observational studies. *Lancet*, 2007;**369**: 1603–1613.

[5] Cook NR, Lee IM, Gaziano JM, Gordon D, Ridker PM, Manson JE, et al. Low-dose aspirin in the primary prevention of cancer: the Women's Health Study: a randomized controlled trial. *JAMA*, 2005;**294**: 47–55.

[6] Gann PH, Manson JE, Glynn RJ, Buring JE, Hennekens CH. Low-dose aspirin and incidence of colorectal tumors in a randomized trial. *J Natl Cancer Inst*, 1993;**85**: 1220–1224.

Single Best Answers

1. Which of the following drugs is *least* likely to cause constipation?

a. Codeine
b. Amlodipine (a calcium channel blocker)

c. Amitriptyline (a tricyclic antidepressant)
d. Aluminium hydroxide (an antacid)
e. Colchicine → NSAID → induced diarrhoea

2. Which of the following combinations of biochemical parameters is most consistent with primary hyperparathyroidism?

a. Calcium ↑, phosphate ↑, ALP ↑, PTH ↑
b. Calcium ↑, phosphate ↓, ALP ↑, PTH ↓
c. Calcium ↑, phosphate ↓, ALP ↑, PTH ↔

d. Calcium ↑, phosphate ↑, ALP ↑, PTH ↓
e. Calcium ↑, phosphate ↑, ALP ↓, PTH ↓

3. Which of the following is not a cardinal feature of bowel obstruction?

a. Abdominal tenderness
b. Colicky abdominal pain
c. Absolute constipation

d. Vomiting
e. Abdominal distension

4. A histology report for a resected colon carcinoma reports that there is invasion through the muscularis propria and involvement of local lymph nodes. What Dukes stage is this tumour?

a. A
b. B
c. C

d. D
e. E

5. The sigmoid colon derives its arterial supply from which branch of the abdominal aorta?

a. Sigmoid artery
b. Left colic artery
c. Inferior mesenteric artery

d. Superior mesenteric artery
e. Coeliac trunk

Diarrhoea

Core case

Read through the sections in the case boxes, covering up the sections that follow so that you don't see the answer. At the end of each case box, try to answer the question before reading on.

> Miss Bowles is an 18-year-old university student referred by her GP to the local hospital because of diarrhoea which has been going on for 5 days. The word 'diarrhoea' means different things to different patients.
>
> **What is the clinical definition of diarrhoea? What are the main causes of diarrhoea?**

Strictly speaking, diarrhoea is an increase in the amount of stool passed daily to over 300 g of stool per day. This is usually accompanied by increased frequency and loosening of the stools. However, many patients will talk of 'diarrhoea' when they actually have *melaena* (dark, tarry stools from digested blood), *steatorrhoea* (pale, floating stools from undigested lipid), *haematochezia* (bright red stools from frank blood), or simply *loose stools* (soft faeces but no increase in frequency or quantity).

Diarrhoea can be caused by:

- Infection of the bowel (infectious diarrhoea)
- Inflammation of the bowel (e.g. inflammatory bowel disease (IBD), diverticular disease)
- Increased bowel motility (e.g. hyperthyroidism, anxiety, irritable bowel syndrome (IBS))
- Malabsorption of nutrients (e.g. coeliac disease, pancreatic insufficiency)
- Obstruction overflow due to a mass allowing only liquid stool to pass beyond it (e.g. constipation—counterintuitively, hard faeces stuck in the bowel are a common cause of overflow diarrhoea in elderly people, colon cancer, ovarian cancer)
- Medications (e.g. laxatives, colchicine, digoxin, metformin, thiazide diuretics, some antibiotics, etc.)

> The GP referral letter explains that for the last 3 days, Miss Bowles has been going to the toilet five times a day and passing soft, watery faeces that do not contain blood and are of normal colour.
>
> **What is your differential diagnosis for diarrhoea in a patient of this age? Try organizing your differential in order of likelihood.**

For a young adult with acute diarrhoea, the most likely diagnoses are shown in Figure 20.1.

Infective diarrhoea
Irritable bowel syndrome (IBS)
Coeliac disease
Crohn's disease
Ulcerative colitis (UC)
Medications (e.g. antibiotics, laxatives)
Hyperthyroidism

Figure 20.1 Differential diagnoses of acute diarrhoea in a young adult.

Would your differential diagnosis look different if the patient was 64 years old?

Yes, it would. In elderly patients, neoplastic disease (villous polyps, colonic adenocarcinoma, pancreatic cancer), diverticular disease, overflow diarrhoea secondary to constipation, ischaemic colitis, microscopic colitis, and bacterial overgrowth (e.g. in patients with diabetes mellitus) are much more likely, whereas coeliac disease is less likely to present for the first time (as it tends to present in younger patients). Curiously, ulcerative colitis (UC) and Crohn's disease are thought to have a bimodal distribution in incidence, with peaks at 15–25 and 50–80 years.

The fact that the GP has referred a patient with diarrhoea to the hospital suggests that they feel the patient is ill enough to warrant in-hospital management and investigations.

Given the 3-day history of diarrhoea, how will you manage this patient before taking a history? Is there anything in particular you are concerned about?

- **Airway, breathing, and circulation (ABC):** always, always, always start the management of a patient with ABC. Although the ABCs will be obviously normal in a large number of patients presenting in a non-emergency setting, you should always keep this in mind when admitting patients to hospital. Note that hypotension is a late and worrying sign in young patients.

- **Dehydration:** in a patient with a 3-day history of diarrhoea, one should be concerned about the possibility of dehydration (hypovolaemia). Dehydration is the main cause of morbidity and mortality in this patient group, so check the heart rate (tachycardia?), the blood pressure (postural drop, narrow mean arterial pressure, or low blood pressure?), mucous membranes (coated tongue, dry lips?), and whether the patient feels thirsty.

- **Electrolyte or pH disturbance:** these can occur either due to excessive loss of ions (e.g. K^+, HCO_3^-) in the faeces, or secondary to the hypovolaemia and ischaemia of tissues (e.g. hyperkalaemia in response to a metabolic acidosis caused by ischaemia). If the patient appears to be *in extremis*, the quickest way to obtain information on both electrolytes and pH is an arterial or venous blood gas. If the patient's respiration appears clinically unimpaired and their oxygen saturations are good (94–98% on air), you can avoid the discomfort (pain!) of inflicting an arterial blood gas on your patient as a venous sample will give you the electrolytes and pH.

Miss Bowles looks unwell: she has dry, pale lips and looks tired. Her airways are clear (she can talk) and her breathing is fast at 20/min with oxygen saturations on air of 98%. Her heart rate is 110 bpm (regular), her blood pressure is 95/70 mmHg, and her temperature is 36.8 °C. Venous blood gas shows:

pH	7.32
HCO_3^-	17 mM
Na^+	134 mM
K^+	3.1 mM
Cl^-	101 mM
Glucose	6.1 mM

How would you interpret these clinical and biochemical findings?

Miss Bowles has:

- **Shock (tachycardic and hypovolaemic).** This patient has diarrhoea, tachycardia and hypotension so she is clinically shocked and therefore critically unwell. Young (especially female) patients can have a naturally low blood pressure, and anxiety can cause a slight tachycardia, but beware—anxiety causing tachycardia would also cause a rise in blood pressure, and anxiety should always be a diagnosis of exclusion made by someone senior.

- **Acidosis (pH <7.35).** Her HCO_3 is low (HCO_3 <22 mM) suggesting consumption of the blood's HCO_3 buffer in an attempt to compensate for the acidosis, by shifting the following equation to the left in an attempt to reduce the amount of H^+:

$$CO_2 + H_2O \rightleftharpoons H^+ + HCO_3^-$$

- This is highly likely to be a **metabolic** acidosis given the aetiology (diarrhoea). In broad terms, metabolic acidosis can be due to either gain of acid (H^+), loss of base (HCO_3^-) or both. Her anion gap ($Na^+ + K^+ - Cl^- - HCO_3^-$) is elevated (>18 mM) suggesting the presence of extra acids (e.g. lactic acid? aspirin? ketone bodies?). It is likely that this patient's tissues are ischaemic due to the hypoperfusion and therefore relying on anaerobic glycolysis for energy, producing lactic acidosis.

- **Hypokalaemia.** This patient probably has hypokalaemia due to K^+ loss in the faeces. It is common for patients with diarrhoea to lose multiple electrolytes in their faeces and thus have low K^+, low Na^+, low Cl^-, and low HCO_3^-. If the patient's kidneys are functioning adequately, these can all be corrected by fluid rehydration with the electrolytes (there is no need for bicarbonate).

How will you manage this patient acutely?

This patient is essentially **dehydrated** due to her ongoing diarrhoea. She therefore needs a cannula placed, bloods taken (so you don't have to bleed her again later), and fluids given. One way to administer fluids is orally, but the fact that she is hypovolaemic after 3 days suggests she is not managing to hydrate orally. The alternative is therefore intravenous (IV) fluid. At this stage, one could give a 'fluid challenge' of 500 mL of a crystalloid solution (e.g. Hartmann's, Plasmalyte, normal saline) and then reassess the patient's blood pressure after 30 minutes. If her blood pressure remains low, she needs more fluids. If her blood pressure has improved you can switch to providing maintenance fluids IV or orally.

The metabolic acidosis will correct with adequate restoration of fluid balance, assuming her kidney function is normal.

Miss Bowles responded well to 2 × 500 mL fluid challenge, with her blood pressure rising to 105/75 mmHg and her heart rate dropping to 98 bpm.

What would you like to know about Miss Bowles' history?

It is tempting to ask a broad and comprehensive set of questions but instead, think of your differential diagnosis and ask questions that will provide important clues pointing you towards or away from each diagnosis.

Characterize the stool

- **Are the faeces mucoid or jelly-like?** This classically suggests infection by *Salmonella* or villous polyps in the colon, but can be seen in any disease causing inflammation of the bowel wall.
- **Are they foul smelling and floating?** This suggests malabsorption, due to coeliac disease, pancreatic duct obstruction (pancreatic cancer, cystic fibrosis), or biliary insufficiency (e.g. recent cholecystectomy).
- **Are the faeces unusually pale?** This suggests lack of bile salts in the faeces due to obstruction of the biliary or pancreatic ducts (e.g. chronic pancreatitis, gallstones).
- **Are the faeces bloody?** (this is rarely the case) If so, can the patient describe their faeces?
  - If the blood is only on the paper when they wipe, or the faeces are streaked with blood, it suggests anal pathology (e.g. anal fissure, haemorrrhoids).
  - If the blood is red and mixed in with the faeces it suggests colorectal pathology (e.g. UC, dysentery, colorectal carcinoma).

Ask about her bowel habit

- **Is there nocturnal diarrhoea?** If so, this suggests an 'organic' aetiology (rather than a 'functional' aetiology as in IBS).
- **Does she ever find herself having to rush to the toilet to pass motions?** Urgency to defecate is suggestive of infectious diarrhoea or IBD.
- **After passing motions, does she ever feel that she hasn't fully evacuated her bowel?** This sensation is called tenesmus and is suggestive of a space-occupying lesion in the rectum (e.g. carcinoma).
- **Has she had a variable bowel habit?** Both IBS (in younger patients) and colorectal cancer (in older patients) can present as an altered bowel habit that alternates between diarrhoea, normal stools and constipation.
- **How often does she suffer from diarrhoea?** Infectious diarrhoea is typically a one-off event (although we will nearly all have had this at some point), whereas other pathologies are usually recurrent. However, remember that chronic diseases still have to present for the first time!

Ask about associated symptoms

- **Has there been any vomiting?** This suggests an infectious gastroenteritis.
- **Has there been any abdominal pain?**
  - Pain in the right iliac fossa associated with diarrhoea is suggestive of terminal ileum inflammation (e.g. Crohn's disease, *Yersinia enterocolitica* infection).
  - Pain in the left iliac fossa associated with diarrhoea is suggestive of diverticular disease.
  - Pain relieved by passing motions is suggestive of IBS.

- **Has she noticed any (significant) weight loss?** Try to quantify this in terms of amount over which time period. Significant weight loss over months suggests a chronic pathological process, e.g. IBD, rather than an acute pathology, e.g. infection.

- **Has she had any eye problems, joint pains, or skin rashes?** Uveitis (painful red eye with loss of vision), scleritis (painful red eye with no loss of vision), episcleritis (uncomfortable red eye with no loss of vision), enteric arthritis, erythema nodosum (painful, dark red nodules on shins), and pyoderma gangrenosum (ulcers with a surrounding purple halo) are all associated with IBD (UC and Crohn's disease).

Ask about risk factors for causes of diarrhoea

- **Has she been abroad recently? Has she eaten anything unusual? Does she know other people with similar symptoms?** Foreign travel and eating certain types of meals (e.g. barbeques, kebabs…) are significant risk factors for infectious diarrhoea. Knowing other people with similar symptoms at the same time is also suggestive of an infectious aetiology.

- **Has she been stressed as of late? What is her diet like?** Stress and a low-fibre diet are associated with IBS.

- **What medications does she take? Have these changed recently?** Remember that diarrhoea is one of the commonest side effects of all oral medications. Look out in particular for antibiotics and proton pump inhibitors (PPIs), which are associated with *Clostridium difficile* diarrhoea.

Ask about her family history

- **Family history of bowel disease?** Is there a family history of Crohn's disease, UC, coeliac disease, or rarer conditions such as hereditary non-polyposis colorectal cancer (HNPCC)?

The questions listed above can help to narrow your differential diagnosis. However, it is also helpful for management to find out whether the patient is still eating and drinking and what medications they have tried for their diarrhoea (e.g. loperamide? oral rehydration salts?).

Miss Bowles is in her first year of university, where she is studying French and Spanish. She says the course is going well. It is the first time she has been away from home but she is not finding it hard. Her main concern is that she will have some illness that will stop her from playing lacrosse with the university team, of which she is vice-captain.

Four days ago she developed pain in her abdomen. The pain was dull and started in the right lower quadrant of her abdomen, before becoming more generalized and giving her cramps that were bad enough to make her curl up in bed. The diarrhoea also came on 3 days ago and has persisted since. She has been passing watery faeces about five times a day. She has had five similar episodes of abdominal pain and diarrhoea over the past year, although they have always been milder and resolved within 2 days. She has been well between episodes, but this episode has left her feeling 'very ill and run down'. She has not vomited, has not noticed any weight loss (although she is fairly slim), and her diarrhoea has always been watery, but never bloody, mucoid, or particularly foul smelling. Passing faeces or wind does not relieve her abdominal pain, which she recalls often starts in her lower right quadrant. She cannot recall eating anything unusual before her symptoms started, and she is a vegetarian who usually cooks for herself. Nobody else in her house or group of friends has been affected at any stage. She has not felt hot or hungry (if anything, she feels 'cold and sleepy'). She has not had any eye problems other than being short-sighted and has not had any joint pains. She has noticed 'a few red marks on my shins when I shave my legs' but thought these were either knocks from lacrosse training or a rash from the shaving cream. She is single and has not been sexually active in the past year.

Miss Bowles has never been to hospital before, and until today, had only ever gone to her GP for 'the usual checks and vaccines'. She takes echinacea drops diluted in hot water when she has a cold but otherwise uses no regular medications. She is not allergic to anything as far as she knows. Her parents and two older brothers are all alive and well, although she thinks her father (aged 52) may have angina. One of her grandmothers is alive but has 'arthritis'; her other grandparents all died of 'old age'.

This history is not suggestive of any one diagnosis in particular, but it does make some pathologies more likely and some less likely.

Try rearranging your original differential diagnosis in order of likelihood given Miss Bowles' history (see Figure 20.2).

Irritable bowel syndrome (IBS)	There is no suggestion of anxiety or depression in the history but this is nonetheless the most common cause of recurrent diarrhoea in young females
Coeliac disease	
Crohn's disease	A strong possibility given the right iliac fossa pain and the suggestion of shin marks which may be erythema nodosum
Ulcerative colitis (UC)	Less likely in the absence of bloody diarrhoea
Infective diarrhoea	Less likely given the relapsing/remitting symptoms over past year
Hyperthyroidism	Less likely as her symptoms are relapsing/remitting

Figure 20.2 Refined differential diagnosis for Miss Bowles.

Is there anything in particular you will look for during your examination of Miss Bowles?

Figure 20.3 shows the features to look for on examination of a patient with diarrhoea.

- **Clubbing?** Crohn's disease, UC, hyperthyroidism, and coeliac disease are causes of nail clubbing although in practice this association is rarely seen as few patients in developed countries with these diseases get unwell enough for long enough to develop clubbing.

- **Iritis** (aka anterior uveitis)? **Episcleritis? Scleritis?** Look for signs of these eye diseases, which are associated with both Crohn's disease and UC.

- **Mouth ulcers?** Crohn's disease produces ulcers anywhere in the gastrointestinal (GI) tract—from mouth to anus.

- **Erythema nodosum?** Both Crohn's disease and UC are systemic inflammatory diseases that can manifest in the skin in the form of erythema nodosum (tender, raised, red nodules) or, less commonly, pyoderma gangrenosum (necrotic ulcers). However, bear in mind that the combined oral contraceptive pill is also a common cause of erythema nodosum in young women.

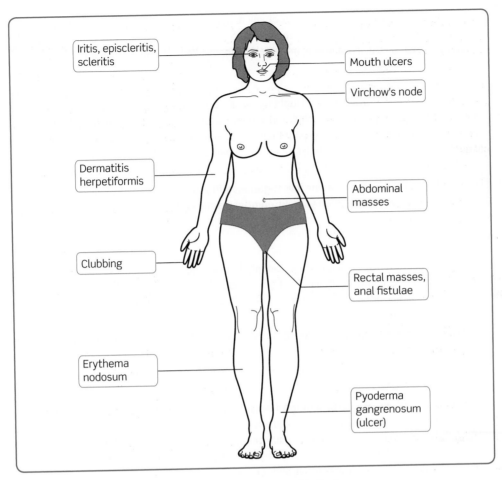

Figure 20.3 Features to look for on examination of a patient with diarrhoea.

- **Dermatitis herpetiformis?** Coeliac disease is often associated with an itchy rash known as dermatitis herpetiformis. The rash is typically found over the extensor surfaces of the limbs and over the scalp. The rash is very itchy, so its papules are usually raw or crusted from the patient scratching them.
- **Virchow's lymphadenopathy?** The stomach and small and large bowel all have lymphatic drainage that travels via the central thoracic duct and joins the venous system in the left subclavian vein. Lymphadenopathy in the left supraclavicular fossa (Troisier's sign) is strongly suggestive of bowel malignancy that has spread.
- **Abdominal masses?** A mass in the right lower quadrant is often found in Crohn's disease (due to inflammation of the terminal ileum). Masses elsewhere in the abdomen, in particular the left lower quadrant, could indicate a malignancy.
- **Anal ulcers or fistulae?** Crohn's disease can cause both ulcers and fistulae around the anus, and the patient may well be unaware of these so be sure to inspect for them.

- **Digital rectal examination.** This is part of any abdominal examination and should be performed in the presence of a chaperone. You are looking for causes of obstruction that could lead to over-flow diarrhoea, specifically a malignant rectal carcinoma. You are also looking at the faeces themselves: are they mucoid or bloody?

> On examination, Miss Bowles has no clubbing, no red eyes, and no mouth ulcers. Her shins have a few red marks that are slightly raised and tender to touch, suggesting they may be erythema nodosum. Her abdomen is tender to palpation throughout but no masses are palpable. A digital rectal examination reveals an empty rectum with no palpable masses, and there are no anal ulcers or fistulae.
>
> **Given this examination, what first-line investigations will you arrange? Think of investigations that can help rule in or exclude items on your differential diagnosis list.**

Blood tests

- **Full blood count (FBC):** coeliac disease, Crohn's disease, and UC can all cause anaemia from malabsorption of iron, folate, or vitamin B_{12}; from GI blood loss caused by the disease (especially UC); or from the chronic disease process per se. They can also cause a high platelet count as this is an inflammatory marker.
- **Erythrocyte sedimentation rate (ESR):** Crohn's disease and UC are systemic inflammatory diseases and usually lead to elevated ESR.
- **C-reactive protein (CRP):** infectious diarrhoea, Crohn's disease, and UC can all cause a rise in CRP levels.
- **Tissue transglutaminase (TTG) and IgA levels:** a positive result has a sensitivity and specificity of over 90% for coeliac disease. You should always check the IgA levels, too, as IgA deficiency can cause false negative results. Antiendomysial antibodies can be used instead of TTG but are more susceptible to IgA deficiency causing false negatives. Antigliadin antibodies have been used to test for coeliac disease but are less sensitive and specific.
- **Thyroid function tests (TFTs):** a low thyroid-stimulating hormone (TSH) and a high tri-iodothyronine/thyroxine (T_3/T_4) level would strongly suggest hyperthyroidism.
- **Urea and electrolytes (U&Es):** the patient may be dehydrated or suffering electrolyte disturbances from the diarrhoea itself (loss of ions) or secondary to acidaemia caused by hypoperfusion and ischaemia.
- **Albumin:** this will be low in patients with chronic diarrhoea and malabsorption, e.g. IBD.
- **Capillary glucose:** a simple bedside blood glucose test will tell you if this patient is diabetic. While diarrhoea would be an unusual presenting complaint for diabetes mellitus, it is easy to exclude.

Faeces tests

- **Faeces microscopy and culture:** infection is still a possibility and should be excluded by the microbiologists. Pus cells may be visible and can indicate inflammation in IBD. Remember that *Giardia* can be very hard to visualize under the microscope even if it is present (i.e. false negative).
- ***C difficile* toxin test:** The patient has no history of antibiotic use that would predispose her to *C. difficile* infection. However, if the patient did have recent antibiotic use, you should consider testing for *C. difficile* toxin.

- **Faecal occult blood test (FOBT):** the patient may not have overt blood in the faeces, but may have blood detectable using a FOBT. This would point towards infection or UC, and away from hyperthyroidism, coeliac disease, and IBS. However, this should only be requested after stopping any drugs that can cause bleeding (e.g. aspirin, warfarin), as these will give a false positive result. If they cannot be stopped, a positive result does not help the diagnosis and therefore you should not order the test.

Miss Bowles is admitted to hospital for fluid resuscitation and observation. Her blood tests on admission reveal:

Haematology		Biochemistry			
Hb	108 g/L	Na	135 mM	TSH	2 mU/L
WCC	8.9×10^9 cells/L	K	3.2 mM	T_4	8 µg/dL
Platelets	300×10^9 cells/L	Urea	10.9 mM		
MCV	98 fL	Creatinine	82 µM		
		Antiendomysial antibodies	Negative		

Her FOBT is negative. Stool is sent off for microscopy and culture.

What is the most likely diagnosis in light of these results? What investigations could be arranged to confirm the diagnosis?

Although infection is still a possibility (pending the results of the stool sample), the raised ESR implies chronicity. Combined with the anaemia and erythema nodosum, this is most consistent with a diagnosis of **IBD** (either Crohn's disease, UC, or indeterminate colitis). The blood tests helped rule out hyperthyroidism and coeliac disease. IBS is largely a diagnosis of exclusion: although statistically the most common cause of recurrent diarrhoea in young females, it would not usually cause diarrhoea severe enough to warrant hospitalization for fluid resuscitation.

In Miss Bowles' case, the lack of bloody diarrhoea and the fact that the abdominal pain often starts in her right lower quadrant are suggestive of **Crohn's disease**. In UC, the pain is usually diffuse and the diarrhoea is often bloody. In addition, patients with Crohn's disease are more likely to suffer with weight loss and failure to thrive between attacks, whereas patients with UC are more likely to be relatively well between acute attacks.

Crohn's disease is believed to be due to mutations in genes responsible for clearing up phagocytosed bacteria. The inability of macrophages to correctly clear the bacteria they ingest leads to them secreting cytokines that make the immune system try to 'wall off' the aberrant situation, forming a granuloma (a situation analogous to what happens in tuberculosis, where macrophages also have difficulty clearing the mycobacteria). The granuloma leads to chronic inflammation. Locally, this leads to diarrhoea, ulcers, strictures of the bowel, and fistulae between the bowel and other compartments (or the outer world). Associated systemic complications include inflammation of the eyes (iritis, episcleritis, scleritis), the joints (arthritis), and the skin (erythema nodosum); as well as anaemia (either through malabsorption or chronic inflammation per se), weight loss, and fatigue.

The next step is to refer Miss Bowles to the gastroenterology team. They can then arrange for **second-line investigations** to confirm or exclude Crohn's disease, such as:

- **Abdominal (plain) radiograph:** this may show signs of bowel inflammation. Abdominal radiographs are essential for patients with severe UC as they are at risk of toxic megacolon (which can perforate), and this can be detected as a large bowel loop that is >6 cm in diameter.

- **Colonoscopy:** this can help visualize the discrete, interrupted lesions of Crohn's disease (or the diffuse, erythematous inflammation of UC) and allows for biopsies to be taken in search of non-caseating granulomas in the bowel mucosa (the hallmark of Crohn's disease).

- **Double-contrast barium enema (DCBE) radiograph:** with the greater availability of colonoscopy, these are now seldom used in the diagnosis of IBD (except when colonoscopy is not possible, or very occasionally if a tight stricture precludes colonoscopy). When performed, this may show discrete lesions and strictures in the colon, suggestive of Crohn's disease.

Miss Bowles' care was taken over by the gastroenterology team. A colonoscopy was arranged and performed during the same admission, and revealed several discrete linear ulcers in the ascending and transverse colon. Histology of biopsies taken at the time of colonoscopy confirmed the presence of non-caseating granulomas and a diagnosis of Crohn's disease was made.

What types of drugs do you think Miss Bowles will be placed on to help manage her Crohn's disease? Will Miss Bowles be able to continue playing lacrosse?

The symptoms of Crohn's disease are due to chronic activation of the immune system in various tissues (e.g. the bowel wall) and its sequelae (e.g. abscesses, fistulae, strictures, adhesions, perforation). Because of this, immunosuppressant medications are used to treat the symptoms of the disease and keep them at bay. Steroid-sparing immunosuppressants such as methotrexate (a folate antagonist), azathioprine (a purine synthesis inhibitor), or newer medications such as anti-tumour necrosis factor-α (anti-TNFα) monoclonal antibodies (e.g. infliximab), are preferred in the longer term. This is both to avoid steroid-related complications (e.g. diabetes, osteoporosis, cataracts) and because steroids do not modify disease or induce sustained mucosal healing. A significant proportion of Crohn's patients ultimately require surgery to resect the most affected portions of their bowel, although the emphasis is on managing the disease medically because surgery is only a temporary solution and other portions of bowel will ultimately become affected, too.

Miss Bowles can continue to play lacrosse. Indeed, provided her disease becomes well managed, it is likely that she will be able to lead her usual active lifestyle.

Short cases

SHORT CASE

Miss Latham is a 25-year-old research scientist who presents to her local Emergency Department at 6 a.m. on a Sunday morning. The previous night she attended a wedding reception and consumed a wide and varied assortment of foods. Within an hour of getting home she was vomiting. She spent all night on the toilet and came in because she feels very unwell. Her only previous episodes of diarrhoea that she can remember were as a child, but she has otherwise been fit and well until today. She looks pale and clammy, but her heart rate is 80 bpm and her blood pressure is 120/90 mmHg.

What is the most likely diagnosis? What management is required?

The history of a single, acute episode of sudden-onset diarrhoea and vomiting after a meal that was potentially undercooked or allowed to stay warm for long periods of time is highly suggestive of an **infectious diarrhoea** (due to the presence of pathogens) or **food poisoning** (due to the presence of toxins). The onset of symptoms within hours of consuming the meal suggests the pathogen had a pre-formed toxin that can affect the bowel, making *Staphylococcus aureus* or *Bacillus cereus* likely candidates.

For the vast majority of infectious diarrhoea, the only management that is required is adequate oral **rehydration**, staying away from work (and out of hospital) until they have had 48 hours without diarrhoea (many patients return sooner out of feeling guilty at not working, but this potentially contributes to spreading of the causative pathogens and hence outbreaks of viral diarrhoea) and good hand hygiene at home to prevent spread to their family. While they are in the Emergency Department, appropriate infection control measures should be followed (e.g. gown and gloves on entering the room, hand washing with soap rather than alcohol gel). Rehydration can be achieved by encouraging the patient to drink water with dissolved **oral rehydration salts**, obtainable at any pharmacy and to be taken 'little and often'. You should emphasize to the patient that these are much better than water because they also contain the electrolytes lost in the diarrhoea, and glucose which helps reabsorb water faster (the glucose importer in the gut co-imports Na^+, which in turn drives water absorption by osmosis). Consider IV fluids only if the patient becomes severely dehydrated or unable to tolerate oral fluids. Most infectious diarrhoeas resolve within 48 hours, and only if they persist should microbiological analysis of the faeces and antibiotics be considered.

SHORT CASE

Miss Webb is a 22-year-old woman who presents for the fourth time in 3 months to her GP practice complaining of recurrent diarrhoea and abdominal pain. You are the locum GP and have never met this patient, so she explains that for the past year she has had bouts of diarrhoea and abdominal crampy pain every couple of weeks. The abdominal pain is diffuse and hard to localize, appearing in different places at different times. It is relieved on defecation. These bouts of diarrhoea and pain are interspersed by weeks where her faeces are often small and hard to pass. Her medical notes reveal that recent investigations have found a normal thyroid function, negative antiendomysial antibodies, a normal FBC and ESR, and no weight loss in the past year. Miss Webb appears anxious and when asked if anything else is wrong, she admits she is finding it hard to get over a break-up with a long-term boyfriend.

What is the most likely diagnosis? How will you manage this patient?

The most likely cause of recurrent diarrhoea in an anxious female patient in the absence of other obvious pathology is **IBS**. The pathophysiology of IBS is unclear, although it is clearly linked to stress, anxiety, and depression. The diagnosis is largely one of exclusion, avoiding over-investigation of the patient and emphasizing that you expect any investigations undertaken to be normal, as they are done to *exclude* other pathologies rather than to diagnose IBS. Diagnosis of IBS is based on the ROME III criteria[*]:

- At least 3 months, with onset at least 6 months previously of recurrent abdominal pain or discomfort associated with two or more of the following:
  - Improvement with defecation; and/or
  - Onset associated with a change in frequency of stool; and/or
  - Onset associated with a change in form (appearance) of stool.

There is no known cure for IBS. Management consists of:

- **Reassurance:** patients benefit greatly from reassurance that they do not have any serious bowel pathology.

- **Antispasmodics:** medications that decrease smooth muscle activity in the bowel (e.g. mebeverine, hyoscine) can alleviate symptoms of IBS. Loperamide is a particularly strong inhibitor of smooth muscle activity in the bowel and should be reserved only for acute episodes of diarrhoea.

- **Antidepressants:** tricyclic antidepressant medications (e.g. amitriptyline) have been found to slow colonic transit time and alleviate symptoms of IBS at doses that are lower than those required for their antidepressive effect, suggesting their effect in IBS is independent of any effect on depression. It is important that the patient understands that using medications that are given at higher doses to other patients for depression does not imply they are depressed.

- **Diet and herbal remedies:** many patients report improvement by avoiding certain foods (e.g. beans that cause bloating), increasing the fibre content in their diet, or by using certain herbal drinks (e.g. peppermint tea).

SHORT CASE

Mrs Adams is an 82-year-old woman who is on a general medical ward at her local hospital, receiving antibiotics for community-acquired pneumonia. She was diagnosed with Alzheimer's disease a year ago. Four months ago she fractured her right neck of femur and had it repaired with a dynamic hip screw. The nurse has called to inform you that Mrs Adams is suffering from 'explosive diarrhoea' and they are having to change her bed hourly. When you arrive, you find a frail old lady who appears delirious. Her lips are dry, her eyes are sunken, her pulse is 100 bpm and her blood pressure is 105/70 mmHg.

What diagnosis should you be worried about? How will you manage this patient?

An elderly (and therefore inevitably immunosuppressed to some extent) patient receiving antibiotics is a high-risk candidate for letting the *Clostridium difficile* that naturally populates our guts grow out of control, become pathogenic, and start producing its toxin. You should be worried that this patient may have developed *C. difficile* **colitis**. Early management is essential and should include:

1 **ABC:** this woman's blood pressure is low for an elderly patient and her mucous membranes are dry, suggesting she is indeed hypovolaemic, which is unsurprising if the nurses are having to change her

[*] © The Rome Foundation

bed every hour due to diarrhoea. She needs IV fluid resuscitation urgently (e.g. 250 mL boluses of IV crystalloid until clinical signs and blood pressure suggest she is no longer hypovolaemic).

2 **Faeces analysis:** send a stool sample off immediately to microbiology for microscopy, culture, and analysis for *C. difficile* toxin.

3 **Isolation:** an obvious, effective, and simple solution to preventing the spread of pathogenic *C. difficile* on the wards, but one that is often hard to implement in many overcrowded and under-resourced hospitals.

4 **Meticulous hygiene:** all staff and visitors should 'glove and gown' and hands must be washed between patients using warm water and soap (alcohol gels will *not* inactivate *C. difficile* which forms highly durable spores).

5 **Antibiotic treatment:** if the faeces analysis is positive for *C. difficile* toxin, you should start appropriate antibiotic therapy without delay. The latest Health Protection Agency (HPA) guidelines from 2012 advise oral metronidazole for 10–14 days as first line, with oral vancomycin reserved for severe, refractory, or recurrent cases. The newer antibiotic fidaxomicin has recently been licensed for treating *C. difficile*, although for cost reasons should normally be reserved for recurrent or refractory illness.

6 **Address precipitants:** HPA guidelines recommend reviewing medications, in particular antibiotic therapy and PPIs, both of which are associated with *C. difficile* infection, to see if they can be stopped.

7 In severe disease (unlike this case), patients should have regular abdominal radiographs (AXR), lactate measurements and daily surgical review to mitigate against the possibility of toxic megacolon and perforation. Colectomy is required in extreme cases.

SHORT CASE

Mr Singh is a 22-year-old web designer who presents to the Emergency Department complaining of bloody diarrhoea. He has had some discomfort in his left iliac fossa over the past 2 days but, since this morning, he has found himself rushing to the toilet four times and then passing 'lots of blood'. He also describes having to remain on the toilet for some time to 'get it all out'. Despite the dramatic nature of his faeces, he admits he feels relatively well, with no fever, malaise, nausea, or vomiting. He has not lost any weight recently, has not travelled abroad, and does not know anybody else who is also suffering from diarrhoea at the moment. He does not smoke or drink alcohol. Examination of the patient is remarkable only for fresh blood in the rectum on digital rectal examination. His observations are heart rate 90 bpm regular, blood pressure 115/80 mmHg, temperature 36.8°C. His initial blood results are:

Haematology		Biochemistry		Clotting	
Hb	143 g/L	Na	136 mM	PT	13.5 s
WCC	9.2×10^9 cells/L	K	4.1 mM	APTT	34 s
Platelets	185×10^9 cells/L	Urea	5.1 mM		
MCV	98 fL	Creatinine	42 µM		
		ESR	78 mm/h		

Blood is sent off for cultures and stool is sent off for microscopy and culture. A colonoscopy is arranged for the next day and reveals a uniformly inflamed rectum and descending colon, with a clear cut-off point between inflamed and normal bowel at the level of the splenic flexure. Biopsies of the inflamed bowel are taken and histology reports 'inflamed crypts, full of fibrin and PMNs [polymorphonuclear leucocytes]'.

What is the likely diagnosis and why? What other conditions are associated with this disease? How is the disease managed?

It is likely that Mr Singh is suffering from **UC**. This is a form of IBD whose aetiology is unknown. The GI tract is affected in a distal to proximal fashion (i.e. from the rectum upwards) and shows gross, uniform inflammation with a clear cut-off point between abnormal and normal bowel. Patients typically present with painless, bloody diarrhoea.

UC, like Crohn's disease, is actually a systemic inflammatory disease that simply happens to manifest most prominently in the bowel. Like Crohn's disease, the systemic inflammation can affect joints (arthritis, sacroiliitis), eyes (uveitis, scleritis, episcleritis), skin (erythema nodosum), and blood (anaemia of chronic disease). Unlike Crohn's disease, UC has a much stronger association with colonic adenocarcinoma (1% risk per year); primary sclerosing cholangitis (obstructive jaundice and liver failure), and cholangiocarcinoma (cancer of the common bile duct).

Management of UC involves three approaches:

1 **Medical therapy:** UC is a systemic inflammatory disease that responds well to anti-inflammatories. Salicylate derivatives (e.g. sulfasalazine, mesalazine), methotrexate, azathioprine, corticosteroids, and anti-TNF antibodies (e.g. infliximab) can all be used to control the inflammation.

2 **Disease monitoring:** due to the high rates of colonic adenocarcinoma in UC, patients are monitored with colonoscopy for early signs of cancer on a regular basis. When acutely unwell, abdominal radiographs are useful in UC for ensuring there is no toxic megacolon (large bowel dilatation >9 cm in diameter).

3 **Surgical therapy:** surgery for UC involves removing the portion of affected bowel. This approach is potentially curative as it removes the main symptomatic focus of the disease and eliminates the risk of colonic adenocarcinoma. However, the removal of the rectum has traditionally resulted in a lifelong end ileostomy which puts many patients off the idea of surgery. The development of the ileal pouch–anal anastomosis (IPAA), whereby a pouch of ileum is used to fashion a rectum and connected to the anus to allow almost normal defecation, has been an important development in surgery for UC patients.

SHORT CASE

Mrs Thompson is a 78-year-old woman who is currently an in-patient at a geriatric psychiatry unit, where she is being managed for her Lewy body dementia. The nurses have reported to the junior psychiatrist on call that Mrs Thompson has become incontinent of faeces over the past few days, with her uncontrolled motions being extremely liquid in nature. Nobody else in the unit is affected with diarrhoea.

Mrs Thompson is unable to give a coherent history or explain how she feels due to her advanced dementia. You look in the notes and see that she has hypertension and osteoporosis for which she is taking indapamide, alendronate, and a combined vitamin D and calcium tablet. Her past medical history is remarkable for hip replacements 3 and 5 years ago, and for osteoarthritis of the right knee. Examination reveals a thin, cachectic-looking woman. Her abdomen is soft and non-tender but there is a palpable mass in her left iliac fossa that is roughly cylindrical and extends a few centimetres longitudinally. Virchow's node is not palpable. Bowel sounds are present. A digital rectal examination reveals a mass of irregular surface on the posterior wall of the rectum and triggers a gush of fluid faeces and flatus. The faeces are positive for blood when tested with a disposable Hemoccult kit.

What is the likely diagnosis? How does that explain her liquid faeces? What key investigations should Mrs Thompson receive?

Mrs Thompson is elderly and suffering with incontinence of liquid faeces. Despite her incontinence, her left iliac fossa (i.e. descending colon/sigmoid colon) feels full to palpation and a digital rectal examination reveals a rectal mass. Tellingly, the digital rectal examination causes a gush of fluid faeces and flatus. Mrs Thompson is most likely suffering from **overflow diarrhoea**. This is caused by an obstruction that allows only fluid and air to bypass, causing a liquid diarrhoea that is hard to control. The obstruction may be due to a mass within the lumen (e.g. solid, impacted faeces due to dehydration and lack of fibre); a mass within the bowel wall (e.g. colonic adenocarcinoma), or a mass outside the bowel wall (e.g. a large ovarian tumour compressing the bowel).

Mrs Thompson's age, the presence of a mass in her rectum on examination, and positive test for occult blood in her faeces should all alert you to the possibility of rectal carcinoma. Mrs Thompson should be investigated by either flexible sigmoidoscopy or rigid proctosigmoidoscopy looking for rectal masses that can be biopsied. She may also be offered a DCBE, which may reveal an 'apple core sign' in the rectal lumen due to the tumour, or CT colonography which has the advantage of being non-invasive and visualizing the surrounding organs for tumour spread. How far to investigate and treat the suspected colorectal carcinoma in this particular patient will to a large extent depend on the patient's previously expressed wishes, her comorbidities, and her realistic life expectancy. In a patient with advanced dementia, it is unlikely that aggressive surgical or oncological management of a rectal cancer (e.g. surgical resection, radiotherapy, chemotherapy) would have any significant impact on life expectancy or be tolerated. However, interventions aimed at symptomatic relief should still be considered (e.g. stenting of a colonic mass).

SHORT CASE

Mr Cox is a 42-year-old zoology researcher who attends his GP complaining of diarrhoea. For the past few weeks, he has found himself going to the toilet up to six times a day and passing fairly loose (albeit not liquid) motions. He used to open his bowels only once a day and his faeces were 'more solid'. He reports being otherwise well although very busy with work. The GP notices that he is wearing only a T-shirt and has come with no jumper or jacket, despite the fact that it is a cold autumn day outside. When asked about weight loss, Mr Cox says he hadn't noticed any but that he has had to wear his belt tighter despite eating rather a lot recently. His past medical history is unremarkable and he takes no medications. He does not smoke and only drinks the occasional pint of ale when socializing with friends. He lives with his wife and their child, who has cystic fibrosis.

The GP asks Mr Cox to take off his T-shirt so that he can be examined. His heart rate is 110 bpm and regular. A resting tremor is noticed when Mr Cox holds his arms out. His eyes look normal but when asked to follow the GP's finger with his eyes, as it descends in front of him, an obvious lid lag is noted. The neck is normal to palpation and the rest of the examination is normal.

What diagnosis should be suspected? What investigations should the GP arrange?

Mr Cox has presented with increased frequency and softer consistency to his stools. He appears to have heat intolerance and may have lost some weight recently, to judge by him wearing his belt tighter than usual. He has a resting tremor, an obvious lid lag and is tachycardic. Feeling hot, losing weight despite increased appetite and eating, increased frequency of bowel motions, tachycardia, tremor, lid lag (due to the eyelids trying to remain wide open when the patient looks down), and a possibility of hyperactivity ('very busy at work') are all suggestive of excessive sympathetic stimulation throughout the body. The likeliest cause is **hyperthyroidism**, as thyroid hormones make tissues more sensitive to sympathetic stimulation.

The GP should take a blood sample and check Mr Cox's TSH, and T_3 and T_4 levels. In hyperthyroidism, one finds elevated T_3 and T_4 but decreased TSH (due to negative feedback by T_3/T_4 on TSH secretion). If hyperthyroidism is confirmed, one should seek a cause. The most common aetiology is Graves' disease, which can be investigated by looking for a raised antithyroid peroxidase (which is not pathogenic but usually correlates with the presence of the pathogenic thyroid-stimulating antibodies) and a raised ESR in the blood. It is unusual to look for the pathogenic thyroid-stimulating antibodies because of the high cost of the test, but this may be requested in pregnant women with hyperthyroidism because these antibodies can cross the placenta, resulting in a thyrotoxic fetus that would require special care at the time of delivery. If these antibody tests are negative, one should arrange for a scan using radiolabelled iodine or technetium, which may reveal one or more nodules in the thyroid gland. Cold nodules are more likely to be malignant thyroid tumours than hot nodules, although both are still more likely to be benign than malignant.

Viva questions

Patients with IBD (Crohn's disease or UC) can experience a number of complications outside the bowel. What are these complications?

- **Nails:** clubbing of finger nails
- **Eyes:** inflammation leading to iritis (anterior uveitis), episcleritis, or scleritis
- **Skin:** erythema nodosum (inflammation of subcutaneous fat nodules leading to raised, red nodules) or pyoderma gangrenosum (inflammatory ulceration and necrosis of the skin)
- **Joints:** inflammation leading to enteric arthritis
- **Blood:** iron-deficiency anaemia (from blood loss in the bowel, especially in UC), folate or vitamin B_{12} deficiency anaemias (from malabsorption due to irritation of the bowel)
- **Biliary system:** primary sclerosing cholangitis (associated with UC), cholesterol gallstones (due to reduced reabsorption of bile salts by the inflamed bowel, leading to precipitation of insoluble cholesterol)
- **Kidneys:** kidney stones, because fat malabsorption leads to (fat-soluble) Ca^{2+} being sequestered in the bowel. The lack of Ca^{2+} (which usually binds to oxalate in the blood) allows oxalate to precipitate and form stones
- **Bones:** the lack of Ca^{2+} (due to malabsorption of fat) can lead to osteomalacia or even osteoporosis
- **Amyloidosis:** chronic systemic inflammatory disorders can lead to deposition of serum amyloid A protein in multiple organs

Why should patients with UC be offered regular colonoscopies?

Patients with UC are at increased risk (fivefold) of colon cancer, and for this reason they are offered regular colonoscopic studies looking for early signs of malignancy. If malignancy is detected, the usual procedure is to excise the entire colon (colectomy). Traditionally, this resulted in the patient needing a permanent colostomy but modern surgical techniques allow for the creation of a new rectum and preservation of anorectal function by performing an ileorectal anastomosis with an ileal pouch.

A common symptom of hyperthyroidism is increased bowel movements, often resulting in frank diarrhoea. Why does hyperthyroidism cause diarrhoea?

T_3 is a hormone that results in cells expressing more adrenergic receptors and modifying the components of the adrenergic response pathway so that they are more sensitive to catecholamine stimulus. The net result is that cells become more sensitive to catecholamines such as adrenaline and noradrenaline, and therefore more sensitive to sympathetic stimulation. Many physiology textbooks claim that sympathetic stimulation of the bowel results in constipation, but as many students nervous before exams will testify, the prolonged effect of catecholamines on the bowel is to increase bowel movements.

What are the most likely infective organisms in each of the following diarrhoea scenarios?

1   An outbreak of vomiting and diarrhoea in an old persons' nursing home
2   An outbreak of bloody diarrhoea at a local primary school
3   A university student with watery diarrhoea a few days after a barbeque
4   A group of guests with sudden-onset diarrhoea a few hours after a wedding reception
5   An 82-year-old man in hospital receiving antibiotics for pneumonia
6   A young woman who has just returned from Ghana and has right iliac fossa pain and diarrhoea

The reality is that it is often hard to predict the pathogenic organism in cases of infectious diarrhoea and microbiological culture often reveals the pathogen to be multiple organisms or an unexpected organism. However, certain patterns are typical for certain pathogens and these are frequently asked about in exams and vivas. Hence:

1   Outbreaks of vomiting and diarrhoea in institutions are usually due to viruses of the small structured round virus (SSRV) type, such as **norovirus.**
2   Outbreaks of dysentery (bloody diarrhoea) are often associated with bacteria of the *Shigella* species or with *Escherichia coli* **strain O157.**
3   In truth, this could be due to a multitude of organisms, but in exams and vivas the answer is that *Campylobacter jejuni* would be a good candidate for a post-barbeque case of diarrhoea.
4   Rapid-onset diarrhoea after a meal suggests that the meal was contaminated with bacteria that have excreted active toxins, hence the rapid onset of symptoms. When the diarrhoea is caused by the pathogen's growth in the bowel, the onset of symptoms is usually much slower. *Staphylococcus aureus* and *Bacillus cereus* are both bacteria that grow on warm food and produce toxins that result in rapid-onset diarrhoea.
5   The diarrhoea could be caused by a multitude of organisms or even the antibiotics per se, but in elderly patients receiving antibiotics you should always be wary of *Clostridium difficile.*
6   Again, the diarrhoea could be simple 'traveller's diarrhoea' caused by an enterotoxigenic strain of *E. coli*, but the right iliac fossa pain should make you suspicious of *Yersinia enterocolitica.*

What is the most important aspect in the management of any of the infectious diarrhoeas mentioned in the previous question?

Fluid balance. Patients with infectious diarrhoea are at risk of dehydration due to the constant watery faeces they pass, and it is dehydration which most commonly kills patients with infective diarrhoea worldwide. Maintaining adequate hydration **with oral rehydration salts** in patients with diarrhoea is more important than establishing the identity of the pathogen or treating it with antimicrobial agents.

What is the difference between (1) a fluid challenge, (2) maintenance fluids, and (3) replacement fluids?

1   **Fluid challenge:** this is an IV bolus of 250–500 mL of crystalloid given over 30 minutes to a patient who is hypovolaemic (thirsty, dry mucous membranes, tachycardic, and with a narrow

CONTINUED ➤

CONTINUED

and/or low blood pressure). After the fluid challenge is given, one must reassess the patient. Three outcomes are possible:

- **No response:** blood pressure remains low. The patient has not received enough fluids or they weren't actually hypovolaemic to begin with. Reassess the patient clinically (to double check they really are hypovolaemic) and repeat a fluid challenge.
- **Transient response (increase) in blood pressure:** the patient was indeed hypovolaemic but you either haven't given them enough fluids *or* they are losing them very rapidly (e.g. haemorrhage). Give them more fluids and consider possible explanations for continuing fluid loss.
- **Sustained response (increase) in blood pressure:** the patient was indeed hypovolaemic and you have restored them to normal fluid balance.

2 **Maintenance fluids:** the average normal adult loses about 2.5 L of fluid every day in urine (1.5 L/day), faeces (200 mL/day), and 'insensible losses' (i.e. those you aren't aware of such as sweating and respiration, 800 mL/day). Lost fluids contain dissolved electrolytes and so the average, normal adult also loses about 100 mM of Na^+ and about 70 mM of K^+ every day. Fluids and electrolytes must be replaced daily to maintain fluid balance, and this is normally achieved by drinking about 2 L of fluids a day and eating normally. If a patient cannot drink, they need maintenance IV fluids to restore their 2.5 L fluid, 100 mM Na^+, and 70 mM K^+ a day.

3 **Replacement fluids:** maintenance fluids (see previous point) will maintain fluid balance in many patients. However, some patients have conditions that result in abnormally high fluid loss and therefore they need extra fluids on top of their maintenance fluids to replace the extra losses. Examples of patients requiring extra, replacement fluids are:

- **Fever:** febrile patients need an extra 500 mL of fluid for every 1 °C above 37 °C.
- **Burns patients:** patients with burns need extra fluids and this can be calculated using formulae such as the Parkland formula, which are readily available online.
- **Stoma patients:** patients with intestinal stomas lose fluids because these exit the bowel before fluids can be reabsorbed. Small bowel stomas obviously result in greater fluid loss than large bowel stomas as more fluid will have been reabsorbed by the time faeces exit a large bowel stoma than a small bowel stoma. The only way to calculate how much excess fluid is being lost is by *measuring and recording* how much fluid a stoma drains, keeping in mind that normal faecal loss of fluid is only 200 mL/day.
- **Third spacing:** traditionally, fluid found in the vasculature is said to be in the 'first space' whereas fluid found in interstitial tissue space is said to be in the 'second space', as both of these 'spaces' contain volumes of fluid that are variable (intracellular fluid is usually fairly constant). The 'third space' refers to areas of the body that accumulate fluid only in disease, thus draining fluids away from the first and second spaces. Thus, patients may have fluid in their peritoneal cavity (e.g. due to ascites in liver cirrhosis or inflammatory exudate around the pancreas in pancreatitis), fluid in their intrapleural space (e.g. pleural effusion as in parapneumonic effusions), build-up of excess fluid in their GI tract (e.g. in small bowel obstruction), etc. Estimating how much fluid has been 'third spaced' in a patient is difficult, and one usually relies on trial and error (giving replacement fluids and then assessing the patient) to work out how much replacement fluid to give.

> **What must you always do (and mention in Objective Structured Clinical Examinations!) with any patient who is receiving IV fluids of any sort?**
>
> If a patient is receiving IV fluids, you must always **document fluid input/output** and **always reassess** the patient clinically and biochemically. That is why, on ward rounds, patients on IV fluids get examined clinically and have bloods taken for (among other things) electrolyte levels.
>
> **Clinical examination** may reveal a patient who is still thirsty, with dry mucous membranes, tachycardia, a narrow pulse pressure, and a urine output <30 mL/h despite IV fluids, suggesting they are not receiving enough fluids. Alternatively, it may reveal the patient who looks puffy (oedematous), has crackles in the bases of their lungs, and a raised jugular venous pressure, suggesting they are receiving too much fluid. Fluid overload is just as common (perhaps even commoner) than inadequate fluid replacement and is a cause of significant morbidity and mortality in elderly patients.
>
> **Blood biochemistry** may reveal a patient who is hyponatraemic or hyperkalaemic.

Single Best Answers

1. **A patient produces stool which is pale in colour, foul smelling, and floats. What is the correct term for this type of stool?**

   a. Diarrhoea
   b. Haematochezia
   c. Melaena

   d. Steatorrhoea
   e. Scybalum

2. **Which of the following features is typical of ulcerative colitis?**

   a. Transmural inflammation
   b. Skip lesions
   c. Cobblestoning

   d. Fistula formation
   e. Mucosal inflammation

3. **Which of the following pathogens does not typically produce bloody diarrhoea?**

   a. *Campylobacter*
   b. *Shigella*
   c. *Giardia*

   d. *Salmonella*
   e. *E. coli* EO157

4. **A patient presents with persistent diarrhoea and weight loss. They are positive for antiendomysial antibodies and tissue transglutaminase. The patient has a number of intensely itchy red vesicles on their elbows. What is the most likely diagnosis for this skin condition?**

   a. Dermatitis herpetiformis
   b. Erythema nodosum
   c. Bullous pemphigoid

   d. Pemphigus vulgaris
   e. Psoriasis

5. **A patient with coeliac disease is noted to be folate deficient. In which part of the intestine is folate absorbed?**

   a. Duodenum
   b. Jejunum
   c. Proximal ileum

   d. Terminal ileum
   e. Ascending colon

Rectal bleeding

Core case

Read through the sections in the case boxes, covering up the sections that follow so that you don't see the answer. At the end of each case box, try to answer the question before reading on.

> Mr McCarthy is a 62-year-old butcher who presents to his local Emergency Department because he has passed blood per rectum.
>
> **What is your first priority when assessing Mr McCarthy?**

As with all acute patients, always start by assessing ABCDE: airways, breathing, circulation, disability, and exposure. In a patient with acute gastrointestinal (GI) haemorrhage (whether upper or lower), assessing their circulation (i.e. haemodynamic status) is a priority. If there are clinical features to suggest haemodynamic instability—such as hypotension, tachycardia, cool peripheries, tachypnoea, or decreased consciousness—then the immediate priority is to resuscitate the patient before proceeding to a thorough history and examination.

> You run through the ABCDE algorithm of assessment, and establish that Mr McCarthy is haemodynamically stable. The next stage is to take a full history of the presenting complaint. Before doing so you should have a mental list of differential diagnoses in mind.
>
> **What is your differential diagnosis for rectal bleeding?**
> You may wish to construct your list anatomically.

The differential diagnosis for rectal bleeding is shown in Figure 21.1.

Anorectal	Colonic	Ileo-jejunal	Upper-GI
• Haemorrhoids	• Diverticular disease	• Peptic ulceration (including Meckel's diverticulum)	• Peptic ulcer
• Rectal tumour	• Angiodysplasia	• Angiodysplasia	• Gastritis/duodenitis
• Anal tumour	• Colitis (inflammatory, ischaemic, infective)	• Arterio-venous malformation	• Varices
• Anal fissure	• Colonic tumour (benign or malignant)	• Crohn's disease	• Tumour
• Anal fistula	• Iatrogenic (endoscopic biopsy, anastomotic leakage)	• Coeliac disease	• Mallory-Weiss tear
• Solitary rectal ulcer	• Vasculitis	• Aorto-enteric fistula	• Osler-Weber-Rendu syndrome
• Radiation proctitis		• Small-bowel tumours	• Aorto-enteric fistula
• Rectal varices			• Dieulafoy lesion
• Trauma			

Figure 21.1 Differential diagnosis for rectal bleeding.

There are a couple of points to note about this differential diagnosis. GI haemorrhage may present as *overt* or *occult* bleeding. This table, and the indications of prevalence within it, refers to *overt* rectal bleeding as *occult* rectal bleeding will not be noticed by the patient. The second point to note is that upper GI sources of haemorrhage may occasionally present with rectal bleeding alone. Although it is more likely that such upper GI sources will also present with haematemesis, you should note that large volumes of blood in the GI tract can act as a cathartic (stimulant of peristalsis) and the resultant rapid transit through the intestine leads to the passage of red blood per rectum.

What questions would you like to ask specifically about the history of the presenting complaint?

- **How much blood has been passed?** This question is directly relevant to your initial haemodynamic status survey. Ask the patient to quantify approximately how much blood they have passed—familiar measures such as a teaspoon, eggcup, or wine glass may be easier for the patient than asking them to provide an estimate in millilitres. Note, however, that it is very easy to overestimate volumes of blood loss if, for example, blood has mixed with water in the toilet bowl. You should additionally enquire about symptoms of hypovolaemia—any light-headedness, collapse, chest pain or breathlessness?

- **What is the duration and frequency of the symptoms?**

- **What did the blood look like?** Generally speaking, the fresher the blood, the more distal the bleed.[†] Substantial bleeding from lesions proximal in the GI tract may present with melaena (jet black, tarry stool caused by bacterial oxidation of haem) or may present as frank blood (haematochezia) if transit times are sufficiently rapid. You may need to specifically ask the patient about melaena. Note that patients may report black stool if they are on iron supplementation.

- **What is the relationship of blood with stool?** This is the key question with regard to potentially localizing the source of bleeding.[†] There are four scenarios:

  - **Blood is mixed with the stool:** this suggests that the lesion is proximal to the sigmoid colon. Stool in the proximal colon is soft (thus facilitating mixing with blood) and there is sufficient transit time to enable mixing.
  - **Blood streaked on stool:** suggests a sigmoid or anorectal source of bleeding.
  - **Blood is separate from the stool:** if the blood is passed immediately after stool, the likelihood is that this is an anorectal condition such as haemorrhoids. If, however, blood is passed on its own, this implies that there has been sufficient bleeding to dilate the rectum and produce a defecation stimulus. Such bleeding is most likely to occur with diverticular disease, angiodysplasia, inflammatory bowel disease, or sometimes a rapidly bleeding cancer (upper GI haemorrhage is another small-print cause).
  - **Blood is only seen on the toilet paper:** this implies relatively minor bleeding from the anal canal, most likely due to haemorrhoids or an anal fissure.

- **Is there any pain or prolapse when opening the bowels?** Most of the conditions resulting in rectal bleeding are non-painful. The most notable exception is an anal fissure (or, very rarely, anal herpes), which produces intense/tearing pain during defecation and perhaps lasting for several hours after defecation; such patients may also complain of an itch or perianal irritation. Colitis may be associated with abdominal cramping, and lower anal cancers may present with pain. Haemorrhoids are not typically associated with pain unless they have thrombosed, but patients may have noticed prolapse.

- **Is there any tenesmus (sensation of incomplete evacuation)?** This question is most specific for rectal cancer, where a luminal mass in the rectum can cause the feeling of incomplete bowel evacuation *after* defecation. It can also be a symptom of colitis.

- **Has there been any change of bowel habit?** The passage of blood per rectum may be associated with diarrhoea (such as with colitis) or mucus (think of colitis, proctitis, rectal cancer, and villous adenomas of the rectum). Extensive haemorrhoids may also be associated with the passage of mucus per rectum.

- **Has the patient lost weight?** In older patients in particular you must retain a high index of suspicion for cancer. Note that rectal cancer may lead to substantial weight loss even in the absence of metastatic spread.

- **Are there any symptoms of anaemia?** The current overt bleed may represent an occult bleed that has been unmasked, for example by anticoagulant drugs. Hence it is useful to ask about symptoms of anaemia such as lethargy and shortness of breath.

As shown in the differential diagnosis in Figure 21.1, diverticular disease, angiodysplasia, haemorrhoids, colitis, anal fissures, and lower GI tumours are the most common causes of rectal bleeding.

Construct a 4 × 2 table that shows how these top diagnoses typically present in terms of (a) relationship of blood and stool and (b) pain or not (Table 21.1).

---

† But note, as discussed under the differential diagnosis, that rapid intestinal transit times can produce a confusing picture.

Table 21.1 Causes of rectal bleeding classified by key characteristics

	Pain	No pain
Blood mixed with stool	Colitis	Colonic tumour
		Colitis
Blood streaked on stool	Anal tumour	Rectal tumour
Blood separate from stool	Colitis	Haemorrhoids
		Diverticular disease
		Angiodysplasia
		Rapidly bleeding colonic or rectal tumour
		Colitis (+ mucus)
Blood on toilet paper	Anal fissure	Haemorrhoids

What is the specific relevance of past medical/surgical history?

There are a number of relevant features in the past medical/surgical history:

- **Previous rectal bleeding?** If so, were these episodes investigated and what was the outcome?
- **Ulcerative colitis?** Increases the likelihood of colonic malignancy… or a flare-up of their ulcerative colitis!
- **Recent bowel trauma?** For example bowel surgery, colonoscopy, or other anorectal procedure such as transrectal prostate biopsy. All may result in rectal bleeding.
- **Aortic surgery?** Non-trivial GI bleeding in a patient who has had previous aortic surgery should make you suspect an aortoenteric fistula until proven otherwise.
- **Radiotherapy to the rectum?** Can induce proctitis.
- **Bleeding tendency?** For example warfarin, haemophilia, platelet dysfunction. In a patient with a known bleeding tendency the degree of blood loss may be disproportionate to that normally expected from a particular lesion.
- **Past medical history that predisposes to upper GI bleeds?** Many diseases that can cause an upper GI bleed (e.g. peptic ulcer disease, chronic liver disease) can very occasionally present as rectal bleeding if the bleeding is profuse enough.

Why is a detailed drug history of particular importance when investigating rectal bleeding?

The drug history is vital as drugs may contribute towards rectal bleeding in four ways:

1 **Increased risk of bleeding.** Anticoagulant and antiplatelet medications can accentuate bleeding from established lesions (a previously occult bleed may become overt). Long-term anticoagulation (as in patients with atrial fibrillation) makes any existing angiodysplasia more likely to bleed. Non-steroidal anti-inflammatory drugs (NSAIDs) are known to increase the likelihood of bleeds from diverticular disease.

2 **Increased risk of peptic ulcers.** NSAIDs, steroids, and bisphosphonates predispose to peptic ulceration.

3 **Increased risk of infectious colitis.** Antibiotic use may predispose to *Clostridium difficile* colitis, as may use of proton pump inhibitors.

4 **Attenuated cardiac response to hypovolaemia.** β-Blockers can stop patients from mounting the usual tachycardic response to hypovolaemia.

Mr McCarthy describes passing 'about a pint' of bright red blood per rectum an hour ago. There was no pain associated with the bowel motion. He says that it looked as if he was passing pure blood—with very little stool mixed in. He was alarmed at the appearance of the toilet bowl and decided to drive straight to his local hospital.

There have been no previous episodes of rectal bleeding. Mr McCarthy has not experienced any tenesmus or recent change in bowel habit. He has not lost weight recently, and reports no symptoms of lethargy or general malaise. Mr McCarthy states that he is otherwise fit and well. He has had no previous operations, no recent bowel trauma, and no radiotherapy to the rectum. His past medical history is unremarkable. He takes simvastatin for his hypercholesterolaemia, and has no known drug allergies. He smokes 10 cigarettes a day, and drinks approximately 20 units of beer each week.

Mr McCarthy will need to be examined.

What are the relevant aspects of the physical examination?

You may wish to consider the examination in three stages: general, abdominal, and rectal.

General examination

- Is Mr McCarthy still **haemodynamically stable?** You must continue to assess Mr McCarthy's pulse and blood pressure for signs of continuing or new bleeding.

- Are there any features suggestive of **chronic blood loss** (signs of anaemia such as extreme pallor or koilonychia) or **malignancy** (such as cachexia or obvious lymphadenopathy)?

Abdominal examination

- You should examine the abdomen for any **focal tenderness** or **masses**—principally looking for signs of GI malignancy (left supraclavicular lymphadenopathy, palpable lesions of the colon, hepatomegaly, ascites).

Rectal examination

- The first step is to **inspect the anus**—you may see an anal fissure ± associated skin tag ± 'sentinel pile', haemorrhoid, or fistula (perhaps associated with inflammatory bowel disease). ▲ All patients presenting with rectal bleeding should have a digital rectal examination (DRE). The only times that a DRE may be omitted are in the presence of a painful anal fissure or abscess. While performing the DRE you should be feeling for **palpable masses**, and then inspecting for **blood on the withdrawn gloved finger**. Note that you won't be able to feel haemorrhoids during a DRE unless they are either prolapsed or thrombosed.

Mr McCarthy is still haemodynamically stable. His pulse is 82 bpm regular, blood pressure 132/87 mmHg, and respiratory rate 14/min. Abdominal examination is unremarkable. A DRE reveals blood in the rectum but no palpable masses.

What are the first-line investigations that you would like to request?

Bloods

- **Full blood count (FBC):** you want to know if the patient is anaemic (due to chronic blood loss) or has low platelets.
- **Clotting:** you want to know if the patient has a bleeding tendency.
- **Group and save** (or cross-match if needed urgently): if there is a suspicion that the patient may need blood replacement or may go to theatre. Mr McCarthy is haemodynamically stable and there is no current indication to request an urgent cross-match. If, however, he was haemodynamically unstable and/or showed signs of continued bleeding a cross-match would be more appropriate.
- **Urea:** a rise in urea is consistent with a recent upper GI bleed (urea is a breakdown product of digested red blood cells).

Endoscopy

- **Proctoscopy ± rigid sigmoidoscopy** should be performed in all such patients unless there are painful anal lesions such as an anal fissure. However, the view of the rectum may be unsatisfactory if there is a lot of blood. Proctoscopy ± rigid sigmoidoscopy will enable the identification of bleeding haemorrhoids or a rectal cancer, and can be performed at the bedside.

A blood sample is taken from Mr McCarthy. He is still haemodynamically stable and there has been no further passage of blood per rectum.
The blood results are reported as:

Hb	136 g/L
RBC	4.8×10^{12} cells/L
WCC	9.3×10^9 cells/L
Platelets	320×10^9 cells/L
MCV	84 fL
PT	12.9 seconds
APTT	36 seconds

How would you proceed to establish the source of haemorrhage?

Figure 21.2 shows a potential algorithm for the investigation of acute rectal bleeding. There are four further main investigations for *acute* lower GI haemorrhage (frank blood per rectum) that may be considered in stable patients in the following order:

1 **Colonoscopy**
   - During an acute bleed it is difficult to achieve a good view of the bowel lumen without copious lavage. If, however, it is possible to fully prepare the bowel, colonoscopy is the investigation of choice in the stable patient.
   - In addition to being diagnostic, colonoscopy affords therapeutic options of controlling local haemorrhage by means of adrenaline injection, argon plasma coagulation, diathermy, or clipping.

- There is an additional role for on-table colonoscopy in those patients who present with profuse haemorrhage and proceed straight to theatre. The colon can be irrigated via a caecal catheter to maximize visualization.

2 **Mesenteric angiography (if available)**
- Useful if haemorrhage obscures the view with colonoscopy, or colonoscopy is not possible. Hence it is often used if patients bleed, then stop, and then re-bleed.
- Not always available, particularly in smaller hospitals and out of hours.
- Mesenteric angiography is particularly useful for detecting angiodysplasia, as evidenced by early filling of vessels and/or bleeding during the capillary phase. In order to demonstrate active bleeding there must be ongoing blood loss of >0.5–1 mL/min.
- Embolization of the bleeding vessel can be performed during the procedure.

3 **CT angiography**
- Gaining popularity as an alternative to conventional mesenteric angiography, particularly as multislice CT can now detect even relatively minor bleeds.
- Involves venous access, thus fewer potential complications than mesenteric (arterial) angiography. In addition, it provides rapid imaging and enables other abdominal pathology (either related or incidental to the rectal bleeding) to be visualized by CT.
- On the down side, there is a lack of therapeutic capability, thus patients with bleeding lesions identified by CT angiography will need to proceed to mesenteric angiography or laparotomy.
- It also involves contrast, thus may be relatively contraindicated in patients with significant renal impairment.

4 **Technetium-99 m-labelled red blood cell scintigraphy (if available)**
- Useful in patients for whom other investigations have failed to identify a source—typically these will be patients who have short-lived intermittent bleeds (such as from a Meckel's diverticulum).
- Rarely available in smaller hospitals or out of hours.
- Lacks the specificity of colonoscopy and mesenteric angiography but is non-invasive. It may be useful if the other two techniques have failed to localize the lesion.
- Can detect bleeding at >0.1 mL/min, and can also be used to detect bleeding lesions up to 24 hours after tracer administration, but has no therapeutic potential (its main role is in guiding surgical resection).
- Also has the advantage of requiring no bowel preparation.

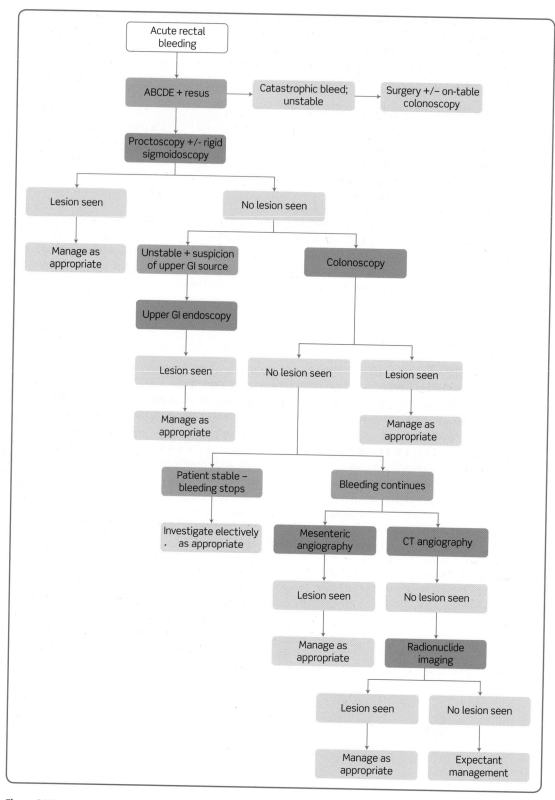

Figure 21.2 Potential algorithm for the investigation of acute rectal bleeding.

Upper GI endoscopy? Some surgeons would advocate upper GI endoscopy in many patients with lower GI haemorrhage, and would certainly do so if there is any indication of haemodynamic compromise. As we have already stated, upper GI haemorrhage may occasionally present as rectal bleeding. Not only is upper GI haemorrhage more common than lower GI haemorrhage (**80% of acute GI haemorrhage is upper**), it is less likely to stop spontaneously and thus more life-threatening.

Small bowel visualization by enteroscopy or video capsule endoscopy? These imaging modalities have limited application in the context of *acute* lower GI haemorrhage. They are only really used if other imaging modalities have failed to find a source of haemorrhage in patients with repeated episodes of haemorrhage. British Society of Gastroenterology guidelines (2007) state that if there is a high index of suspicion for a GI bleed despite a negative gastroscopy and colonoscopy, a second endoscopy should be undertaken before a capsule endoscopy. Push enteroscopy should only be undertaken once a bleeding site has been identified on capsule endoscopy.

It is worth noting that the investigations may all come back negative, either because the source of bleeding cannot be found (yet there is evidence of bleeding) or because the bleeding has stopped. Angiodysplasia and a Dieulafoy lesion (a ruptured submucosal artery, most commonly at the oesophagogastric junction, but also in the small bowel and rectum) are two 'classic' causes of intermittent bleeds that can be very difficult to visualize.

Mr McCarthy passes another ~200 mL of bright red blood per rectum. His observations are still stable.

Proctoscopy does not reveal any obvious source of bleeding. Rigid sigmoidoscopy is not done as the ongoing bleeding would obscure the view. The endoscopist on call performs an oesophagogastroduodenoscopy because of a suspicion of possible upper GI bleeding, but it shows no stigmata of haemorrhage in the upper GI tract. The endoscopist decides that colonoscopy is likely to give inadequate views of the bowel lumen due to the continued rectal bleeding. A mesenteric angiogram is therefore performed and shows an actively bleeding area of angiodysplasia in the ascending colon which is successfully embolized by the radiologist.

What is angiodysplasia?

Colonic angiodysplasia is a submucosal arteriovenous malformation that is believed to be acquired. The cause of these lesions is unknown, but the predominance of lesions in the right colon raises the possibility that high wall tension may be a contributory factor. Typically, lesions are less than 1 cm in diameter, but they can bleed out of proportion to their size. In contrast to haemorrhage from colonic diverticular disease (which is arterial, from the vasa recta), angiodysplasia results in venous blood loss. Angiodysplasia produces a characteristic 'cherry red spot' appearance at endoscopy (although blood will frequently obscure the field of view during acute haemorrhage). The diagnosis has become more common since the advent of mesenteric angiography. It may present with frank rectal bleeding or may result in occult blood loss and subsequent anaemic symptoms. Treatment options include embolization, surgical resection, or endoscopic laser electrocoagulation.

Short cases

Mr Barnes is a 37-year-old gardener who presents to his GP following an episode of rectal bleeding. Mr Barnes tells you that this is his first episode of rectal bleeding. He says that he passed a stool a few hours earlier in the day. After wiping his rear, he noticed fresh blood on the toilet paper. Upon inspecting the toilet bowl he saw drips of blood lining the side of the bowl. He describes blood in the water, but estimates that the amount was very small. To the best of his knowledge, his stool was not bloodstained. He has not experienced any abdominal or rectal pain, and has not noticed any prolapse. There has not been a change in bowel habit and he is otherwise fit and well. He has not experienced anything similar before and has no significant past medical history.

General and abdominal examination of Mr Barnes is unremarkable. He consents to a DRE. There are no perianal lesions on inspection. DRE reveals no palpable masses in the anal canal, but the gloved finger is streaked with blood when it is withdrawn.

Mr Barnes is referred to the general surgeons as a non-urgent outpatient, and they subsequently perform proctoscopy and rigid sigmoidoscopy. Proctoscopy revealed two smooth lesions in the anal canal below the dentate line—at positions corresponding to 3 o'clock and 7 o'clock when viewed with Mr Barnes in the left lateral position. Rigid sigmoidoscopy was unremarkable.

What is the diagnosis and what management options exist for Mr Barnes?

Mr Barnes is suffering from **internal haemorrhoids**.‡

There are a variety of treatment strategies, including conservative, medical, and surgical management:

Lifestyle modification

- Increased dietary fibre, which may soften faeces and minimize straining at stool (although study evidence is somewhat lacking)
- Keep well hydrated
- Avoid straining at stool.

Medical management

- Local anaesthetic creams can be used to relieve soreness and itching
- Steroidal creams/suppositories can be used to reduce local inflammation
- Evidence of efficacy for both is limited
- Appropriate laxative therapy where constipation causes straining, hard stool and ultimately bleeding, and conservative (lifestyle) measures have been unsuccessful.

‡ You should note, however, that the presence of haemorrhoids does not exclude the possibility of an additional and more proximal—and more sinister—culprit lesion (see Viva questions).

Surgical management

There are numerous surgical options, the suitability of which may differ according to patient and the haemorrhoid characteristics:

- Rubber band ligation
- Injection sclerotherapy
- Infrared coagulation/photocoagulation
- Haemorrhoidectomy
- Stapled haemorrhoidopexy
- Doppler-guided haemorrhoidal artery ligation and rectoanal repair (DG-HAL-RAR).

SHORT CASE

Dr Sloane is a 63-year-old retired psychiatrist who presents to her GP complaining of rectal bleeding. She reports that she has noticed small amounts of blood on the toilet paper over the last couple of months, and that the water in the toilet is sometimes bloodstained. Until recently, there has never been enough blood for her to worry. However, over the past few weeks there has been more blood than normal for her. Direct questioning reveals that this blood is not bright red, but it is not melaena either. Dr Sloane remarks that she 'may not remember much from her days as a junior doctor, but I'd never forget the sight or smell of melaena!'. Instead, the blood is dark red and is mixed with the stool. The passage of blood has not been associated with any pain, and Dr Sloane denies any tenesmus. She has, however, noticed a change in her bowel habit, with looser motions over the past 6 weeks. On direct questioning, she concedes she has lost a little weight recently and has been feeling rather 'washed out'.

Dr Sloane says she has suffered with haemorrhoids since the birth of her second child 30 years ago, for which she was treated with rubber band ligation on two occasions. However, she says that neither of these treatments has been particularly successful, and she still suffers from intermittent anal itching and minor bleeds. There is no other remarkable past medical history. She takes no regular medications and has no allergies. She has never smoked and drinks approximately 14 units of wine with meals each week.

On examination, Dr Sloane is in sinus tachycardia (107 bpm, regular). Abdominal examination reveals no masses or tenderness. A DRE reveals a small amount of dark red blood, but no masses. The GP sends bloods for FBC, urea and electrolytes (U&E), and clotting.

Her blood results are as follows:

Haematology		Biochemistry		Clotting	
Hb	91 g/L	Na	136 mM	PT	13.7 seconds
RBC	4.1×10^9 cells/L	K	4.1 mM	APTT	39 seconds
WCC	7.6×10^9 cells/L	Urea	6.2 mM		
Platelets	278×10^9 cells/L	Creatinine	71 μM		
MCV	72 fL	Ferritin	8 μg/L		

What is the most likely diagnosis? How would you proceed to investigate Dr Sloane?

While it is possible that a recurrence of her haemorrhoids could account for the blood which is streaked onto the toilet paper and dripping into the toilet pan, haemorrhoids would not account for the appearance of dark red blood which is mixed with the stool. Given the additional details of a 6-week history of altered bowel habit and weight loss you should have **colorectal carcinoma** at the top of your differential diagnosis. Dr Sloane is also suffering from iron deficiency anaemia (microcytic red blood cells, and a low ferritin), most likely caused from occult bleeding in her GI tract.

She should **urgently** be referred to the colorectal surgeons where she will be investigated using proctoscopy, rigid sigmoidoscopy, and colonoscopy. In addition, it would be useful to request additional blood tests that give some insight into the possibility of liver or bone metastases: liver enzymes (although Dr Sloane's prothrombin time is normal), calcium, alkaline phosphatase.

SHORT CASE

Mr Potter is a 72-year-old retired factory worker who attends the Emergency Department following the passage of 'profuse' amounts of blood per rectum. He is immediately assessed and is deemed to be haemodynamically stable.

On further questioning, Mr Potter reports that he felt the urge to defecate while gardening at home. He went to the toilet but realized that he was not passing anything solid. On inspecting the toilet bowl he realized that he had passed 'bright red' blood and what looked to him like a few clots. His vague estimate was that a pint of blood had been passed. There was no pain associated with the bowel movement, and Mr Potter reports that he has felt very well recently. He is specifically asked about any previous episodes of rectal bleeding, tenesmus, change in bowel habit, or weight loss—and denies any of these symptoms.

Regarding his past medical history, Mr Potter suffered an ischaemic stroke 4 years ago and has hypertension, atrial fibrillation, and osteoarthrosis of the wrist. He takes warfarin, bisoprolol, atorvastatin, bendroflumethiazide, diclofenac, and omeprazole. He is a non-smoker and is teetotal. *abstinent of alcohol*

The Emergency Department team keep Mr Potter under observation and restrict him to his bed, fearing that if he gets up to go to the toilet he may pass more blood and collapse. His INR is 2.3 and he has profuse rectal bleeding, so he is given 2 mg vitamin K intravenously and his warfarin is stopped. The colorectal surgeons take over Mr Potter's care. They arrange for his bowel to be prepared for colonoscopy, which takes place the following day. Colonoscopy reveals mural outpouchings throughout the left colon, with stigmata of haemorrhage (but no active bleeding) within such lesions in the sigmoid.

What is the most likely diagnosis? How would you like to manage Mr Potter?

The history of a relatively large, non-painful, bright red rectal bleed with no other associated symptoms is most suggestive of either diverticular disease or angiodysplasia. The colonoscopy findings confirm that Mr Potter is indeed suffering from **diverticular disease**. The absence of any previous episodes of left iliac fossa pain, a characteristic feature of diverticulitis, is not surprising given that diverticulitis does not increase the risk of bleeding diverticular disease and it is rare for the two pathologies to coexist. Colonic diverticula are most common in the left colon and sigmoid, but it is notable that right-side diverticula (which are usually only seen when left-sided lesions are also present) have a greater propensity to bleed.

The first priority when managing Mr Potter is to establish that he is haemodynamically stable. Once this has been confirmed you can think about stopping the bleeding and preventing recurrence. Bleeding stops spontaneously in as many as 75% of patients with symptomatic diverticular disease, but there is a ~25% chance of a second bleed. In the case of Mr Potter, he received vitamin K to reverse his warfarin and his haemorrhage then stopped without further intervention, but his chance of future bleeds can be substantially reduced by stopping his diclofenac. NSAIDs are known to increase the risk of diverticular haemorrhage, and thus he may wish to discuss other means of controlling his arthritis with his GP. Whether to restart warfarin should involve discussion with a cardiologist to weigh up the risk of stroke from his atrial fibrillation (which can be calculated using the CHADS-VASc score) versus the risk of future bleeds from his diverticulosis (one might use the HAS-BLED score to assess his bleeding risk at 1 year).

If the rectal bleeding had not stopped, Mr Potter would likely have been taken to theatre where the portion of colon affected by bleeding diverticula would have been removed. Traditionally, patients undergo a Hartmann's procedure to resect the abnormal bowel. Some surgeons now advocate primary anastomosis at the time of resection (see Figure 21.3).

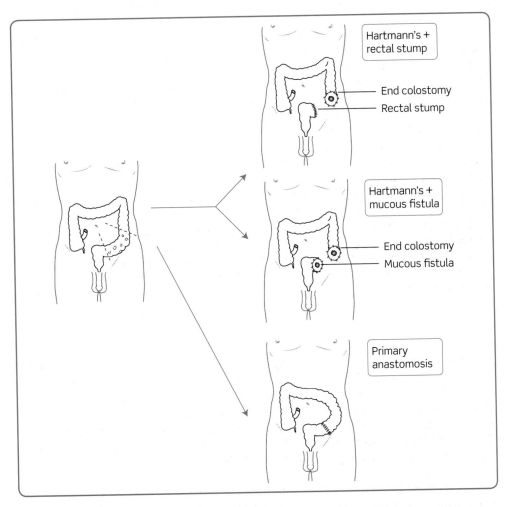

Figure 21.3 Surgical options for diverticular disease.

SHORT CASE

Mrs Chapoutier is a 26-year-old nursery worker who presents to her GP complaining of rectal bleeding. She describes how she has noticed bright red blood on the toilet paper after wiping herself. This has happened after every bowel motion for the past week. She adds that it is exquisitely tender for her to wipe herself and thus she does so with great care. She says defecation produces a tearing sensation in her back passage that may take up to an hour to subside. On further questioning, she says she has not noticed any blood in the toilet bowl, and has had no previous episodes of bleeding. There has been no change of bowel habit and no other symptoms.

She is otherwise fit and well, with no significant past medical history and no medications or allergies. The GP examines Mrs Chapoutier in the left lateral position. A small, posterior, midline anal crack is visible. The examination is painful for Mrs Chapoutier and the GP does not attempt a DRE.

What is the likely diagnosis? What options exist for treating Mrs Chapoutier?

The history of a persistent tearing pain following defecation, accompanied by fresh red blood on wiping and examination findings of a posterior midline crack, indicate that Mrs Chapoutier has an **anal fissure**.

Most anal fissures are shallow and will heal spontaneously within a few weeks. Deep fissures have poor healing because sphincter spasm impairs the anal blood supply. The main aim of treatment is to relieve anal sphincter spasm and tearing of the anal mucosa, in addition to promoting healing. This can usually be achieved with medical therapy, although surgery may be needed for refractory cases:

Medical management

- A high-fibre diet coupled with laxatives and/or non-constipating analgesics (i.e. avoid opioids) may prevent further damage (caused by hard stool) and relieve pain.
- Topical anaesthetics (e.g. lidocaine gel) can help with the pain.
- Topical glyceryl trinitrate (GTN) may increase local blood flow and relax the internal anal sphincter, thus promoting healing, but GTN often causes headaches. Topical diltiazem (calcium channel blocker) has been advocated for use when topical GTN has been ineffective, but the evidence base is weak.
- Botox injections into the anal sphincter can relieve spasm and promote healing in patients with chronic fissures.

Surgical management

- Lateral internal sphincterotomy is very effective at reducing sphincter spasm in those patients who have failed to respond to medical therapies. The integrity of the external anal sphincter must be checked with an ultrasound scan before surgery because cutting the internal sphincter in the presence of a damaged external sphincter (e.g. following childbirth) would cause disastrous faecal incontinence. Indeed, previously, both anal sphincters used to be manually dilated under general anaesthetic but this is no longer done as, unsurprisingly, it resulted in anal incontinence for many patients.
- Anal advancement flap (in which adjacent well-vascularized tissue is advanced into the defect left following fissure excision) is also used by some specialists.

Viva questions

What is the anatomical definition of 'lower' GI haemorrhage?

'Lower' GI haemorrhage refers to bleeding that arises distal to the ligament of Treitz at the duodenojejunal junction.

How do you classify internal haemorrhoids?

The most commonly used grading system for internal haemorrhoids reflects the degree of prolapse and reducibility, but does not necessarily reflect symptom severity:

- First degree: bleed but do not prolapse
- Second degree: prolapse but reduce spontaneously
- Third degree: prolapse and do not reduce spontaneously, but can be manually reduced
- Fourth degree: prolapse and are irreducible

What is the anatomical significance of the dentate line?

The dentate or pectinate line represents an anatomical watershed that separates zones of different epithelial cell types, arterial supply, venous drainage, lymphatic drainage, and nervous supply (see Figure 21.4 and Table 21.2).

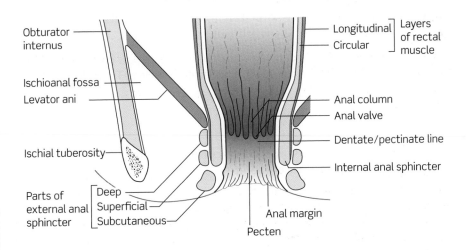

Figure 21.4 Anatomy of the anal canal.

This figure was published in *Clinical Anatomy*, Monkhouse WS, Fig. 11.37, p. 138, Copyright Elsevier 2007.

CONTINUED ➤

CONTINUED

Table 21.2 Zones of the anal canal

	Above dentate line	Below dentate line
Epithelium	Columnar (mucosa)	Stratified squamous (skin)
Arterial supply	Branches of inferior mesenteric, e.g. superior rectal artery	Branches of internal iliac, e.g. inferior rectal artery
Venous drainage	Portal circulation via inferior mesenteric veins	Systemic circulation via internal iliac veins
Lymphatic drainage	Mesenteric nodes	Inguinal nodes
Innervation	Autonomic (stretch only)	Somatic (normal skin sensation)

What is the difference between diverticulosis, diverticular disease, and diverticulitis?

- **Diverticulosis** refers to the presence of diverticula (outpouchings of the mucosa) in the intestine.
- Symptomatic diverticulosis (e.g. bleeding, producing pain) is referred to as **diverticular disease.**
- **Diverticulitis** refers to diverticular inflammation.

[As an aside, colonic diverticula are not actually 'true' diverticula (outpouchings covered by all layers of the bowel wall, as in a Meckel's diverticulum). Since colonic diverticula lack the outer coat of muscularis propria they are 'false' diverticula.]

A patient presents to you with a known diagnosis of haemorrhoids. He is now suffering acute anal pain. What is your differential diagnosis?

Uncomplicated haemorrhoids are not normally painful, thus acute pain in the anal region suggests either a complication of haemorrhoids or an additional pathology. The differential diagnosis includes:

- Thrombosed external haemorrhoid
- Anal fissure
- Proctalgia fugax (a poorly understood stabbing/cramp-like sensation in the anus, that may last up to 30 minutes, and is more common at night)
- Anal abscess
- Lower anal cancer

What are the known risk factors for colorectal carcinoma?

The risk factors with the strongest evidence base include:

- Increasing age
- Male sex (only for rectal carcinoma)

CONTINUED ➤

CONTINUED

- Central obesity
- Colorectal disease:
  - Inflammatory bowel disease (especially ulcerative colitis, but also Crohn's)
  - Previous history of colorectal cancer
  - Colorectal polyps
  - Colorectal irradiation
- Familial conditions including:
  - Familial adenomatous polyposis (FAP)
  - Hereditary non-polyposis colorectal cancer (HNPCC)
  - Peutz–Jeghers
  - Juvenile polyposis
  - Cowden's disease
  - *MYH*-related polyposis
- Sedentary lifestyle (lack of regular exercise)

Dietary factors such as red meat, high fat, and low fibre may also be risk factors, but the evidence base for these is weaker (see Viva questions in Chapter 19).

How do serum ferritin and total iron-binding capacity (TIBC) help distinguish between iron deficiency anaemia and anaemia of chronic disease? What is the role of C-reactive protein (CRP)?

Ferritin is an acute-phase reactant and may be elevated by infection, inflammation, or malignancy, and is also increased by excess alcohol consumption. By requesting CRP in addition to ferritin you can establish the significance of a raised ferritin level. The only way of identifying iron deficiency anaemia in the presence of a raised CRP level is by also looking at the TIBC. See Table 21.3.

Table 21.3 Summary of ferritin, TIBC, and CRP in anaemias

	Ferritin	TIBC	CRP
Iron deficiency anaemia	Low	High	Normal
Anaemia of chronic disease	High	Low	Normal or high
Iron deficiency anaemia + inflammation/infection	High	High	High

---

A 61-year-old patient presents to their GP with rectal bleeding, and internal haemorrhoids are identified as a probable culprit lesion. Should the patient also be referred for colonoscopy with a view to excluding colorectal carcinoma?

The presence of haemorrhoids does not exclude the possibility of an additional and more sinister culprit lesion such as malignancy, but the dilemma is in deciding which patients warrant further investigation. NICE has published guidelines (2005) for the urgent referral of patients with suspected lower

CONTINUED ➤

CONTINUED

GI malignancy. Although these guidelines were intended for use by GPs, they also serve as a useful reference for investigation of inpatients. It is recommended that patients are referred for urgent specialist investigation in the following instances:

- Aged 40 years and older, reporting rectal bleeding with a change of bowel habit towards looser stools and/or increased stool frequency persisting 6 weeks or more.
- Aged 60 years and older, with rectal bleeding persisting for 6 weeks or more without a change in bowel habit and without anal symptoms.
- Aged 60 years and older, with a change in bowel habit to looser stools and/or more frequent stools persisting for 6 weeks or more without rectal bleeding.
- Any age with a right lower abdominal mass consistent with involvement of the large bowel.
- Any age with a palpable rectal mass (intraluminal and not pelvic; a pelvic mass outside the bowel would warrant an urgent referral to a urologist or gynaecologist).
- Men of any age with unexplained iron deficiency anaemia (Hb ≤110 g/L).[†]
- Non-menstruating women with unexplained iron deficiency anaemia (Hb ≤100 g/L).[†]

† Unexplained in this context means a patient whose anaemia is considered on the basis of a history and examination in primary care not to be related to other sources of blood loss (for example, ingestion of NSAIDs) or blood dyscrasia.

Single Best Answers

1. **A patient presents to their GP having noticed some blood dripping into the toilet pan after they have passed stool. The GP examines the patient's anus and notes two prolapsed anal cushions at the 3 and 7 o'clock positions. The GP is able to reduce these haemorrhoids with his finger. What grade would these haemorrhoids be classified as?**

    a. 1
    b. 2
    c. 3

    d. 4
    e. 5

2. **Investigation of a patient with rectal bleeding reveals that they have a microcytic hypochromic anaemia. Which of the following combinations of biochemical parameters is most consistent with iron deficiency anaemia?**

    transferrin carries Fe.

    a. Fe ↓, ferritin ↓, transferrin saturation ↑
    b. Fe ↓, ferritin ↓, transferrin saturation ↓
    c. Fe ↓, ferritin ↑, transferrin saturation ↓

    d. Fe ↓, ferritin ↑, transferrin saturation ↑
    e. Fe ↑, ferritin ↓, transferrin saturation ↓

3. **Which of the following investigations would enable a bleeding lesion in the sigmoid colon to be biopsied?**

    a. Proctoscopy
    b. Rigid sigmoidoscopy
    c. Flexible sigmoidoscopy

    d. Double contrast barium enema
    e. Mesenteric angiography

4. **A patient with known diverticular disease presents to hospital with profuse rectal bleeding. Which of the following drugs from their medication list may have provoked this bleeding?**

    a. Metoprolol
    b. Ramipril
    c. Simvastatin

    d. Allopurinol
    e. Diclofenac

5. **A radiologist performs selective mesenteric angiography on a patient with rectal bleeding. At which vertebral level does the inferior mesenteric artery branch from the abdominal aorta?**

    a. T12
    b. L1
    c. L2

    d. L3
    e. L4

Poor urinary output

Core case

Read through the sections in the case boxes, covering up the sections that follow so that you don't see the answer. At the end of each case box, try to answer the question before reading on.

> Mr Chowdhury is a 68-year-old man who is recovering from surgery. You have been bleeped at 1 a.m. and informed by the duty nurse that Mr Chowdhury has not passed any urine into his catheter bag in the last 3 hours.
>
> **What should you ask the nurse while they are on the phone?**
>

You should ask the nurse:

- What the trend is in urine output—has it been gradually decreasing, or suddenly stopped? If the latter, have they checked if the urinary catheter is blocked by flushing it? This is a rapidly reversible cause of poor urinary output.

- What the observations are for the patient. Ask for the heart rate, blood pressure, respiratory rate, oxygen saturations, and temperature, so you can get an idea of how unwell the patient is. This will help you prioritize how soon you need to see the patient.

> The nurse tells you that the output has been decreasing gradually, and that she already checked that the urinary catheter is not blocked. The patient is sleeping and his observations are stable, with a heart rate of 70 bpm, respiratory rate of 12/min, temperature of 36.8 °C, blood pressure of 115/65 mmHg, and oxygen saturations of 97% on air.
>
> **How much urine should Mr Chowdhury be passing? Why does he need your attention?**

Healthy adults have a urine output of about 1 mL/kg/hour. **Oliguria** refers to a reduced urine output and is defined variously as <400 mL/day, <0.5 mL/kg/hour, or <30 mL/hour. **Anuria** refers to the complete absence of urine output.

Decreased urine output should be taken very seriously as it may be the first (and only) sign of impending acute renal failure. Untreated, patients may die from hyperkalaemia, profound acidosis, or pulmonary oedema due to the kidneys not performing their usual physiological role.

> As you walk over to the surgical ward to see Mr Chowdhury, you run through the possible diagnoses causing poor urine output.
>
> **What are the possible causes for poor urine output?**

Normal urine output requires:

- adequate blood supply to the kidneys
- functioning kidneys, and
- flow of urine from the kidneys, down the ureters, into the bladder, and out via the urethra.

Pathology affecting any of these requirements can result in poor urine output, which is why the differential diagnosis for poor urinary output is often classified as shown in Figure 22.1.

Pre-renal (i.e. inadequate blood supply to the kidneys)	Renal (i.e. damage resulting in impaired kidney function)	Post-renal (i.e. obstruction to urinary flow)
• **Hypovolaemia** (decreased circulating volume due to e.g. dehydration, haemorrhage) • **Hypotension** (decreased vascular resistance due to e.g. sepsis, pancreatitis) • Heart failure • Reduced local perfusion of kidneys (e.g. dissecting aneurysm, renal emboli)	Tubular causes • **Acute tubular necrosis** Glomerular causes • Glomerulonephritis Interstitial causes • Interstitial nephritis (usually caused by drugs, e.g. NSAIDs, antibiotics) Vascular causes • Vasculitides • Haemolytic uraemic syndrome • Thrombocytic thrombocytopenic purpura • Disseminated intravascular coagulation • Malignant hypertension • Scleroderma Infectious • Malaria • Legionnaires' disease • Leptospirosis Complex mechanism • Multiple myeloma	Ureter • Abdominal/pelvic mass (e.g. tumour) compressing ureters • Complication of pelvic surgery • Bilateral calculi • Retroperitoneal fibrosis Bladder • Neuropathic bladder • Anticholinergic or sympathomimetic drugs • Bladder stones or tumour • Uterovaginal prolapse (women) Urethra • **Benign prostatic hyperplasia (BPH)** • **Blocked catheter** • Prostate cancer • Urethral stricture • Posterior urethral valve • Trauma • Infection (e.g. herpes simplex making it painful to pass urine)

Figure 22.1 Differential diagnosis for poor urinary output.

In practice, as a junior doctor **you want to diagnose and treat the prenal and postrenal causes**. If you come to the conclusion that it is a renal cause (by exclusion), call the renal physicians for an expert opinion.

> You arrive on the ward and find Mr Chowdhury fast asleep and with normal observations apart from his anuria. You decide to look at Mr Chowdhury's notes before waking him up.
>
> **What clues in the notes might help you establish the cause of Mr Chowdhury's poor urinary output?**

Fluid balance chart

This is *crucial* in determining the diagnosis:

- **Adequate intake?** Remember that an adult of average size will require about 3 L of fluid intake per 24 hours (30–50 mL/kg/day). Febrile patients will require an extra 500 mL for every 1 °C above 37.0 °C to compensate for increased loss of fluids from evaporation and increased respiratory rate.

- **Positive balance?** Ensure that there is at least as much fluid going into the patient (orally or via intravenous (IV) fluids) as there is coming out (urine, fluid faeces, nasogastric (NG) tubes, vomit, stomas, drains). Don't forget to look through the notes carefully for charts because fluid balance is often documented in various separate places (e.g. NG tube output is sometimes documented separately).

Surgical operative notes

- **Type of surgery?** Pelvic surgery may result in damage to the urinary tract. Surgery to the urinary tract itself can cause damage (e.g. perforation of the bladder during a transurethral resection of a bladder tumour). Laparotomies (especially those of long duration) can result in dehydration by evaporation of water from the open peritoneal cavity and this loss of volume will not be recorded in the fluid balance charts.

- **Blood loss?** Inadequately replaced blood loss may cause a patient to be sufficiently hypovolaemic that their kidneys cannot filter blood properly as they do not have sufficient renal perfusion pressures across Bowman's capsule. Blood loss that has been adequately replaced may nonetheless have resulted in temporary ischaemic damage to the underperfused kidneys (ischaemic acute tubular necrosis) so that the kidneys no longer function properly.

Drug chart

- **Nephrotoxic drugs?** Some drugs are potentially damaging to the kidneys, in particular non-steroidal anti-inflammatory drugs (NSAIDs), angiotensin-converting enzyme (ACE) inhibitors, diuretics and some antibiotics (e.g. gentamicin, vancomycin). Stop these drugs in any patient with oliguria or a worsening renal function, as you risk making any renal failure much worse. Consider switching to an alternative antibiotic if appropriate. Also consider whether the patient has had IV contrast for a recent scan and whether the timing of this coincides with that of the renal injury.

Blood test results

- **Haemoglobin?** Compare pre- and postoperative results in case of pre-existing anaemia. However, note that acute blood loss results in a delayed drop in haemoglobin. This is because haemorrhage results in loss of haemoglobin and serum in equal measure, whereas the haemoglobin calculated by the lab is a measure of concentration rather than the actual volume. This will fall in due course as serum is replenished more rapidly than red blood cells.

- **Renal function?** Again compare pre- and postoperative results, as the patient may have long-standing renal impairment. A 50% increase in baseline creatinine is said to constitute acute kidney injury (AKI). The presence of AKI points towards a pathology resulting in renal hypoperfusion (prerenal) or potentially a renal aetiology.

Past medical history

- **Comorbidities?** Patients with pre-existing cardiac disease, for example, may be more vulnerable to developing acute renal failure. This can provide clues as to the aetiology (e.g. more likely to be prerenal in patients with heart failure).

The surgical notes show that Mr Chowdhury underwent an elective laparoscopic right hemicolectomy 16 hours ago for colorectal carcinoma. The procedure lasted 180 minutes and the estimated blood loss was 150 mL. The patient received 1 L of crystalloid during the operation. An indwelling urinary catheter was placed in theatre during induction of anaesthesia. He had bloods taken at a preoperative assessment but has had none postoperatively; these are requested for the morning.

Haematology		Biochemistry	
Hb	124 g/L	Na	141 mM
WCC	5.5 × 10⁹/L	K	4.4 mM
Platelets	201 × 10⁹/L	Urea	7.0 mM
		Creatinine	104 µM

The nursing notes contain Mr Chowdhury's fluid chart (Table 22.1).

Table 22.1 Mr Chowdhury's fluid chart

Name   Janesh Chowdhury   Hospital number   13265844
Date   01/03/2010
Nil by mouth?   YES/NO   Previous day's balance:

| Time | INTAKE (mL) | | | | OUTPUT (mL) | | | |
| | Oral | | Intravenous | | Urine | | Other | |
	Vol. given	Running total	Vol. given	Running total	Vol. measured	Running total	Vol. Measured	Running total
0100								
0200								
0300								
0400								
0500								

CONTINUED ➤

CONTINUED

Time								
0600								
0700								
0800								
0900								
1000								
1100								
1200								
1300								
1400								
1500		1000	1000		550	550		
1600								
1700					200	750		
1800								
1900								
2000								
2100					200	950		
2200								
2300					50	1000		
2400								
TOTAL								

The drug chart shows that Mr Chowdhury is on 1 gram paracetamol q.d.s. and 100 mg tramadol p.r.n., max 6 hourly, for analgesia. He has also been prescribed compression stockings for both legs to prevent deep vein thrombosis.

Mr Chowdhury is now awake despite the late hour as the nurse has just given him paracetamol with a cup of water. You ask the nurse how much water he has been drinking and she estimates that he has probably had one full glass of water since arriving on the wards. The bag of crystalloid has about 50 mL of fluid left in it.

What is Mr Chowdhury's fluid balance status? What has happened to his urinary output over time?

Mr Chowdhury's fluid intake/output can be tabulated as shown in Table 22.2.

It would appear that Mr Chowdhury has a positive fluid balance of 2050 − 1150 = 900 mL. While this is positive, it may not be sufficient as there are insensible losses and the blood loss is an estimate. Do not be surprised by the fact that Mr Chowdhury's limited oral intake has not been documented in the fluid balance chart: it is hard to find perfectly kept charts on any busy ward.

Mr Chowdhury's urinary output has been dropping over time, suggesting a gradual onset of pathology (e.g. gradual dehydration) rather than a sudden one (e.g. bladder stone blocking the outlet, blood clot blocking the catheter), as shown in Table 22.3.

Table 22.2 Mr Chowdhury's fluid intake/ouput

Input	Output
1 L crystalloid	150 mL blood loss (estimated)
950 L crystalloid	1 L urine
100 mL of oral water (rough estimate)	
Total: 2050 mL	Total: 1150 mL

Table 22.3 Change over time in Mr Chowdhury's urinary output

Time period	Output	Rate
13:00–15:00 (2 hours)	550 mL	275 mL/hour
15:00–17:00 (2 hours)	200 mL	100 mL/hour
17:00–21:00 (4 hours)	200 mL	50 mL/hour
21:00–23:00 (2 hours)	50 mL	25 mL/hour (oliguria)
23:00–01:00 (2 hours)	0 mL	0 mL/hour (anuria)

What questions will you ask Mr Chowdhury?

Remember that it is 1 a.m. and the patient is likely to be sleepy, so keep your questions to a targeted minimum. A good approach is to think of questions which might identify some of the more likely diagnoses.

Prerenal disease (e.g. hypovolaemia)

- **Does he feel thirsty?** A symptom of dehydration and hypovolaemia.

Renal disease (e.g. nephrotoxic drugs, glomerulonephritis)

You have already looked at the drug chart for nephrotoxic medications.

- **Does he have any pre-existing renal disease?** This may not be in the notes and it is worth asking.
- **Does he have any symptoms of conditions that cause renal disease?** Ask in particular about haematuria (?glomerulonephritis), swollen ankles or frothy urine (?nephrotic syndrome), or rashes and arthralgias suggestive of a multisystem vasculitis or SLE.

Postrenal obstruction (e.g. BPH, blocked catheter)

He is catheterized, making postrenal obstruction very unlikely. Indeed, rather than asking the (uncatheterized) oliguric patient questions that are not that sensitive or specific, once you have excluded prerenal causes you would catheterize them to see if obstruction was the problem.

Were the patient not catheterized, you would ask about lower urinary tract symptoms (LUTS), e.g. hesitancy, frequency, strangury, poor stream, terminal dribbling.

Mr Chowdhury says he is thirsty. He has pain around the surgical incision but not by his bladder. He has never stopped passing urine before. You examine Mr Chowdhury.

What are you looking for on examination?

- **Check the catheter bag:** you are looking to see if there has been any more urine output since the last entry in the fluid balance chart, and also for blood in the bag which would suggest the possibility of clot retention (clot formation in the bladder following haematuria, with the clot subsequently occluding the catheter). The colour of the urine can also be very informative. Highly concentrated/dark urine is suggestive of an underfilled patient.

- **Signs of dehydration:** dry lips, mouth, and tongue. If the patient is becoming hypovolaemic, you may also find tachycardia, a narrow pulse pressure, and eventually a low blood pressure, prolonged capillary refill time (>2 seconds), and cool peripheries. A lying versus standing blood pressure showing a significant postural drop has traditionally been thought of as a reliable sign of hypovolaemia but most evidence suggests that postural changes in blood pressure and heart rate are poor at predicting the degree of dehydration because many patients will naturally have a postural drop (without any dehydration or symptoms) and, conversely, many moderately dehydrated patients will often compensate and show no postural changes. What is more useful is whether the patient feels dizzy on standing, irrespective of any measurement . It is important to be aware of the signs of intravascular hydration status versus extravascular hydration status—the former is the critical parameter in this instance, and the relevant markers are pulse, blood pressure, capillary refill time, and jugular venous pressure (JVP). Remember that it is perfectly possible for a patient to be overloaded with fluid in the extravascular compartment, but to be fluid depleted intravascularly, e.g. in septic shock. You may also see an increased respiratory rate, particularly in children.

- **Signs of heart failure (i.e. fluid overloaded):** raised JVP; displaced apex beat; gallop rhythm (third heart sound); bilateral and basal lung crepitations; dependent oedema (sacrum if in bed). Beware oedematous patients though, as their intravascular volume may be depleted, with the potential for renal hypoperfusion.

- **Signs of urinary retention due to postrenal obstruction:** palpable, distended bladder that is dull to percussion (as it is filled with fluid). Pressing may stimulate the urge to urinate.

On examination, Mr Chowdhury is obviously tired. The urinary catheter bag contains dark urine from earlier in the day. His lips are moist (as he has just had water to take his medication). His heart rate is 100 bpm, regular. His blood pressure is 115/85 mmHg. His JVP is not raised and his apex is undisplaced. He does not have any dependent oedema but there are faint crackles in the bases of both lungs. His abdomen is tender around the laparoscopic port sites but his bladder is neither palpable nor tender.

What do your findings suggest so far?

- **Hypovolaemia.** Mr Chowdhury has experienced a gradual decrease in urinary output. While he has a positive fluid balance, this is before insensible losses and assumes the blood loss estimate is accurate. Clinically, he is thirsty, his urine is dark, and he is borderline tachycardic with a narrow pulse pressure. This all suggests that Mr Chowdhury has become progressively dehydrated and hypovolaemic, and this may well account for the gradual decrease in urinary output.

- **?Atelectasis.** Mr Chowdhury has bilateral basal lung crackles. Although these could be pulmonary oedema due to heart failure, there is no other evidence for this. It is more likely that they are due to postoperative atelectasis: small areas of alveolar collapse that are common after surgery (particularly abdominal surgery with poor postoperative analgesia).

You suspect that Mr Chowdhury has reduced urinary output due to hypovolaemia, a fairly common scenario in postoperative patients.

What investigations will you arrange?

- **Check that the catheter has been flushed.** It is possible that Mr Chowdhury's urinary catheter has become blocked. Although this would typically cause a sudden drop in urinary output (rather than a gradual one as is the case here) you should always check that the urinary catheter is patent. Using aseptic technique, gently flush 50 mL of normal saline up the catheter. You should not meet any resistance—if you do, it suggests a blockage and you should replace the catheter.

- **Venous blood gas:** this is a quick way of getting his electrolyte balance (particularly potassium), acid–base status, and haematocrit.

- **Bloods:** for the latest renal function and haemoglobin in particular. If the urea is raised, it suggests hypovolaemia. If the creatinine is also raised, it suggests renal injury (e.g. acute tubular necrosis). You should interpret the results in the context of previous investigations.

- **Fluid challenge:** if you suspect the cause of oliguria/anuria is hypovolaemia, give the patient a bolus of 250–500 mL of a crystalloid solution, 'stat' (i.e. under gravity, fast flowing). Monitor the urine output and basic observations (pulse, blood pressure, etc.) closely. If his observations and urine output improve over the next hour and stay like that, you have solved the problem. If they improve but fall back again, the patient was indeed hypovolaemic but needs even more fluids—try another fluid challenge. If it does not increase, consider the possibility that the patient is not hypovolaemic (or that they are woefully underfilled!). If the patient becomes short of breath and his JVP rises, it suggests fluid overload, i.e. congestive heart failure.

- In patients who are not catheterized (i.e. unlike Mr Chowdhury), you should consider an **ultrasound** to exclude postrenal obstruction, which would be suggested by the finding of dilated ureters (hydroureter) or renal pelvis/calyces (hydronephrosis).

Mr Chowdhury's catheter can be easily flushed with 50 mL of normal saline, suggesting no obstruction at all. His venous blood gas and urinalysis are unremarkable. You send bloods to the lab. Meanwhile, you start Mr Chowdhury on a 250 mL bolus of crystalloid, stat. You ask the nurse to record his observations and urine output every 30 minutes. You return to assess Mr Chowdhury an hour later and see from his fluid chart that he passed 40 mL of urine during the first 30 minutes and 20 mL of urine during the next half hour. Mr Chowdhury's heart rate is now 90 bpm and his blood pressure is 115/70 mmHg. The blood results are now available and show:

Haematology		Biochemistry	
Hb	114 g/L	Na	143 mM
WCC	7.1 × 10⁹ cells/L	K	3.6 mM
		Urea	11.8 mM
		Creatinine	103 µM

What is the reason for Mr Chowdhury's poor urinary output? How will you manage him?

Mr Chowdhury has experienced a gradual decrease in urinary output that responds transiently to a fluid bolus. In addition, he has shown clinical signs of hypovolaemia and has a raised urea. This suggests that the reason for Mr Chowdhury's poor urinary output is **prerenal hypovolaemia**, probably due to insufficient fluid replacement. This case illustrates the importance of always assessing and reassessing the patient clinically when working out fluid balance in a patient, rather than relying on fluid charts which can be helpful but often incorrect (due to estimations and inadequate clerking).

The fact that the fluid bolus corrected the situation only transiently suggests Mr Chowdhury is still dehydrated. You should correct the dehydration with further fast IV fluids until his observations normalize and remain so. You then need to remember to keep him on maintenance fluids.

Ideally, maintenance fluids should be given orally (or via a correctly sited nasogastric feeding tube); a recent National Confidential Enquiry into Patient Outcome and Death (NCEPOD) has highlighted the significant morbidity and mortality associated with IV fluid therapy. If enteral fluids are not possible, he will need parenteral fluids and this will usually involve IV fluids, but in some patients (e.g. demented patients who repeatedly pull out their cannula), subcutaneous fluids can be just as effective. It was common practice until recently to prescribe adults who couldn't drink 3 L of maintenance fluids per day divided as 2 × 1 L of normal saline plus 1 L dextrose (5%) all containing 20 mM of KCl. This recipe has fallen out of favour as it leads to fluid overload in many patients (e.g. elderly patients with low BMI) and disturbances in pH (metabolic acidaemia) and electrolytes (hypernatraemia, hyperchloraemia) from the use of these non-physiological fluids. NICE guidelines (2013) recommend using the following as a guide to maintenance:

Volume: 25–30 mL/kg/day (based on ideal weight if the patient is obese)

Electrolytes: 1 mmol/kg/day of K, Na, and Cl

Glucose: 100 g/day (simply to prevent starvation; this will not meet their feeding requirements).

There are numerous fluid regimes that can achieve the targets above and to some extent what you prescribe will depend on what is locally available. You will obviously have to adjust this for individual patients based on the urea and electrolyte (U&E) results, any oral intake, any additional ongoing losses (e.g. drain output), or any fever (add 100 mL/day per 1 °C above 37 °C).

Mr Chowdhury's urine output remained adequate and he was eventually discharged home.

Short cases

Mr Garcia is a 76-year-old retired teacher who presents to his local hospital complaining that he has been unable to pass any urine for the last 8 hours. He has the urge to pass urine intermittently every half hour or so, and his lower abdomen is very painful. He is not constipated, having opened his bowels once a day regularly up to and including last night. He has had a poor stream and frequency for many months but never sought help as he assumed it was just him 'getting old'. On examination, his bladder is palpable and tender in the suprapubic area of the abdomen. An enlarged, smooth, symmetrical prostate with a central sulcus can be palpated on digital rectal examination and his rectum contains some soft faeces.

What is the likely diagnosis? How should Mr Garcia be managed?

Mr Garcia has presented with a painful desire but inability to urinate: **acute urinary obstruction**. You know it is acute or acute-on-chronic as he has pain, and chronic obstruction is painless. This is almost certainly due to his enlarged prostate, which is probably **benign prostatic hyperplasia (BPH)** given its smooth and symmetrical nature. However, prostate cancer is also a possibility.

Management of Mr Garcia will consist of:

1 **Catheterization and IV fluids:** if you cannot pass a standard 16G urinary catheter due to an enlarged prostate, try gently with a larger and more rigid catheter. Catheterization will void the bladder (the patient will be very grateful) and give you a clue about the pathogenesis: if the volume voided is >1 L, it suggests this is an acute-on-chronic urinary retention, as acute retention alone rarely gets to such a large volume. IV fluids should be set up in advance to compensate for the expected diuresis that often follows relief of the urinary obstruction and which can otherwise lead to substantial hypotension.

2 **Assess renal function:** assess renal function by monitoring blood urea, creatinine, and electrolytes, and by monitoring urine output over the subsequent 12–48 hours with the catheter. If the creatinine is raised you should anticipate a diuresis. Depending on the degree of derangement, you may also want to refer to the renal physicians for follow up.

3 **Assess cause of obstruction:** the most likely cause is BPH, as Mr Garcia is not constipated. However ensure the urine is dipped to exclude a urinary tract infection (UTI). Prostate cancer should be kept in mind, particularly since the digital rectal examination revealed an enlarged prostate. Suspected prostate cancer should be investigated with a urology referral where relevant. Do *not* request a prostate-specific antigen (PSA) as this is raised in acute urinary retention and therefore would not be useful at this time.

4 **Trial without catheter (TWOC):** if the patient voided <1 L upon catheterization and has normal renal function, they are suitable for a TWOC. The patient is started on an α-blocker (to relax the internal urinary sphincter) and given a single dose of antibiotics (to prevent UTI after the catheter is removed) and then one simply waits to see if the patient can urinate. As one only has the urge to urinate when the bladder is full, a TWOC is normally undertaken by the nurses at midnight (so the patient's bladder is full by the morning) or early morning (so their bladder is full during the course of the day). Undertaking a TWOC in the afternoon or evening is not advisable as then the patient's

bladder will only be full during the night. If they are unable to void they will potentially run into trouble overnight when fewer staff are available to help them.

- If they can urinate, they are discharged on an α-blocker or 5α-reductase inhibitor but warned that the risk of recurrence is very high (up to 70% over a year).
- If they cannot urinate, in addition to an α-blocker or 5α-reductase inhibitor, they are discharged with an indwelling catheter and booked for a later attempt in an outpatient TWOC clinic. If this fails, they may require a surgical solution to their problem, most likely a transurethral resection of the prostate (TURP).
- Note that if their creatinine was raised on presentation, they would not be a candidate for a TWOC and need to have a TURP.

SHORT CASE

Mrs Janeway is a 52-year-old woman who is well known to her local Emergency Department. She has attended 125 times over the last 10 years, usually because of back pain or other musculoskeletal pain and demanding opioid analgesia. She is the principal carer for her husband, who is disabled due to multiple sclerosis.

Mrs Janeway was lifting her husband out of bed the day before when she suddenly developed lower back pain. The pain was excruciating at first but gradually became more bearable as the day went by and she took some ibuprofen and paracetamol. However, she has not been able to pass any urine for 12 hours. She has a strong urge to go and finds her bladder painful. She last opened her bowels before the onset of back pain but usually only passes faeces a few times a week anyway. She has not noticed any loss of sensation or power in her lower limbs.

On examination, the range of movement in Mrs Janeway's lower spine is severely restricted due to pain. Her lower limbs have reduced power (4/5 on the MRC power scale) and reduced knee and ankle reflexes. Her plantar reflexes are downgoing, and both coordination and sensation in the lower limbs appear normal. On digital rectal examination there is marked perianal numbness and lax anal tone. Throughout the clerking, Mrs Janeway begs for Entonox (nitrous oxide gas and air) for the pain and for something to 'let her pee'. A urinary catheter is placed and she voids 860 mL of urine, much to her relief.

Which diagnosis should you be worried about? What should the next step in management be?

Mrs Janeway has presented with lower back pain, urinary retention (it would be difficult to voluntarily retain >500 mL of urine), signs of a lower motor neuron lesion affecting both lower limbs, perianal numbness, and lax anal tone. Until proven otherwise radiologically, this is **cauda equina syndrome**. This is a medical emergency whereby the lumbosacral nerve roots that form the cauda equina in the spinal canal become compressed (usually by a centrally prolapsing intervertebral disc). This results in a lower motor neuropathy affecting the bladder sphincters, bowel sphincters, and lower limbs.

Cauda equina syndrome needs urgent attention from spinal surgeons. Mrs Janeway needs an urgent MRI scan of her back to investigate the possibility of cauda equina compression and, if this is confirmed, she will need an urgent surgical intervention to decompress the affected nerve roots (Figure 22.2). The longer treatment is delayed, the less likely she is to recover any loss of function.

Figure 22.2 MRI scan showing cauda equina syndrome due to an intervertebral disc prolapse.
With kind permission from Dr J. Teh.

SHORT CASE

Mr Bodden is 64-year-old man who presents to his GP because of problems passing urine. For some months now, he has noticed his urine 'spraying' when he goes to the toilet. However, for the past few weeks he has found it hard to pass urine, having to spend minutes at a time in the toilet as his urine painfully drips out slowly. He is worried that this is related to his bladder cancer. He has not noticed any discharge from his urethra and declares that he otherwise feels fit and well.

His medical notes reveal that he has had transitional carcinoma of the bladder, papillary type, for the last 6 years. For this, he receives regular cystoscopies to resect the low-grade tumour and to inject bacille Calmette–Guérin (BCG) into the bladder. His last cystoscopy was 6 weeks ago.

What is the likely diagnosis? What is the next step?

It is likely that Mr Bodden has developed a **urethral stricture** due to the repeated trauma to his urethra over the years of cystoscopies. The next step is to refer Mr Bodden to the urological surgeons and visualize the actual stricture if it exists (using, ironically, cystoscopy). If a urethral stricture is found, treatment options include dilating the urethra, a urethral stent, a cystoscopic urethrotomy (a small incision to relieve the stricture), or surgery to remove the affected portion of urethra altogether.

SHORT CASE

Mrs Potter is a 68-year-old woman recovering on an orthopaedic ward from a replacement of her total hip replacement prosthesis, which kept dislocating. She is a type 2 diabetic patient on metformin, ramipril, aspirin, and atorvastatin. You have been called because her urine output has consistently been <20 mL/hour since the operation 18 hours ago. The operative notes suggest the surgery resulted in significant blood loss and estimate that she lost 2 L of blood. She required vasopressors at numerous points during the operation to keep her blood pressure above 80 mmHg systolic and she received four units (~1.2 L) of blood during the operation, plus a further 2 L of Hartmann's solution over the last 16 hours on the ward.

Mrs Potter looks pale and lethargic. A catheter is in place that has been flushed. She is not thirsty but does feel short of breath. Her heart rate is 90 bpm and her blood pressure is 150/80 mmHg. Her JVP is visible at about 6 cm above the manubriosternal angle and there are faint crackles at the bases of her lungs. Her oxygen saturations are 94% on 4 L/min of oxygen but drop to 86% on air.

The latest bloods (taken postoperatively) for Mrs Pottter reveal:

Na	131 mM
K	4.8 mM
Cl	104 mM
Urea	11.4 mM
Creatinine	280 µM (with a baseline of 164 µM)

What is the likely diagnosis? What is the next step?

Mrs Potter has oliguria (urine output <0.5 mL/kg/hour) and AKI (oliguria for >6 hours and rise in creatinine >50% of baseline). She is essentially in renal failure. Possible reasons are:

Prerenal cause?

A prerenal cause of oliguria (e.g. hypovolaemia, heart failure leading to reduced cardiac output and renal hypoperfusion) is unlikely. Although Mrs Potter was likely hypovolaemic during the surgery, she is currently fluid overloaded (high JVP, pulmonary oedema clinically).

Postrenal cause?

A postrenal cause of oliguria (e.g. ureter damage, urinary tract obstruction) is unlikely in this case, as Mrs Potter is catheterized and has been passing urine since the operation, although it must be ruled out. If a postrenal cause is suspected, Mrs Potter should be referred to the urological surgeons.

Renal cause of oliguria?

A renal cause of oliguria (e.g. nephrotoxic medications, acute tubular necrosis due to previous hypovolaemia) is most likely in Mrs Potter by default, given that prerenal and postrenal causes appear unlikely. She is an elderly patient with type 2 diabetes, placing her at increased risk of renal failure, and has just suffered hypovolaemia during her surgery. It is likely her kidneys have suffered **acute tubular necrosis** from the transient hypovolaemia during her operation. As a renal cause is suspected, Mrs Potter should be referred to the renal physicians.

Next steps?

- **Stop her IV fluids.** She is already fluid overloaded.

- **Assess the need for dialysis.** Any of hyperkalaemia, severe acidosis, fluid overload, or hyperuricaemia, refractory to medical management, is an indication for urgent dialysis. Mrs Potter has pulmonary oedema so she warrants **immediate referral to the renal physicians for consideration of emergency dialysis.**

- **Check her drug chart** for nephrotoxic drugs that can be stopped. In this case, you should stop her ACE inhibitor. You should also stop her metformin while she is in renal failure as she at risk of metformin-induced lactic acidosis.

- **Blood tests:** A low Ca^{2+} and high inorganic phosphate (P_i) are suggestive of chronic renal failure, but can sometimes occur in acute renal failure, too.

- **Renal tract ultrasound** to confirm intact ureters and rule out hydronephrosis due to obstruction. Small kidneys with poor corticomedullary differentiation suggest long-standing renal impairment that may have suddenly decompensated.

- **Urine analysis.** Haematuria may suggest renal tract damage. Its absence makes a glomerulonephritis less likely. A raised urine albumin:creatinine ratio can suggest nephrotic syndrome.

Viva questions

What are the main complications of urethral bladder catheterization?

- UTI, particularly with *Proteus mirabilis* which is a highly motile bacterium that can swim up the catheter
- Urethral trauma, including creation of a false passage
- Urethral scarring and stricture
- Bladder perforation

What are the main complications of chronic urinary retention?

- Urinary incontinence due to overflow. The patient may not be able to void the bladder completely but will 'dribble' small amounts of urine uncontrollably
- UTI (upper or lower) due to urinary stasis in the bladder
- Bladder stones due to urinary stasis
- Hydroureters and hydronephrosis (dilatation of the ureters and kidney calyces)
- Renal failure (secondary to the hydronephrosis)
- Acute-on-chronic urinary retention (painful, unlike chronic urinary retention)
- Bladder wall hypertrophy (trabeculation) and outpouchings (diverticula)

What are the principal physiological mechanisms for regulating serum volume and serum osmolarity?

Volume is primarily regulated by the **renin–angiotensin–aldosterone** axis. Renin is released by the kidneys in response to signals from the body that circulating volume is low. Amongst other effects, it stimulates the production of angiotensin I in the liver and its conversion to angiotensin II by the ACE produced in the lungs. Angiotensin II has many effects (aimed at increasing blood pressure), including vasoconstriction and stimulating the release of aldosterone from the adrenal cortex. Aldosterone acts on the distal tubule to increase sodium (and hence water) uptake into the blood.

  Osmolarity is primarily regulated by **antidiuretic hormone** (ADH, vasopressin), released by the posterior pituitary. ADH increases water (but not sodium) reabsorption in the distal tubule, concentrating the urine and diluting the serum.

Which nerves, neurotransmitters, and receptors are responsible for bladder control and micturition? How is this applied in the pharmacological treatment of continence problems?

Urine is continuously produced but its release (micturition) is controlled by the bladder. The first urge to void is normally felt at around 200 mL (total bladder capacity is 300–500 mL), conveyed by afferent stretch fibres in the bladder wall. These relay information to the pons, which is responsible for the micturition reflex.

  The sympathetic, parasympathetic, and somatic nervous systems are all involved in bladder control (Figure 22.3):

CONTINUED ➤

CONTINUED

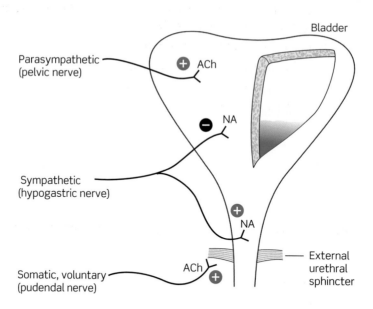

Figure 22.3 The neuronal control of micturition. The diagram represents a bladder with a section missing to show urine inside.

- The smooth muscle (detrusor) of the bladder wall is under joint control of the parasympathetic and sympathetic nervous systems. The parasympathetic system, via the pelvic nerve and muscarinic acetylcholine receptors, stimulates detrusor muscle contraction. Antimuscarinics, e.g. tolterodine and oxybutynin, are used in individuals with incontinence due to an overactive bladder. The sympathetic system, via a branch of the hypogastric nerve and using noradrenaline as a neurotransmitter, inhibits the detrusor muscle.

- The internal urethral sphincter is made of smooth muscle and is therefore under sympathetic control, mediated by the action of noradrenaline on alpha receptors. The input arises from another branch of the hypogastric nerve. α-Adrenergic blockers, e.g. doxazosin and prazosin, act on these receptors to block sphincter contraction and so are used to alleviate outflow obstruction.

- The external urethral sphincter is made of striated muscle and is under voluntary control, i.e. the somatic nervous system, via the pudendal nerve. The neuromuscular junction contains nicotinic acetylcholine receptors.

- The pelvic floor and striated muscle of the urethra are also under voluntary control.

  Micturition occurs when bladder pressure exceeds urethral pressure.

Which drugs commonly cause urinary retention?

Any drug with antimuscarinic effects can cause urinary retention, particularly:

- Antihistamines (e.g. chlorpheniramine, cetirizine)
- Tricyclic antidepressants (e.g. amitriptyline, imipramine)
- Drugs used to treat urinary incontinence (e.g. tolterodine, oxybutynin)

What are the indications for dialysis in the acute setting (e.g. at 3 a.m.)?

If the patient is in acute renal failure (i.e. oliguria or anuria with deranged renal function) and has any or all of the following, they are a candidate for dialysis:

- Severe hyperkalaemia ≥6.5 mM (despite maximal medical therapy)
- Severe acidosis pH ≤7.2 (despite maximal medical therapy)
- Severe pulmonary oedema (despite maximal medical therapy)
- Urea ≥30 mM and creatinine ≥1000 μM
- Uraemic encephalopathy

A 55-year-old man requests that his PSA levels be tested to check whether he has prostate cancer. Is the PSA test any good for screening for prostate cancer in asymptomatic men?

When considering whether to offer PSA testing to asymptomatic men, there are two main issues to consider:

1 How good is the test?
2 Is there an effective treatment?

How good is the test?

A lot of patients will enquire about the usefulness of the PSA test for detecting prostate cancer. Figure 22.4 shows what would happen if you screened a population of 1000 asymptomatic men aged 50–70 using the PSA test.

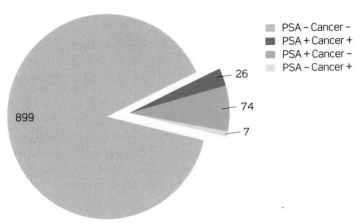

Figure 22.4 Incidence of prostate-specific antigen (PSA) test positives and true cancers in men aged 50–70 years.

CONTINUED ➤

CONTINUED

As you can see, the vast majority of those with a raised PSA will *not* have prostate cancer on transrectal biopsy of the prostate. The vast majority of men with a raised PSA will actually have either BPH or prostatitis. However, the usefulness of the PSA test for diagnosing prostate cancer can be increased somewhat by setting various cut-off values, rather than simply reporting 'positive' or 'negative':

PSA <3 ng/mL	Very low risk of prostate cancer (~0.7%)
PSA 3–10 ng/mL	Moderate risk of prostate cancer
PSA >10 ng/mL	High risk of prostate cancer
PSA >40 ng/mL	High risk of metastatic prostate cancer
PSA >100 ng/mL	Almost certainly metastatic prostate cancer

Thus, the PSA test is useful if it is <3 ng/mL (prostate cancer unlikely, but still possible) or >10 ng/mL (prostate cancer likely). Unfortunately, most patients with a positive PSA lie in the 3–10 ng/mL range and will need referring, according to 2011 NICE guidelines for referring suspected cancer (which use age-related PSA levels). For these patients, one needs to keep in mind that:

- The majority of patients with a PSA of 3–10 ng/mL will *not* have prostate cancer.
- Finding out which of them has cancer involves a transrectal prostate biopsy. This involves a rectal probe that inserts several (up to 12) needles through the rectal wall, into the prostate. The procedure is uncomfortable, often painful, and can cause prostatitis, sepsis, rectal bleeding, and (very rarely) death.

So, is the PSA test useful for detecting prostate cancer?

- **Yes,** if the patient has possible **symptoms** of prostate cancer (prostatism, bone pain) as a diagnosis of prostate cancer will then dictate treatment that can help with symptoms.
- **Yes**, if the PSA turns out to be **>10 ng/mL** as a diagnosis of prostate cancer is then likely and detecting prostate cancer at an early stage improves prognosis.
- **No**, if the PSA turns out to be 3–10 ng/mL as the patient will then be anxious about prostate cancer, may undergo a significant procedure (biopsy), and may be diagnosed with a prostate cancer that would never have caused any problems (as a significant proportion of prostate cancers cause no problems).

Is there an effective treatment for prostate cancer?

Prostate cancer is *very* common (60% of men over 80 years), usually asymptomatic (90% of cases), and usually not fatal (75% of cases). The management of prostate cancer depends on the stage and grade of the prostate cancer. Current strategies for the management of prostate cancer are summarized in Table 22.4. Please refer to local and national guidelines as relevant.

CONTINUED ➤

CONTINUED

Table 22.4 Management of prostate cancer

Prostate cancer	Preferred treatment	Alternatives
In situ, low risk[a]	Active surveillance[d]	Radical treatment (prostatectomy or radiotherapy with hormonal therapy[e])
In situ, intermediate risk[b]	Radical treatment	Active surveillance Brachytherapy (radiation implants) as adjunct to radiotherapy
In situ, high risk[c]	Radical treatment if realistic prospect of long-term disease control	Brachytherapy as adjunct to radiotherapy
Locally invasive	Radical treatment ± pelvic radiotherapy	
Metastatic	Bilateral orchidectomy or hormonal therapy	Docetaxel, dexamethasone, palliative care

[a] Low risk is defined as a PSA of <10 ng/ml *and* a Gleasons score of ≤6 *and* clinical stage T1–T2a.

[b] Intermediate risk is defined as a PSA of 10–20 ng/ml *or* a Gleasons score of 7 *or* clinical stage T2b.

[c] High risk is defined as a PSA of > 20 ng/ml *or* a Gleasons score of 8–10 *or* clinical stage T2c–T4

[d] Active surveillance involves regular (every 3–6 months) review of symptoms, PSA testing, and digital rectal examination, as well as a transrectal ultrasound ± biopsy every few years.

[e] Hormonal, or androgen deprivation, treatments are usually LHRH agonists (e.g. goserelin) or antiandrogens (e.g. cyproterone acetate, bicalutamide), although there are newer agents.

Single Best Answers

1. **A patient has a transurethral resection of the prostate (TURP) for his benign prostatic hyperplasia (BPH). Shortly after his return to the ward he is noted to be anuric and clot retention is suspected to be the most likely cause. Which of the following catheters is the appropriate choice for irrigating the bladder of such a patient?**

   a. Suprapubic
   b. Fogarty
   c. Swan–Ganz

   d. Three-way Foley
   e. Foley

2. **Which of the following may cause poor urinary output by a postrenal mechanism?**

   a. Cervical adenocarcinoma
   b. Retroperitoneal fibrosis
   c. Benign prostatic hyperplasia (BPH)

   d. Bladder transitional cell carcinoma
   e. All of the above

3. **Which of the following can commonly cause acute tubular necrosis?**

   a. Aminoglycoside antibiotics
   b. Myeloma
   c. Rhabdomyolysis

   d. Contrast reagents
   e. All of the above

4. **Which of the following diagnoses is most likely to explain the phenomenon of new onset renal failure and seizures?**

   a. Wegener's granulomatosis
   b. Thrombotic thrombocytopenic purpura (TTP)

   c. Myeloma
   d. Retroperitoneal fibrosis
   e. Goodpasture's

Polyuria

23

Core case

Read through the sections in the case boxes, covering up the sections that follow so that you don't see the answer. At the end of each case box, try to answer the question before reading on.

Mr George is a 74-year-old retired taxi driver who presents to his GP complaining that he is going to the toilet 'all the time'.

What would you ask to work out whether this is polyuria or high urinary frequency?

In both polyuria and high urinary frequency the patient will be passing urine more often than before. But in polyuria, patients will pass **abnormally large volumes** of clear urine each time. In urinary frequency, the volume voided each time will be normal or reduced. The only way of knowing objectively whether this is the case is by collecting a 24-hour urine sample (>3 L = polyuria). As this is usually impractical outside of hospital, one must rely on the patient's recall, with the caveat that many patients find it difficult to estimate urine output. In the history, then, ask them whether they feel they are passing a larger volume every time they go to the toilet.

Remember that it is important to be as sure as you can that you are dealing with polyuria and not urinary frequency or nocturia, as the differential diagnoses are quite distinct.

You ask Mr George and his responses indicate he has polyuria.

What is the differential diagnosis for polyuria? See Figure 23.1.

> Diabetes mellitus (type 1 or type 2)
> Diuretics (e.g. diuretic medication, caffeine, alcohol, lithium)
> Heart failure
> Hypercalcaemia
> Hyperthyroidism
> Primary polydipsia
> Hypokalaemia
> Hyperuricaemia
> Diabetes insipidus (cranial or nephrogenic)

Figure 23.1 Differential diagnosis for polyuria.

CORE CASE

Chronic renal failure and hypercalcaemia (e.g. due to bone metastases) cause polyuria by inducing nephrogenic diabetes insipidus. Similarly, steroids and Cushing's syndrome can cause polyuria by causing diabetes mellitus.

> The history can help to separate out some of the causes.
>
> **What questions in the history will narrow down the differential?**

- **Temporal pattern of urine output** (number of times in the day and at night), especially **nocturia**. At night, the kidneys concentrate urine in order to retain fluid (as intake is zero), removing the need to urinate during sleep. Thus nocturia (in the absence of other causes of nocturia, e.g. benign prostatic hyperplasia (BPH)) is often one of the earliest signs of a loss of concentrating ability. This symptom makes primary polydipsia less likely.
- **Fatigue, weight loss, recurrent infections**. All can be features of diabetes mellitus.
- **Lower urinary tract symptoms (LUTS)**, e.g. frequency, urgency, hesitancy, terminal dribbling, incomplete voiding. These symptoms indicate pathology in the bladder or the outflow tract, e.g. prostatism in men, detrusor instability and prolapse in women. Not strictly speaking polyuria.
- **Pain, frequency, change in urine colour and smell**. These are all symptoms suggestive of a urinary tract infection (UTI), which would cause increased *frequency* but not polyuria.
- **Past medical history**. Look for any history of renal problems or conditions that may precipitate chronic renal failure (e.g. vasculitides, hypertension, chronic urinary retention). In older patients, ask about cancer and known bony involvement, as this is one of the most common causes of hypercalcaemia. Primary polydipsia is more common in patients with a history of psychiatric disorders (although hyponatraemia from polydipsia may itself cause mania).
- **Drug history**. Diuretics are a potential and obvious cause of polyuria. Always ask about any recent changes in medications or new over the counter drugs. Don't forget that lithium (used for managing bipolar disorder) can cause polyuria by inducing a nephrogenic diabetes insipidus.
- **Family history**. There is a hereditary component to diabetes mellitus and some forms of cancer. Familial forms of diabetes insipidus (both nephrogenic and cranial) present very early in life.

> Mr George tells you he has been passing urine on average 10 times a day for the past week, and has to get up three or four times every night to pass urine, which is bothering his partner. He has not been particularly fatigued, or had any weight loss or recent infections.
>
> His past medical history is notable for chronic back pain over the past 18 months and occasional heartburn, for which he takes paracetamol, naproxen, and omeprazole. He takes no other medications and has no drug allergies. His parents both died in their eighties but he cannot remember what from. His brother is alive and well, and Mr George knows of no conditions running in his family.
>
> On inspection, Mr George looks well. There are no signs of cachexia to suggest malignancy or hyperthyroidism and, on testing his visual fields there is no bitemporal hemianopia to suggest a (rare) pituitary tumour (a cause of even rarer cranial diabetes insipidus).
>
> **What investigations should the GP request?**

First and foremost the GP should do some simple tests:

- **Capillary blood glucose**, to look for diabetes mellitus.
- **Urinalysis** with a dipstick, to exclude a UTI. This would give urinary frequency without polyuria, but it is important to exclude given the different management pathways and the fact that patients

often confuse urinary frequency with polyuria. Urinalysis can also detect glucosuria and ketonuria, other signs of diabetes mellitus.

As a next step, the GP should request the following investigations:

- **Fasting plasma glucose**. If the capillary blood glucose is towards the upper limit of normal (or indeed above), the GP should request a fasting plasma glucose to exclude diabetes mellitus. This also allows you to calculate serum osmolarity.

- **Urine osmolality**. There are two different mechanisms that lead to polyuria, with differing effects on urine osmolality:
  - Inability to reabsorb solutes by the kidneys. The solutes (e.g. glucose, urea) remain in the urine and keep water with them, leading to *high urine osmolality* (>300 mOsm) and volume.
  - Inability to reabsorb water due to distal tubule pathology or a deficient antidiuretic hormone (ADH) pathway. This results in *low urine osmolality* (<250 mOsm).

- **Electrolytes**. In primary polydipsia, serum sodium will be dilute due to excessive water intake. In all other pathologies, serum sodium will be concentrated as the patient is dehydrated. These abnormalities will be mirrored in the other electrolytes. You will also need the potassium if you want to calculate serum osmolarity.

- **Urea, creatinine, and estimated glomerular filtration rate (eGFR)**. This will help to exclude chronic kidney failure.

- **Serum calcium**. Although Mr George's clinical picture doesn't suggest hypercalcaemia, it is still worth excluding with a simple blood test.

- **Thyroid function**. Hyperthyroidism is the cause of polyuria in about as many cases as hypercalcaemia (~1/100 cases).

The GP tests Mr George's capillary blood glucose, which is 5.2 mM. Urinalysis is unremarkable. He then proceeds to request a fasting plasma glucose, urine osmolality, serum sodium, serum calcium and thyroid function. The biochemistry results come back:

Glucose (fasting)	5.4 mM	Na	144 mM	Ca (corrected)	2.51 mM
		K	3.7 mM	TSH	3.2 mU/L
		Urea	7.2 mM		
		Creatinine	130 µM		
		eGFR	110 mL/min		
Urine osmolality	242 mOsm				

What is the most likely diagnosis? How does this cause the diuresis?

The polyuria, absence of symptoms of diabetes mellitus, and normal blood and urine glucose suggest this is not diabetes mellitus. The low urine osmolality and normal serum sodium indicate that the kidney is failing to reabsorb water. The most likely diagnosis is a problem with the ADH pathway: **diabetes insipidus**. As a result the kidneys do not concentrate the urine and the patient, unable to retain fluid, passes large quantities of urine.

The next step is to determine which subtype of diabetes insipidus Mr George is suffering from.

What is the difference between the subtypes of diabetes insipidus?

What test can you use to distinguish them, and what are the principles behind this test?

There are two subtypes of diabetes insipidus that have a different underlying mechanism:

1   **Cranial/central**. ADH secretion is either reduced or absent due to a defect in the hypothalamic–pituitary axis. Consequently the signal to the kidneys to concentrate the urine is weak or absent. Causes include head injury, pituitary tumours, craniopharyngiomas or metastases, surgery, a vascular lesion, and meningitis.

2   **Nephrogenic**. The kidneys become less sensitive to ADH, and therefore do not respond to signals to concentrate the urine. This insensitivity may follow renal damage caused by low potassium, high calcium, drugs such as lithium, pyelonephritis, hydronephrosis, or may be inherited.

The **water deprivation test** can be used to distinguish between these two. As the name implies, the patient is fluid restricted. The normal response to water deprivation is release of ADH from the pituitary causing the kidneys to concentrate the urine. In diabetes insipidus, the urine remains abnormally dilute. However, if desmopressin, an artificial ADH analogue, is given, those with cranial diabetes insipidus (but normal kidneys) will be able to concentrate their urine. Those with nephrogenic diabetes insipidus will continue to have dilute urine. This is a very labour-intensive test, so before you start, you should confirm there is *true polyuria* by ensuring a 24-hour urine collection is >3 L. The test is also potentially dangerous in patients with diabetes insipidus as the deprivation of water intake can cause hypovolaemia, so patients must be weighed throughout and the test must be stopped if there is body weight loss of >3%.

The approach to the patient with polyuria outlined here is summarized in the flowchart in Figure 23.2.

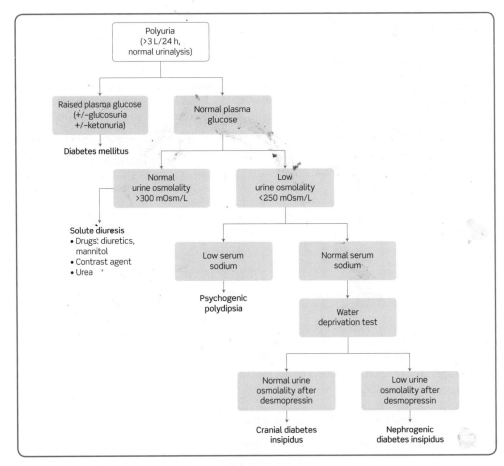

Figure 23.2 The diagnostic approach to polyuria.

A water deprivation test is performed, with the results shown in Figure 23.3.

Figure 23.3 Result of Mr George's water deprivation test.

What is the diagnosis?

Mr George has diabetes insipidus, as indicated by his inability to concentrate urine despite water deprivation. The correction on administration of the ADH analogue desmopressin demonstrates that this is due to a lack of ADH, i.e. he has cranial diabetes insipidus.

Given Mr George's diagnosis, how should he be managed?

Mr George's management should consist of the following:

1 **Adequate fluid intake**. This may be enough if his condition is mild. However, patients should be wary of dehydration.

2 **Investigation of the underlying cause**. Where no obvious cause is present (e.g. intracranial surgery), a MRI scan of the head should be performed to look for a pituitary lesion (about 25% of cases are due to intracranial tumours). Mr George should also be referred to an endocrinology unit.

3 **Replacement ADH**. If no reversible cause for the cranial diabetes insipidus is found (e.g. a pituitary tumour), patients will have to take replacement ADH for life.

Other medications are sometimes used in nephrogenic diabetes insipidus (e.g. chlorpropamide, carbamazepine) but not in cranial diabetes insipidus.

Short cases

Jane is a 17-year-old who presents to her GP complaining of increasing urinary frequency and thirst over the last month. She believes that over this month she has been passing a greater volume of urine every day. She has had no dysuria and there has been no change in the smell or colour of her urine. She has been drinking copious amounts of water in keeping with her thirst. The polydipsia has been going on since she started passing more urine, which makes sense to her. She hasn't felt particularly tired but has been losing weight—about 5 kg in the last 6 months. She has had two chest infections and a UTI in the last year, which she feels is unusual as she had always considered herself very healthy.

She has had eczema and childhood asthma in the past but is currently well and takes no medications other than the oral contraceptive pill. Her parents are alive and well with no medical history of note, but her older sister was diagnosed with Hashimoto's syndrome 2 years ago.

What is the most likely diagnosis? Which investigation(s) will you request, and what are the diagnostic criteria?

Jane presents with polyuria, polydipsia, weight loss, and recurrent infections. With her young age and family history, the most likely diagnosis is **type 1 diabetes mellitus**. Type 1 diabetes mellitus is caused by a reduction in pancreatic β cells and lack of insulin synthesis, making the patient insulin dependent. It is thought to be an autoimmune condition: anti-glutamic acid decarboxylase (GAD) autoantibodies are found in a large number of patients who are diagnosed early. There is some evidence that autoimmune destruction of islet cells may follow one or more environmental triggers such as a virus. There is also a genetic susceptibility (10 times increased risk if a first-degree family member is affected with type 1 diabetes mellitus).

A urinalysis and capillary glucose can be done as a screening test in the GP's surgery. However, the diagnosis of diabetes mellitus is based on measures of serum glucose. The **World Health Organization (WHO) criteria** for the diagnosis of diabetes mellitus are either:

- Fasting plasma glucose ≥ 7.0 mM
- Plasma glucose ≥ 11.1 mM when taken 2 hours after ingesting 75 g of glucose ('oral glucose tolerance test')

These criteria must be met on two separate occasions or on one occasion in the presence of symptoms suggesting diabetes mellitus. The diagnosis may be supported by an elevated glycated haemoglobin (HbA1c > 6.5%). The degree of glycation of haemoglobin reflects its exposure to glucose over the preceding months, thus this provides a medium term measure of blood glucose levels. In this case, as her symptoms have lasted only a month, it is likely that her HbA1c will be normal and thus of no diagnostic value.

Jane's diagnosis is confirmed and she is started on insulin replacement therapy. Six months later she is brought in to see you in a drowsy state. Her mother tells you that earlier in the evening she was complaining of abdominal pain and had been sick. Her mother insists that she has been compliant with her insulin therapy and new diet but concedes that they have not been very good about measuring her capillary glucose regularly as she doesn't like needles. Everything else has been unremarkable, although the mother mentions that Jane came down with a cold a couple of days ago and has been off school. During this time she has been unusually irritable.

On examination, Jane is indeed drowsy with a Glasgow Coma Scale (GCS) score of 12 (Eyes = 3, Verbal = 4, Motor = 5). Her heart rate is 105 bpm, blood pressure 102/64 mmHg, temperature 37.6 °C, respiratory rate 22/min, and saturations of 100% on air. She looks flushed but her tongue is dry. Respiratory and abdominal examinations are unremarkable. There are no other positive examination findings.

What has happened to Jane, and why? Why is she hyperventilating?

She has most likely suffered one of the complications of type 1 diabetes mellitus, **diabetic ketoacidosis** (note: type 2 diabetics do *not* suffer this complication as ketogenesis is inhibited with even a tiny amount of insulin, and the problem in type 2 diabetes is not lack of insulin production, but lack of sensitivity to insulin by target tissues). Common causes include previously undiagnosed type 1 diabetes mellitus, non-compliance (sometimes deliberate, but often forgetfulness), and illness, the latter being the most likely in Jane's case. During an illness, the body makes more corticosteroid in response to the physiological stress. Cortisol acts to antagonize the action of insulin, thus the normal insulin requirements go up during illness. Type 1 diabetics should therefore increase their insulin doses when they are unwell, and should monitor their capillary glucose to ensure they get the balance right. When you speak to Jane's mother, she tells you that they have been giving the same dose throughout and hadn't felt her cold was bad enough to warrant extra insulin. With more regular capillary glucose measurement this might have been evident.

Jane's breathing pattern is what is described as **Kussmaul breathing**: rapid, deep inspiration ('air hunger' to observers). It is caused by the ketoacidosis. The decrease in pH stimulates the respiratory centre. This then goes into overdrive to try to correct the acidosis (remember that by hyperventilating, you 'blow off' CO_2 and generate a respiratory alkalosis).

SHORT CASE

Mrs Jeffrey is a 73-year-old woman who presents to her GP with thirst and polyuria which has been present for 6 weeks. On further questioning, it emerges that she has also had constipation, for which she has been taking two sachets of Movicol a day. Throughout this period, she has felt nauseated and fatigued.

Her past medical history is notable for several months of low back pain and atrial fibrillation, for which she takes paracetamol, naproxen, bisoprolol, and warfarin; and vaginal prolapse, which the gynaecologists manage with pessaries. On examination, she is afebrile but appears dehydrated, with a dry tongue. There are no other positive findings.

The GP requests blood tests, which show:

Haematology		Biochemistry			
Hb	94 g/L	Na	138 mM	Glucose	4.8 mM
WCC	8.0×10^9 cells/L	K	4.1 mM		
Platelets	210×10^9 cells/L	Urea	9.1 mM		
MCV	92 fL	Creatinine	202 µM		

Urinalysis is negative for glucose, ketones, leucocytes, or nitrites.

What do the blood tests show? What is the most likely diagnosis? How does this explain her symptoms and blood results? What other blood tests would you like to request?

This patient has presented with polyuria, constipation, fatigue, and back pain. She has a **normocytic anaemia** (low Hb with normal MCV) and **renal impairment** (raised urea and creatinine). The other results shown (WCC, platelets, glucose, and electrolytes) are within the normal ranges. Although this could simply be chronic renal impairment combined with NSAID use, you must exclude **hypercalcaemia due to bone malignancy**, which could also explain this constellation of symptoms and blood results. High calcium levels reduce activation of voltage-gated sodium channels, thus reducing neuromuscular excitation and causing constipation. The high calcium also causes a nephrogenic diabetes insipidus (mechanism unknown), hence the polyuria. The anaemia (due to chronic malignancy or bone marrow infiltration) would explain the fatigue, and the bone malignancy (metastasis or multiple myeloma) would explain the bone pain.

The blood tests not shown above that you should request include **serum calcium**, to confirm the hypercalcaemia. If this is high, the GP should then arrange:

- **Alkaline phosphatase (ALP)**. This will be raised in bone metastasis (which activates ALP-producing osteoblasts) but not in multiple myeloma (which activates only osteoclasts).

- **Serum and urine electrophoresis**, looking for paraprotein (an oligoclonal band) found in multiple myeloma.

- **Lumbar radiograph**, looking for lytic lesions where she has the pain.

The results of these tests suggested that Mrs Jeffrey had multiple myeloma, which was confirmed with a bone marrow biopsy.

SHORT CASE

Mr Salvatore is a 23-year-old fisherman who lives at home with his parents and has schizophrenia. For the past 4 weeks his parents note that he has been drinking and passing large quantities of water. They are worried that this may be related to his medications, as they know there can be many different side effects. Mr Salvatore himself is not bothered by his symptoms although he agrees that he has been drinking and peeing a lot. There is nothing of note on examination (and notably, no signs of dehydration), although he displays disordered thought in conversation. He takes olanzapine for his schizophrenia and his parents say he has been compliant with this, although they add he's been a bit more muddled than usual over the past few days.

The results of his initial blood tests are as follows:

Haematology		Biochemistry			
Hb	137 g/L	Na	121 mM	Glucose	4.0 mM
WCC	5.0×10^9 cells/L	K	3.2 mM	T_4	8 µg/dL
Platelets	265×10^9 cells/L	Urea	2.1 mM		
MCV	89 fL	Creatinine	42 µM		

Urinalysis is negative for glucose, ketones, leucocytes, or nitrites.
Urine osmolality is 201 mOsm/L.

What do the blood results show? What is the most likely diagnosis? What test should you order next?

The patient has normal blood glucose, ruling out diabetes mellitus. He also has both a dilute serum (low electrolytes including hyponatraemia) and a dilute urine (201 mOsm/L), but no signs of dehydration. The patient is basically overhydrated—a sign of **primary polydipsia**. This patient should undergo a **water deprivation test** to confirm the diagnosis (his urine osmolality will increase as his body is deprived of water), and be referred for specialist management by psychiatry.

The diagnosis of primary polydipsia is most commonly seen in schizophrenics, although the reason for this is unknown. The management involves fluid restriction, and in some people certain antipsychotics can be helpful (e.g. clozapine).

Viva questions

What are the long-term complications of diabetes mellitus?

Diabetes mellitus affects the vascular system, thus the common complications can be divided into macrovascular and microvascular:

- Macrovascular (affecting any of the three major vascular beds)
  - Ischaemic heart disease
  - Cerebrovascular disease
  - Peripheral vascular disease
- Microvascular
  - Retinopathy
  - Neuropathy (e.g. 'glove-and-stocking' paraesthesia, autonomic dysfunction, mononeuritis multiplex)
  - Nephropathy (nephrotic syndrome)

In addition, diabetics can get lipohypertrophy around injection sites, and a variety of other skin complications have been described.

What is the pathology of hyperosmolar hyperglycaemic state (HHS)

HHS (previously known as HONK) is a life-threatening complication of type 2 diabetes mellitus. It is characterized by severe hyperglycaemia in the absence of any ketosis. The hyperglycaemia may be precipitated by any number of factors, including illness, dehydration, and/or non-compliance with diabetic medications. As the patient is a type 2 diabetic, they still produce insulin – but the amount produced is insufficient to control the hyperglycaemia. However, because only a small amount of insulin is needed to inhibit ketogenesis, this is sufficient to prevent ketosis.

The hyperglycaemia has two deleterious complications:

1 Fluid shifts under osmosis from the extravascular (including interstitial) compartment to the intravascular compartment. Thus, there is cellular dehydration.
2 There is an osmotic diuresis, with subsequent water loss in the urine. This can result in hypovolaemia.

If the hypovolaemia becomes severe, patients become vulnerable to shock, thrombosis, and neurological impairment.

Where is ADH produced, where does it act, and what does it do?

ADH is produced in the posterior pituitary in response to even slight increases in serum Na concentration. It acts in the collecting duct of the nephron in the kidney, where it causes an increase in the number of aquaporin channels. Normally the membrane of the collecting duct is relatively impermeable to water, preventing the water in the dilute 'urine' from passing down the osmotic gradient into the 'plasma'. By causing the insertion of aquaporin channels in the membrane, ADH makes it more permeable to water, which then diffuses across, leaving more concentrated urine.

CONTINUED ➤

CONTINUED

Thus, ADH is crucial for retaining fluid, e.g. when dehydrated or overnight (when we drink less). The nocturnal increase in ADH stops most people needing to urinate overnight and is the reason that ADH analogues (e.g. desmopressin) are sometimes used as a last resort in managing children with nocturnal enuresis (bedwetting).

What is the mechanism of action of the following diabetic drugs: biguanides (e.g. metformin); glitazones (or thiazolidinediones, e.g. rosiglitazone); sulphonylureas (e.g. gliclazide); meglitinides (e.g. nateglinide); gliptins (e.g. sitagliptin); α-glucosidase inhibitors (e.g. acarbose)?

- **Biguanides** (metformin) decrease hepatic glucose production and increase peripheral glucose uptake by an unknown mechanism(s)
- **Glitazones** (or thiazolidinediones) activate peroxisome proliferator-activated receptor gamma (PPAR-γ), a nuclear transcription factor that increases lipoprotein lipase (LPL), and fatty acid transporter protein 1 (FATP1) transcription, amongst other genes involved in lipid metabolism, to increase peripheral insulin sensitivity (and hence glucose uptake by peripheral tissues, e.g. muscle and adipose tissue)
- **Sulphonylureas** and **meglitinides** increase insulin secretion by blocking the K_{ATP} channel in pancreatic β cells, causing depolarization and calcium entry, stimulating insulin secretion
- **Gliptins** competitively inhibit dipeptidyl peptidase-4 (DPP-4), an enzyme that normally inactivates glucagon-like peptide 1 (GLP-1), an incretin that stimulates insulin secretion and inhibits glucagon release
- α-**Glucosidase** inhibitors decrease glucose absorption in the intestine

Single Best Answers

1. **Which of the following oral hypoglycaemic agents is the most appropriate initial therapy for a newly diagnosed type 2 diabetic with normal renal function and a body mass index (BMI) of 34?**

   a. Gliclazide
   b. Metformin
   c. Acarbose

   d. Rosiglitazone
   e. Repaglinide

2. **A patient with type 2 diabetes is taking a combination of oral hypoglycaemic agents. Since the introduction of a new medication they have reported embarrassing levels of flatulence. Which of the following drugs is the most likely culprit?**

   a. Gliclazide
   b. Metformin
   c. Acarbose

   d. Rosiglitazone
   e. Repaglinide

3. **Which of the following electrolyte abnormalities can result in nephrogenic diabetes insipidus?**

   a. Hypercalcaemia
   b. Hypernatraemia
   c. Hypokalaemia

   d. a and b
   e. a and c

4. **Which of the following tumours is most likely to cause cranial diabetes insipidus?**

   a. Meningioma
   b. Prolactinoma
   c. Glioblastoma multiforme

   d. Craniopharyngioma
   e. Ependymoma

5. **A patient is admitted with HHS (hyperosmolar hyperglycaemic state). Other than correcting their hyperglycaemia and dehydration, which of the following steps is an essential part of their management?**

   a. CT head
   b. IV diazepam
   c. Prophylactic anticoagulation

   d. IV adrenaline
   e. Echocardiogram

Groin lump

Core case

Read through the sections in the case boxes, covering up the sections that follow so that you don't see the answer. At the end of each case box, try to answer the question before reading on.

> Mr Harcourt is a 36-year-old firefighter who is referred to the general surgical outpatient clinic by his GP because he has a groin lump.
>
> **What is your differential diagnosis for a groin lump? Try to think of the anatomical structures in the groin region, and any pathology that may arise from those structures.**

Considering the anatomy and associated pathology in a systematic fashion, the lump may represent:

- **Psoas sheath** → psoas abscess or psoas bursa
- **Femoral nerve** → neuroma
- **Femoral artery** → femoral aneurysm or pseudoaneurysm
- **Femoral vein/long saphenous vein** → saphena varix (dilated great saphenous vein due to incompetence at the saphenofemoral junction)
- **Lymph nodes** → lymphadenopathy (infectious or malignant)
- **Hernial orifices** → inguinal hernia, femoral hernia
- **Testicular apparatus** → ectopic testis, undescended testis, hydrocele of cord
- **Skin/subcutis** → lipoma, infected abscess (e.g. from intravenous (IV) drug use), sebaceous cyst.

> **Which of these diagnoses are most common? Try to arrange them in order of prevalence.**

See Figure 24.1 for the main causes of groin lumps arranged in order of prevalence.

Indirect inguinal hernia
Direct inguinal hernia
Femoral hernia
Inguinal lymphadenopathy
Saphena varix
Psoas abscess/bursa
Lipoma
Sebaceous Cyst
Neuroma
Femoral aneurysm/pseudoaneurysm
Ectopic testis
Unde scended testis
Hydrocele of cord

Figure 24.1 Groin lumps according to prevalence.

What questions should you ask about the lump itself that might help you characterize it?

In common with lumps anywhere on the body, you will need to establish:

- **How long has the lump been there?** Many of the diagnoses listed in Figure 24.1 will develop rather insidiously, but there are some that may have a rather shorter history. For example, a patient may develop a femoral artery pseudoaneurysm (a collection of blood outside the vessel lumen) following angiography, a direct inguinal hernia may be precipitated by a period of heavy lifting, or inguinal lymphadenopathy may follow a lower limb infection. Ectopic or undescended testes would be present from birth, but it is extremely unlikely that a man would reach adulthood in the Western world without having had this defect corrected by orchidopexy (orchid = testis, -pexy = fixation in correct position) or orchidectomy (orchid = testis, -ectomy = removal).

- **Is the lump always there? Does it reduce when the patient lies down?** This question relates to hernias and saphena varix. Increases in intra-abdominal pressure, for example during coughing or straining at stool, may cause hernias to increase in size. A saphena varix may increase in size if the patient stands for long periods of time as retrograde flow through incompetent venous valves will allow blood to pool. A saphena varix will disappear completely when the patient lies down.

- **Has the lump got bigger, smaller, or stayed the same size?** Almost all of the pathologies on our differential (with the possible exception of ectopic/undescended testes) may change in size over time. Rapid changes in size may hint at an infective process such as a psoas abscess or lymphadenopathy.

- **Is the lump painful?** Reducible and incarcerated hernias may or may not be painful (they are more often mildly uncomfortable), whereas a strangulated hernia will be acutely painful. A groin abscess, infected sebaceous cyst, or infected pseudoaneurysm may also be painful.

- **Are there any other lumps?** There may be another lump in the other groin (about 20% of inguinal hernias are bilateral). Equally, inguinal lymphadenopathy may occur in conjunction with more widespread lymphadenopathy (e.g. lymphoma, primary HIV infection, systemic lupus erythematosus (SLE)).

What questions should you ask if you suspect a hernia?

If the history is suggestive of a hernia, you should ask:

- **Has there been any abdominal pain?** The main risks of hernia formation are bowel obstruction (when the flow of bowel contents is interrupted) and bowel strangulation (when the blood supply to a section of bowel is compromised and thus ischaemia ensues). Hernias may present as an emergency due to either of these problems, but even with an elective presentation (following the discovery of a groin lump) it is possible to have a history of intermittent episodes of subacute obstruction as bowel moves in and out of a hernial orifice. Such episodes of obstruction would result in colicky abdominal pain, together with abdominal distension, vomiting, and absolute constipation if the obstruction was prolonged.

- **Has the patient been straining at stool, struggling to pass urine, or suffering from a chronic cough? Does their job or a leisure activity involve heavy lifting?** All of these factors will increase intra-abdominal pressure and increase the likelihood of hernias.

- **Has the patient had any prior operations in the groin?** Previous surgery can of course predispose to incisional hernias. More importantly, a history of inguinal or femoral hernias may raise such diagnoses to the top of the differential list, and may dictate a different approach to repair (for example, laparoscopic hernia repair may be indicated for recurrent inguinal hernias).

What questions should you ask if you suspect an infective process or malignancy?

Questions that are more relevant to lymphadenopathy include:

- **Has there been any trauma or infection in the lower limbs or groin?** You may need to specifically ask about injecting drug use, as not all patients will admit to this. Also ask about minor injuries such as insect bites or infected toenails, as patients may consider these to be so trivial that they don't initially volunteer the information. Sexually transmitted diseases can cause inguinal lymphadenopathy (although the groin lump is not usually the presenting complaint), so a sexual history and questions about genital rash and discharge may be appropriate.

- **Have there been any indicators of anal, scrotal, or cutaneous malignancy?** For instance, new or changing lumps/bumps or marks in the surrounding region. Inguinal lymphadenopathy may represent metastatic spread from anal cancer, scrotal cancer, or melanoma.

- **Does he have a fever?** Febrile symptoms make an infective pathology such as a psoas abscess or lymphadenopathy more likely. Note that fever is also one of the 'B symptoms' of lymphoma along with weight loss, night sweats, and anorexia—one of the important differential diagnoses for lymphadenopathy.

- **Has there been any weight loss, night sweats, or pruritus?** The former two are general features of malignancy while pruritus is another symptom of lymphoma.

Mr Harcourt explains that the lump has probably been in his right groin for a couple of months. He can't remember exactly when or why he first noticed it, but says that he was first aware of a rather dull ache in his groin. The lump appeared relatively insidiously. On further questioning he explains that the lump isn't always there. It will invariably be present if he's had an active day at work, but may not make an appearance if he's just lounging around at home. When the lump appears it is always the same size. It has never extended into his scrotum. He says that it is never truly painful, but will ache at the end of the day.

He has no previous surgical history, and is otherwise fit and well. He takes no medications. The next stage is to examine Mr Harcourt.

How would you approach the examination of a groin lump?

The first step is to ensure that the patient is *adequately exposed*—and this means being able to fully inspect both groins and the abdomen. You will also need to examine the external genitalia, but to preserve the patient's dignity it is best to leave the genitalia covered until you need to examine them.

It is fine to start with the patient lying down, but you will also need to repeat the groin examination with the patient *standing up*.

Look at *both sides* of the groin for any masses or scars from previous surgery.

> **What particular features of the lump should you characterize during palpation?**

There are a number of key features that you will need to establish during palpation:

Site

- **Where is the lump?** It is crucially important that you are familiar with the anatomy of the inguinal region, as knowing the normal surface landmarks for structures will enable you to establish the origin of a lump (see Figure 24.2). A saphena varix will lie over the saphenofemoral junction.[†] As far as hernias are concerned, try to establish whether the **neck of the swelling** is:
  - Superior and medial to the pubic tubercle (inguinal hernia)
  - Inferior and lateral to the pubic tubercle (femoral hernia)

(*Note that the anatomical relations refer to the neck of the hernia and not the swelling itself.*)

- **Which tissue layer does the lump lie within?** Is it cutaneous, subcutaneous (lipoma), or associated with the deeper tissues?

- **Does the lump extend into the scrotum?** If so, this is almost certainly an indirect inguinal hernia (rarely a direct inguinal hernia).

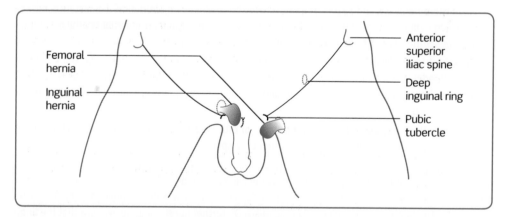

Figure 24.2 Diagram of anatomy of inguinal (patient right) versus femoral hernias (patient left).

[†] The site of the saphena varix corresponds with the saphenofemoral junction, 2–3 cm inferolateral to the pubic tubercle. Another way of thinking about this is to remember that the femoral vein (hence saphenofemoral junction) lies just medial to the femoral artery—which is itself located at the mid-inguinal point.

Size

How big is the lump? This might not affect the management, but it is part of a complete characterization of any lump and surgeons will always ask for this information.

Is the lump tender and/or warm?

- The skin overlying a strangulated hernia is likely to be red and inflamed, and there may be signs of a systemic inflammatory response (if there is bowel necrosis) and signs of bowel obstruction.
- Reducible hernias may be tender to palpation.
- Groin abscesses, reactive lymph nodes, or infected pseudoaneurysms may also be warm and tender to palpation, and associated with overlying erythema.

Is the lump solid or fluctuant?

Swollen lymph nodes are solid. A hernia, saphena varix, femoral aneurysm/pseudoaneurysm, psoas bursa, or hydrocele of the cord will be softer and may be fluctuant.

Is the lump pulsatile?

A truly pulsatile lump can only be a femoral aneurysm (either a true aneurysm or pseudoaneurysm). Remember, however, that you may detect a transmitted pulse if, for example, a swollen lymph node overlies the femoral artery.

Does the lump have a cough impulse?

This means that the lump expands and increases in tension during coughing—and is thus diagnostic of hernias as these will expand in response to increased intra-abdominal pressure, pushing more of the contents through the abdominal wall defect, unless incarcerated. It does not mean that the lump moves in response to coughing. To detect this you should put your hands over the lump (or where the patient says the lump appears) and ask the patient to cough. Direct inguinal hernias will typically expand outwards (through the defect in the posterior wall of the inguinal canal) whereas indirect inguinal hernias will tend to expand along the path of the inguinal canal in an inferomedial direction.

Is the lump reducible? If so, in which direction does it reduce?

- The only reducible groin lumps are hernias or a saphena varix. Saphena varix is rare—it is a soft, bluish swelling that is only seen when the patient stands. It will empty with minimal palpation and fill upon release of the pressure.
- The direction of reducibility is most useful for distinguishing between direct and indirect inguinal hernias. The former tend to reduce superiorly and posteriorly whereas the latter reduce superolaterally and posteriorly (indirect hernias tend to reduce along the length of the inguinal canal). You will often find that patients themselves can show you the most comfortable way to reduce their hernia.
- Remember that not all hernias are reducible.

What further information will percussion and auscultation of the lump add?

Percussion of a groin lump will not, in clinical practice, provide any reliable information about its contents. Auscultation can be useful as a groin lump with audible bowel sounds is more likely to represent herniated bowel.

Mr Harcourt is initially examined lying on the bed. No groin swellings are visible on general inspection but a mass with a cough impulse is felt in the right groin when Mr Harcourt is asked to cough. The lump does not reduce spontaneously. It is oval shaped, 4 cm long, and fluctuant. The neck of the lump is medial and superior to the pubic tubercle.

His abdomen is palpated while he is lying down, and nothing abnormal is noted. The external genitalia are normal.

Mr Harcourt is asked to stand and the groin examination is repeated. The lump does not appear until Mr Harcourt is asked to cough. He is able to comfortably reduce the swelling when he is lying down.

Why was the rest of Mr Harcourt's abdomen examined?

Which diagnosis do you think is most likely?

The rest of Mr Harcourt's abdomen was examined to check for any abdominal masses (such as ascites, a tumour, or gross faecal loading) which could increase intra-abdominal pressure and predispose to hernia formation.

The history and examination findings are highly suggestive of a **reducible inguinal hernia**—a fluctuant mass, with a cough impulse, that has its origin superior and medial to the pubic tubercle.

Is there a simple bedside test that will help you to distinguish between a direct or indirect hernia?

The key lies in appreciating the origins of direct versus indirect inguinal hernias (Figure 24.3).

With direct inguinal hernias, the hernial sac protrudes through a defect in the transversalis fascia which forms the posterior wall of the inguinal canal. By contrast, the sac of an indirect inguinal hernia protrudes through the deep inguinal ring at the lateral end of the inguinal canal. As such, it should be possible to control a reduced indirect inguinal hernia by applying pressure to the deep inguinal ring. To

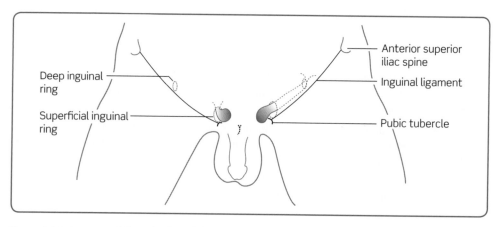

Figure 24.3 Anatomy of direct (patient right) versus indirect (patient left) inguinal hernias.

do this you will need to reduce the hernia and then place a finger over the deep ring (at the midpoint of the inguinal ligament). Now ask the patient to cough. If the hernia reappears while your finger is still occluding the deep ring then the hernia must be direct (or you have your finger in the wrong place!). An indirect hernia will reappear only when pressure over the deep ring is released.

About 75% of adult hernias are indirect and about 25% are direct. Note that it is possible for direct and indirect hernias to coexist as a 'pantaloon hernia'.

In truth, the correct diagnosis of direct versus indirect inguinal hernia is often only made in the operating theatre as clinical examination is only correct about 50% of the time! Indirect inguinal hernias have their origin lateral to the deep inferior epigastric artery (which lies medial to the deep inguinal ring) while direct hernias have their origin medial to the deep inferior epigastric artery.

Once Mr Harcourt has reduced the groin swelling, the examiner places his hand over the right deep inguinal ring and asks Mr Harcourt to cough. The lump does not reappear. The examiner then removes his hand, asks the patient to cough again, and observes that the lump appears.

What is the diagnosis and how should Mr Harcourt be managed?

The examination evidence is consistent with a **right reducible indirect inguinal hernia**.

Indirect hernias have a higher risk of strangulation than direct hernias as the hernial sac passes through a smaller defect (compared with the hole in the transversalis fascia that direct hernias pass through)—this also explains why direct hernias have a greater tendency to spontaneously reduce when patients lie down.

Appropriate management would be an elective surgical repair.

Short cases

Mrs Taylor is a 72-year-old woman who presents to her GP with a lump in her groin. She first noticed the lump a week ago. The lump has been present for the whole of the last week—it has never disappeared and does not appear to have changed in size. Mrs Taylor reports that it is slightly tender. She is not aware of any other lumps and says that she is otherwise fit and well.

She takes a calcium channel blocker for hypertension, calcium-vitamin D tablets and a bisphosphonate for osteoporosis. She has got three children, one of whom was born by Caesarean section. She had a cholecystectomy in her forties.

On examination, Mrs Taylor has a fluctuant lump of diameter 2 cm in her left groin, the neck of which is inferior and lateral to the pubic tubercle. There is the impression of a weak cough impulse. It is not possible to reduce the lump with gentle pressure. The lump is not tender to palpation, and there is no overlying erythema.

The right groin and abdominal examination are unremarkable.

What is the most likely diagnosis?

How urgently would you refer Mrs Taylor to the surgeons?

Mrs Taylor's history and examination are consistent with the diagnosis of a **femoral hernia** as she has a fluctuant mass, the neck of which sits inferior and lateral to the pubic tubercle. Femoral hernias are more common in women than in men. However, inguinal hernias are still more common than femoral hernias in women.

Femoral hernias have a higher risk of strangulation than inguinal hernias (as they have a narrower neck). She should be **referred to the surgeons for operative repair without delay**. A truss should never be used for femoral hernias.

Mrs Taylor is referred to the surgeons. Three days after her original GP consultation she returns to the surgery. She says that for the past 6 hours the lump in her groin has been far more painful. The overlying skin is also warm and red. Following further questioning by her GP she says that she has had colicky abdominal pain for the past 4 hours. She hasn't been to the toilet but is unsure whether she has passed any flatus. She has not vomited.

On examination, there is a tender red swelling in her left groin. She is febrile (38.2 °C), her pulse is 106 bpm regular, and her blood pressure is 137/86 mmHg.

What has happened to Mrs Taylor?

What is the next course of action?

It is likely that Mrs Taylor's **hernia has strangulated**. There are local signs of inflammation (a red and tender lump), together with systemic signs (tachycardia and fever). Additionally, the colicky abdominal pain hints that she is developing small bowel obstruction. The other features that we expect to see with intestinal obstruction—namely vomiting, absolute constipation, and abdominal distension—may not have developed yet as the history is still quite short and she has a *distal* obstruction.

Mrs Taylor must now be **seen by the surgeons as an emergency** as there is a risk of bowel necrosis and perforation. The operative mortality for strangulated hernia repairs is almost 10 times higher than that for elective hernia repairs.

SHORT CASE

Mr Johnson is a 52-year-old publican who presents to his GP with a lump in his right groin. He says that the lump has been there 'for ages', but that he has not been concerned about it as it gives him no pain and hasn't changed in size or location. His wife thinks that it is a hernia and wants him to get it checked. Her brother has recently had an inguinal hernia repair and she wonders whether the same may be suitable for her husband as she worries about his ability to cope with lifting beer barrels around the pub. Mr Johnson explains that he only ever notices the lump when he is standing up. Following further questioning he states that he has had no abdominal pain and is not aware of any other lumps.

His past medical history is significant for a right-sided hip replacement 2 years ago. His stay in hospital was complicated by a deep vein thrombosis (DVT) in his right thigh that was treated with 3 months of warfarin therapy. He says that he is otherwise fit and well. He takes symbicort and salbutamol inhalers for asthma, allopurinol for gout, and sildenafil for Mrs Johnson.

Mr Johnson is asked to remove his trousers and pants and is examined standing up. On inspection, Mr Johnson is noted to have marked varicosities over the inferomedial aspect of his right thigh. Examination reveals a fluctuant swelling in his right groin, approximately 2 cm inferior and lateral to the pubic tubercle. The lump points down the leg, is approximately 1.5 cm × 1 cm, and has a bluish tinge. It is non-tender to palpation and there is an expansile cough impulse. The lump easily reduces with light palpation, and reappears as soon as the examiner's finger is removed. No bowel sounds are audible over the lump, and it is non-pulsatile. Mr Johnson is asked to lie down and the lump disappears within seconds. Examination of the rest of the abdomen and external genitalia is unremarkable.

Which diagnosis is most likely?

The differential diagnosis for a non-tender, fluctuant groin lump with a cough impulse is a hernia or saphena varix. The position of the swelling inferior and lateral to the pubic tubercle narrows the differential to a femoral hernia or saphena varix. The fact that this swelling has a bluish tinge, is easily reduced, and disappears as soon as the patient lies flat, makes **saphena varix** more likely. The history of a DVT and examination findings of other venous varicosities in the right leg add further support to this diagnosis.

SHORT CASE

Mr Guscott is a 78-year-old retired headmaster who presents to his local Emergency Department at 8 p.m. with sudden-onset crushing chest pain that radiates to his left arm. He had a myocardial infarction aged 60, and two-vessel coronary artery bypass graft when he was 63, and has been admitted to hospital twice over the last year with acute coronary syndrome. He takes aspirin, clopidogrel, carvedilol, ramipril, atorvastatin, and nicorandil. He smokes 30 cigarettes a day, and says that his exercise tolerance is 'nil'.

A medical student clerks Mr Guscott once his condition has stabilized. As part of a thorough examination the student notes that he has a prominent swelling in his right groin. The swelling is fluctuant, has a cough impulse, and points towards the pubic tubercle. The neck of the swelling is superior and medial to the pubic tubercle. The swelling does not extend into the scrotum. It is not tender and the overlying skin is normal. It reduces with ease and reappears as soon as Mr Guscott is asked to stand up. He is encouraged to reduce the swelling, and does so, but pressure applied by the student over the deep inguinal ring fails to control the hernia, which reappears as soon as Mr Guscott is asked to cough. The rest of the abdominal examination is unremarkable and the external genitalia are normal. Mr Guscott says that he has had the lump for years, and that it hasn't given him any trouble.

The student presents his clerking on the ward round the following morning. He describes the lump and suggests that Mr Guscott has a general surgical review as part of his management plan.

What is the most likely diagnosis for the groin lump? How should it be managed?

The examination suggests that this is a **direct inguinal hernia**. The location of the neck of the hernia medial and superior to the pubic tubercle distinguishes this from a femoral hernia. The fact that the swelling appears as soon as the patient stands, coupled with the fact that pressure over the deep inguinal ring fails to control the lump, is highly suggestive of a direct hernia.

Although indirect hernias are still more common than direct hernias in elderly people, direct hernias are more common than they are in the younger population. As direct hernias have a wider neck than indirect hernias they are at less risk of strangulation. This affords a more conservative approach to their management. Options include:

- **Doing nothing**—and reassuring the patient that this is a common and relatively benign condition. If the patient is overweight you may advise them to lose some weight as this will help to reduce intra-abdominal pressure. The patient can be advised to re-present if the hernia becomes symptomatic.

- Recommending that the patient **wears a truss** to prevent bowel obstruction. There is limited evidence that they work, perhaps because of compliance issues, but they remain very popular with elderly patients. Note that you should never put a truss over an irreducible hernia.

- **Surgical repair.**

The significance of Mr Guscott's past medical history affects his fitness for a general anaesthetic. Spinal anaesthesia is contraindicated due to his antiplatelet therapy (which the cardiologists are unlikely to allow to be stopped, given his recent episodes of acute coronary syndrome). Some surgeons advocate the use of local anaesthesia for elective surgical repair in such patients, but the patient needs to be relatively slim to make this feasible. Many would favour conservative management (particularly in this case, given that Mr Guscott is asymptomatic from his hernia).

SHORT CASE

Mr Pemberton is a 26-year-old artist. He first noticed a firm lump in his left groin 1 week ago, and now presents to his GP. He is certain it wasn't there before. The lump is non-tender, and has not changed in size or location. He has been checking his groin several times a day, and also while in bed at night, and reports that the lump is always present. He says that he feels otherwise well. He has no significant past medical history and is taking no medications.

Examination reveals a firm rubbery lump, 1.5 cm in diameter, in the left groin crease. The lump is relatively mobile and does not appear to be tethered to underlying structures. It is not possible to reduce the lump. Examination of the right groin, abdomen, and external genitalia is unremarkable.

What is the most likely diagnosis? What can cause such a lump? How would you proceed to investigate the possible underlying cause?

This lump is consistent with **inguinal lymphadenopathy**.

When considering the causes of inguinal lymphadenopathy it is usual to divide our differential into local versus systemic, and infective versus neoplastic causes (Table 24.1).

Table 24.1 Causes of inguinal lymphadenopathy

	Systemic	Local
Infective	HIV Tuberculosis	Non-specific lymphadenopathy from groin/lower limb infection/ sexually transmitted disease Others, e.g. lymphogranuloma venereum (very rare in the West)
Neoplastic	Lymphoma Leukaemia	Metastases: from primary in lower limb, external genitalia,[a] or perianal region (e.g. squamous cell carcinoma, melanoma)

[a] Remember that the testes drain to para-aortic and not inguinal lymph nodes.

The first step in investigating the potential cause of inguinal lymphadenopathy is to take a more detailed history. You may have to specifically enquire about:

- Any recent lower limb trauma or infection, including sexually transmitted diseases
- Potential exposure to specific pathogens such as tuberculosis/HIV
- Any preceding ulcers?—the painful lymph nodes seen with lymphogranuloma venereum are preceded by an ulcer
- Symptoms of anal cancer such as bleeding
- Symptoms of systemic malignancy—night sweats, fever, weight loss, pruritus.

The majority of cases of inguinal lymphadenopathy will be a response to non-specific groin or lower limb infection. It is thus very important that you also examine the leg for signs of an infective or malignant (e.g. melanoma) source. If the history and examination findings raise any other suspicions, there are a number of further investigations that can be carried out:

- Full blood count and blood film: looking for features of leukaemia.
- HIV test: guideline is that this should be done in any acutely unwell patient in high-prevalence areas (>2:1000, i.e. virtually all of London) and does not need formal consent. In reality very few patients object; if they do, they can be reassured that HIV has a good prognosis now if treated.
- Fine needle aspirate: sending samples for cytology (lymphoma) and microbiology (infection). Note that it is often very difficult to diagnose low-grade lymphoma by fine needle aspiration, and core biopsy may be required.
- An open excisional biopsy may be required if a diagnosis has still not been made.

Viva questions

Define a 'hernia', 'fistula', 'sinus', and 'stoma'

- A **hernia** is the abnormal protrusion of the contents of a cavity through the wall that normally contains it.
- A **fistula** is an abnormal communication between two epithelial surfaces, such as two hollow organs or between a hollow organ and the exterior.
- A **sinus** is a blind-ended tract between an epithelial surface and a cavity lined with granulation tissue.
- A **stoma** is the artificial opening of an internal tube (e.g. gastrointestinal (GI) tract, ureter) that has been brought to the surface. See Figure 24.4.

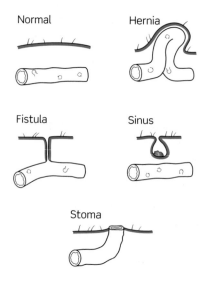

Figure 24.4 Diagram comparing the normal state with a hernia, fistula, sinus, and stoma.

What is the most common type of hernia in women?

Indirect inguinal hernias are the most common hernias in men and women. Don't fall into the trap of saying femoral hernias—while it is true that femoral hernias are the only hernia that is more common in women than in men, indirect inguinal hernias are still more common.

What is the difference between reducible, irreducible, incarcerated, obstructed, and strangulated hernias?

- A **reducible hernia** can be pushed back into the right place.
- An **irreducible hernia** cannot be pushed back into the right place. This is not a problem for the patient per se, but is at risk of causing problems. A hernia may be irreducible because it is:

CONTINUED ➤

CONTINUED

- **Incarcerated:** stuck in the abnormal position because either there are adhesions between the hernial sac and surrounding structures, or there are adhesions between structures within the sac such that the sac is now wider than its neck and no longer able to pass through the wall defect.
- **Obstructed:** the neck of the hernial sac provides an obstruction to the passage of flow through the bowel (but the blood supply of the bowel is intact).
- **Strangulated:** if the bowel becomes so constricted by the neck of the hernial sac that the blood supply is compromised it is referred to as a strangulated hernia. This is a major problem for the patient as their bowel will necrose rapidly from ischaemia.

What are the contents of the inguinal canal?

If you watch a hernia operation it is almost guaranteed that somebody will ask you to name the contents of the inguinal canal. The male canal contains the ilioinguinal nerve and spermatic cord, while the female canal contains the ilioinguinal nerve and round ligament. Perhaps the easiest way to remember the contents of the spermatic cord is to think of structures arising in sets of three. Hence there are:

- Three layers of fascia:
  - external spermatic fascia (from the external oblique aponeurosis)
  - cremasteric fascia (from the internal oblique aponeurosis)
  - internal spermatic fascia (from the transversalis fascia)

- Three arteries:
  - the gonadal artery (arising directly from the aorta)
  - the cremasteric artery (arising from the inferior epigastric artery)
  - the artery of the vas (arising from the inferior vesical artery)

- Three veins, which mirror the arteries:
  - testicular vein/pampiniform plexus
  - cremasteric vein
  - vein of the vas

- Three nerves:
  - ilioinguinal nerve (which lies outside the spermatic cord)
  - sympathetic supply from T10 and T11
  - genital branch of the genitofemoral nerve

- Three other things:
  - vas deferens
  - lymphatics
  - patent processus vaginalis (if present)

What are the boundaries of Hesselbach's triangle and what is its significance?

Whether an inguinal hernia is direct or indirect is defined according to its relationship to Hesselbach's triangle (Figure 24.5). The borders of the triangle are as follows: medially, rectus sheath; inferiorly, inguinal ligament; superiorly, deep inferior epigastric artery. An inguinal hernia that arises within

CONTINUED ➤

Hesselbach's triangle is direct, whereas indirect hernias arise lateral to the deep inferior epigastric artery and thus lateral to the triangle.

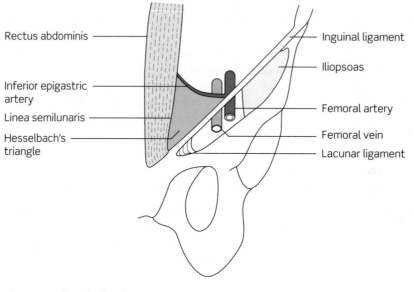

Figure 24.5 Hesselbach's triangle.

What are the boundaries of the inguinal canal?

- **Anterior:** skin, superficial fascia, external oblique aponeurosis, and internal oblique for lateral third.
- **Posterior:** conjoint tendon medially and transversalis fascia laterally.
- **Roof:** arching fibres of internal oblique and transversus abdominis.
- **Floor:** inguinal ligament. See Figure 24.6.

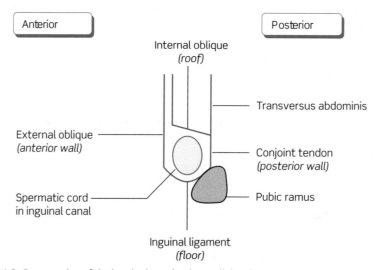

Figure 24.6 Cross-section of the inguinal canal at its medial end.

What are the boundaries of the femoral canal?

- **Anterior:** inguinal ligament
- **Posterior:** pectineal ligament and pectineus
- **Medial:** lacunar ligament
- **Lateral:** femoral vein

What is the difference between herniotomy, herniorrhaphy, and hernioplasty?

- A **herniotomy** refers to the surgical excision of a hernial sac.
- **Herniorrhaphy** involves the repair of a hernia using locally available tissues (for example, a sutured repair such as the Bassini).
- **Hernioplasty** involves the repair of a hernia using synthetic material such as a mesh.

The inguinal hernias that typically occur in childhood are due to a patent processus vaginalis and thus the repair is usually a herniotomy as there is rarely a weakness in the inguinal canal which needs repairing. By contrast, adult hernias are due to a defect in the boundaries of the inguinal canal and are thus usually repaired by herniotomy in conjunction with herniorrhaphy/hernioplasty.

What are the potential complications of a surgical hernia repair?

When asked to list complications for any procedure you should take a systematic approach. Thus you may recognize complications of surgery in general, including anaesthetic complications, and complications peculiar to the particular procedure:

1. Potential **complications of surgery in general:**
   - Haemorrhage[†]
   - Infection[†]
   - Thromboembolism (DVT or pulmonary embolism (PE))
   - Anaesthetic complications (e.g. inadequate analgesia, respiratory depression, urinary retention, cardiac depression)
   - Death

2. Potential **complications of hernia repair:**
   - Hernia recurrence
   - Ischaemic orchitis/testicular atrophy
   - Bruising of scrotum and penis
   - Cutaneous anaesthesia or hyperaethesia (but note that there is considerable overlap in the cutaneous areas supplied by the iliohypogastric, ilioinguinal, and genitofemoral nerves).

CONTINUED ➤

---

† Haemorrhage following hernia repair may be seen as scrotal haematoma. Infection is more likely if a mesh repair is performed.

CONTINUED

Note that it is important to be familiar with complications so as to be able to explain the risks to patients in the process of soliciting their consent. Indeed, only surgeons who are familiar with the procedure and its complications should seek consent from patients.

What is the difference between the *mid-inguinal point* and the *midpoint of the inguinal ligament*?

- The **mid-inguinal point** is half-way between the anterior superior iliac spine (ASIS) and the symphysis pubis. It represents the surface landmark of the *femoral artery*.
- The **midpoint of inguinal ligament** is half-way between the ASIS and the pubic tubercle. It represents the surface landmark of the *deep inguinal ring*.

Figure 24.7 summarizes these differences.

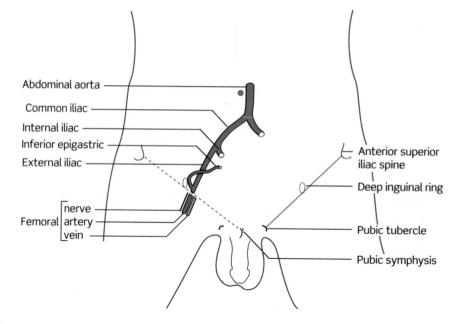

Figure 24.7 The mid-inguinal point versus the midpoint of the inguinal ligament.

Single Best Answers

1. Which is true of the relative positions of the femoral nerve, artery, and vein in the inguinal region?

a. Nerve is medial to artery
b. Nerve is medial to vein
c. Vein is lateral to artery

d. Vein is medial to artery
e. Artery and vein are lateral to nerve

2. A patient undergoes surgery for a presumed femoral hernia. At operation, it is noted that only part of the wall of the small bowel has been strangulated in the defect. What type of hernia is this?

a. Richter's
b. Spigelian
c. Maydl's

d. Littré's
e. Obturator

3. Which artery is used as an intraoperative landmark to differentiate between direct and indirect inguinal hernias?

a. External iliac
b. Deep circumflex iliac
c. Cremasteric

d. Superficial epigastric
e. Deep inferior epigastric

4. What is the most common type of hernia in women?

a. Indirect inguinal
b. Direct inguinal
c. Femoral

d. Obturator
e. Lumbar

5. Why are smokers more likely to develop hernias?

a. Chronic cough
b. Smokers are more likely to be obese
c. Impaired connective tissue metabolism

d. There is no association
e. None of the above

Scrotal mass

Core case

Read through the sections in the case boxes, covering up the sections that follow so that you don't see the answer. At the end of each case box, try to answer the question before reading on.

> Mr Collons is a 36-year-old Pilates instructor who presents to his GP because he has noticed a lump in his scrotum.
>
> **Before you examine Mr Collons it would be prudent to establish a few more details about this 'lump'. What else what you like to know?**

In common with lumps anywhere on the body, you will need to establish:

- **Is the lump painful?** This is an absolutely critical question. An acutely swollen and tender scrotum is testicular torsion until proven otherwise, which is a surgical emergency. Most cases of testicular malignancy are not painful.
- **How long has the lump been there?** A testicular torsion will only have been present for hours whereas a testicular tumour may have been present for weeks/months.
- **What made the patient first notice the lump?** It may be that Mr Collons checks his testes regularly, but it is equally likely that this is a chance finding, perhaps following some minor trauma to his scrotum.
- **Has the lump got bigger, smaller, or stayed the same size?**
- **Is the lump always there?** This is not such a strange question as it may sound. An inguinal hernia may extend into the scrotum in response to increases in intra-abdominal pressure, such as during periods of exertion or after prolonged periods of standing. Varicoceles can vary in size throughout the day, and will typically disappear when the patient lies flat.
- **Are there any other lumps?** The pathology may not be confined just to the testicles.
- **Does he have any other symptoms?** You should ask about symptoms of urinary tract infection (dysuria, polyuria, suprapubic pain, offensive-smelling urine, urgency, strangury, haematuria) and symptoms suggestive of sexually transmitted infections (such as purulent urethral discharge) in order to identify possible sources of infection which may have ascended into the testis and/or epididymis.
- **Has there been any trauma to the testes?**

There is one further question that can be particularly informative regarding scrotal swellings:

- **Does the testis feel heavy?** While there are no symptoms that are truly pathognomonic for testicular cancer, this symptom should raise suspicions… if clinical examination supports the diagnosis.

On further questioning you establish that Mr Collons' partner first noticed the swelling in his scrotum 2 weeks ago. He doesn't usually check himself for lumps, but following this discovery he has been checking his scrotum daily while having his morning shower. The lump is always there and hasn't changed size. Like many men, he didn't want to rush to the doctor to have his testicles examined, but says that his partner kept urging him to get it checked out. Furthermore, he admits that he has become progressively more anxious that something isn't quite right.

When quizzed about pain, he says that he hasn't had any true pain, but his left testicle has a bit of a dull ache and just doesn't feel right. He has otherwise felt well and has had no urethral discharge or features of urinary tract infection.

You will need to examine Mr Collons. Other than tenderness, what are the four key characteristics of a scrotal mass that will enable you to narrow your differential diagnosis?

- **Can you get above it?** Meaning, is the swelling confined to the scrotum or does it extend proximally into the groin? Extension of the mass into the groin is consistent with an inguinoscrotal hernia.

- **Is it possible to palpate the testis separately from the swelling/lump?** While examining the scrotal contents you should make every effort to ensure that you can clearly identify the spermatic cord, epididymis, and testis. If you can't distinguish these separate structures due to the presence of a lump or swelling, you should aim to establish which of the remaining structures you can palpate.

- **Does it transilluminate?** When you shine a torchlight into the mass it will glow if full of fluid, but will be opaque if it is a solid structure.

- **Is the mass tender?**

What is your differential diagnosis of scrotal masses? Can you organize the above four questions into a flowchart that helps you sort out your differential diagnosis?

Figure 25.1 shows a flowchart for differential diagnosis of scrotal masses. Diagnoses listed in a smaller font are rare.

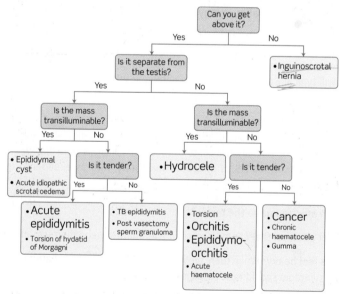

Figure 25.1 Diagnostic approach to a scrotal mass.

A cautious but wise maxim is to consider any acutely swollen and tender scrotum as testicular torsion until proven otherwise. As this condition rapidly progresses to irreversible testicular ischaemia it must be treated as an emergency (see Chapter 16).

Upon examination of Mr Collons' scrotum, you can discern a mass in the left hemiscrotum. It is possible to palpate the testis, and the mass is within the testis and confined to it (i.e. you can get above it). More precisely, the mass is on the lower pole of the testis—it is approximately 1 cm in diameter, protrudes beyond the natural curvature of the testis, but has a smooth surface. The mass is not fluctuant and does not transilluminate. The epididymis and spermatic cord can be palpated as distinct from the mass. The testes are not tender to palpation. The overlying scrotum appears normal and there is no erythema.

What is the most likely pathology?

The history and examination findings are highly suggestive of a **testicular tumour**—a non-tender solid mass within the testis, associated with abnormal testicular sensation. Tumours may present as a 'nodule' within the testis, or as an ill-defined circumferential swelling.

If the swelling had been circumferential, rather than projecting beyond the natural curvature of the testis, then the differential would also include a chronic haematocele or a gumma (syphilitic infection of the testis). A chronic haematocele may develop following an acute bleed that is noticed but ignored, or following a bleed that the patient is oblivious to. The clotted blood within the tunica vaginalis contracts and hardens around the testis, producing a mass that is clinically indistinguishable from a tumour. Figure 25.2 shows the different types of scrotal mass.

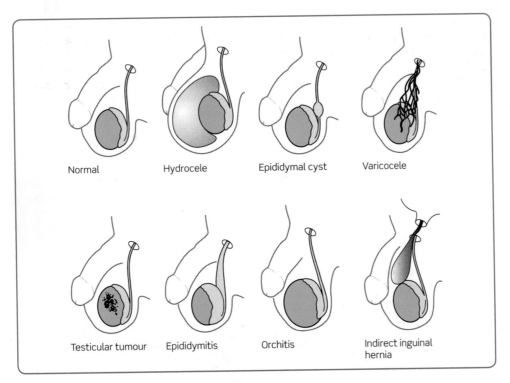

Figure 25.2 Line drawing showing different types of scrotal mass.

Reproduced from Judge RD *et al.*, *Clinical diagnosis: a physiologic approach*, 5th edition, Little Brown & Co, Boston, 1989, with permission from Wolters Kluwer Ltd.

Are you aware of any risk factors for this disease?

The single biggest risk factor is a history of undescended or maldescended testes. As many as 10% of patients will give a history of orchidopexy (surgical placement of the testis within the scrotum).

Bearing in mind the maxim that solid testicular lumps are tumours until proven otherwise, the GP prepares to refer Mr Collons for urgent urological review. Prior to doing so he will wish to assess whether there is any evidence for metastatic spread.

Which lymph nodes should the GP palpate?

Remember that the testes themselves drain to para-aortic nodes whereas the scrotal skin drains to inguinal nodes. There was no evidence of scrotal skin involvement and so the GP should focus his examination on the para-aortic nodes (palpating for a mass in the centre of the abdomen, above the umbilicus) and the supraclavicular nodes. However, in reality, unless these para-aortic notes are very large they will be impossible to palpate even in slim patients.

What are the systemic symptoms of malignancy?

The systemic symptoms that you should enquire about in anyone with suspected malignancy are weight loss, fatigue, and night sweats. You could ask more specific questions relating to particular sites of metastases—including respiratory symptoms, back pain, or neurological symptoms.

Mr Collons is urgently referred to a urologist.

Which investigations are likely to be requested?

In the first instance, the most appropriate investigation is an **ultrasound scan** of both testes. Indeed, ultrasound is the investigation of choice for any scrotal mass. In experienced hands this test has a sensitivity of almost 100%.

If the ultrasound scan is highly suggestive of a tumour, the next stage is to request **tumour markers**. The role of tumour markers is threefold: aiding diagnosis (in conjunction with histology), monitoring response to treatment, and monitoring for relapse. α-Fetoprotein (AFP) is expressed by 50–70% of teratomas but is not usually expressed by seminomas. β-Human chorionic gonadotropin (β-HCG) is expressed by 40–60% of teratomas and about 30% of seminomas. Lactate dehydrogenase (LDH) is a less specific marker—it is present in most tissues and is released during tissue breakdown, so is elevated in many cancers—but is more commonly raised in seminomas. Blood samples are taken prior to, during, and following treatment.

Staging scans will also be requested—the most suitable being a plain chest radiograph and CT scan of chest/abdomen/pelvis.

Shortly after his appointment with the urologist Mr Collons underwent a radical left orchidectomy. Sperm was collected for storage prior to the procedure, as a safeguard against any reduction in fertility following surgery and subsequent radiotherapy. Histology showed the tumour to be a seminoma with no evidence of metastatic spread. Fortunately, seminomas are highly radiosensitive and Mr Collons is expected to have very good survival prospects following his postoperative radiotherapy.

Short cases

Dr Barlow is a 43-year-old engineering lecturer who presents with a mass in his scrotum. He says that he has been checking his testicles regularly over the past year, prompted by media coverage of testicular cancer, but is slightly unsure what is normal. He reports that he has felt some sort of lump in his right scrotum for much of the past year, but as it was small and painless he had not presented to his GP. However, he now feels that the lump may have grown slightly and it is becoming mildly painful. He is otherwise fit and well, with no significant past medical history.

Examination reveals an irregularly shaped fluctuant mass superior and posterior to the right testis. It is possible to get above the mass. The mass transilluminates and is tender to palpation. It is approximately 15 mm in diameter and feels multilocular. The right testis is palpable and feels normal, as does the left testis. The overlying scrotal skin is normal.

What is the most likely diagnosis?

The examination findings are consistent with the diagnosis of an **epididymal cyst**. These are fluid-filled swellings, derived from the epididymal collecting tubules, and are relatively common in middle-aged and elderly men. The characteristic features are that the swelling is:

* Distinct from the testis (strictly superior and posterior to it).
* It is possible to get above the swelling, thus differentiating it from an inguinoscrotal hernia.
* The swelling is cystic and is thus fluctuant and transilluminable.

Epididymal cysts are frequently multiple or multilocular, and may be bilateral. Although epididymal cysts are usually painless they may sometimes be tender. It is possible for the cysts to reach quite impressive sizes—sometimes >5 cm in diameter. Epididymal cysts are often confirmed by ultrasound and are not usually removed unless they are symptomatic (e.g. they may chafe the legs or cause unsightly bulges in the trousers).

It is worth noting that spermatoceles are a subtype of epididymal cyst that contains milky fluid rather than the usual clear fluid. As it is only possible to make this distinction following removal or aspiration of the cyst it is best to avoid using the term spermatocele.

Mike is a 22-year-old rower who presents with a lump in his scrotum. The lump has got progressively larger over the past 6 months and is starting to cause him some discomfort. He complains of a dull ache in his scrotum following training sessions—particularly after lifting heavy weights. He is otherwise fit and well, with no significant past medical history.

Mike is examined while standing up. The lump feels like 'a bag of worms', and sits below and behind his left testis. It is possible to get above the lump.

What is the most likely diagnosis? Why was Mike examined while standing up? What treatment would you offer him?

The 'bag of worms' is a classic description of the dilated tortuous veins that comprise a **varicocele**. In common with varicose veins elsewhere in the body, these varicosities of the pampiniform plexus are responsive to changes in venous pressure and may thus increase in size at the end of the day (due to venous pooling) or following strenuous exercise.

The veins should empty when the patient lies down and thus a varicocele will only be palpable if the patient is standing up.

As many as 10–25% of men will have a varicocele, and this figure may be as high as 40% in infertile men, although it is controversial as to whether there is any causative link. The first step when offering Mike treatment is to **reassure him** that varicoceles are incredibly common. **Scrotal support**, by means of a jockstrap or tighter pants may relieve him of some of the discomfort. If his varicocele becomes painful he may wish to consider treatment. Options include **embolization**, **surgical ligation**, or **sclerotherapy** of the veins draining the testis.

SHORT CASE

Mr Hoff is a 53-year-old pub singer who presents because he is concerned that his testicle is growing in size. He has no pain or discomfort, and was initially rather proud of his large appendage but is now concerned that it might not stop growing. He has no history of testicular cancer, trauma, or infection. He is otherwise fit and well.

Examination reveals a large fluctuant mass of 7 cm diameter in his right hemiscrotum. It is possible to feel the spermatic cord above the lump, but it is not possible to clearly distinguish the right testis as it is within the swelling. The mass transilluminates brightly and is non-tender.

What is the most likely diagnosis? What is the significance of a negative history of testicular cancer, trauma, and infection?

This is a **hydrocele**—a collection of fluid within the tunica vaginalis. The key features in the examination are that there is fluid (hence the lump is fluctuant) surrounding the testis and thus it is not possible to palpate the testis itself. If this were an epididymal cyst, the testis would still be palpable. It is possible to feel the spermatic cord above the swelling—thus distinguishing this from an inguinoscrotal hernia (the situation is rather more complicated with childhood hydroceles). Hydroceles may reach impressive sizes and contain as much as 500 mL of fluid.

The significance of a negative history of trauma, infection, or testicular cancer is that there are two sorts of hydrocele: primary (idiopathic), and secondary to the aforementioned testicular insults. Secondary hydroceles usually present in men in their twenties to forties, as this age group is most susceptible to the initiating pathologies. Treatment options differ according to whether the hydrocele is primary or secondary. With secondary hydroceles, treatment is of the underlying condition. With primary hydroceles, options are to do nothing, aspirate the fluid collection (most will recur), or undergo surgery.

SHORT CASE

Mr Blofelt is a 32-year-old club rep who has just returned from a season in Ibiza. He presents with a 10-hour history of pain and swelling in his scrotum. He has had a headache and rigors, and believes that he has a temperature. On direct questioning he admits to having had some penile discharge and painful micturition over the previous 3 days. He says that he was 'very' sexually active while on his recent travels.

Examination reveals a swollen, red, tender, warm right hemiscrotum. The right epididymis and right testis are very tender to palpation. Prehn's sign (relief of pain upon elevating the scrotum) is positive, and the cremasteric reflex (elevation of the testes upon stroking the inner thigh) is present (although neither sign is pathognomonic). There is no visible urethral discharge. His temperature is 38.3 °C, pulse 105 bpm regular, and blood pressure 147/82 mmHg.

What is your differential diagnosis? Which diagnosis is most likely? What investigations would you like to order?

Remember that an acutely painful testis in a young man should always make you suspect testicular torsion. Although we must consider torsion in this instance the history and examination are more suggestive of **epididymo-orchitis**. Mr Blofelt has had systemic symptoms, is febrile, and provides a history that is suggestive of a sexually transmitted infection. Acute infections of the testis and epididymis usually ascend via the vas, having arisen in the urinary tract or as sexually transmitted infections.

It would be wise to request the following tests:

- **Blood cultures** as he is septic. These should be taken before antibiotics are started, provided they don't delay treatment, as they can help guide antimicrobial therapy if positive. An **HIV test** should be performed. Guidance from the British Association for Sexual Health is that in areas where HIV prevalence exceeds 2:1000 (e.g. nearly all of London), *all* acutely unwell patients should be routinely tested (without specific consent). This man is particularly at risk. Doctors often find it uncomfortable to bring up the issue of HIV testing with patients but you should remember that HIV is now a manageable disease (but with fatal consequences if not managed). A **full blood count (FBC)** is usually done at the same time and, although this won't change management (he already meets criteria for sepsis/systemic inflammatory response syndrome (SIRS)), if he fails to respond to treatment and the blood cultures are negative, a rising white cell count may prompt you to change antibiotics whereas a falling count may support a switch to oral therapy.

- **Urine dipstick** (looking for positive leucocytes and nitrites), **microscopy, culture, and sensitivities (MC&S)** (looking for culprits of the infection).

- You should advise a **urethral swab** and **genitourinary medicine (GUM) screen**, which is often best done by referring him to the sexual health clinic. Here they can also offer lifestyle advice and undertake contact tracing if appropriate (e.g. *Chlamydia* or *Gonococcus* infection).

Treatment is likely to involve bed rest, scrotal elevation, and appropriate antibiotics for at least a month. HIV status is particularly important as atypical organisms are more common with HIV (e.g. cytomegalovirus (CMV) or *Cryptococcal* infection), which may not be covered by standard antimicrobial therapy.

Your threshold for investigating a possible testicular torsion should be low and some surgeons advocate surgical exploration of any acutely painful testis (particularly in children). Surgical investigation provides an immediate and certain answer and avoids missing torsion, which has grave consequences—although this advantage must be balanced with the risks of surgery (bleeding, infection, anaesthetic risk). Sometimes, with a low pre-test probability of torsion, duplex ultrasound can be helpful in avoiding unnecessary surgical exploration.

Viva questions

Why is a radical orchidectomy performed via an inguinal incision rather than a scrotal incision?

Removing a malignant testis via a scrotal incision would potentially risk seeding malignant cells into the scrotum during the procedure. The significance of this lies in the lymphatic drainage of the testes and scrotum—the former drain to para-aortic nodes whereas the scrotum drains to inguinal nodes.

Does orchidopexy reduce the cancer risk of previously undescended testes?

Orchidopexy does not reduce the cancer risk of undescended or maldescended testes per se. It does, however, mean that the testes (which are abnormal and hence have an inherently higher cancer risk) can now be checked easily and hence cancer can theoretically be detected at an earlier stage.

What are the most common types of testicular tumour?

The two most important types to know about are seminomas and teratomas as these combined represent 90% of testicular tumours. Teratomas typically affect men aged 20–30 whereas seminomas classically affect men in their thirties to fifties.

Are varicoceles more common on the right or left? Why is this?

Almost 98% of idiopathic varicoceles present on the left. Various theories have been put forward, but the most consistent explanation relates to the anatomy of the venous drainage of the testes. The right gonadal vein drains directly into the inferior vena cava, and does so at an oblique angle. By contrast, the left gonadal vein drains into the left renal vein at a 90° angle. It is believed that this draining arrangement contributes to the development of varicosities.

Bilateral varicoceles occur in about a third of patients.

What might you consider if a left-sided varicocele appears suddenly in a previously normal scrotum?

The sudden appearance of a left-sided varicocele is a rare, but important, presentation of renal tumours (e.g. renal cell carcinoma) as these tumours may invade the left renal vein and hence compromise drainage of the left gonadal vein. As such, the sudden appearance of a left-sided varicocele in an older patient should prompt consideration of underlying pathology.

Which pathogens are most likely to cause epididymo-orchitis in patients <35 years and >35 years?

In men <35 years of age sexually transmitted infections are the most likely source of ascending infection, thus consider *Chlamydia trachomatis* and *Neisseria gonorrhoeae*. In men >35 years of age, urinary tract pathogens such as *Escherichia coli* are most likely.

Of note, patients who engage in anal intercourse have increased risk of epididymitis due to exposure to coliforms.

Which pathogen might you consider in a boy who presented to his GP with a swelling adjacent to the angle of his jaw 8 days ago, and now presents with a swollen testis?

You should consider the mumps virus. Mumps orchitis is a blood-borne infection and may present without any previous history of parotid swelling.

What is idiopathic scrotal oedema?

This is a condition that primarily affects prepubescent boys, peaking around 6–7 years. The boy presents with acute-onset erythematous, oedematous scrotal swelling, which is often bilateral and may extend into the groin. A key feature which helps distinguish idiopathic scrotal oedema from other causes of the 'acute testis/scrotum' is that the child is often unconcerned about the swelling (they may be slightly tender to palpation) and will often be running around the Emergency Department completely bemused by the amount of attention being paid to his nether regions. This is in stark contrast to a boy with testicular torsion, hydatid torsion, or epididymo-orchitis—all three of which would result in pain.

Idiopathic scrotal oedema will resolve over 48–72 hours and needs no further management other than reassurance (of parents and child) and analgesia.

Single Best Answers

1. **A 24-year-old man is diagnosed with testicular cancer. Based solely upon the patient's age, what is the most likely histological diagnosis?**

   a. Teratoma
   b. Leydig cell tumour
   c. Choriocarcinoma

   d. Seminoma
   e. Yolk sac tumour

2. **What is the most useful first-line investigation for a suspected testicular tumour?**

   a. Tumour markers
   b. CT chest/abdomen/pelvis
   c. Plain abdominal radiograph

   d. MRI pelvis
   e. Testicular ultrasound

3. **A patient presents to his GP with a left-sided scrotal swelling that is intermittently present. The patient reports a dull ache in the left hemiscrotum at the end of the day, and following periods of physical exertion. On examination, an irregular cystic mass, separate from the testis, is palpable. The mass is only palpable when the patient is standing. What is the diagnosis?**

   a. Epididymal cyst
   b. Hydrocele
   c. Varicocele

   d. Gumma
   e. Inguinoscrotal hernia

4. **When examining a testicular swelling, which of the following questions should the examiner address?**

   a. Is it possible to get above the swelling?
   b. Is the testis palpable?
   c. Does the swelling transilluminate?

   d. Is it tender?
   e. All of the above

5. **An adult patient presents with a swelling in his scrotum that transilluminates. On examination, it is not possible to get above the swelling. What is the most likely diagnosis?**

   a. Epididymal cyst
   b. Vaginal hydrocele
   c. Indirect inguinal hernia

   d. Direct inguinal hernia
   e. Femoral hernia

Limb weakness

Core case

Read through the sections in the case boxes, covering up the sections that follow so that you don't see the answer. At the end of each case box, try to answer the question before reading on.

> Mr Walker is a 62-year-old farmer who has been brought into the Emergency Department by ambulance after waking up that morning with left arm weakness.
>
> **What things might be confused with limb weakness?**

The definition of weakness is important, because many patients who self-describe a 'weak limb' will actually have a clumsy limb (**ataxia**), a numb limb (**reduced sensation**), or a limb that is too **painful** to move.

> The two key things to establish clinically with any acute limb weakness are the *time course* and the likely *location* of the neurological lesion.
>
> **What does the time course tell you about the possible cause of limb weakness?**

The time course of the onset of the symptoms in general reflects the time course of the underlying pathology:

- **Sudden onset** (seconds to minutes) usually implies either trauma (e.g. displaced vertebral fractures due to major trauma) or certain vascular insults (e.g. stroke, transient ischaemic attack (TIA)).
- **Subacute onset** (hours to days) suggests a progressive demyelination (e.g. Guillain–Barré syndrome, multiple sclerosis) or a slowly expanding haematoma (e.g. subdural haematoma).
- **Chronic onset** (weeks to months), is consistent with pathologies such as a slow-growing tumour or motor neuron disease (progressive degeneration of motor neurons).

As only acute and subacute limb weakness will present acutely to generalists in hospital (chronic onset cases will most likely be referred to neurology from primary care), we have limited the chapter to these cases.

> **What are the possible anatomical locations for the lesion causing Mr Walker's limb weakness?**

Limb movement requires an intact pathway from the cerebral cortex, down the corona radiata, internal capsule, and pons, along the corticospinal tract of the spinal cord, out along a nerve root, and down a peripheral nerve to the neuromuscular junction and muscle itself (see Figure. 26.1). If a patient has limb weakness, there must be a lesion somewhere in this pathway.

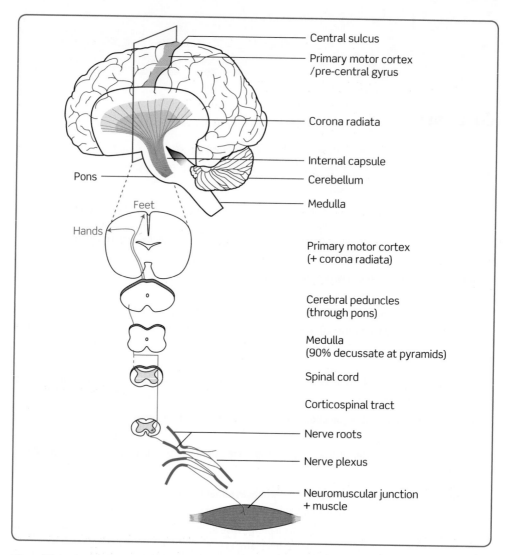

Figure 26.1 The motor tract from primary cortex to muscle.

What is your differential diagnosis for limb weakness? Try to classify your diagnoses based on time course and location.

Figure 26.2 gives the differential diagnosis for limb weakness.

	Sudden onset (seconds to minutes)	Subacute onset (hours to days)	Gradual onset (weeks to months)
Brain	**Ischaemic stroke** **Transient ischaemic attack (TIA)** Haemorrhagic stroke Hemiplegic migraine Todd's palsy (post seizure paralysis) Hypoglycaemia	**Multiple sclerosis** Haematoma (e.g. subdural, extradural) Tumour Abscess	
Spinal cord	Spinal disc prolapse Spinal cord transection Spinal cord infarction	**Multiple sclerosis** Tumour Transverse myelitis	**Spinal canal stenosis** Vitamin B$_{12}$ deficiency
Nerve root	Spinal disc prolapse Vertebral fracture	Guillain-Barré syndrome Poliomyelitis	
Peripheral nerve or nerve plexus	Acute limb ischaemia (e.g. peripheral artery embolus). Traumatic nerve injury (e.g. laceration)		Diabetes mellitus Vasculitis
Neuromuscular junction		Botulism Tetanus	Myasthenia gravis Lambert-Eaton syndrome
Muscle			Myositis

Figure 26.2 Differential diagnosis for limb weakness.

Mr Walker tells you that he went to bed as usual at 11 p.m. last night without any symptoms. He awoke at 6 a.m. this morning and found his left arm was paralysed and he couldn't get out of bed without help from his wife. His wife dialled 999 and an ambulance was sent immediately.

What else do you want to know about Mr Walker's history?

Mr Walker has presented with **rapid onset of left-sided arm weakness**. Key clues in the history to elicit include:

- Exact **time of onset**? This is critical in suspected strokes because the window of time in which to confirm the diagnosis and administer thrombolysis (if appropriate) is only 4.5 hours from onset of symptoms (after that, you risk doing more harm than good to the patient). If you suspect a stroke in a patient within that time frame, call the thrombolysis team immediately. In this case, all we can say is that the onset was at some point in the 7 hours between 11 p.m. (when he went to sleep) and 6 a.m. (when he woke up), so we cannot confidently say the onset was within 4.5 hours.

- Any **speech disturbance** or **visual disturbance**? If a patient has a deficit in speech or vision as well as limb weakness, it immediately tells you that the problem is likely to be in the brain rather than the spine or peripheral nervous system.

- Any **headache** with his symptoms? A headache is unusual in stroke or TIA. A sudden-onset, terrible headache might make you suspect a subarachnoid haemorrhage. A unilateral headache preceding the limb weakness might make you suspect a hemiplegic migraine. A gradual-onset headache preceding the limb weakness might make you suspect an intracranial mass (e.g. slowly expanding subdural haemorrhage).

- Any **seizure** or **loss of consciousness**? Seizures and loss of consciousness are *not* typical features of strokes and should make you consider the diagnosis of stroke mimics such as Todd's paresis (post seizure) or hypoglycaemia.

- Any **neck or back pain**? If present, suspect spinal pathology such as a spontaneous disc prolapse, traumatic injury to the spine, discitis or spinal abscess. Guillain–Barré syndrome usually presents less suddenly than Mr Walker's symptoms, but of interest, is often accompanied by back pain.

- Any **trauma** to the head in the last few months? Slowly expanding subdural haemorrhages in elderly patients often present several days or weeks after a relatively minor head injury.

- Any **risk factors for stroke** or TIA? The three main risk factors for stroke that one can elicit on history are previous stroke or TIA, atrial fibrillation and atherosclerotic risk factors (smoking, family history, hypertension, diabetes mellitus, dyslipidaemia). Migraine with aura and systemic lupus erythematosus (SLE) are also risk factors for ischaemic stroke.

> Mr Walker denies any headache, neck or back pain, trauma to his head, visual disturbance, or speech problems. His past medical history is remarkable only for the lack of a distal phalanx on the little finger of his right hand due to an accident on the farm. When asked, he admits he occasionally gets some chest pain if he over-exerts himself. He has smoked two packs of cigarettes a day since he was 16. He drinks a single pint of ale every evening at his local pub. He lives with his wife and one of his two sons on a local farm. His family history is unremarkable, with both of his parents dying of 'old age' in their late seventies; his only sister is alive and well. He takes no medications and has no allergies.
>
> **What will you look for on examination to help you locate the likely anatomical site of his neurological deficit?**

Upper motor neuron vs lower motor neuron lesion

In an upper motor neuron (UMN) lesion, the pathology causing the muscle weakness lies within the central nervous system (CNS; spinal cord and brain). In a lower motor neuron (LMN) lesion, the pathology is peripheral, i.e. between the spinal cord and the muscle. The signs that distinguish between UMN and LMN lesions are shown in Table 26.1, but the brisk reflexes and increased tone found in UMN lesions actually take some days to develop.

Table 26.1 **Differences between UMN and LMN signs**

UMN signs	LMN signs
↑ Tone	↓ Tone
↑ Reflexes	↓ Reflexes
↑ Plantars (Babinski reflex)	Fasciculations (sometimes)
Clonus (sometimes)	Wasting

Language defects

These suggest pathology in the **cortex of the dominant hemisphere** (usually the left, even if the patient is left-handed). Look specifically for:

- **Receptive dysphasia.** The patient speaks fluently (although often with jumbled words and phrases) but cannot comprehend language. This suggests a lesion to Wernicke's area (in the temporal lobe) of the dominant hemisphere.

- **Expressive dysphasia.** The patient can comprehend language and follow instructions, but cannot find words or speak fluently (classically with correct phrases but like a telegram with missing 'link words'). This suggests a lesion to Broca's area (in the frontal lobe) of the dominant hemisphere. Indeed, Broca's original patient could only say the word 'tan'.

Attention defects

If a patient appears to be ignoring half of their sensory world (e.g. only responding to cues on one side of the bed), you should suspect a lesion to the **parietal cortex**.

Eye signs

Depending on the specific defect, these suggest a lesion at different points of the visual pathway. There are many potential lesions and defects, but those that arise most commonly in the context of limb weakness include:

- **Complete blindness** in one eye. The lesion is likely to be in the optic nerve (e.g. optic neuritis) or globe itself.

- **Homonymous hemianopia,** or loss of the same half of the field of vision in both eyes. It suggests a lesion (ischaemia, mass) at some point between the optic chiasm and the visual cortex, on the contralateral side... but beware that visual neglect due to lesions to the parietal cortex can mimic homonymous hemianopia.

- **Eye deviation.** If the eyes deviate away from the weak side, this suggests a cortical lesion. If the eyes deviate towards the weak side, this suggests a brain-stem lesion.

There are other higher cortical functions you can test for (e.g. graphaesthesia, astereognosis, apraxia, acalculia), to see if the lesion is cortical rather than lying in deeper brain structures (e.g. the internal capsule), but it is unusual to do so in the acute setting.

Sensory symptoms

These include paraesthesia or loss of one or all of the sensory modalities. In a weak limb with LMN signs, sensory signs can help distinguish between a nerve root or peripheral nerve lesion (sensory signs present) and a neuromuscular or muscular lesion (absent). In limb weakness with UMN signs, sensory loss can indicate damage to specific tracts in the spinal cord: spinothalamic (pain and temperature) versus dorsal columns (light touch, vibration, position sense or proprioception). This helps distinguish types of spinal cord pathology (e.g. an anterior spinal artery infarct spares dorsal columns).

You examine Mr Walker. On inspection you note that the left corner of his mouth is drooping and his left arm is lying completely still, although he is moving his right arm normally.

Examination of his left arm reveals decreased tone, power 0/5 on the MRC scale (for definition of the MRC scale see the Viva questions), decreased reflexes, and decreased (but still present) sensation to both pinprick and vibration. The left lower limb shows decreased tone, power 3/5 on the MRC scale, present patellar reflex, and upgoing plantar reflex and normal pinprick and vibration sensation. There are no abnormalities on examination of the right upper and lower limbs.

Examination of his cranial nerves reveals several positive findings. Visual field testing reveals a loss of the left field of vision in both eyes (homonymous hemianopia). On examination of his facial movements, the patient is unable to blow out his cheek or grin on the left side. However, he is still able to wrinkle both sides of his forehead and blink normally. His tongue deviates towards the side of the limb weakness (left). His speech is spontaneous and fluent but slightly slurred.

Cardiovascular examination reveals a regular heart rate of 80 bpm, blood pressure 170/100 mmHg, and a bruit in his right carotid. Peripheral pulses are all present. Respiratory examination is unremarkable except for tar stains on his fingers.

What has the examination told you about: the pattern of weakness; whether there are UMN or LMN signs; the presence of other localizing signs; and consequently, the most likely site(s) of the lesion?

From the examination you can deduce the following about the location of the lesion:

- **Pattern of weakness:** Mr Walker is unable to blow out his cheek or grin on the left, but note that forehead wrinkling and blinking is present bilaterally (we will come to this shortly). Therefore he has a left-sided facial weakness. This confirms that he has a **full-body, left-sided weakness**. Note that the arm and face weakness is greater than the leg weakness, where there is some residual movement (3/5 on the MRC scale).

- **UMN versus LMN:** the decreased tone in his limbs is consistent with either a LMN lesion or the acute phase of an UMN lesion. But the intact knee reflex and upgoing plantar reflexes and the ability to wrinkle his forehead on both sides confirm that it is an **UMN lesion**. Sparing of forehead wrinkling and blink distinguishes UMN facial weakness from LMN facial nerve palsy: in a LMN lesion the final common pathway to the frontalis and orbicularis muscle is destroyed, but these muscles have obligate bilateral cortical representation and are therefore spared in a unilateral UMN lesion.

- **Other localizing signs:** Mr Walker has **homonymous hemianopia** (loss of the left half of his visual field in both eyes). This suggests a lesion in the **right cortex** affecting the optic radiation as well as the motor pathway. There are no language impairments other than dysarthria, which is most likely due to acute tongue and facial muscle weakness.

- **Likely location of lesion:** clinically, Mr Walker has got signs of an UMN lesion, suggesting the lesion is somewhere in the CNS. He also has a homonymous hemianopia, suggesting the lesion is in the cerebral cortex (rather than the spinal cord) and is affecting the optic tract (between the optic chiasm and lateral geniculate nucleus), both optic radiations (between the lateral geniculate nucleus and occipital visual cortex), or the occipital visual cortex. The left-sided hemiparesis and left-sided homonymous hemianopia suggest the lesion is on the right side. Thus, Mr Walker has a lesion in his **right cerebral cortex**.

What is the differential for this type of lesion? Are there any clues to the aetiology from the examination above?

The possibilities include those shown in Figure 26.3.

Stroke (infarct or haemorrhage)

Cerebral mass (e.g. tumour, abscess – potentially with a bleed into it)

Hemiplegic migraine

Hypoglycaemia (can present with localized signs although it is unclear how)

Figure 26.3 Likely differential diagnosis for Mr Walker based on information so far.

The weakness is greater in the arm and face than the leg. From neuroanatomy we know that the most medial part of the primary motor cortex maps to the lower limb, whereas the more lateral areas map to the upper limb and face (see Figure. 26.4). Moreover, we know that the medial primary motor cortex is primarily supplied by the anterior cerebral artery (ACA), whereas the rest of the primary motor cortex is supplied by the middle cerebral artery (MCA; see Figure 26.4). The MCA also supplies the right posterior parietal cortex, where damage can cause a contralateral hemineglect.

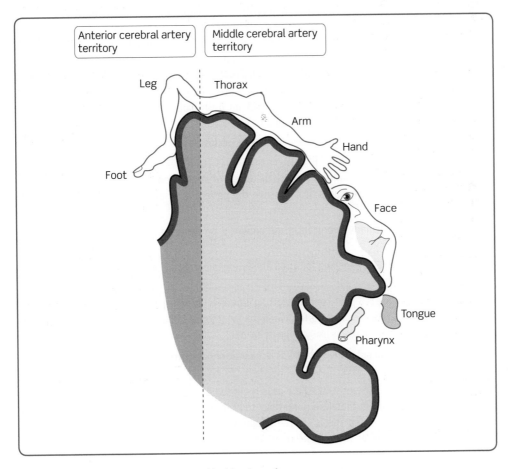

Figure 26.4 The primary motor cortex and its blood supply.

Thus, Mr Walker's pattern of weakness and the acute time course is suggestive of a right MCA stroke, either resulting from an infarct or mimicked by haemorrhage. On examination, there was a right carotid bruit, which could represent the source of emboli causing an infarct. Strictly speaking, if his symptoms and signs resolve entirely within 24 hours of onset, this will have been a TIA (i.e. occlusion of a cerebral artery/arteriole that has fully resolved without leaving any infarcted brain tissue) rather than a stroke. However, the vast majority of TIAs last less than 1 hour. Those that last >1 hour and resolve fully within 24 hours usually show rapid signs of improvement (which isn't the case in Mr Walker) and on diffusion-weighted MRI often show signs of minor infarction, meaning many are retrospectively found not to be true TIAs but actually minor strokes from which the patient has recovered rapidly. The fact that Mr Walker's symptoms and signs are not resolving rapidly within 1 hour of presentation makes it very unlikely that this will prove to be a TIA (rather than a stroke) by the time 24 hours have elapsed.

Having decided that a right-sided MCA stroke is the most likely diagnosis, what first-line investigations will you arrange?

- **CT head scan.** Although stroke is a clinical diagnosis, you must determine whether this is an ischaemic stroke or a haemorrhagic stroke. A non-contrast CT head scan should be performed immediately on all patients with suspected stroke presenting within 4.5 hours of onset of symptoms, and within 24 hours for stroke patients presenting outside the 4.5-hour thrombolysis window. A CT will also help rule out alternative diagnoses such as a space-occupying lesion in the right hemisphere. Although MRI is more sensitive at picking up the initial stages of ischaemia, CT is better at viewing haemorrhages (fresh blood is bright white/highly attenuating), and is quicker and more readily available than MRI. Note that while CT can pick up fresh blood straight away, it can take up to 24 hours for infarction to become apparent on a CT scan.

- **Full blood count:** this may reveal a cause for arterial occlusion (e.g. polycythaemia, thrombocytosis) or haemorrhage (e.g. thrombocytopenia).

- **Blood glucose:** although you have made a diagnosis of stroke, you must rule out hypoglycaemia as a cause for the limb weakness—it is possible the patient has not only had a stroke but is also hypoglycaemic.

- **Blood clotting:** particularly important if the patient is on warfarin and also to exclude a haemophilia or coagulopathy.

- **Electrocardiogram (ECG):** looking for atrial fibrillation, a potential cause of emboli.

Mr Walker's blood glucose is 5.3 mM and his clotting is normal (international normalized ratio (INR) 1.1). His ECG is normal. A CT head scan is performed in the Emergency Department and excludes a haemorrhage, suggesting that the stroke is likely to be ischaemic.

Why is it important to find out if the stroke was ischaemic or haemorrhagic?

Ischaemic strokes (about 80% of strokes) are usually caused by embolism or *in situ* thrombosis occluding a cerebral artery and are therefore potentially treatable by thrombolysis (e.g. with tissue plasminogen activator, tPA), provided this is started within 3–4.5 hours of onset of symptoms, as well as antiplatelet therapy. However, antiplatelet treatment and particularly thrombolysis are likely to make a haemorrhagic stroke worse!

The main treatment for the approximately 20% of strokes that are haemorrhagic is supportive therapy to aid rehabilitation and risk factor reduction to prevent further episodes.

Your consultant agrees with the diagnosis of right-sided MCA ischaemic stroke.

How should Mr Walker be managed acutely?

Mr Walker has presented outside the 4.5-hour window of opportunity for possible thrombolysis. However, there is still much that can be done for him that will significantly improve his outcomes (and as you will see in the Viva questions, there is debate about the role of thrombolysis in any case).

- **Antiplatelet drugs.** Antiplatelet drugs (typically aspirin) have been shown to improve outcomes in ischaemic stroke, probably from early secondary prevention. They are given as soon as a haemorrhagic stroke has been excluded by imaging but are delayed 24 hours if the patient receives thrombolysis.

- **Stroke unit/specialist ward.** Mr Walker needs transferring to a specialist stroke unit where he can be looked after by a **multidisciplinary team** consisting of specialist nurses (e.g. who will manoeuvre the patient regularly to avoid bedsores), specialist speech and language therapists (SALT) who are experts at assessing, for example, whether a patient is safe to swallow food and liquids without choking, specialist occupational therapists (e.g. who will assess how a patient can start to mobilize and gain independence again), specialist physiotherapists (who will help patients start to mobilize again), and social workers (e.g. who will consider the financial and community care needs of the patients after their discharge).

- **Venous thromboembolism (VTE) prophylaxis:** stroke patients are largely immobile and therefore at increased risk of thromboembolic events (deep vein thrombosis and/or pulmonary embolus) due to blood stasis. However, compression stockings such as those used to prevent clots in postoperative patients have not been found to be of any benefit in stroke patients. Low molecular weight heparin can be used if a haemorrhagic stroke has been excluded and the patient is deemed low risk of the ischaemic stroke becoming haemorrhagic and there are no other contraindications. Alternatively, intermittent pneumatic compression devices to the calves can be used.

There is still not enough evidence that any **neuroprotective agent** is safe or beneficial to patients, although they have attracted much media attention.

What second line investigations should Mr Walker have on the stroke unit?

For patients like Mr Walker who have had an ischaemic stroke, and for those who have had a TIA (i.e. the neurological deficit has resolved in <24 hours), the following investigations should be performed:

- **Carotid Doppler ultrasonography:** an ultrasound of the carotid arteries will identify or exclude carotid artery atheromas that could be the source of emboli causing the stroke. Clinical examination for carotid bruits is not a sensitive way of detecting carotid artery stenosis.

- **Echocardiogram:** an echocardiogram will help identify a cardiac source of emboli such as an atrial thrombus (e.g. indicated by atrial fibrillation, a recent myocardial infarction, an abnormal ECG, a heart murmur, ischaemic events affecting more than one cerebral artery territory) or a patent foramen ovale.

Note that patients can have 'dual pathology', e.g. both carotid stenosis and atrial fibrillation. Finding one potential cause should not preclude a search for another.

Thinking beyond the acute setting, what medical complications of stroke should you be worried about? What actions can you take to minimize the likelihood of these occurring?

- **Pressure ulcers:** patients who are immobile are at risk of developing bedsores (very quickly), which can then become infected. Bedsores can be prevented by regularly moving the patient and/or having them on a special inflatable mattress which periodically varies the area of the body that is resting most heavily on the mattress.

- **Aspiration pneumonia:** stroke patients often have difficulty swallowing and are therefore at risk of aspirating food, fluids, or gastric secretions, leading to pneumonia. This can be prevented by carrying out a swallowing assessment and, if necessary, feeding the patient via a nasogastric (NG) tube.

- **Venous thromboembolism (VTE)** and **recurrent ischaemic stroke:** as discussed earlier under acute management.

> In patients with a suspected stroke you should always assess disability, as this is critical in establishing the level of care and support they need on the ward.
>
> **Which elements should form part of your disability screen? Why is each important?**

You should assess the patient in terms of the following:

- **Glasgow Coma Scale (GCS) score:** the GCS will have been recorded as part of the initial survey (under D for disability, after ABC). Remember that the GCS score reflects the patient's best response. Thus, because this patient can move his right side normally he scores 15/15, indicating no impairment of consciousness. The GCS is used to monitor progress and/or inform a decision to intervene (e.g. intubating). The GCS score on admission also gives an indication of prognosis.

- **Swallow:** an assessment is required to see if the patient is safe to swallow solids and/or fluids. If not, they are at risk of aspiration and may need a secure airway and/or NG tube. It will also determine how they are given fluids and nutrition.

- **Speech and language:** you will have assessed this as part of your neurological examination, but a speech and language therapist may be additionally involved to aid communication between the patient, staff, and family.

- **Visual fields:** a patient with severely impaired visual fields will need care to avoid tripping over, to avoid food or water being placed outside their field of vision, etc.

- **Gait:** it is vital to determine whether a patient is safe to walk or not. If they cannot walk, they will need prophylaxis for deep vein thrombosis and pressure sores secondary to immobility.

> A week after his admission, Mr Walker is recovering. He is somewhat low in mood but is determined to 'get back to normal'. His left facial palsy is still present, but improving. His left arm has developed a spastic weakness but power is now 3/5 and he can grab objects, albeit clumsily. The tone in his left leg is almost normal and although power is still only 4/5, the occupational therapist is keen that he should attempt walking soon.
>
> **How should Mr Walker be managed now that the acute phase is over?**

- **Risk factor reduction:** Mr Walker has two modifiable risk factors that should be addressed before discharge:
  - **Carotid artery disease:** Mr Walker's right carotid bruit suggests carotid artery stenosis due to atherosclerotic disease. It is quite probably the source of the embolus responsible for his right-sided MCA stroke. Mr Walker should have a duplex ultrasound of his carotid arteries within a week of the onset of his stroke. If this shows a stenosis of >70%, and Mr Walker is deemed

to have made a good functional recovery, he may benefit from a carotid endarterectomy and should be referred to the vascular surgeons without delay (the evidence for this comes from the NASCET and ECST trials[1,2,3]).

- **Smoking:** Mr Walker should be advised to stop smoking, as this is a significant risk factor for all atherosclerotic disease, including strokes. It should be made clear to him that although quitting is not easy, there is lots of help available from the NHS and that his chances of successfully quitting are much greater if he gets help.

- **Drug prophylaxis:** patients who have suffered an ischaemic stroke benefit from three lifelong medications:
  - Daily antiplatelet prophylaxis (e.g. clopidogrel) to reduce the chances of further thrombotic events. This should be started before discharge.[4]
  - Daily statin, even if cholesterol levels are normal.[5]
  - Daily angiotensin-converting enzyme (ACE) inhibitor and/or thiazide diuretic, aiming for a blood pressure of <130/85 mmHg (or <120/80 mmHg if diabetic).[6]

- **Discharge with community care:** Mr Walker is now probably fit enough for discharge to an intermediate community hospital. This will allow him to continue to recover and adapt to his new circumstances in an environment that is still supportive (with nurses, occupational therapists, physiotherapists, and access to physicians) but hopefully closer to his home. In time, pending a full assessment from the individuals in his multidisciplinary team (e.g. occupational therapist, physiotherapist) and in the context of his social circumstances (e.g. is there anyone who could help care for him or will he need carers?), Mr Walker will hopefully return home.

- **Follow-up:** it is important that his GP monitors him for any of the stroke risk factors picked up in hospital and continue to manage these as relevant.

Acute management of stroke is summarized in Figure 26.5.

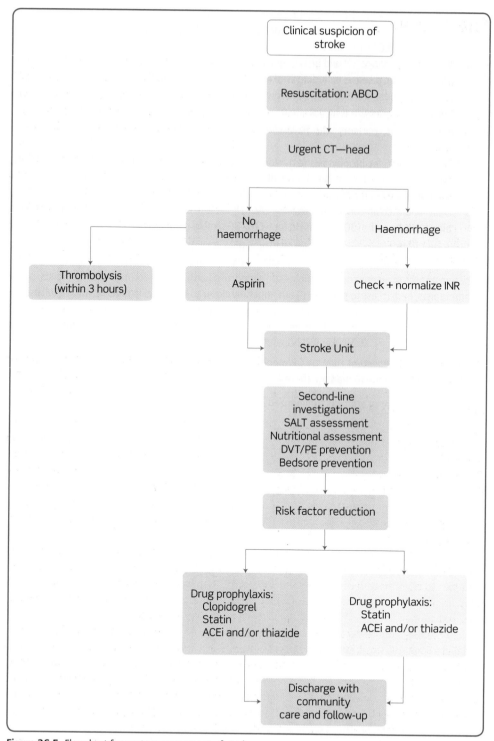

Figure 26.5 Flowchart for acute management of stroke.

ABCD, airways, breathing, circulation, and disability; INR, international normalized ratio; SALT, speech and language therapists; DVT, deep vein thrombosis; PE, pulmonary embolism; ACEi, angiotensin-converting enzyme inhibitor.

Short cases

Mrs Nindecass is a 72-year-old woman who has been rushed into the Emergency Department by ambulance. She was having tea with some friends in her village when one of them noticed the right side of her face was drooping. She promptly dropped the cup of tea she was holding in her right hand and one of her friends who is with her says she has been 'talking gibberish' ever since. An ambulance was called via 999 and her friend does not understand why it bypassed the nearest district general hospital and instead drove an extra 40 miles (>60 km) on 'blues and twos' to the larger city hospital. She has arrived within 90 minutes of the onset of symptoms. On examination, Mrs Nindecass has a patent airway, normal vital signs and is conscious but she has a dense, right-sided, flaccid paralysis to her face, arm and leg. She can obey simple commands with her left arm and leg but her speech is an unintelligible string of random words that appears to be frustrating her enormously. Her blood glucose is 6.4 mM and her friend confirms that at no stage has Mrs Nindecass fainted, had a seizure, or complained of a headache.

What is the likely diagnosis? What is the single most important investigation to be performed as soon as possible? Why didn't the ambulance take Mrs Nindecass to the nearest hospital?

Mrs Nindecass has presented with sudden-onset right-sided body weakness and expressive dysphasia that started within the last 2 hours. Her glucose is normal and there is no suggestion of headache, trauma, seizure or syncope. We must assume this is an **acute stroke** that has presented within the **thrombolysis window** (4.5 hours).

The single most important investigation at this stage is an *immediate* CT scan of her head to rule out a haemorrhagic stroke. If this is ruled out, the consultant on call for thrombolysis will then decide whether Mrs Nindecass is a candidate for thrombolysis to break up the clot that is causing her stroke. Thrombolysis carries a significant risk of haemorrhage so the decision will be based on weighing up the severity of her stroke symptoms and signs versus any contraindications to thrombolysis (see Viva questions). Remember—**time is brain**, and acute strokes must be treated with the same urgency as acute myocardial infarctions. However, see the first Viva question for some debate about the role of thrombolysis in stroke.

The ambulance correctly drove Mrs Nindecass to a hospital designated as a hyperacute stroke unit (HASU). This is done for the same reason that patients suffering major trauma or myocardial infarctions are taken to major trauma centres and hospitals with 24-hour cardiology angioplasty services. It is a recognition that these patients do better if they are in hospitals that see a large volume of these conditions and are equipped to offer 24-hour specialty consultant-delivered care.

Unfortunately, Mrs Nindecass' level of consciousness started to drop en route to her CT scan, which revealed a large, left-sided, intracerebral haemorrhagic stroke with midline shift. This ruled out any possibility of thrombolysis and within half an hour of her CT scan, she was unconscious. There was nothing that could be done to reverse the bleeding as her clotting, platelets, and blood pressure were all within normal limits. Her case was discussed with the neurosurgeons who felt, upon urgent review of her CT images and the patient, that a surgical intervention would not change the poor outcome in her case. She was admitted for palliative therapy and died within 6 hours of admission.

Despite advances in stroke management, it is still the case that 14% of patients presenting with a stroke will die within 1 year from complications of their stroke.

Mr Browne is a 67-year-old investment banker who has been attending a ball to celebrate his daughter's engagement. At the ball, Mr Browne remembers feeling unusually short of breath dancing the twist, and took a break to have a cocktail. He suddenly dropped the cocktail he was holding and found himself unable to move his right arm. His daughter noticed that his speech was slurred. They called for an ambulance but by the time Mr Browne arrived to the Emergency Department (40 minutes later), his speech was back to normal. On examination, his right arm has regained its strength and has a power of 5/5 with normal sensation. The remainder of the neurological examination is unremarkable. His heart rate is irregularly irregular and his blood pressure 164/105 mmHg. An ECG showed no P-waves, confirming his heart was in atrial fibrillation.

Mr Browne's past medical history includes an appendicectomy and hypertension, for which he takes amlodipine. He admits feeling unusually short of breath playing cricket over the past few weeks. He has never smoked and drinks only socially (he insists this is less than 10 units a week). He lives at home with his second wife and although he still works part-time, they are both hoping to retire to the south of France soon.

How would you assess Mr Browne in terms of the framework above (i.e. time course, deficit, location, disease, aetiology)? What is the most likely diagnosis? How should he be managed in the Emergency Department?

- **Time course:** acute onset, short-lived, and self-resolving.
- **Deficit:** right hemiparesis and dysarthria on history (but no UMN/LMN signs on examination).
- **Location:** ?left primary motor cortex.
- **Disease:** reversible vascular insult, i.e. **TIA**.
- **Aetiology:** emboli from either the left atrium, as he is in **atrial fibrillation**, or the carotids. His **uncontrolled hypertension** is additionally a risk factor for atherosclerosis, which may be a source of emboli, and small vessel haemorrhages.

TIAs are usually caused by small emboli lodging in cerebral arteries and causing cerebral ischaemia. Unlike in stroke, the clots in TIAs dissolve naturally under the action of the plasmin system before any lasting neurological defect can develop. Hence TIAs resolve spontaneously (80% within 1 hour, 100% within 24 hours) and leave no long-term deficit.

Management

Although TIAs self-resolve, the management is as for stroke: you need to establish the likely source of the emboli. If you don't and the cause is left untreated, about 25% will have a further TIA, a stroke, or a fatal cerebrovascular event within 90 days. This risk is highest early on (especially the first 24 hours), then decays. All patients with a TIA are started on 300 mg daily aspirin and referred to a specialist TIA clinic. The urgency with which they are seen in TIA clinic depends on their ABCD2 score (see Figure 26.6), which predicts the risk of stroke in the 48 hours after a TIA. The aim of the clinic is to identify and treat reversible causes of TIA and stroke (see next short case).

Mr Browne has an ABCD2 score of 5 and was seen the next morning in his local TIA clinic.

The ABCD2 score

Age:	1 point for age >60 years
Blood pressure:	1 point for >140/90 mmHg
Clinical features:	1 point for speech disturbance without weakness
	2 points for unilateral weakness
Duration of symptoms:	1 point for 10–59 minutes
	2 points for >60 minutes
Diabetes:	1 point

Figure 26.6 The ABCD2 scoring system, used to stratify the risk of stroke after TIA. A score of ≥4 is considered high risk and warrants TIA clinic within 24 hours.

Reprinted from *The Lancet*, 369, 9558, S Claiborne Johnston *et al.*, 'Validation and refinement of scores to predict very early stroke risk after transient ischaemic attack', pp. 283–292, Copyright 2007, with permission from Elsevier.

SHORT CASE

Mr Browne (from the previous case) attends his TIA clinic the very next day. He has had no recurrence of symptoms overnight. His BP in clinic is 152/87 mmHg. His ECG shows that his heart remains in atrial fibrillation. Examination of his cranial nerves and peripheral upper and lower limb nerves is normal. He has no carotid bruits or heart murmurs on auscultation.

What investigations will the TIA clinic arrange? What medications is Mr Browne likely to be recommended?

The main aim of the TIA clinic is to ensure the TIA has truly resolved, has not recurred and to search for reversible causes of future strokes. Patients with a TIA such as Mr Browne's, where a large portion of the cerebral cortex must have been affected, will usually have a **brain MRI** to look for any residual infarction which may not be apparent clinically. The main modifiable risk factors looked for are:

- **Smoking**. This is not the case with Mr Browne (see previous short case).
- **Hypertension.** Mr Browne has hypertension despite being on amlodipine. After asking whether he really takes his medication regularly, it will be worth either increasing his dose of amlodipine or (if a maximum dose has been reached), adding a second antihypertensive medication such as an ACE inhibitor.
- **Hyperlipidaemia.** Mr Browne will require a fasting lipid profile to see if there is any hyperlipidaemia that can be treated (e.g. with a statin).
- **Diabetes mellitus.** Mr Browne will require at the very least a random capillary glucose to rule out diabetes mellitus. As he is having a fasting lipid profile done, he might as well have a fasting laboratory glucose and HbA1c level done at the same time.

- **Carotid artery stenosis.** Mr Browne will require imaging of his carotid arteries to rule out any stenosis that is amenable to a surgical carotid endarterectomy. A Doppler ultrasound is usually the first-line investigation for this. Clinical examination alone (i.e. the lack of carotid bruits) is not sensitive enough to rule out significant stenosis.

- **Atrial fibrillation.** Mr Browne has a new diagnosis of atrial fibrillation. He will need referral to cardiology (for initial assessment and echocardiogram to rule out mitral valve pathology as the cause) and his GP may wish to consider starting him on medication to control his heart rate (e.g. bisoprolol), as his heart will be prone to episodes of fast ventricular response (tachyarrhythmia). From a TIA/ stroke point of view, his atrial fibrillation is the main modifiable risk factor as it increases his risk of stroke fivefold. To reduce this, the TIA clinic will consider whether Mr Browne is suitable for anticoagulant therapy with either warfarin or a non-vitamin-K-antagonist such as apixaban, dabigatran, or rivaroxaban.

Note that there is an important difference between **anticoagulants** (which affect the clotting cascade) and **antiplatelets** such as aspirin or clopidogrel (which affect platelet aggregation). Clots that form through blood stasis (such as those that form in deep veins or fibrillating atria, where a pool of static blood can form) are rich in fibrin and erythrocytes ('red clots') and are thus more effectively prevented using drugs that inhibit fibrin mesh formation. Clots that form through endothelial activation of platelets (such as those that form upon atherosclerotic plaque rupture) are rich in platelets ('white clots') and are thus more effectively prevented using drugs that inhibit platelet activation. This is why anticoagulants (e.g. warfarin, ribaroxaban) are used to prevent venous thromboembolism and atrial clots, whereas antiplatelets (e.g. aspirin, clopidogrel) are used to prevent myocardial infarctions and primary ischaemic strokes (i.e. those not caused by atrial clots). This is also why the 2014 NICE guidelines no longer recommend using aspirin to prevent strokes caused by atrial fibrillation. The 300 mg aspirin that all TIA patients are initially started on is not aimed at preventing strokes from atrial fibrillation, but rather those from atherosclerotic plaque rupture or embolization.

Although anticoagulants decrease the risk of embolic stroke, they increase the risk of haemorrhage. NICE recommends the use of two scoring systems to help determine the benefit (CHA_2DS_2-VASc score) versus the risk (HAS-BLED score) of starting a patient with atrial fibrillation on anticoagulation. The simplest way to use these scores is via a free online calculator (such as <http://www.sparctool.com>), which conveniently tells you (and the patient) the number of patients needed to treat with a particular anticoagulant before you see benefit versus harm. Note that neither NICE nor HAS-BLED makes any mention of 'falls risk' as a reason to not anticoagulate a patient. It has been common practice until now to stop anticoagulation in frail, elderly patients who suffer frequent falls under the belief that this puts them at serious risk of suffering a major bleed during one of their falls, but the current evidence does not (counterintuitively) support using falls as a criterion for determining risk when using anticoagulants. This view may change as more studies are performed.

Mr Browne has a CHA_2DS_2-VASc score of 2 (hypertension, age) and a HAS-BLED score of 2 (hypertension, age). His brain MRI did not suggest any infarction or haemorrhage. Using <http://www. sparctool.com> we can see that his annual risk of stroke from atrial fibrillation is 3% (cf. 0.7% for control population) but can be reduced to 1% using anticoagulation. However, we can also see that anticoagulation will increase his risk of major haemorrhage from 0.6% to 3%. Mr Browne decided with the stroke physicians that, on balance, he feared a disabling stroke more than a potentially treatable bleed. Mr Browne was thus started on lisinopril (in addition to his amlodipine), bisoprolol, and warfarin (with LMWH cover until his INR was 2–3). His aspirin was stopped, as there is no added benefit to aspirin in stroke prevention for patients started on anticoagulants.

SHORT CASE

Mr Bell is a 62-year-old man who is referred to his local hospital because of a recent onset of leg weakness. He first noticed his legs becoming weak about a fortnight ago, when he found himself struggling to get out of the armchair or his car. The weakness progressed to the point where he had to use his wife's walking frame to get around the house, but for the last 2 days he has been unable to walk at all.

A year ago Mr Bell had a right coronary artery stent after a myocardial infarction, but has no other past medical history of note. He currently takes aspirin, clopidogrel, and simvastatin. His family history is remarkable for three of his five siblings developing colorectal cancer in their early sixties. He is a retired police officer who lives with his wife in a bungalow. He smoked two packs of cigarettes a day for most of his adult life, giving up only 2 years ago at the insistence of his daughter. He has not had any alcohol for some years.

On examination, both of Mr Bell's legs have increased tone and clonus, reduced power (2/5 on hip flexion and knee flexion), brisk patellar reflexes and ankle reflexes, upgoing plantar reflexes, and coordination which is difficult to test accurately due to the weakness. He has lost vibration sensation below the hips and pinprick (pain) sensation below the umbilicus. His anal sphincter tone and perianal sensation are normal on digital rectal examination. Examination of his upper limbs, cranial nerves, cardiovascular, and respiratory systems is unremarkable and he is apyrexial.

How would you assess Mr Bell in terms of the framework above? What is the most likely diagnosis? What investigation(s) should be arranged in light of his history and examination?

- **Time course:** gradual onset (weeks).
- **Deficit:** spastic (UMN) paraparesis (bilateral leg weakness) + bilateral sensory loss in the lower limbs.
- **Location:** ?spinal cord lesion around T10 in the cord (corresponds to a vertebral level around T6). There are UMN signs, thus it must be in the spinal cord or brain. The weakness is bilateral, and two cortical lesions are less likely than a single spinal lesion. The loss of pain sensation below the umbilicus, a landmark for the T10 dermatome, suggests a lesion around T10. Because the spinal cord is shorter than the spinal column, the vertebral level will be around T6.
- **Disease:** the most likely cause is **cord compression**.
- **Aetiology:** cord compression may be due to disc herniation, spondylolisthesis, or any other space-occupying lesion, i.e. a tumour, abscess, cyst, or haematoma. The subacute onset argues against e.g. haematoma.

Investigations

You should order an investigation to confirm your clinical suspicion, which in this case would be a **spinal MRI**. This will provide more information about the type of lesion (e.g. spondylolisthesis, tumour, etc.).

SHORT CASE

Mrs Bean is a 26-year-old postdoctoral laboratory researcher who presents to her GP complaining of a weak left leg. She describes that she first noticed an odd tingling sensation spreading up her leg about a week ago, which is still present. A few days after the tingling, she found herself tripping over several times in a single day. By this morning, she was limping and could not manage the stairs at home alone.

Nothing like this has ever happened before and she does not recall any trauma. She has never been admitted to hospital before but says that about a year ago she had some eye problems while travelling in Africa. She recalls that her right eye became painful and that she had blurred vision for almost a week, before it gradually resolved. She did not seek medical help at the time as she was 'in the middle of nowhere' and put it down to 'some weird infection'. She currently takes the combined oral contraceptive pill and sumatriptan for her occasional migraines. Her family history is unremarkable. She does not smoke and drinks only very occasionally. She lives with her husband and their 2-year-old child.

There are a number of notable features on neurological examination: when you get Mrs Bean to *rapidly* move her eyes from extreme right gaze to extreme left gaze, you notice that the right eye is slow to adduct relative to the left and there is abnormal nystagmus of the left eye. Adduction on convergence is normal. In addition, there is a relative afferent pupillary defect (Marcus Gunn pupil) on the right. On examination of her limbs you find that despite the tingling in her left leg, sensation in both legs is objectively intact. However, her left leg has increased tone, decreased power (3/5 on hip flexion and knee flexion), a brisk patellar reflex, an upgoing plantar reflex, but normal coordination. Although she has not noticed anything in her right leg, this too has decreased power considering the patient's young age (4/5 on hip flexion and knee flexion), although tone, reflexes, and coordination are normal on the right.

How would you assess Mrs Bean in terms of the framework above? What is the most likely diagnosis? What investigations should you order to support this diagnosis?

- **Time course:** gradual (1 week), ?previous episode.
- **Deficit:** spastic (UMN) paraparesis (bilateral leg weakness) with a relative afferent pupillary defect (RAPD) and internuclear ophthalmoplegia (INO; slow adduction of her right eye during saccadic movements and leading eye nystagmus with preserved adduction on convergent gaze).
- **Location:** ?spinal cord lesion. The UMN signs mean it must be in the spinal cord or brain, and the bilateral nature makes the spinal cord more likely. However, INO indicates an additional lesion in her right medial longitudinal fasciculus. The previous episode of loss of vision suggests a further lesion in the optic nerve (at an earlier time).
- **Disease:** multiple lesions at different times over a period of months or years are consistent with a demyelinating disorder. The UMN signs and involvement of vision indicate central (rather than peripheral) demyelination, i.e. **multiple sclerosis**. Stroke is unlikely given her age, the gradual onset, and the bilateral pattern of weakness with additional lesion(s).
- **Aetiology:** the underlying cause of multiple sclerosis is unknown.

Multiple sclerosis characteristically causes central nervous lesions that are disseminated in space and time, and is strongly associated with both optic neuritis and INO. The earlier acute episode of a painful eye with blurred vision that spontaneously resolved after a week is highly suggestive of inflammation of her right optic nerve (optic neuritis). The right RAPD adds further weight to a diagnosis of a previous right optic nerve lesion.

Multiple sclerosis is, at least in part, an autoimmune disease in which Tc cells destroy the myelin sheath around neurons in the CNS at unpredictable locations and times, with some demyelination being reversible but some being permanent.

Investigations

Various investigations can help confirm a clinical diagnosis of multiple sclerosis, but should only be made by an experienced neurologist because of the great fear and misunderstanding that it causes in many patients:

- **Lumbar puncture,** looking for oligoclonal bands. In multiple sclerosis, it is characteristic to find elevated levels of multiple IgG antibodies in the cerebrospinal fluid (CSF) compared with the blood serum. These are known as oligoclonal bands because the various different antibodies arise from multiple B-cell clones (oligoclonal) and appear as dark 'bands' on a protein gel used to visualize the proteins found in the CSF or the serum. These antibodies should be matched with a serum sample in order to elucidate whether they originate in the CSF or are features of a systemic immune response. Note that oligoclonal bands are a non-specific sign of multiple sclerosis.

- **MRI of the brain and spinal cord,** looking for plaques. As its name implies, multiple sclerosis causes many sclerotic (demyelinated) plaques to appear throughout the CNS. These can be visualized using MRI and help confirm a diagnosis of multiple sclerosis.

- **Visually evoked potentials:** optic neuritis leads to demyelination of the optic nerve and therefore slower electrical conduction along this nerve. It is possible to measure the activation of both visual cortices (occipital areas of both brain hemispheres) in response to visual stimulation. Delayed response indicates slow electrical conduction and a lesion along the optic pathway that may not be apparent clinically.

Viva questions

Why don't all patients with ischaemic strokes receive thrombolysis treatment? What is the evidence to support thrombolysis? What are the contraindications to thrombolysis?

The role of thrombolysis in stroke is currently a source of much debate among physicians despite a large drive in recent years to have all stroke patients assessed for thrombolysis potential and NICE guidelines recommending it for patients meeting certain strict criteria. Of the 12 large clinical trials looking at the role of thrombolysis in acute ischaemic strokes, only two (NINDS-2[7] and ECASS-3[8]) showed any positive outcome (decreased dependency at 3 months but at a cost of increased mortality from haemorrhage in the first few weeks), and only if thrombolysis was given within 4.5 hours of onset of symptoms. Of the other 10 trials, 6 found no difference in thrombolysis vs placebo[9,10,11,12,13,14] and 4 had to be stopped early due to increased harm from thrombolysis.[15,16,17,18]

The list of contraindications for stroke thrombolysis is long:

* Onset cannot be confirmed as within 4.5 hours
* Acute intracranial haemorrhage on CT scan
* Seizure at onset of stroke
* Symptoms suggestive of subarachnoid haemorrhage
* Stroke or serious head injury in the preceding 3 months
* Major surgery or serious trauma within 2 weeks
* Previous intracranial haemorrhage
* Intracranial neoplasm
* Arteriovenous malformation or aneurysm
* Gastrointestinal or urinary tract haemorrhage in the preceding 3 weeks
* Lumbar puncture in the preceding week
* Platelets $<100 \times 10^9/L$
* INR >1.7
* Glucose <2.7 mmol/L or >22 mmol/L
* Positive pregnancy test
* Rapidly improving neurological signs (suggests a TIA)
* Systolic BP >185 mmHg, diastolic BP >110 mmHg or continuous IV antihypertensives required to lower BP below this range
* Suspected acute pericarditis in addition to the stroke

With such a long list of contraindications, you won't be surprised that as little as 1– 11% of patients presenting with stroke are actually candidates for thrombolysis.

A young man is rushed to his regional major trauma centre after crashing his motorbike at high speed. Advanced trauma protocols are promptly followed by the trauma team, and the patient is found to be suffering from no life-threatening injuries. The team proceeds to examine the patient's limbs.

The patient has sustained a comminuted, closed, supracondylar fracture of the distal metaphysis of his right humerus. The patient has lost sensation over the ulnar aspect of his right hand on both the dorsal and palmar side and has weakness in finger adduction and abduction. The patient can still extend and flex his wrist, and has strong thumb abduction. However, abduction in his other fingers is weak and Froment's sign is positive.

What lesion has this patient most likely sustained during his accident that can explain the pattern of weakness?

Figure 26.7 A hand with ulnar palsy.

Reproduced from Warrell DA, Cox TM, and Firth DJ, *Oxford Textbook of Medicine*, Vol. 3, 4th edition, 2003, Figure 2, page 1185, with permission from Oxford University Press.

The complex, distal fracture of his right humerus has probably injured his **ulnar nerve**. This would explain the weakness of the *intrinsic interossei* muscles of his right hand (responsible for abduction and adduction of the fingers) and the loss of sensation over the medial third of this hand (Figure 26.7).

Brown–Séquard syndrome is a rare neurological condition most commonly due to intrinsic cord lesions, e.g. multiple sclerosis, but classically seen in penetrating trauma to the spine or spinal fractures during road traffic accidents. Although rare, it is a favourite topic of examiners because it illustrates the neuroanatomy of the spinal cord.

Can you explain the features of Brown–Séquard syndrome anatomically?

Each half of the spinal cord contains (among many other things):

- UMNs innervating the *ipsilateral* side of the body.
- Dorsal column neurons (vibration, proprioception, fine touch) innervating the *ipsilateral* side of the body.

CONTINUED ➤

CONTINUED

- Spinothalamic neurons (pain, temperature, light touch) innervating the *contralateral* side of the body.

Thus, section of half of the spinal cord results in loss of power (paralysis) and loss of vibration, proprioception, and fine touch on the same side of the body below the lesion, but loss of pain and temperature on the opposite side of the body (usually a few vertebral levels below the lesion, as spinothalamic neurons do not cross immediately upon entering the spinal cord).

What scale is used to grade limb weakness?

Power (and therefore weakness) in muscles is graded using the MRC scale for power*:

Grade 5: normal power
Grade 4: can move limb against gravity and some resistance exerted by examiner
Grade 3: can move limb against gravity
Grade 2: movement only if gravity is eliminated
Grade 1: flicker is perceptible in the muscle
Grade 0: no movement

* Reproduced from *Aids to the investigation of the peripheral nervous system*. London: Her Majesty's Stationary Office; 1943. © Medical Research Council.

What do the terms hemiparesis, hemiplegia, paraparesis, paraplegia, quadriplegia all mean? Where are the neurological lesions likely to be for each of these terms?

The pattern of weakness is described using a combination of the terms as follows:

- The prefix mono- implies one limb
- The prefix hemi- implies half of the body
- The prefix para- implies the lower limbs
- The prefixes tetra- or quadra- imply all four limbs
- The suffix -paresis implies weakness (can still move)
- The suffix -plegia implies complete paralysis.

So, for example, a patient with a weak left arm and leg (with or without a weak left face) would be described as having a left hemiparesis, whereas a patient with paralysed legs has a paraplegia. The types of lesions that can give rise to these patterns of weakness are summarized in Table 26.2.

Table 26.2 Different patterns of weakness and possible lesion sites

Pattern of weakness	Site of lesion
Full body hemiparesis	Contralateral cerebral motor cortex (e.g. widespread stroke) Contralateral corona radiata, internal capsule, or pons (e.g. stroke)
Limb hemiparesis	Contralateral cerebral motor cortex (e.g. stroke) Contralateral corona radiata, internal capsule, or pons (e.g. stroke) Ipsilateral spinal lateral motor tract (e.g. cervical disc prolapse)
Isolated limb weakness (arm or leg)	Contralateral cerebral motor cortex (e.g. localized stroke) Contralateral corona radiata, internal capsule, or pons (e.g. stroke) Ipsilateral peripheral nerve root (e.g. osteophyte) Ipsilateral peripheral nerve plexus (e.g. trauma to brachial plexus) Ipsilateral peripheral nerve *per se* (e.g. angiogram sheath injury to the femoral nerve)
Paraparesis	Bilateral cerebral motor cortex (e.g. parasagittal meningioma) Bilateral motor spinal tracts (e.g. cord compression) Cauda equina (e.g. lumbar intervertebral disc prolapse) Bilateral lumbosacral plexus (e.g. Guillain–Barré syndrome)
Tetraplegia	Bilateral motor tracts of cervical spinal cord (e.g. traumatic spinal cord transection at C5) Peripheral nerves (demyelinating disease, i.e. Guillain–Barré syndrome)
Proximal muscle weakness	Neuromuscular junction (e.g. myasthenia gravis, Eaton–Lambert syndrome) Muscle (e.g. polymyositis, dermatomyositis) or secondary to other conditions (e.g. hyperparathyroidism) or drugs (e.g. statins)
Several episodes separated in time and space	Various sites in central nervous system (e.g. multiple sclerosis)

References

1   North American Symptomatic Carotid Endarterectomy Trial Collaborators. Beneficial effect of carotid endarterectomy in symptomatic patients with high-grade carotid stenosis. *New Engl J Med*, 1991;**325**: 445–453.

2   European Carotid Surgery Trialists' Collaborative Group. Randomised trial of endarterectomy for recently symptomatic carotid stenosis: final results of the MRC European Carotid Surgery Trial (ECST). *Lancet*, 1998;**351**: 1379–1387.

3   Barnett HJ, Taylor DW, Eliasziw M, *et al.* Benefit of carotid endarterectomy in patients with symptomatic moderate or severe stenosis. North American Symptomatic Carotid Endarterectomy Trial Collaborators. *New Engl J Med*, 1998;**339**: 1415–1425.

4   Diener HC, Cunha L, Forbes C, Sivenius J, Smets P, Lowenthal A. European Stroke Prevention Study. 2. Dipyridamole and acetylsalicylic acid in the secondary prevention of stroke. *J Neurol Sci*, 1996;**143**: 1–13.

5   Collins R, Armitage J, Parish S, Sleight P, Peto R. Effects of cholesterol-lowering with simvastatin on stroke and other major vascular events in 20536 people with cerebrovascular disease or other high-risk conditions. *Lancet*, 2004;**363**: 757–767.

6   Hankey GJ. Angiotensin-converting enzyme inhibitors for stroke prevention: is there HOPE for PROGRESS After LIFE? *Stroke*, 2003;**34**: 354–356.

7   The National Institute of Neurological Disorders and Stroke rt-PA Stroke Study Group. Tissue plasminogen activator for acute ischemic stroke. *N Engl J Med*, 1995;**333**: 1581–1587.

8   Hacke W, Kaste M, Bluhmki E. Thrombolysis with alteplase 3 to 4.5 hours after acute ischemic stroke. *N Engl J Med*, 2008;**359**: 1317–1329.

9   Hacke W, Furlan AJ, Al-Rawi Y. Intravenous desmoteplase in patients with acute ischaemic stroke selected by MRI perfusion-diffusion weighted imaging or perfusion CT (DIAS-2): a prospective, randomised, double-blind, placebo-controlled study. *Lancet Neurol*, 2009;**8**: 141–150.

10 Davis SM, Donnan GA, Parsons MW. Effects of alteplase beyond 3 h after stroke in the Echoplanar Imaging Thrombolytic Evaluation Trial (EPITHET): a placebo-controlled randomised trial. *Lancet Neurol*, 2008;**7**: 299–309.

11 Multicentre Acute Stroke Trial–Italy (MAST-I) Group. Randomised controlled trial of streptokinase, aspirin, and combination of both in treatment of acute ischaemic stroke. *Lancet* 1995;**346**: 1509–1514.

12 The European Cooperative Acute Stroke Study. Intravenous thrombolysis with recombinant tissue plasminogen activator for acute hemispheric stroke. *JAMA*, 1995;**274**: 1017–1025.

13 Second European-Australasian Acute Stroke Study Investigators (ECASS-II). Randomised double-blind placebo-controlled trial of thrombolytic therapy with intravenous alteplase in acute ischaemic stroke. *Lancet*, 1998;**352**: 1245–1251.

14 The IST-3 collaborative group. The benefits and harms of intravenous thrombolysis with recombinant tissue plasminogen activator within 6 h of acute ischaemic stroke: a randomised controlled trial. *Lancet*, 2012;**379**: 2352–2363.

15 The Multicenter Acute Stroke Trial–Europe Study Group (MAST-E). Thrombolytic therapy with streptokinase in acute ischemic stroke. *N Engl J Med*, 1996;**335**: 145–150.

16 Australian Streptokinase (ASK) Trial Study Group. Streptokinase for acute ischemic stroke with relationship to time of administration. *JAMA*, 1996;**276**: 961–966.

17 Clark WM, Wissman S, Albers GW, Jhamandas JH, Madden KP, Hamilton S. Recombinant tissue-type plasminogen activator (Alteplase) for ischemic stroke 3 to 5 hours after symptom onset. The ATLANTIS (B) Study: a randomized controlled trial. Alteplase Thrombolysis for Acute Noninterventional Therapy in Ischemic Stroke. *JAMA*, 1999;**282**: 2019–2026.

18 Clark WM, Albers GW, Madden KP, Hamilton S. The rtPA (alteplase) 0- to 6-hour acute stroke trial, part A (A0276g): results of a double-blind, placebo-controlled, multicenter study. Thrombolytic therapy in acute ischemic stroke study investigators. *Stroke*, 2000;**31**: 811–816.

Single Best Answers

1. **A patient is unable to move their leg, but the quadriceps muscles are observed to flicker when the patient is asked to lift their leg off the bed. How would you grade this on the MRC scale?**

   a. 0

   b. 1

   c. 2

   d. 3

   e. 4

2. **Which nerve roots are chiefly responsible for the ankle jerk?**

   a. S1/S2

   b. S2/S3

   c. S3/S4

   d. L1/L2

   e. L3/L4

3. **Which peripheral nerve provides motor supply to biceps and sensory innervation to the lateral forearm?**

   a. Axillary

   b. Radial

   c. Musculocutaneous

   d. Ulnar

   e. Median

4. **A patient presents to hospital with a suspected acute stroke. Which of the following must you not do in every such patient?**

   a. Check their blood pressure

   b. Check their blood glucose

   c. ECG

   d. CT head

   e. Start anticoagulant/antiplatelet treatment

5. **A patient reports an episode of transient limb weakness. On further questioning, they describe how their vision was disturbed for 20–30 minutes, during which time they saw wiggly lines and stars. Once their vision had cleared they started to feel their right arm tingling. The tingling started in the fingers and gradually spread up the arm. This tingling was followed by a period of arm weakness which the patient estimates lasted a few minutes. By the time of presentation to the Emergency Department 1 hour later, all symptoms have resolved. What is the most likely diagnosis?**

   a. Hypoglycaemia

   b. Migraine

   c. Epileptic seizure

   d. TIA

   e. Stroke

Acute joint pain

Core case

Read through the sections in the case boxes, covering up the sections that follow so that you don't see the answer. At the end of each case box, try to answer the question before reading on.

> Mr Sullivan, a 54-year-old magazine editor, presents to the Emergency Department with knee pain that has been present since he woke up. He denies any recent trauma to the joint.
>
> **What diagnosis must you exclude in a patient with acute joint pain and why?**

The 'must exclude' diagnosis is **septic arthritis**. Not only can it destroy articular cartilage within days if not treated (hence permanently reducing joint function), but it is also associated with a mortality of about 10% due to underlying bacteraemia.

> Joint pain can be due to pathology in the joint or from structures outside the joint (i.e. not a true arthritis).
>
> **What are the articular causes of a single, acutely painful joint (i.e. monoarthritis)? What periarticular and non-articular pathologies can cause pain around a joint?**

Remember that pain may be referred from elsewhere. For example, hip pathology may present as knee pain, and lumbar spine pathology may present as hip pain.

The causes of a single, acutely painful joint include those shown in Figure 27.1, with larger font size highlighting those that are more common.

Articular	Peri-articular	Non-articular
• **Trauma** (resulting in e.g. fracture, meniscal tear) • **Gout** • **Pseudogout** • **Septic arthritis** • Seronegative spondyloarthropathy • Transient synovitis • First presentation of chronic mono-/poly-arthritis (e.g. osteo-, rheumatoid) • Haemarthrosis • Sarcoidosis • Amyloidosis • Vasculitis • SLE • Rheumatic fever	• **Ligament injury** • **Tendinitis** • Bursitis • Fasciitis • Epicondylitis • Periostitis	• Nerve entrapment • Radiculopathy • Bone malignancy • Vasculopathy • Osteomyelitis • Neuroma

Figure 27.1 The main causes of a single, acutely painful joint in an adult.

What questions in the history will help you narrow down the differential?

- **Pain.** You should characterize the pain as for any other pain along the lines of **SOCRATES** (see Chapter 1). Pain that worsens with movement and improves with rest is likely to be non-inflammatory. An acute onset (hours) is consistent with septic arthritis, gout/pseudogout, and trauma. A more insidious onset is more common in conditions like bursitis and tendonitis, where the relevant anatomical structure becomes inflamed with overuse. Chronic onset suggests osteoarthritis (note that some rheumatologists prefer the term osteoarthrosis to reflect the fact that the inflammation is not the primary pathology). The severity of pain can usefully be assessed by asking about joint function—for example, can the patient weight bear?

- **Trauma.** Mr Sullivan has already said he does not remember there being any trauma, but you must always ask and make sure. Even the slightest of knocks can cause significant pain. However, this does not exclude other diagnoses—trauma can precipitate infection or gout, for example.

- **Common risk factors for gout.** There are many potential causes of gout, but the more common ones that you should ask about include use of thiazide diuretics, recent heavy alcohol intake, chronic renal failure, and chemotherapy (high cell apoptosis, leading to degradation of DNA and excess urate). A history of renal stones or previous episodes of gout also makes gout more likely.

- **Common risk factors for septic arthritis.** Again there are many possible risk factors, but the key ones are immunosuppression (e.g. diabetes, HIV, steroid use) and any prosthetic joints.

- **Risk factors for haemarthrosis.** Typically due to a coagulopathy (e.g. classically haemophilia), anticoagulant use (typically warfarin) or trauma (e.g. a ruptured anterior cruciate ligament in the knee).

- **Past medical history**
  - **Recent gastrointestinal (GI) or urethral infection?** Reactive arthritis can develop after either of these types of infection. You should take a sexual history as a gonococcal infection may be asymptomatic, and can lead to septic (rather than reactive) arthritis (via haematogenous spread).
  - **Previous episodes?** Think first of recurrent conditions like crystal arthropathies and overuse injuries.
  - **Rheumatological disease?** This is as relevant for joint pathology as a past surgical history is for abdominal pathology.
- **Other joints.** The involvement of several joints *sequentially* is characteristic of gonococcus or rheumatic fever. The involvement of several joints *simultaneously* suggests a first presentation of a chronic polyarthritis such as rheumatoid or psoriatic arthritis. If you suspect the latter, you should ask about cutaneous psoriatic plaques.
- **Drug history.** A variety of drugs (e.g. thiazides, low-dose aspirin, or ciclosporin) can predispose to gout. Steroids predispose to osteoporosis, with subsequent pathological fractures, although pathological fractures are usually in the spine and very rarely in the knee.

Mr Sullivan tells you the pain in his left knee is a sharp pain and is severe. It was there when he woke up this morning and is still present when you clerk him mid-afternoon. He's tried paracetamol and ibuprofen but they have had no effect. He does not think he has had a fever.† He says his knee is red, hot, slightly swollen, and tender. There are no breaks in the skin.

Mr Sullivan is partial to wine and drinks half a bottle to a bottle with meals most nights. He has eczema and hay fever but no other ailments currently or previously. He uses an emollient cream for his eczema, steroid nasal spray, and cetirizine tablets. He is married and has not had sex with another partner for over 5 years. No other joints are involved.

Any monoarticular pain requires examination of the relevant joint.

Describe how you would approach your examination of Mr Sullivan's knee. What features would help you distinguish articular from periarticular pain?

† Note that fever is not a very useful symptom, as it is neither specific nor sensitive enough to diagnose or exclude septic arthritis.

You should examine the relevant joint *and* one joint above and below, as pain may be referred from these joints. In Mr Sullivan's case, this means the knee, hip, and ankle—and the other knee for comparison.

Your joint examination should be based around 'look, feel, move':

- **Look:** inspect the joint for erythema, scars, swelling, muscle wasting, bony deformities. Make the most of symmetry and compare left with right, as in some individuals it may be difficult to tell if a joint is swollen or in some other way abnormal.
- **Feel:** for any effusions; for tenderness on the bones, ligaments, tendons, or along the joint line; for temperature (in case of infection or inflammation); and for neurovascular status. Checking neurovascular status is crucial, as a neuropathy or vasculopathy (either causing the pain or secondary to joint damage) may rapidly lead to irreversible damage and loss of function.
- **Move:** being careful and gentle with the painful joint, test the full range of passive and active movement.

- **Articular conditions** are more likely to present with a diffusely inflamed joint (red, hot, painful) and pain on passive as well as active motion.
- **Periarticular conditions** tend to have a focal point of tenderness on palpation (in bursitis this would be over the bursa; in tendonitis, over the tendon) and pain is usually much worse on active movement than on passive movement.

Many conditions causing acute monoarticular pain may have signs beyond the joint.

What would you look for on examination beyond the joint(s)?

You should keep an eye out for the following:

- Skin:
  - **Tophi**: deposits of urate crystals that can be found anywhere on the body usually around joints and bones. They are hard lumps that sometimes break through the skin with a chalky appearance (Figure 27.2). If present, they suggest chronic gout.
  - **Rheumatoid nodules**: subcutaneous nodules, classically found on elbows and ears, which are pathognomonic of rheumatoid arthritis.
  - A variety of **rashes** are seen in conditions that can also cause arthritis e.g. psoriasis, systemic lupus erythematosus (SLE).
- **Nails**: look for pitting, subungual hyperkeratosis, and onycholysis—all signs of psoriasis, associated with psoriatic arthritis.

Figure 27.2 Gouty tophi.

Reproduced from Warrell DA, Cox TM, and Firth DJ, *Oxford Textbook of Medicine*, Vol. 3, 4th edition, 2003, Figure 4, page 71, with permission from Oxford University Press.

- **Uveitis** (inflammation of the middle layer of the eye), evidenced by a painful red eye with diminished vision, and sometimes an irregularly shaped pupil. This is often associated with HLA-B27-positive inflammatory arthropathies.

- **Mouth ulcers** which may be evidence of inflammatory bowel disease (particularly Crohn's disease), itself associated with arthropathy.

- Lung signs suggestive of **fibrosis** (e.g. fine crackles at the end of inspiration, clubbing), as pulmonary fibrosis is associated with various inflammatory arthropathies (e.g. rheumatoid arthritis) and their treatments (e.g. methotrexate).

Do not focus unduly on these, as beyond the skin and nail signs these are relatively rare in someone presenting with acute joint pain (and indeed, outside of a rheumatology clinic).

> You examine Mr Sullivan. He has patches of eczema on his forearms and knees. He does not appear systemically unwell and is afebrile. His left knee is swollen and red compared with his right. On palpation it is warm and there is no effusion. You find he is diffusely tender to palpation around the joint, but not especially along the joint line, the patellar ligament, or patella. His dorsalis pedis and posterior tibial pulses are present, and sensation is normal throughout his lower leg. Active and passive knee flexion are markedly reduced due to pain (as a result, you cannot test for strength). His right hip and ankle are not tender and have a normal range of movement.
>
> **Taking this information into account, what is the differential and how will you proceed?**

The diagnosis is still not clear despite the history and examination—both septic arthritis and crystal arthropathies remain equally likely. In such cases you *must* perform **arthrocentesis** to exclude septic arthritis, given the seriousness of this condition. Arthrocentesis is the most useful diagnostic tool for discriminating between septic arthritis and other causes of acute monoarticular pain. It has the added benefit of offering some symptomatic relief. Unfortunately the signs and symptoms of septic arthritis—fever, joint pain, and swelling—are non-specific and do not help distinguish it from some of the other causes of monoarticular pain

> The registrar in the Emergency Department aspirates Mr Sullivan's left knee using local anaesthetic and a strict aseptic technique. The aspirate is yellowish but clear. The sample is sent to the laboratories and the microbiology technician on call is asked to review the sample urgently. **What are the possible findings and what do they mean?**

You will want the microbiology laboratories to perform microscopy (cell count and crystals), Gram stain, and culture on the joint fluid aspirate. Gram stain and microscopy are the most urgent tests, as culture results will typically take at least 24 hours to come back. There are several possible findings:

- **Crystals.** Present in gout (urate crystals—negatively birefringent and needle shaped) and pseudogout (calcium pyrophosphate crystals—positively birefringent and rhomboid). Detected by microscopy (Figure 27.3).

- **Infection.** Cloudy aspirate with elevated white blood cell count, a high neutrophil component, and bacteria visible on microscopy, with positive cultures a few days later, indicate septic arthritis. Note, however, that the white cell count may also be elevated in crystal arthropathies. Also note there is a false negative rate of about 20–25% in gonococcal septic arthritis. If you suspect gonococcus, you should request additional tests (see later).

- **Blood.** Haemarthrosis is seen in trauma with or without a fracture. If fat globules are present, it strongly suggests a fracture (the fat comes from the bone marrow).

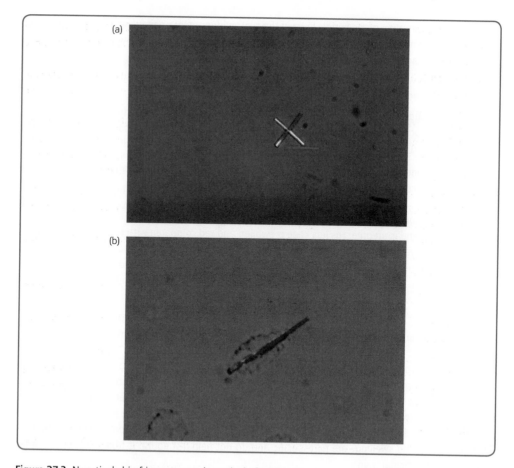

Figure 27.3 Negatively birefringent crystals, typical of gout.

Reproduced from Isenberg *et al.*, *Oxford Textbook of Rheumatology*, 3rd edition, 2004, Plate 189, with permission from Oxford University Press.

- **White cells.** In the absence of crystals, blood, and infection (all of which cause inflammation as well), inflammation as evidenced by white cells could be due to reactive arthritis (Reiter's syndrome), enteric arthropathy (due to inflammatory bowel disease), rheumatoid arthritis, psoriatic arthritis, and rheumatic fever. Non-inflammatory aspirate (clear and with a normal white cell count) usually suggests trauma or osteoarthritis.

Arthrocentesis is usually the only first-line investigation indicated. However, there are a number of other investigations that you may consider depending on the history and findings from arthrocentesis:

- **Cultures:** take swabs of skin lesions, or of throat, urethra, cervix, and rectum if gonococcal arthritis is a possibility. Blood cultures should be requested if there is a clinical suspicion of sepsis, although results may be negative in early infection.
- **Bloods:**
  - **Full blood count (FBC), C-reactive protein (CRP), and erythrocyte sedimentation rate (ESR):** these will reveal any widespread inflammatory and/or infectious process. Osteomyelitis will also result in deranged inflammatory markers (e.g. ESR and CRP) but not always a raised white cell count.

- **Prothrombin time (PT)** and **activated partial thromboplastin time (APTT)**: if arthrocentesis reveals a haemarthrosis in the absence of trauma sufficient to explain the injury, these should be requested to screen for a coagulopathy.
- **Rheumatological investigations**: if you suspect rheumatological disease, you may want to request rheumatoid factor, anticyclic citrullinated peptide (anti-CCP) antibodies, antinuclear antibody (ANA), and other autoantibodies.
- **Serum urate?** Patients who develop gout have often had hyperuricaemia for years, although during acute gout their serum urate is often normal or low. For this reason it should *not* be ordered in the acute setting. Also note that asymptomatic hyperuricaemia is fairly common in the population and thus a finding of elevated urate is not very helpful in diagnosis.

- **Plain radiographs:** These can be useful in the diagnosis of an acutely painful joint as they may show:
  - An unsuspected fracture, such as a tibial plateau osteochondral defect from a twist injury to the knee or a metastatic lytic lesion to the humeral head
  - Atraumatic avascular necrosis of the femoral head (Perthe's disease) or navicular (Köhler's disease) in children
  - An effusion that is not clinically obvious, such as an elbow effusion
  - Erosion of joint surfaces (e.g. in the hand or wrist) from an aggressive septic arthritis or an inflammatory, autoimmune arthropathy
  - Chondrocalcinosis, i.e. the deposition of calcium pyrophosphate crystals in large joint cartilage (typically the knee) in pseudogout.
- **MRI:** MRI is very useful if you suspect a soft tissue injury (e.g. meniscal tear in the knee) or bony pathology that isn't showing up on a plain radiograph (e.g. osteomyelitis). Unfortunately, MRI is time consuming in terms of both data acquisition and data review and as such it is rarely available in the acute setting or out-of-hours.

As with all presentations, resist the temptation to request a 'standard' panel of investigations as they may misdirect you. This is particularly the case with investigations such as ANA, which are relatively non-specific.

> The microbiology technician calls you 45 minutes later and reports 'negatively birefringent crystals', 10 white cells per high power field (which is high) of which 75% are 'PMNs'. The Gram stain microscopy is negative for microbes. Cultures are pending.
>
> **What is the diagnosis? Why is the Gram stain result important?**

Urate crystals are negatively birefringent, needle-shaped crystals. There are lots of white cells (predominantly polymorphonuclear cells (PMNs)—seen in acute inflammatory processes) in the aspirate suggesting an acute inflammation, but a negative miscroscopic Gram stain suggesting no obvious microbes. The presence of urate crystals and PMNs is pathognomic for **acute gout.** Gout most commonly affects the big toe (podagra), but the knee is the second most common joint affected and thus Mr Sullivan's presentation is not atypical. Calcium pyrophosphate crystals seen in pseudogout are positively birefringent, rhomboid-shaped crystals.

Even in the presence of crystals, it is crucial to exclude septic arthritis, which may coexist with a crystal arthropathy. Hence Gram staining, and cultures, remain crucial to the diagnosis.

> **What are the options for managing Mr Sullivan? What contraindications might drive your management?**

Treatment of gout can be divided into **acute** and **chronic.**

Acute management

During the acute episode of gout, the following medications can be helpful:

- **Colchicine,** if administered within 24 hours, can provide dramatic relief. However, it is contraindicated in patients with renal or hepatic impairment and can cause severe GI side effects unless used in low doses.
- **Non-steroidal anti-inflammatory drugs (NSAIDs),** which can be given in combination with colchicine. NSAIDs are contraindicated in patients with peptic ulcer disease, acute or chronic renal failure, heart failure, or pregnancy. Asthma is a relative contraindication for NSAID use as it can trigger exacerbations in some asthmatics, but many mild asthmatics have learnt from personal experience that NSAIDs don't trigger exacerbations in them and NSAID use is appropriate in these patients as long as they are warned to look out for exacerbations and know to stop the medication and seek immediate medical attention if this occurs.
- **Corticosteroid injections** either injected into the joint, or given systemically, are useful in patients who cannot take NSAIDs or colchicine.

Interestingly, aspirin is contraindicated in gout because low doses can cause hyperuricaemia by impairing urate excretion. However, this effect appears to be dose dependent, such that daily, low-dose aspirin used for preventing cardiovascular events increases urate levels far less than full-dose aspirin. For this reason, many patients with gout and significant cardiovascular risk factors continue to be prescribed low-dose aspirin, as a single acute cardiovascular event is arguably a worse outcome than occasional episodes of gout, which may (or may not) be caused by the low-dose aspirin in any case.

Chronic management

In the longer term, you will want to investigate Mr Sullivan for hyperuricaemia. If present, this can be treated using three strategies, although none of these will work in the acute setting:

- **Decrease urate production: allopurinol** and **febuxostat** are inhibitors of xanthine oxidase and limit the production of urate during the degradation of nucleic acids. The dose of allopurinol is titrated to the serum or urinary levels of urate until these are reduced to normal levels. The dose must be reduced in patients with renal or hepatic impairment and must be stopped if it causes a rash, as this tends to pre-empt more serious side effects. *Colchicine must always be co-prescribed with allopurinol for the first 6 weeks because the initial doses of allopurinol can paradoxically result in acute gout.*
- **Increase urate excretion: sulfinpyrazone** and **probenecid** are drugs that inhibit the reuptake of urate at the proximal convoluted tubules in the kidneys, thereby increasing urate excretion. They are useful for patients who cannot tolerate allopurinol.
- **Increase degradation of urate: rasburicase** is a uricase enzyme that can be administered to patients with severe hyperuricaemia due to chemotherapy. **Pegloticase** is another uricase enzyme for those who do not respond to xanthine oxidase inhibitors, but is currently not NICE approved primarily on cost effectiveness grounds.

Short cases

Mrs Hanbury is a 32-year-old school teacher who presents with an acutely tender left elbow that she knocked while gardening at the weekend. She took ibuprofen and paracetamol at night to alleviate the pain but was unable to sleep and has come to the Emergency Department because it is getting worse. She says it hurts 'no matter what I do' and is tearful. She drinks the occasional glass of white wine, has had no recent medical problems, and is on the combined oral contraceptive pill but nothing else.

You examine Mrs Hanbury's left elbow. It appears swollen compared with the right elbow and is red and tender. You also note the presence of lots of scratches on the skin over her elbow, which she explains are from her gardening. Sensation and capillary refill are normal in her left hand. However, she finds active and passive motion exquisitely painful. Her pulse is 88 bpm, blood pressure 110/58 mmHg, temperature 38.4 °C, respiratory rate 14/min, and saturations 99% on room air.

The radiologist performs arthrocentesis of the affected elbow under ultrasound guidance. The aspirate, which is yellow and turbid, is sent off to the laboratories for appropriate analysis.

What diagnosis should you be worried about? How should Mrs Hanbury be managed while you wait for the results of the arthrocentesis?

Mrs Hanbury has a very painful joint that developed acutely, with evidence of trauma to the skin (possible route of entry for infection, although most septic arthritis is due to haematogenous spread). The joint is clinically inflamed (red, hot, swollen, tender) and painful to both active *and* passive motion. She is also pyrexic, and has a yellow, turbid aspirate that would be consistent with pus. The diagnosis you should be worried about is **septic arthritis**.

If you suspect septic arthritis you should immediately start **analgesia**, take **blood cultures** to help identify the responsible pathogen, and start **broad-spectrum empirical antibiotics** (in accordance with local guidelines, to be adjusted when sensitivities are known). If the diagnosis is confirmed—which it should be very shortly by the microbiologist on call performing a Gram stain—she will need **joint aspiration and lavage**, either arthroscopically or as an open surgical procedure. She should therefore be referred immediately to the **orthopaedic surgeons**. Keep in mind that most septic arthritis is not from local trauma but from haematogenous spread of bacteria in the blood, so do not be falsely reassured by the lack of obvious trauma to the joint—this is, in fact, usually the case.

Mrs Jones is a 48-year-old shop assistant at a supermarket who presents to the Minor Injuries Unit with pain in her right shoulder that has been ongoing for some days but is getting worse and is limiting her activities. She gets the pain around the front of the shoulder, and it occurs when she tries to move the joint. She is a keen tennis player and has been playing a lot recently, so thought it might be a strain. As a result she has tried resting the arm in a sling (from her first aid box) and applying ice with some relief. There has been no trauma and no redness or swelling although her shoulder is tender. Her past medical history is notable for anxiety, for which she takes citalopram, and asthma, which is managed using a salbutamol inhaler as required. She dislocated the same shoulder when she was 22 and although she hasn't dislocated it since, she feels 'it isn't right'. Her job involves shifts of stacking shelves, which is very repetitive. She has not had a cold and is not sexually active. She does not drink and is a vegetarian.

She is apyrexial and comfortable at rest, and is wearing a self-fashioned sling. You expose both her arms, and on inspection her right and left shoulders look the same. However, her right shoulder is tender over the bicipital groove, unlike her left. Shoulder flexion reproduces the pain, although abduction, adduction, and internal and external rotation are normal. Special tests of the rotator cuff muscles are also normal. On examination of the elbow, you find elbow flexion and forearm supination cause pain.

What is the most likely diagnosis? What investigation would you consider for this lady? How might you manage her?

Mrs Jones has **bicipital tendonitis**, an overuse injury particularly common in those performing repetitive lifting activities (such as stacking shelves). It usually coexists with other shoulder pathology including rotator cuff damage and shoulder instability. Mrs Jones probably has the latter, having dislocated her shoulder and reporting it feels like it 'pops out a bit' at times. Tenderness over the bicipital groove suggests inflammation of the long head of the biceps tendon that passes through that groove. Pain on shoulder flexion, elbow flexion, and supination is classic in this condition.

She should be managed with **analgesia** (regular paracetamol and cautious use of anti-inflammatories such as NSAIDs because of her asthma) and **rest**. If the pain is severe or persists, it is sometimes helpful to administer a **corticosteroid injection** into the affected space (e.g. the bicipital groove) but *never* into the tendon itself, as this can cause it to rupture.

If her symptoms do not resolve, the investigation of choice would be **MRI** given that this is a soft tissue injury. This is particularly the case given her history of shoulder problems, as you will want to check the rotator cuff and other structures for damage as well.

SHORT CASE

Mr Taylor is a 27-year-old fitness instructor who presents with a 3-day history of a painful, stiff left knee and difficulty walking. The pain is always there and has not improved despite rest and analgesia. There has been no trauma to his knee. He says he has had some trouble recently with a sore, red eye. He also suffers from mouth ulcers, and has a couple at present. On direct questioning, he tells you that he has developed a rash on his glans penis and has had urethral discharge for the past 2 weeks with dysuria. He has had a number of male sexual partners over the last couple of months and has not yet been to the sexual health clinic, which he insists he was planning to do. There is no history of gout or other illness, and he takes no medications. He enjoys wine but does not drink heavily.

On examination, he has a temperature of 37.6 °C and a hot, red, swollen, and very tender knee. All active and passive movements of his left knee are painful. In addition, you note that the conjunctiva of his right eye is red but his visual acuity is 3/3 (normal) bilaterally.

Arthrocentesis reveals a clear fluid with no blood or crystals. Gram stain and cultures are pending, as are urethral, rectal, and pharyngeal swabs and bloods.

Based on the history and examination findings, what is the most likely diagnosis? If you are correct, what is the management?

Mr Taylor's history of urethral and eye symptoms, and the clinical finding of a red eye (conjunctivitis) in addition to an inflamed joint, are highly suggestive of **reactive arthritis (Reiter's syndrome)**.

Reiter's syndrome is an inflammatory arthropathy that typically affects patients with the HLA-B27 genetic allele and follows an episode of either gastroenteritis (*Salmonella* spp., *Campylobacter* spp., *Shigella* spp.) or sexually transmitted urethritis (*Chlamydia trachomatis*). The syndrome classically causes a triad of uveitis, urethritis, and arthritis (remembered as '*can't see, can't pee, can't climb a tree*').

You should consider all of the following in your management plan:

- Analgesia: regular, multimodal analgesia in the form of regular paracetamol, regular NSAID and a weak opioid (codeine, tramadol) as required.
- Relative rest of the affected joint. He needs to avoid exercises that cause pain to his knee but he also needs to keep the knee as mobile as pain allows to avoid it stiffening up and to avoid wasting of the quadriceps muscle, which can occur within days if a limb is not used.
- IV antibiotics until cultures are back to exclude a septic arthritis.
- If you suspect *Chlamydia* (or gonorrhoea, although this typically causes a septic arthritis), treat as per local antibiotic guidelines.
- Ophthalmology referral (as an in-patient).
- Testing for HIV as an in-patient (explain to the patient this is an appropriate test for any young patient presenting with his constellation of symptoms).
- Ask the patient to self-refer to a sexual health clinic on discharge (for contact tracing, advice, and screening for sexually transmitted diseases).
- Arrange rheumatology follow-up in outpatients (as there is a risk of chronic arthritis).

Viva questions

Describe the pathophysiological circumstances in which serum urate might be elevated.

Remember that urate is the major end product of the degradation of purine (a component of nucleic acids). Thus there are a number of causes of hyperuricaemia:

- Primary (90%):
  - Enzyme defects resulting in overproduction of urate ± underexcretion of urate
- Secondary (10%):
  - Increased nucleic acid turnover, e.g. leukaemia, polycythaemia, cytotoxic drugs
  - Underexcretion, e.g. chronic renal disease, drugs (diuretics particularly thiazides, excess alcohol which competitively inhibits urate excretion), starvation.

When is a rheumatological referral warranted for patients with painful joints?

You should consider referring patients with:

- suspected inflammatory polyarthritis, or
- recurrent monoarthritis unresponsive to treatment.

What are the most likely infective organisms in a native joint compared with a prosthetic joint?

- **Native joint infection:** *Staphylococcus aureus* is the most common infective organism of joints in all patients. In immunosuppressed patients one might find *Mycobacterium tuberculosis*. In patients with a possible or proven sexually transmitted disease one might find *Neisseria gonorrhoeae*. In patients with sickle cell disease one might find *Salmonella* spp.
- **Prosthetic joint:** *Staphylococcus epidermidis* is commonly implicated in infection of prosthetic joints. This probably reflects its ability to attach itself to artificial surfaces and its abundance (it is a major component of everyone's skin flora).

What are the features of osteoarthritis on a plain radiograph?

An osteoarthritic joint has a characteristic radiograph (Figure 27.4) that may include some or all of the following features. These can be easily remembered using the mnemonic LOSS:

Loss of joint space
Osteophyte formation
Subchondral sclerosis
Subchondral cysts

CONTINUED ➤

continued

Figure 27.4 Radiograph of knee with osteoarthritic changes.

Single Best Answers

1. **Which of the following drugs must not be given during an acute attack of gout?**

  a. Naproxen

  b. Diclofenac

  c. Colchicine

  d. Allopurinol

  e. Steroids

2. **A patient presents with a red swollen joint that is painful to passive movement. Which of the following investigations is most crucial?**

  a. Serum urate

  b. Temperature

  c. White cell count

  d. Arthrocentesis

  e. Plain radiograph joint

3. **A joint aspirate is reported to show positively birefringent rhomboid-shaped crystals. What is the diagnosis?**

  a. Gout

  b. Pseudogout

  c. Rheumatoid arthritis

  d. SLE

  e. Septic arthritis

4. **A patient with acute joint pain is noted to have numerous areas of pitting on his nails, and areas of onycholysis underneath the nail. Which of the following diagnoses becomes more likely?**

  a. Rheumatoid arthritis

  b. SLE

  c. Pseudogout

  d. Psoriatic arthritis

  e. Behçet's disease

5. **A previously fit and well young male patient presents with a hot swollen joint and septic arthritis is diagnosed. What is the most likely pathological organism?**

  a. *Salmonella* spp.

  b. *Neisseria gonorrhoeae*

  c. TB

  d. *Staphylococcus aureus*

  e. *Staphylococcus epidermidis*

Core case

Read through the sections in the case boxes, covering up the sections that follow so that you don't see the answer. At the end of each case box, try to answer the question before reading on.

Mrs McDonald is a 48-year-old cleaner who presents to a local hospital Emergency Department complaining of a swollen right calf that has appeared over the last few hours.

What is your differential diagnosis for an acutely swollen calf?

The main causes of an acutely swollen calf are shown in Figure 28.1.

> ## Deep vein thrombosis (DVT)
> ## Cellulitis
> ## Ruptured Baker's cyst
> ## Muscular strain (e.g. torn gastrocnemius)
> Septic arthritis (knee, ankle)
> Allergic response e.g. to insect bite
> Compartment syndrome

Figure 28.1 Main differential diagnosis for an acutely swollen calf.

Note that it is possible for different pathologies to coexist: a patient may present with a deep vein thrombosis (DVT) and ruptured Baker's cyst, for example. Also, many patients will get a swollen leg following surgery to that leg, but this shouldn't present much of a diagnostic challenge (although you must obviously exclude DVT if the symptoms and signs warrant this) and therefore this is not included in the list in Figure 28.1.

Would your differential diagnosis be different if *both* of her legs were swollen?

Yes, because most of the diseases listed in Figure 28.1 are local diseases and it would be highly unlikely for the patient to have two similar events in both legs at the same time. Instead, it would be more likely that the patient has either a systemic problem or a problem affecting central vessels. However, it is worth remembering that a DVT can arise in a patient with pre-existing bilateral leg oedema, so don't rule out a DVT just because both legs are swollen. Figure 28.2 gives the main causes of bilateral swollen legs.

> Right heart failure (in isolation or together with left heart failure)
> Lymphoedema
> Venous insufficiency
> Pregnancy
> Vasodilators (e.g. calcium-channel blockers)
> Hypoalbuminaemia: from renal failure (nephrotic syndrome), liver failure, malabsorption/malnutrition, or sepsis
> Pelvic tumour (e.g. ovarian) compressing the inferior vena cava
> Fluid overload (iatrogenic)

Figure 28.2 Main causes of bilateral swollen legs.

What specific questions would you ask Mrs McDonald during your history-taking? Think of questions that will provide key clues to help rule in or rule out particular diagnoses.

- Are there any risk factors for venous thrombosis? Consider Virchow's triad:
  - **Hypercoagulable blood?** Trauma, major surgery within the last 3 months, pregnancy and post-partum state (women are at increased risk of a venous clot for 6 weeks after birth and the risk is actually higher during the first few weeks after birth than during pregnancy itself), inflammatory bowel disease, active cancer, obesity (body mass index (BMI) >30 kg/m²), combined oral contraceptive pill or hormone replacement therapy (HRT), family history or past medical history of DVTs.
  - **Stasis?** Bed rest (>3 days) or long-haul travel (the actual length of flight that qualifies as 'high risk' is controversial).
  - **Vessel injury?** Trauma, surgery.
- **Has she felt breathless, had any chest pain, or coughed up any blood?** If DVT is high on your differential list, it would be wise to enquire about symptoms of a possible pulmonary embolism (PE).
- **Has she had any cuts, insect bites, or other wounds to her right leg?** If the patient has recently had a wound in her right leg, infective diseases such as cellulitis and septic arthritis become much more likely.
- **Is the swelling getting bigger?** Cellulitis can spread fairly rapidly along the affected limb, whereas the other pathologies are more likely to remain confined in the short term.
- **Has she had any abdominal pain? Has she noticed any blood in her faeces? Has she had any unusual vaginal bleeding? Has she noticed any weight loss, fever, or malaise?** If you are considering a pelvic malignancy as the cause of the limb swelling, you can ask for symptoms that are suggestive of colon, ovarian, or uterine malignancies.
- **Has she recently had radiotherapy or surgery to her right leg or abdomen?** Radiotherapy or surgery may have damaged the lymphatic drainage from her affected limb, causing the accumulation of lymph (lymphoedema).
- **Does moving the joints in her leg elicit the pain?** Patients with septic arthritis will tell you that movement of the affected joint brings on *excruciating* pain in the joint.

Mrs McDonald is in town visiting her daughter, who is getting married next week. She arrived yesterday after a 10-hour overnight bus journey and noticed that her right calf started swelling within a few hours of arriving. She can still walk on her affected limb, which is only slightly painful but 'feels very hot'. She thinks the swelling has been the same for the past few hours. She has not noticed any cuts, bites, or wounds in her right leg. She has not had any recent surgery, but started taking HRT last month to help with the unbearable hot flushes that she was getting from her menopause—her last period was 5 months ago and she has had no vaginal bleeding since. She has never had any cancer or radiotherapy, but had her appendix removed when she was a teenager. Her past medical history is otherwise unremarkable. She has been trying to lose weight recently in preparation for her daughter's wedding but admits to limited success in her efforts as her BMI is still >30 kg/m^2.

Can you identify risk factors for any of your differential diagnoses in the history?

- **Long-distance travel:** several studies have shown an increased risk of venous thrombosis in people who are immobilized through travelling for more than 8 hours non-stop. It is important to realize that what matters is the prolonged immobility, and not the type of transport used. Thus, most lay people will (wrongly) associate DVTs with all forms of flying (irrespective of duration) but will not consider long-haul bus, train, or car journeys as a risk for DVT. Also, it is important to note that most studies suggest that the increased risk of DVT associated with long-distance journeys applies only to people with other predisposing risk factors for DVT, although patients may not be aware of these at the time of travelling.

- **Oestrogen- and progesterone-based therapies:** several studies have shown that medications involving oestrogen and/or progesterone analogues (e.g. contraceptive pills in fertile women, HRT for menopausal women, tamoxifen in breast cancer patients) increase the risk of venous thrombosis. However, it is important to note that most people taking oestrogen/progesterone-based medications will have a low baseline risk of venous thrombosis, and so increasing that risk only moderately will still result in a risk that is still low overall.

- **Obesity:** obesity also increases the risk of thrombotic disease.

Having taken a history, you examine Mrs McDonald.

Is there anything in particular you will look for on examination that might help you sort out your differential diagnoses?

- **Cuts, bites, wounds, or superficial infections:** patients often haven't noticed small cuts, puncture wounds, or insect bites so look carefully for these all over the affected limb. Also check between the toes for fungal infection as a portal of entry.

- **Location of the swelling:** septic arthritis is likely to produce inflammation that is principally over a joint (e.g. the ankle, the knee). Compartment syndrome is likely to produce inflammation which is confined to the calf or thigh muscle compartments but spares the joints. A ruptured synovial sac in the knee ('Baker's cyst') would emerge from the popliteal fossa and track down into the calf.

- **Extent of swelling:** measure the extent of swelling using a tape measure to compare the circumference of both limbs at the same point (e.g. 10 cm below the tibial tuberosity). Also, mark the area of swelling and/or erythema with a pen so that you can monitor progression.

- **Lymphadenopathy:** check for swollen lymph nodes in the popliteal fossa and in the groin, as lymphadenopathy would be highly suggestive of an infection in the limb.

- **Abdominal masses:** an abdominal mass in the right lower quadrant would suggest a tumour that could be compressing the right iliac vein.

- **Neurovascular status of the limb:** it is imperative that you check and document the sensation, motor function, and pulses of the affected limb distal to the swelling. These can be affected by compartment syndrome, and compromise of neurovascular status is a surgical emergency.
- **Pain on gentle passive movement:** septic arthritis will elicit pain in the affected joint whereas pain in the calf is suggestive of compartment syndrome. Note that the joint should be moved gently and slowly to avoid dislodging any DVTs into the circulation.
- **Is she febrile?** It is possible to have a low-grade pyrexia with a DVT, but a significantly raised temperature points strongly towards an infective aetiology.

Mrs McDonald looks systemically well but her right calf is indeed swollen (pitting oedema), red, warm, and tender from just below the knee to just above her ankle. Her right calf is 3.5 cm greater in circumference than her left calf. No wounds are visible on her leg and no lymph nodes palpable in her right leg or right groin. Palpation of the popliteal fossa reveals no swelling. Slow, passive movement of the ankle and toes does not elicit any pain, only mild discomfort in her right calf. Her sensation to light touch is preserved throughout her right limb. Her posterior tibial pulses are present. Dorsalis pedis is not palpable on either leg, but capillary refill time in the toes of both feet is <2 seconds. Power on dorsiflexion, plantar flexion, and big toe dorsiflexion (extensor hallucis longus) is 5/5 on the MRC scale for both feet. No abdominal masses are palpable.

Do you know of any scoring systems to help you decide how this patient should be investigated?

The diagnosis to exclude in this context is DVT. The pre-test probability of a patient having a DVT can be estimated using the Wells scoring system (note that there are different Wells scores for DVT and PE) (Table 28.1).

Table 28.1 The Wells scoring system for DVT

Criteria	Points
Entire leg swollen	1
Calf swollen >3 cm (circumference) compared with the other leg	1
Pitting oedema confined to the leg (affected side)	1
Paralysed or immobilized leg	1
Bed rest for >3 days or major surgery within the last 12 weeks	1
Tenderness along the course of deep veins of the leg	1
Collateral superficial veins visible on leg (non-varicose)	1
Active cancer (treatment within last 6 months or palliative)	1
Previous DVT	1
Alternative diagnosis at least as likely as DVT[a]	−2
Score ≤1 = unlikely DVT	
Score ≥2 = likely DVT	

[a] This refers to patients in whom the clinical history and examination strongly point towards a particular diagnosis for a swollen limb that is not a DVT. Thus, a patient with a rapidly spreading, shiny, red swelling over the calf and an obviously purulent puncture wound over the sole of the foot is quite likely to have cellulitis.

Reprinted from *The Lancet*, Vol. 345, P.S. Wells *et al.*, Accuracy of clinical assessment of deep-vein thrombosis, 1326–1330, Copyright 1995, with permission from Elsevier.

Mrs McDonald has a Wells score of 3 (pitting oedema, calf swollen >3 cm, and tender along course of deep veins).

Given Mrs McDonald's Wells score, what investigations and acute management will you arrange?

Table 28.2 is useful for deciding the investigations in suspected DVT using the Wells score. Note that the main role of the D-dimer blood test is to help exclude, rather than diagnose, DVT.

Table 28.2 Diagnostic approach for a suspected deep vein thrombosis (DVT)

Wells score	D-dimer	Ultrasound scan
<2	Negative	Not required as DVT excluded
< 2	Positive	1 required
≥ 2	Negative	1 required
≥ 2	Positive	2 required (2nd after 1 week if initial scan negative)

- **Doppler ultrasound of the proximal leg veins:** this is the most sensitive, rapid, and non-invasive way of visualizing a DVT in the lower limb. Ultrasound will also enable a ruptured Baker's cyst to be diagnosed.

- **Serum D-dimer levels:** D-dimers (fibrin degradation products) can be elevated by DVTs and PE, but also in various other situations such as cellulitis, acute coronary syndromes, atrial fibrillation, pneumonia, vasculitis, sickle cell crises, superficial phlebitis, malignancies, and disseminated intra-vascular coagulation. Elevated D-dimers have >90% sensitivity for DVT, but only 30–40% specificity. An elevated D-dimer is therefore not useful in positively diagnosing a DVT. However, a normal D-dimer level is useful because it helps to rule out a DVT in someone with a low Wells score without the need for an acute ultrasound. Also, an elevated D-dimer in someone with a high Wells score is an indication for performing a repeat ultrasound after 6–8 days (rather than a single investigation, if the first ultrasound scan is negative). Ultimately, however, it is the ultrasound that will positively diagnose the DVT.

- **Full blood count (FBC) and clotting studies:** a FBC may reveal a high white cell count (WCC; you still haven't ruled out cellulitis) or a high red blood cell count (RBC; polycythaemia—a rare cause of DVT) and clotting studies may reveal deranged coagulation.

- **Anticoagulation:** the gold standard is for patients to receive their ultrasound within 4 hours of request. In reality, many patients who are suspected of having a DVT and who are low risk for bleeding are given a treatment dose of low molecular weight heparin (LMWH) or novel oral anticoagulant while awaiting their scan the following day.

Mrs McDonald has a Wells score of 3 (tender calf, swollen calf and pitting oedema), a positive D-dimer and a normal FBC. Irrespective of the D-dimer, her Wells score (≥2) suggests she needs an ultrasound scan to rule out a DVT so she is given an injection of subcutaneous (SC) LMWH and referred to the next day DVT clinic. In clinic, the Doppler ultrasound of Mrs McDonald's leg shows an occlusion in the right femoral vein consistent with a DVT.

How will you manage Mrs McDonald?

Mrs McDonald has had a diagnosis of **DVT** confirmed by Doppler ultrasound. Her management should include:

- **Anticoagulation.** This is to prevent clot extension, PE, and recurrence. Acutely, patients should be given LMWH or fondaparinux. If they have significantly impaired renal function, or are at risk of bleeding (e.g. postoperative patients), unfractionated heparin is used. LMWH is administered via a SC injection and is dosed according to the patient's weight. Options for ongoing anticoagulation are either rivaroxaban or warfarin (or ongoing LMWH if underlying malignancy). If warfarin is chosen the patient should be counselled and have their international normalized ratio (INR) measured. The parenteral anticoagulant should be continued for 5 days or until the INR is in range for >24 hours, whichever is longer. The optimal duration of anticoagulation therapy is debated and varies with a number of factors such as location (above/below knee), previous DVTs, and the presence of risk factors. Mrs McDonald will require 3 months of anticoagulation.

- **Compression stockings.** Offer a below-knee graduated compression stocking (ankle pressure >23 mmHg) to be worn 1 week after diagnosis or after leg swelling has reduced (assuming no contraindications). The stocking should be worn for 2 years on the affected limb, and replaced 2–3 times per year.

- **Lifestyle advice.** Lifestyle advice, e.g. considering cessation of HRT or the combined oral contraceptive pill, weight loss. These are risk factors for DVT that you should address.

Note that as there is a clear predisposing factor for the DVT in this instance (prolonged travel/stasis), there is no requirement to search for another cause. In other words, the DVT is 'provoked'.

Short cases

Mr Bullen is a 34-year-old gardener who is on the Trauma Unit of his local hospital because he has broken his right tibia. He presented yesterday morning having been hit by a car while attempting to cross the road. He was diagnosed with a closed, transverse, minimally displaced fracture of the right tibial shaft which required internal fixation.

You have been bleeped by the nurse on the Trauma Unit. Mr Bullen is complaining that his leg is 'excruciatingly painful' and that he cannot feel his toes. You attend and confirm that his analgesic requirements have been progressively increasing over the past few hours. He cannot feel you touching his toes, which protrude from the cast. You immediately cut and remove the cast to reveal a right calf that is red, tender, swollen, and with skin that looks tense and shiny. There is no pitting oedema. Passive movement of his right toes or ankle causes severe pain. Sensation to light touch is diminished over the distal portion of his right calf, over the dorsum of his right foot, and over his toes. His right posterior tibial pulse is palpable but his dorsalis pedis is not, although it is palpable on the left leg.

What is the diagnosis? How will you manage this patient?

Mr Bullen has features that are very strongly suggestive of **compartment syndrome**: a tense, shiny, swollen limb that is painful to passive movement and has now progressed to neurovascular compromise. Inflammation due to trauma (accidental or iatrogenic) is the most common cause of compartment syndrome. Limbs have muscle groups surrounded by tight inelastic fascia. The inflammation in a confined compartment can occlude the deep veins, impeding venous drainage of the limb, which therefore starts to swell, further occluding the deep veins. Pressures in the affected limb can become high enough to cause ischaemia and necrosis of all the tissues in the limb, leading to an irreversible atrophy of the limb known as **Volkmann's contracture**.

Compartment syndrome is a **surgical emergency** requiring urgent decompression via **fasciotomies**. The skin, subcutaneous tissue, and tight fascia surrounding the affected limb are all divided and left open. Two longitudinal incisions are made in the leg in order to decompress all four compartments (anterior and lateral compartments via an anterolateral incision, and superficial and deep posterior compartments via a medial incision). Note that in this patient there is no role for compartment pressure monitoring—the diagnosis of compartment syndrome has been made clinically and the patient is already showing signs of neurovascular compromise—he should be transferred to theatre without delay.

Miss Patel is a 21-year-old student who has just returned from celebrating the end of her university studies with her friends at a Mediterranean coastal resort. A few days after her return, her left ankle started to swell. She has presented because the swelling has been spreading up her leg and into her foot. She does not use the contraceptive pill. She has never had a 'blood clot in her legs or lungs' before, and has not had any recent surgery. Her past medical history is unremarkable. Her flight back from Catalunya lasted only 2.5 hours.

Inspection reveals a red, swollen distal calf, ankle, and dorsum of the foot; although a tape measure reveals that the swelling is actually only 1 cm more than her right limb. The swelling is warm, soft, and tender to touch but has no pitting oedema nor visible superficial veins. A small punctum is visible just next to her lateral malleolus, and she explains that it is a mosquito bite that was particularly itchy. Passive movement of her ankle and toes does not elicit any pain, although it is uncomfortable because of the swelling. No other lumps or bumps are palpable in the leg or abdomen. The patient is apyrexial.

What is the most likely working diagnosis and how will you manage this patient?

It is likely that Miss Patel has either **cellulitis** or an **inflammatory response to the mosquito bite** over her left ankle. Her Wells score is −2 and therefore a DVT is unlikely. A D-dimer won't be any help as it is likely to be high due to the inflammation. Ultimately, there is no reason to suspect a DVT clinically given the lack of risk factors, the history and the examination. She has no signs of septic arthritis or compartment syndrome.

Management of Miss Patel should include:

- **FBC:** looking for signs of bacterial infection (a neutrophilia).
- **Antibiotics:** an antibiotic that covers both streptococci and staphylococci should be used, such as flucloxacillin, as per local hospital protocols.
- **Demarcation:** the erythema should be marked with a pen to allow monitoring of progression/ response to treatment.
- **Elevation:** will help to reduce swelling and aid patient comfort.
- **Topical steroids and oral antihistamines:** given the story suggesting that the mosquito bite may have triggered the episode, you should also consider that the swelling may simply be an inflammatory response to the mosquito bite (essentially an allergic response to the mosquito bite). If so, the inflammatory response will benefit from topical steroids (to dampen the immune response) and antihistamines (as histamine release by mast cells is likely to be driving the inflammation).

SHORT CASE

Mr Leroy is a 72-year-old man who limps into the Emergency Department using a walking stick. He complains of a painful, swollen right calf since he woke up this morning. He has a past medical history of osteoarthrosis in his right knee and low-grade (papillary) bladder cancer for which he has received a cystoscopic resection and for which he receives ongoing, regular irrigation of his bladder with BCG (Bacille Calmette–Guérin, which is usually used for tuberculosis vaccination). He states that he has been aware of a small swelling behind his right knee 'for some time'. On examination, his right calf is swollen (2 cm), pitting, warm, red, and tender all over (not specifically along the veins), with the inflammation extending up into the popliteal fossa. There are no other masses palpable in his leg or abdomen. His right foot has normal sensation, power, and pulses. Passive movement of his ankle and toes brings on mild pain in his calf. Suspecting a DVT because of his Wells score (pitting oedema, active cancer = 2), a Doppler ultrasound of his leg is arranged but no occlusion of any deep veins can be seen. His D-dimer is negative, so a single ultrasound is good enough to rule out a DVT.

What is the most likely diagnosis and how should the patient be managed?

This patient probably has a **ruptured Baker's cyst**. This is caused by rupture of a synovial sac protruding from the knee in the popliteal fossa, usually in patients with arthropathy of the knee. The fluid from the ruptured synovial sac (Baker's cyst) can then track down into the calf, producing signs that are clinically indistinguishable from a DVT. However, the Doppler ultrasound helps to rule out a DVT, making the diagnosis of ruptured Baker's cyst the more likely one.

Treatment can include **elevation of the affected limb, aspiration of the fluid** and **injection of corticosteroids** into the knee, to reduce the inflammation and alleviate the pain.

Viva questions

A concerned patient comes to his GP to seek advice on how to prevent DVTs while travelling, because his brother suffered from a DVT after a long-haul flight last year. The patient explains that he will be flying from London to Istanbul, before taking a bus to the Cappadocia region of Turkey. The patient wants to know if he should take aspirin and wear compression stockings during the flight.

Several studies have shown that the risk of DVT while travelling is only increased if the patient is immobile for >8 hours and has other risk factors for DVT (although the patient may not be aware of these). The flight from London to Istanbul will take less than 8 hours and therefore poses little risk of DVT for this patient. However, the bus journey from Istanbul to Cappadocia is likely to take >8 hours and involve far less opportunity to mobilize than during the flight, so the patient may wish to wear compression stockings during the bus journey, rather than the flight. There is no evidence that aspirin prevents DVT in the context of long-haul travel. NICE recommends the following approach to preventing DVT when travelling:

- **No risk factors for DVT:** General advice about mobilizing as often as possible.

- **Moderate risk factors for DVT** (pregnancy, 1 month post-partum, obese, heart failure, previous DVT/PE, family history of DVT/PE, polycythaemia, phlebitic varicose veins of legs, lower limb fracture in cast): **graduated compression stockings** provided there is no peripheral vascular disease.

- **High risk factors for DVT** (active cancer, major surgery in past 3 months, known thrombophilia): **graduated compression stockings** (provided there is no peripheral vascular disease) and consideration of **LMWH** injections in discussion with local haematology team.

Several congenital mutations, acquired diseases, and drugs can all make a patient's blood more likely to clot. Can you name them?

Congenital mutations

- Factor V Leiden mutation (5% of Caucasians)
- Prothrombin G20210A mutation (2% of Caucasians)
- Antithrombin III deficiency (0.4% of Caucasians)
- Protein C deficiency (0.5% of Caucasians)
- Protein S deficiency (0.5% of Caucasians)

Diseases

- Any form of malignancy
- Antiphospholipid syndrome
- Disseminated intravascular coagulation
- Polycythaemia

CONTINUED ➤

CONTINUED

Drugs

- Combined oral contraceptive pill
- HRT
- Heparin-induced thrombocytopenia (HIT), which can counterintuitively cause thrombosis by an unknown mechanism but which can fortunately be prevented by using LMWH instead of full-length heparin
- Procoagulant and antifibrinolytic drugs? One might expect that drugs that promote clotting (e.g. aprotinin) or delay clot breakdown (e.g. tranexamic acid) would increase the risk of DVT but the evidence so far suggests this is not the case.

What components of the clotting cascade does warfarin interfere with? What additional drug should all patients starting on warfarin be placed on and why?

Warfarin is a competitive antagonist of vitamin K, the cofactor used by liver hepatocytes to synthesize factors II, VII, IX, X, protein C, and protein S.

Warfarin can take a few days to have an effect on clotting because it inhibits the synthesis of coagulation factors, and these have to become depleted. Also, warfarin can initially cause a paradoxical increase in clotting because of the depletion of protein C and protein S (anticoagulant) before the depletion of other clotting factors (procoagulant). For this reason, patients are started on LMWH for up to 5 days or until the INR is in target range for >24 hours.

What are the main contraindications and side effects of warfarin therapy? What advice would you give a patient starting on warfarin?

Contraindications

- Pregnancy (warfarin is teratogenic)
- Severe hypertension (risk of haemorrhagic stroke)
- Peptic ulcer disease (risk of bleeding ulcer)

Side effects

- Haemorrhage
- Nausea, vomiting, diarrhoea, rash (like most drugs!)
- Purple toes and skin necrosis
- Hepatic dysfunction, jaundice
- Pancreatitis

Advice for patients

- Avoid alcohol, cranberry juice and St John's wort
- Check with GP before taking any other medication
- Consult GP if faeces or urine go dark or bloody.

A patient who has been diagnosed with having a right femoral DVT is placed on LMWH and warfarin, but continues to throw off clots and suffer from small PEs. Is there any further treatment that can be offered?

You may wish to consider placing an inferior vena cava (IVC) filter using a venous catheter, to catch any clots that become dislodged.

A 19-year-old woman who uses the oral contraceptive pill presents to the Emergency Department with a swollen left calf. She has a past medical history of non-Hodgkin's lymphoma for which she received chemotherapy until 2 months ago. A Doppler ultrasound of her leg confirms occlusion of a proximal deep vein by a DVT. She is placed on LMWH and warfarin and admitted to hospital for observation in view of the proximal nature of her DVT (and thus higher risk of dislodging). That night, she suffers a thromboembolic stroke. What may have happened?

This patient is very young for thromboembolic strokes. It is possible that her blood is in a highly coagulable state due to underlying malignancy and that this has predisposed to clot formation, but even then it would be hard to explain a clot forming in the fast-flowing arteries that supply the brain. It is more likely that the clot has formed in the slow-flowing veins and somehow reached the arteries supplying the brain without getting lodged in the lungs. The most plausible anatomical explanation is that the patient has a patent foramen ovale between her atria which has allowed for the dislodged DVT to cross into the systemic circulation and reach her brain.

This is not as far-fetched as it may sound. Echocardiographic studies show that 10% of the population have a patent foramen ovale. About 35% of embolic strokes have no identifiable source and of these, 20% of patients have a patent foramen ovale, which is presumed to have allowed for the 'paradoxical embolus' to reach the brain.

When are D-dimer levels useful in suspected DVT or PE?

D-dimer is the breakdown product of fibrin and is therefore elevated in any inflammatory process, e.g. infection, cancer, thrombosis, trauma. It is very sensitive but non-specific and thus has a high negative predictive value (i.e. if negative, a venous thromboembolism (VTE) is unlikely, but not impossible). In the context of suspected DVT or PE it is **used together with the Wells score to help stratify patients as either low risk or high risk, which in turn guides their investigations**.

Single Best Answers

1. Which of the following statements is true regarding DVTs and D-dimers?

a. D-dimer is always elevated if there is a DVT
b. D-dimer is specific for DVT
c. Elevated D-dimer is diagnostic of DVT
d. Patients should be treated based upon D-dimer alone
e. D-dimer is useful for excluding DVT if the pre-test probability of DVT (Wells) is low (<2)

2. What is the target INR range in a patient with a proven DVT?

a. 1–2
b. 1.5–2.5
c. 2–3
d. 2.5–3.5
e. 3–4

3. What is the most common heritable thrombophilia?

a. Factor V Leiden
b. Prothrombin G20210A
c. Antithrombin III deficiency
d. Protein C deficiency
e. Protein S deficiency

4. Which pathogen is most commonly responsible for cellulitis?

a. *Staphylococcus aureus*
b. *Staphylococcus epidermidis*
c. *Streptococcus pyogenes*
d. *Pseudomonas aeruginosa*
e. *Clostridium perfringens*

5. A patient presents with a red, warm, swollen calf. They are in considerable pain, which appears disproportionate to the appearance of their calf. They have a high fever and appear very unwell. The patient reports that the area of redness has rapidly increased in size. On examination, blistering and dark purple patches have started to appear at the margins of the redness. Which diagnosis must you consider as a priority?

a. Cellulitis
b. Erysipelas
c. Necrotizing fasciitis
d. Gas gangrene
e. Herpes zoster

Leg ulcer

Core case

Read through the sections in the case boxes, covering up the sections that follow so that you don't see the answer. At the end of each case box, try to answer the question before reading on.

Mrs Swanson is a 72-year-old woman admitted to hospital overnight because of increasing confusion secondary to pneumonia. On the ward round the next morning, the nurse points out that Mrs Swanson also has an ulcer over her right ankle that will need investigating.

What is your differential diagnosis for a leg ulcer?

Figure 29.1 illustrates the differential diagnoses for a leg ulcer, with font size indicating prevalence.

Venous ulcer
Mixed arterial/venous ulcer
Arterial (atherosclerotic) ulcer
Pressure ulcer
Neuropathic ulcer
Lymphoedema ulcer
Traumatic ulcer
Malignant ulcer (e.g. a Marjolin ulcer: a squamous cell carcinoma in a long-standing ulcer)
Vasculitic ulcer (e.g. rheumatoid arthritis, pyoderma gangrenosum)
Infective ulcer (e.g. tuberculosis, syphilis, leprosy)
Haemolytic anaemia (sickle cell, hereditary spherocytosis)

Figure 29.1 Differential diagnosis for leg ulcers.

Venous ulcers account for by far the majority (about 70%), with mixed arterial/venous (about 10%) and arterial (about 10%) most of the remainder. Pressure ulcers have become increasingly common because of the increase in elderly, frail, and relatively immobile patients. The other causes are relatively rare with the exception of neuropathic ulcers in patients with diabetes mellitus.

Note that many leg ulcers may have a multifactorial aetiology, i.e. they may involve more than one of the pathologies listed in Figure 29.1.

What do you want to know about the history of the ulcer itself, and how would each of the main types differ?

The first thing is to ask about the ulcer. You should consider:

- **Is the ulcer painful?**
  - **Venous ulcers** are caused by venous stasis in the leg and are thus *less painful when elevated* and drained of blood. However, only about 30% of venous ulcers are painful.
  - **Arterial (atherosclerotic) ulcers** are caused by ischaemia to the leg and are thus *more painful when elevated* and drained of blood. Patients often say the ulcers are painful enough to wake them up at night and that they obtain relief by lowering their leg over the side of the bed.
  - **Neuropathic ulcers** are caused by loss of sensation (which predisposes to constant trauma) and are thus *not painful.*
  - **Pressure ulcers** are caused by, as the name suggests, prolonged pressure on the affected site. They tend to be exquisitely *tender* but not necessarily painful if no pressure is being applied.

- **How long has the ulcer been there?**
  - **Venous ulcers** are less painful and can therefore present late. They often have a long and recurring history.
  - **Arterial ulcers** tend to present relatively early because of pain. They often occur secondary to trivial trauma.
  - **Neuropathic ulcers** are associated with a loss of sensation and thus often present late.
  - **Pressure ulcers** can develop surprisingly rapidly (e.g. days in immobile patients if they are not turned regularly during their admission, even hours in patients who suffer a long lie following a fall), but can have a more indolent course depending on how much pressure is put on for how long. Thus the time course is not especially helpful.
  - A long history should arouse suspicion of a **Marjolin ulcer**, which only occurs in long-standing ulcers.

The pathologies causing ulcers are not limited to the ulcer but will be evident in other symptoms. These will vary depending on the pathology.

What other symptoms occur in the most common pathologies causing ulcers (and therefore which symptoms should you ask about)?

The associated symptoms you should ask about are:

- **Venous ulcers:** chronic venous insufficiency may lead to varicose veins and may also lead to pruritic stasis eczema, and discoloration of the surrounding skin (any of haemosiderin deposition, stasis dermatitis, or lipodermatosclerosis can occur). These same patients may develop ankle oedema (due to impaired venous return), leading to complaints of swollen ankles and a sensation of 'heavy feet'.

- **Arterial ulcers:** atherosclerosis is likely to be manifest systemically, thus ask about symptoms of peripheral arterial disease, and also coronary artery or cerebrovascular disease. These include claudication, night pain, rest pain (increased with limb elevation), cold extremities, angina or shortness of breath on exertion, and a history of stroke or transient ischaemic attack (TIA). It is unusual to develop arterial ulcers without a preceding history of severe claudication and night pain, thus asking patients how far they can walk without pain in their calves can be very informative.

- **Neuropathic ulcers:** these are associated with sensory loss, and patients may also have an unsteady gait. There is often secondary infection, and if this is by anaerobes the patient may comment on a foul smell.

> The probability of each type of ulcer is affected by the presence or absence of risk factors.
>
> **What risk factors should you ask about in the history?**

You should make a note of the following risk factors:

- **Venous ulcers** usually occur in patients with varicose veins, especially those who are immobile (reduced venous drainage of legs) and/or malnourished (reduced healing). They may also occur in patients with recurrent deep vein thrombosis (DVT), a pelvic mass (compressing the iliac veins), or arteriovenous malformations (increasing venous pressure). Major joint replacement (e.g. of a hip or knee) is also a risk factor, as up to about 25% of such operations are associated with subclinical DVTs.

- **Arterial ulcers** invariably occur in patients with risk factors for atherosclerosis (smoking, diabetes mellitus, hypertension, hyperlipidaemia, strong family history of atherosclerotic disease, male) and/ or evidence of other atherosclerotic disease: coronary artery disease (angina, myocardial infarction), cerebrovascular disease (TIA, stroke), peripheral arterial disease (claudication, impotence, abdominal aortic aneurysm (AAA)).

- **Neuropathic ulcers** mostly occur in patients with diabetes mellitus or alcohol overuse.

- **Pressure ulcers:** Pressure ulcers can develop within hours due to a part of the body being under constant pressure, causing ischaemia to the tissue. Patients who are bedridden due to frailty or sickness or who are immobilized (e.g. anaesthesia, intensive care, paramedic scoops) are at very high risk of developing pressure sores as they cannot move to relieve the pressure and discomfort. Poorly applied splints, braces, and plaster casts can also cause pressure ulcers.

The key points from the history, covering the most common ulcers, are summarized in Table 29.1.

Table 29.1 Key points in an ulcer history

	Venous	Arterial	Neuropathic	Pressure
About the ulcer	Moderately painful, better on elevation. Present relatively late as not overly painful	Severe pain, worse on elevation. Present early due to pain	Painless and therefore present late	May be tender but often not painful
Associated symptoms	Varicose veins, stasis eczema (itchy), heavy legs, swelling around ulcer	Claudication, night pain, rest pain, impotence, cold feet, angina	Loss of sensation in feet, contractures of feet	Immobility
Risk factors	Varicose veins, DVT/ pulmonary embolism, pelvic masses (compressing iliac veins), arteriovenous malformations, major joint replacement	Smoking, diabetes mellitus, hypertension, hypercholesterolaemia, angina, myocardial infarction, TIA, stroke, claudication, impotence, AAA	Diabetes mellitus, poor foot care	Nil specific, but consider bedridden patients, and use of splints, plaster casts, etc.

After 24 hours antibiotics for her pneumonia, Mrs Swanson's delirium improves and she is able to give you a history. She tells you that her ulcer is not really painful but that her legs often 'feel heavy' if she has been standing for a while. Her right ankle has been very itchy lately. She does not get pain in her calves when walking, but her mobility is limited by osteoarthrosis of her hips. She never gets chest pain or suffers from shortness of breath. Her past medical history is remarkable for bilateral hip osteoarthrosis, well-controlled hypertension, a presumed TIA 2 years ago, and chronic glaucoma in her right eye. She takes regular paracetamol and naproxen (with omeprazole to protect her stomach) for her hip pain, timolol and latanoprost for her glaucoma, and aspirin, simvastatin, and ramipril because of her hypertension and previous TIA. She smoked a packet of cigarettes every day from her twenties until her fifties. She has lived at home alone since the death of her husband 2 years ago.

What will you look for on examination?

Think of what features might distinguish the most common types of leg ulcers. Also think about other signs associated with the underlying pathology that you can look for.

- **Site of the ulcer** (see Figure 29.2):
  - **Venous ulcers** occur where venous pressures are highest, which is the gaiter area of the legs (i.e. the area covered by a long sock). The most commonly affected area is just above the medial malleolus because this is the site of the medial calf perforators.
  - **Arterial ulcers** occur where arterial blood supply is worst, which tends to be the distal areas of the foot (e.g. between toes) and those that are frequently compressed (e.g. ball of foot, lateral malleolus, and bony prominences).
  - **Neuropathic ulcers** are caused by repetitive trauma in a foot that has lost sensation, and thus occur in pressure areas where the foot rubs on poorly fitting footwear (e.g. beneath the metatarsal heads).
  - **Pressure ulcers** are caused by constant pressure and are therefore usually found on bony prominences such as the heel or overlying the malleoli in immobile, bedridden patients (and other pressure points typically not on the legs, e.g. sacrum).

Figure 29.2 Typical locations of venous, arterial, neuropathic, and pressure ulcers.

- **Characteristics of the ulcer:**
  - **Venous ulcers:** shallow, wet, and with irregular borders that look white and fragile
  - **Arterial ulcers:** deep, punched-out, dry, and often elliptical
  - **Neuropathic ulcers** and **pressure ulcers** often have very thick, keratinized, raised edges surrounding them (this thickened skin is referred to as callus)
  - **Pyoderma gangrenosum** (a type of ulcer associated with inflammatory bowel disease or haematological malignancies) often has a characteristic dark blue/purple halo around it.

- **Associated signs:**
  - **Venous ulcers** are due to increased hydrostatic (venous) pressure, which can also cause oedema, extravasation, and death of erythrocytes (skin pigmentation from haemosiderin staining) and eventually scarring of the skin ('atrophie blanche') and underlying tissue ('lipodermatosclerosis'). Superficial varicose veins or a collection of small, dark, engorged superficial veins ('ankle flare') may be visible. In extreme cases, severe lipodermatosclerosis may lead to an 'inverted champagne bottle' appearance to the leg.
  - **Arterial ulcers** are due to limb ischaemia and are therefore associated with cold, pale limbs with poor capillary refill, venous guttering, absent or weak pulses, and atrophic skin changes (dry, shiny, hairless). Buerger's test may reveal blanching of the foot on elevation to 45° and reactive hyperaemia on lowering the leg, suggesting arterial insufficiency. They usually occur in patients with widespread atherosclerotic disease. Thus, ensure that you palpate and document the presence or absence of all lower limb pulses, utilizing a handheld Doppler if pulses are not palpable and calculating the ankle-brachial pressure index accordingly. You should also specifically check for popliteal and abdominal aortic aneurysms.
  - **Neuropathic ulcers** are due to loss of sensation. Typically, vibration and proprioception are lost before other modalities. In the majority of these patients you will encounter a 'glove and stocking' distribution of peripheral sensory neuropathy. Foot deformities may be present due to motor neuropathy or repetitive joint trauma secondary to sensory neuropathy (Charcot joints).
  - **Pressure ulcers** are due to immobility and constant pressure. If you find one on the legs, you should look at other pressure areas such as the sacrum and buttocks.
  - **Inguinal lymphadenopathy:** check for this if you suspect infection or malignancy as the cause of the ulcer.

Ulcer examination is summarized in Table 29.2.

Table 29.2 Summary of ulcer examination

	Venous	Arterial	Neuropathic	Pressure
Site	Gaiter area (especially medial)	Ball of foot, between toes, tips of toes, lateral malleolus	Pressure areas of foot	Heel, malleoli
Ulcer characteristics	Irregular, sloping, white edges	Well-defined, deep, punched-out edges	Raised callous edges	Raised callous edges
Associated signs	Oedema, stasis eczema, skin pigmentation, lipodermatosclerosis, ankle flare, atrophie blanche	Cold, hairless, dry-skinned limb with weak or absent pulses. Poor capillary refill. Venous guttering. Buerger's positive test. Carotid bruits. Abdominal aortic and/or popliteal aneurysms	Decreased sensation (especially vibration), contractures of foot	Immobile patient, pressure ulcers on sacrum or buttocks

Mrs Swanson has a single 5 × 5 cm ulcer just above the medial malleolus of her right leg. The ulcer looks wet, has fragile-looking irregular borders, and the surrounding skin is deeply pigmented. Her feet (and hands) feel slightly cold but dorsalis pedis and posterior tibial pulses are palpable in both feet. Her capillary refill time is 2 seconds in both feet. The rest of her cardiovascular exam is normal. Sensation is intact in both of her legs.

What is the most likely diagnosis? What first-line investigations will you arrange?

Mrs Swanson is an elderly woman with limited mobility who has a wet, irregular ulcer on the medial aspect of her right leg (gaiter area). Sensation is intact. There is surrounding skin pigmentation and no suggestion of arterial insufficiency on examination. The most likely diagnosis is a **venous ulcer**. Nonetheless, you should arrange the following investigations in case there is coexisting arterial disease, diabetes mellitus, or infection, as these will influence your management:

- **Bloods:** full blood count (FBC, for anaemia exacerbating any ischaemia and contributing to delayed healing), fasting lipids (for hyperlipidaemia, contributing to any atherosclerosis). In Mrs Swanson's case inflammatory markers will be unhelpful as her underlying pneumonia will cause these to be deranged. Similarly, her albumin will fall due to the pneumonia and intravenous fluids she is given, so will not be helpful as a marker of nutritional status in the acute setting.

- **Capillary glucose:** a quick and reliable way of assessing whether Mrs Swanson has undiagnosed diabetes mellitus. Remember that up to 50% of type 2 diabetes mellitus is undiagnosed.

- **Urinalysis:** looking for glucose (diabetes mellitus affecting healing). It is not applicable in this specific case, but if vasculitis is considered you should look for haematuria/proteinuria on urinalysis.

- **Venous duplex ultrasound:** this is the gold standard investigation to assess the competence of the saphenofemoral and saphenopopliteal junctions, and state of the perforators and deep venous system.

- **Ankle–brachial pressure index (ABPI):**[†] measured to exclude arterial disease as the cause. It is measured using a manual sphygmomanometer and portable Doppler probe (for dorsalis pedis and posterior tibial pressure). The ABPI is the ratio of the ankle systolic pressure (the best of either dorsalis pedis or posterior tibial) over the brachial artery systolic pressure. Even if you are clinically convinced that an ulcer is venous, it is important to measure the ABPI because if the ABPI is <0.8, the patient must *not* have a pressure bandage applied as this suggests the ulcer is actually a mixed venous/arterial ulcer and compression will make the arterial ischaemia worse. If the ABPI is <0.5, or there has been a sudden change, the patient needs urgent referral to a vascular surgeon. (In reality, you could be excused for not performing ABPIs in Mrs Swanson's case as she has palpable pedal pulses and thus will almost certainly have ABPIs >0.8.)

- **Swabbing** an ulcer for microscopy, culture, and sensitivities (MC&S) is not routinely performed as all ulcers will have some growth. Swabbing may, however, be useful in the case of spreading cellulitis.

- **Biopsy?** There is no routine role for tissue biopsy in the majority of cases, unless you expect an unusual aetiology such as Marjolin's ulcer.

---

† Beware: patients with diabetes mellitus or chronic renal failure can have calcified (hard) arteries that give falsely high ABPI readings even in the presence of significant limb ischaemia. Oedema may also result in erroneous readings.

Mrs Swanson's admission blood results show leucocytosis and a raised C-reactive protein (CRP), as expected in a patient with pneumonia. An ABPI is not performed as she has palpable pedal pulses.

How should Mrs Swanson's ulcer be managed?

Mrs Swanson almost certainly has a **venous ulcer**. This is the result of prolonged venous stasis in her lower limb, and thus management involves:

- **Adequate nutrition,** vital for any healing process but especially relevant for venous ulcers as they tend to occur in elderly patients who may be malnourished or deficient in key vitamins and minerals (e.g. vitamin C, zinc).
- **Lifestyle modification:** encourage patients to mobilize (to encourage venous blood flow in the legs). Obese patients should be encouraged to lose weight in the longer term.
- **Leg elevation** whenever possible, to reduce venous stasis in the lower limb.
- **Compression bandages** applied and frequently changed by an experienced nurse, to reduce the pooling of venous blood in the lower limb. This can be done safely if her ABPI is >0.8.
- **Graduated class I or II elastic stockings** will be helpful once the venous ulcer has healed to prevent recurrence.
- **Varicose vein surgery** may also be helpful in preventing recurrence if there is venous duplex evidence of an incompetence superficial venous system and there is no deep vein incompetence (see Viva question).

With this management, about 80% of venous ulcers will heal within 6 months. Note the time course involved—it is very important to give patients realistic expectations of how long they are likely to require dressings. Those that fail to heal in this way may be candidates for split skin grafting by the plastic or vascular surgeons, although success rates are not fantastic in these patients.

Short cases

Mr Griffin is a 58-year-old man who presents to his GP because of an ulcer on his left foot which has been present for 2 weeks. The ulcer causes him constant 'sharp pain' that is worse at night unless he sleeps with his foot dangling over the edge of the bed. Mr Griffin gets a stabbing pain in both calves if he walks too fast, but denies any chest pain, shortness of breath, or impotence. He also denies any itch, heaviness, or loss of sensation in his legs. He does not recall any trauma that could have caused the ulcer. His past medical history is remarkable for type 2 diabetes mellitus. He takes metformin, gliclazide, aspirin, simvastatin, and ramipril. He has smoked two packets of cigarettes a day for most of his adult life. His family history is unremarkable.

On examination, a well-demarcated, deep, dry ulcer is found over the ball of his left foot. His legs are pale, smooth, and hairless. Both feet are cold and have a capillary refill time of 5 seconds. On the right, dorsalis pedis is palpable but the posterior tibial pulse is not. On the left, neither pulse is palpable. Buerger's test is positive on both legs. The ABPI is 0.45 on the left and 0.65 on the right. Sensation in his lower limb is normal for all modalities. Examination of the rest of his cardiovascular system is unremarkable. His heart rate is 85 bpm (regular) and his blood pressure is 128/76 mmHg.

What is the diagnosis of Mr Griffin's ulcer? How should it be managed?

Mr Griffin has significant risk factors for atherosclerosis (lifelong smoker, diabetes mellitus) and a history of claudication on exercise. He has a well-demarcated, deep, dry ulcer on his left foot. His feet have poor capillary refill, weak or impalpable pulses, a positive Buerger's test, and an ABPI <0.8. This all suggests that Mr Griffin has an **arterial (atherosclerotic, ischaemic) ulcer** on his left lower limb. Furthermore, Mr Griffin has **critical limb ischaemia**—he has rest pain, tissue loss (the ulcer), and an ABPI <0.5 in the left leg—and therefore needs urgent referral to a vascular surgeon.

Management should involve:

- **Investigations:** remember that atherosclerosis is a systemic disease.

    - Arterial **duplex ultrasonography of his lower limbs** (or magnetic resonance angiography if his vessels are highly calcified) to assess the patency of the arteries and potential for revascularization or bypass surgery. Alternatively, **percutaneous angiography** can be performed to allow for assessment and treatment (angioplasty) to be done all in one. Note that Mr Griffin is taking metformin: many interventional radiologists will advise that this is withheld for 48 hours prior to contrast angiography (particularly in the setting of a raised creatinine) because of the risk of lactic acidosis. In some centres, prehydration, *N*-acetyl cysteine (orally), and/or sodium bicarbonate (IV) are given before and after a significant contrast load, particularly in patients with renal impairment.
    - **Electrocardiogram (ECG)**
    - **Fasting serum lipids, fasting glucose, and HbA1c levels,** to see if Mr Griffin's lipid and glucose control are adequate
    - **FBC**, as anaemia will exacerbate any ischaemia.
- **Interim management:**
    - **Dressing of the ulcer** to prevent infection, but take care to avoid the bandage being tight as this will worsen the ischaemia. It should also be pointed out that under no circumstances should

such a patient be prescribed compression stockings such as those used to prevent deep vein thrombosis.

- **Analgesia**
- **Antibiotics:** only if there are any signs of infection.

- Surgical intervention:
  - **Angioplasty ± stenting** can be performed if an artery is stenotic or there is a short occlusion and there is a patent artery downstream of the occlusion.
  - **Bypass surgery** using a venous graft or artificial conduit can be performed if angioplasty is not possible (but again requires distal run-off).
  - **Amputation**. If there is no suitable target for angioplasty, and insufficient distal run-off onto which the vascular surgeons can anastomose a bypass graft, then some patients with intractable pain and ulceration will be offered an amputation.

SHORT CASE

Mr Griffin is admitted to hospital and has an arterial duplex scan that shows moderate stenosis of both the left and right external iliac arteries and severe stenosis (about 80%) of the left superficial femoral artery. He is placed on the waiting list for angioplasty and stenting. On the second night of Mr Griffin's admission the nursing staff bleep the duty junior doctor and ask her to come and see Mr Griffin. He states that he was awoken 2 hours ago because the pain from the ulcer in his left foot had suddenly spread to affect his entire left leg below his knee. He describes the pain as sharp and 8/10 in severity, with a tingling sensation confined to the foot.

On examination, Mr Griffin's left leg is significantly colder than the right. Both legs have typical Anglo-Saxon pallor but the sole of his left foot is ghostly white compared to his right. His popliteal pulse, dorsalis pedis, and posterior tibial are all impalpable on the left. On the right, dorsalis pedis is palpable but the posterior tibial pulse is not (as per his GP's findings). Sensation is diminished over the left foot.

What has happened to Mr Griffin? What is your next step?

Mr Griffin is a patient with known atherosclerotic disease of both lower limbs who has presented with the cardinal features of **acute limb ischaemia** which can be remembered as the six Ps: a painful, pale, pulseless, paralysed, perishingly cold leg with paraesthesia. Note that not all 6 Ps have to be present (paraesthesia and paralysis are later signs). This is likely to represent either thrombosis at the site of known stenosis or embolism.

Acute limb ischaemia is a **surgical emergency** that requires urgent intervention by the vascular surgeons to avoid losing the limb from irreversible ischaemic necrosis. For this reason, the next step should be to discuss Mr Griffin with the vascular surgeon on call *immediately*. The vascular surgeons will then decide whether to heparinize Mr Griffin and whether to attempt an embolectomy, percutaneous thrombolysis, revascularization angioplasty, bypass surgery, or amputation of the affected limb.

SHORT CASE

Mr Cleveland is a 52-year-old man who has attended his local Endocrinology Department for a routine follow-up of his type 1 diabetes. During the consultation, Mr Cleveland points out that he has developed a painless ulcer on his right foot and his community nurse has urged him to get it checked. After removing the bandage for inspection, there is a small ulcer over the lateral aspect of the fifth metatarsophalangeal joint. The ulcer has surrounding callus and is deep. After removing some pus, it is obvious that the ulcer extends down to the bone. Mr Cleveland's feet are warm and well perfused. All pulses are palpable in Mr Cleveland's lower limbs and there is no eczema, varicose veins, or lipodermatosclerosis. However, Mr Cleveland has, for several years now, had diminished sensation to vibration in both feet. The registrar confirms that this is still the case, and that Mr Cleveland is now starting to lose his proprioception in both feet as well.

What is the likely cause of Mr Cleveland's ulcer? How should the ulcer be managed? What complication should you be concerned about?

Mr Cleveland is a patient with known diabetes mellitus who has presented with an ulcer on his foot. Diabetes mellitus increases one's risk of arterial (atherosclerotic) ulcer. However, this ulcer is directly over a pressure site (where shoes often rub), has surrounding callus, and is painless. Mr Cleveland has signs of peripheral neuropathy in both feet, whereas there are no signs of arterial disease. This is therefore a **neuropathic ulcer**.

Neuropathic ulcers in diabetics are due to repeated trauma and pressure plus a reduced ability to heal skin breaks and fight infection. For this reason, treatment involves:

- **Foot care:** avoid tight-fitting shoes until the ulcer is healed. Always wear soft, comfortable shoes thereafter and examine the feet daily. All such patients should have appropriately fitting shoes made by the orthotics team and should have regular podiatry review.
- **Manage diabetes:** make sure diabetic control is optimized, as uncontrolled hyperglycaemia will hinder ulcer repair and fighting infections.
- **Debridement:** ulcers in diabetics tend to build up necrotic tissue. This needs debriding either using special bandages (e.g. hydrogel sheets) or surgically.
- **Treat infections:** if there are clinical signs of infection.

The major complication to worry about in diabetic foot ulcers is infection. Given that Mr Cleveland's ulcer extends down to the bone you need to exclude **osteomyelitis**. In practice, a plain film of the foot is the first investigation as it can be done quickly and will show any bony deformity, gas in the soft tissues, and signs of osteomyelitis (e.g. osteolysis = reduced opacity, periosteal reaction = formation of new bone from the cortex outwards). If the plain film is inconclusive an MRI scan is far more sensitive for osteomyelitis. Many hospitals will have dedicated 'diabetic foot clinics', consisting of endocrinologists, vascular surgeons, orthopaedic surgeons, podiatrists, and orthotics technicians, and Mr Cleveland is likely to require such a multidisciplinary approach. Ultimately he is likely to require surgical debridement and/or amputation.

SHORT CASE

Mrs Glenn is an 82-year-old woman who has been referred to the surgeons at her local hospital because of a large ulcer on her right shin. Mrs Glenn lives in a nursing home because she has advanced Alzheimer's dementia. Her GP referral letter states that Mrs Glenn has had a long-standing venous ulcer (flat, wet, with irregular borders), on her right shin for the past 3 years. Management has been attempted with alginate-based compression dressings changed regularly by the nursing home staff, but the GP has noticed that the ulcer has recently changed: its central area has become raised and indurated, the ulcer smells far worse than usual, and its borders have spread and become raised.

On inspection, there is a large fungating ulcer on the right shin, surrounded by an area of lipodermatosclerosis and skin pigmentation.

What has most likely happened to Mrs Glenn's ulcer? How should it be investigated? What is the prognosis?

Mrs Glenn has had a long-standing venous ulcer over her right pretibial region, as suggested by the lipodermatosclerosis, the skin pigmentation, and the GP's letter. The ulcer is now fungating, suggesting malignancy or infection. It is likely that Mrs Glenn's chronic venous ulcer has transformed into a squamous cell carcinoma—also known as a **Marjolin ulcer**.

Investigation involves biopsies of the *peripheral* area of the ulcer in order to obtain histological confirmation (as the central area is likely to contain necrotic tissue which is hard to visualize for a histological diagnosis).

Management of a Marjolin ulcer is by wide excision and split skin grafting, but the prognosis is poor and she may not be a candidate for surgery given her age and advanced, irreversible dementia.

SHORT CASE

Miss Takenawa is a 32-year-old woman who has been admitted to hospital for intravenous corticosteroid therapy for a particularly bad flare-up of her ulcerative colitis. During a teaching ward round, a medical student notices that Miss Takenawa has a small ulcer over the lateral aspect of her right leg. Miss Takenawa states that she was bitten by a midge several weeks ago while hiking in Scotland and assumes the ulcer has arisen because of the high-dose steroids she is currently receiving. The ulcer has a purplish halo at its border. She says it has been painful although it is now improving.

What type of ulcer has Miss Takenawa developed? How should it be managed?

Miss Takenawa is a patient with known ulcerative colitis who has developed an ulcer on her leg that has a purple halo around it. In the absence of any other obvious cause for her ulcer this is consistent with **pyoderma gangrenosum**, a complication of systemic inflammatory diseases (e.g. Crohn's disease, ulcerative colitis, rheumatoid arthritis) or haematological malignancies.

Management of pyoderma gangrenosum is with good nursing care (bandages to prevent infection and promote healing) and treatment of the underlying disease. As Miss Takenawa is already on intravenous corticosteroids, it is likely that the ulcer will improve as her ulcerative colitis settles.

SHORT CASE

Mrs Lowenbrau is a frail 81-year-old woman with vascular dementia who lives with her husband. She has carers who come in four times a day and for the past few weeks she has largely become confined to her bed due to increasing frailty and poor mobility. Her carers have noticed that she has become more sleepy and more confused than usual and she has been sent to her local Emergency Department for assessment. The triage nurses, as part of their routine checks for elderly patients, notice that Mrs Lowenbrau has an area of ulcerated skin on the heel of her right foot and an area of bruising on the heel of her left foot. She also has an area of ulceration on her sacrum. Her feet are both somewhat cold and pale, but dorsalis pedis is palpable bilaterally and she appears to have grossly intact sensation and no pain. She is not diabetic. Ultimately, Mrs Lowenbrau is found to be dehydrated and suffering from a urinary tract infection. She is admitted under the care of the elderly care physicians.

What type of ulcers does Mrs Lowenbrau have? How should they be managed?

Mrs Lowenbrau is a frail elderly patient who spends most of her day in bed or in a recliner chair. She has ulcers on areas of her body that are under constant pressure most of her day: the sacrum and the heels of her feet. It is most likely that she has **pressure ulcers**, caused by ischaemia to the delicate tissues from the constant pressure. More mobile patients don't get these ulcers because they will (usually subconsciously, and even when asleep) move every time a part of their body starts getting uncomfortable due to constant pressure. Patients who can't move can develop pressure ulcers within an hour, so beware of patients who are immobile due to anaesthesia, sedated on intensive care, immobilized after trauma, or too frail to move.

Management of pressure ulcers involves:

- **Record the ulcer:** grade the ulcer using the European Pressure Ulcer Advisory Panel classification (quite a mouthful!) from 1 to 4 in severity (see Viva questions), measuring its dimensions, documenting its location and asking medical photography to take photographs of the ulcer. This information may seem tedious but is the only way of assessing for improvement or deterioration in the ulcer reliably because although these ulcers form very rapidly, they heal (or deteriorate further) more slowly and it can be hard to notice any change over time.

- **Relieve the ulcer:** dress the ulcer using a soft, moist, padded, modern ulcer dressing (e.g. hydrocolloid, hydrogel, foam). Provide the patient with a pressure relieving mattress, ensure the patient is moved regularly if they cannot do so themselves and consider limiting the amount of time they spend sitting in chairs to <2 hours at a time. Involve physiotherapy and occupational therapy to maximize the patient's mobility.

- **Reduce further ulcers:** optimize patient nutrition and educate carers and family members.

- **Reassess the ulcer:** this should be done regularly and using objective parameters such as those described earlier.

- **Involve the tissue viability team:** these specialist nurses are experts at wound care and can advise on specific dressings and further management (such as when to refer for surgical debridement).

Viva questions

What are the indications for surgery of varicose veins?

Patients with any of the following should be considered for surgery of their varicose veins under the UK National Health Service (NHS):

- Symptomatic primary or symptomatic recurrent varicose veins
- Venous leg ulcers that have not healed within 2 weeks
- Lower limb skin changes (pigmentation, lipodermatosclerosis)
- Superficial vein thrombosis with venous incompetence
- Healed venous leg ulcers

The above criteria are based on the current (2013) NICE guidelines. As one can see, cosmetic reasons alone do not qualify for surgery under the NHS. These guidelines represent quite a departure from previous guidelines, which suggested that most patients underwent a trial of compression hosiery. The new guidelines suggest that patients in the above categories who have confirmed varicose veins and truncal reflux on venous duplex should be offered endothermal ablation (or foam sclerotherapy if unsuitable) and should only be offered compression hosiery if interventional treatment is unsuitable.

NICE guidelines recommend prophylactic surgery of varicose veins to prevent recurrence of healed venous ulcers. Is there any evidence that surgery for varicose veins can reduce the recurrence of venous ulcers?

The ESCHAR trial[†] compared the long-term outcomes for patients with venous ulcers who were managed either with compression bandages alone or compression bandages plus surgery for any superficial varicose veins. The trial found that surgery did not accelerate ulcer healing times but almost halved the rate of recurrence at 4 years. The trial therefore suggests that it is better to surgically treat *superficial* varicose veins in patients who have had a venous ulcer as soon as possible, rather than waiting for a recurrent and unresolving ulcer to develop. The same benefit has not yet been found for *deep* venous disease.

[†] Gohel MS, Barwell JR, Taylor M, Chant T, Foy C, Earnshaw JJ *et al.* Long term results of compression therapy alone versus compression plus surgery in chronic venous ulceration (ESCHAR): randomised controlled trial. *BMJ*, 2007;**335**: 83.

What surgical options are there for treating varicose veins?

- **Avulsion/phlebectomy:** small incisions are made along the varicose vein and it is then pulled out with forceps.
- **Stripping:** small incisions are made at the ends of the varicose vein and an endoluminal hook and wire is used to pull the vein out.

CONTINUED ➤

CONTINUED

- **Injection sclerotherapy:** this involves sealing the vein from within by injecting an irritant sclero-sant. Unfortunately, the procedure is associated with skin discoloration in about 10% of patients and a 30% risk of recurrence if there is valvular incompetence, and is thus being used less often. A variant of injection sclerotherapy involves injecting a foam that blocks the vein, but there is a (very small) risk of the foam embolizing into the venous system.
- **Radiofrequency ablation:** an endoluminal catheter is inserted into the long saphenous or short saphenous vein and a tip used to deliver high-energy radio waves (VNUS) that seal the vein from within. A similar procedure involves using a laser (EVLT) rather than radio waves to achieve the same effect.

What are the risks of percutaneous angioplasty for arterial ischaemic limb disease?

Whenever you are asked about risks, try to have a structure to help you answer the question:

General risks (common to any procedure)

- Infection of puncture site
- Haemorrhage from puncture site
- Haematoma
- Reaction to the sedative used during the procedure

Specific risks (particular to this procedure)

- Thrombosis or embolization, potentially leading to loss of the limb
- Perforation of the artery, requiring further surgical intervention
- Aneurysm or pseudoaneurysm of the artery at the site of dilatation and stenting or at the puncture site
- Reaction to the contrast dye used in the angiography.

What are the main types of dressings for ulcers?

- **Low-adherence dressings:** useful only if there is little exudate that needs soaking up because they have little adherence, but they can often be left in place for 7 days.
- **Hydrogel dressings:** as the name implies, they are useful for *hydrating* dry ulcers (e.g. arterial) and for encouraging debridement of dead tissue (e.g. diabetic neuropathic ulcers).
- **Hydrocolloid dressings:** these contain a gel that covers the ulcer and keeps it moist and protected. They are useful to cover pressure ulcers.
- **Foam dressings:** useful for covering pressure ulcers in areas that are likely to have ongoing pressure (e.g. the heels).
- **Alginate dressings:** like the dry algae they are based on, they mop up water and are thus useful for wet ulcers (e.g. venous ulcers, fungating ulcers) that need drying.
- **Antibacterial dressings:** these prevent growth of bacteria by incorporating silver, honey, iodine, or metronidazole.

What is meant by a grade 4 pressure ulcer?

This grading system is advocated by the European Pressure Ulcer Advisory Panel (EPUAP). There are four grades*:

1 Non-blanching erythema of intact skin

2 Partial thickness skin loss or blistering

3 Full-thickness skin loss. Subcutaneous fat may be visible, but not underlying tendon, bone, muscle, etc.

4 Full-thickness tissue loss with involvement of bone/muscle/tendon. May be covered with thick slough or eschar.

* Adapted from European Pressure Ulcer Advisory Panel and National Pressure Ulcer Advisory Panel. Prevention and treatment of pressure ulcers: quick reference guide. Washington, DC: National Pressure Ulcer Advisory Panel; 2009, with permission. Available online at <http://www.epuap.org/guidelines/Final_Quick_Prevention.pdf>

Single Best Answers

1. **An elderly woman is seen at home by a health visitor who notes an ulcer on the patient's shin. The ulcer is foul-smelling and appears overgrown, with everted edges. The surrounding skin is scarred and shows features of long-standing venous insufficiency. The patient admits that the ulcer has been present 'for some years'. What is the most likely diagnosis?**

   a. Venous ulcer
   b. Arterial ulcer
   c. Pyoderma gangrenosum
   d. Basal cell carcinoma
   e. Squamous cell carcinoma

2. **Which of the following is not a feature of venous insufficiency?**

   a. Venous guttering
   b. Lipodermatosclerosis
   c. Haemosiderin staining
   d. Atrophie blanche
   e. Venous eczema

3. **A diabetic patient presents with a small ulcer on the dorsum of their foot. The ulcer is punctate and surrounded by pale atrophic skin. There are no other skin changes in the leg. Foot pulses are impalpable. What is the most likely diagnosis?**

   a. Venous ulcer
   b. Neuropathic ulcer
   c. Arterial ulcer
   d. Mixed arterial/venous ulcer
   e. Pyoderma gangrenosum

4. **What is the most important factor for the healing of chronic venous ulcers?**

   a. Skin grafting
   b. Antibiotics
   c. Endovascular intervention
   d. Compression
   e. Optimal glycaemic control

5. **Which of the following factors can impair ulcer healing?**

   a. Diabetes mellitus
   b. Anaemia
   c. Smoking
   d. Malnutrition
   e. All of the above

Appendix

Single Best Answer questions: answers and feedback

Chapter 1: Headache

1 **a. Feedback:** Raised intracranial pressure, meningitis, and subdural haematoma are all potentially acutely life-threatening. Sinusitis can be serious but is not acutely life-threatening.

2 **a. Feedback:** NICE guidance is very clear on this: paracetamol, NSAIDs, opioids, and oral triptans are not indicated. Verapamil is only indicated for prophylaxis and will not help acutely. Oxygen should be administered through a non-rebreathe bag at a rate of at least 12 L/min.

3 **b. Feedback:** The second nerve is the optic nerve; the third, fourth, and sixth nerves control eye movements. A fourth nerve palsy results in torsional and downgaze diplopia, causing patients to tilt their head. A sixth nerve palsy causes a failure of abduction in the affected eye. Neither cause ptosis. In Horner's syndrome, damage to the sympathetic supply to the eye causes unilateral partial ptosis, miosis, and anhydrosis. It is easily confused with a third nerve palsy, but in the latter the pupil is dilated (mydriasis) and the ptosis is complete.

4 **e. Feedback:** All of these conditions can cause a ring-enhancing lesion on CT, although it is most classically seen in tumours, abscesses, and toxoplasmosis (less so in multiple sclerosis).

5 **d. Feedback:** In T2-weighted MRI, fluid and fluid-filled tissues appear brightest (H_2O is bright in T2). This is not the case for either CT without contrast or T1-weighted MRI. When contrast is used with CT, it is injected intravenously and thus blood appears bright, but the ventricles do not as they are filled with cerebrospinal fluid (except in the case of haemorrhage).

Chapter 2: Confusion

1 **e. Feedback:** There are many possible causes of confusion, including all of those listed. You need to start with a wide screen when approaching patients with confusion.

2 **b. Feedback:** Broca's and Wernicke's areas are found in the dominant hemisphere (left in 99% of right-handers and 95% of left-handers), with Broca's area in the frontal lobe and Wernicke's in the temporoparietal area. Damage to Wernicke's area leads to receptive dysphasia, whereas damage to Broca's area leads to an expressive dysphasia. Brodmann numbered all the different parts of the brain, thus there is no single 'Brodmann's area' but Brodmann areas 1, 2, 3, etc.

3 **c. Feedback:** Opiates are the only drugs listed in the options that give you pinpoint pupils (organophosphates, found in agricultural products, are another common toxin that can do this). The remainder all cause dilated pupils.

4 **e. Feedback:** Haloperidol and lorazepam are occasionally used to sedate patients with acute behavioural disturbance, but these should be a last resort. Chlordiazepoxide is a long-acting benzodiazepine used in diminishing doses to help wean the patient off alcohol and prevent symptoms of alcohol withdrawal. Rehydrating the patient with saline is often necessary in alcoholics, but the only drug listed that prevents Wernicke–Korsakoff syndrome is thiamine.

5 **c. Feedback:** This patient is most likely to be dehydrated and to have lost sodium as a result of her diarrhoea. Thus you would expect her to have a hypovolaemic hyponatraemia.

Chapter 3: Blackout

1 **c. Feedback:** Strokes cause a variety of symptoms but not typically a loss of consciousness (although this may occur if the patient subsequently falls and hits their head, for example, or with brainstem strokes). ACE inhibitors, like all antihypertensives, can cause postural hypotension with cerebral hypoperfusion on standing. Heart block, like other arrhythmias, can also result in a brief spell of cerebral hypoperfusion and loss of consciousness.

2 **d. Feedback:** Although metformin is used as an oral antidiabetic agent, one of its principal benefits is that it does not cause hypoglycaemia (unlike other antidiabetic agents). Ramipril is an ACE inhibitor and blood pressure-lowering agent that can cause hypotension and subsequent loss of consciousness.

3 **c. Feedback:** This is an extradural haematoma, with the characteristic history of trauma followed by a lucid interval then a loss of consciousness, and the convex shape on CT. Damage to the middle meningeal artery results in the build-up of blood between the skull and the dura and increasing intracranial pressure ultimately leading to loss of consciousness. Death can follow if surgery is not undertaken promptly.

4 **d. Feedback:** Congenital bicuspid valves are a more common cause amongst younger patients as calcification takes a long time. Rheumatic fever is thankfully very rare in the UK but may be a more common cause abroad. Infective endocarditis typically causes valve damage and regurgitation rather than stenosis. Connective tissue disorders can also cause aortic regurgitation but not stenosis.

5 **a. Feedback:** Brugada syndrome is one of several (rare) syndromes associated with sudden cardiac death. Dressler's syndrome describes pericarditis occurring 2 or more weeks after an acute myocardial infarction. Eisenmenger syndrome is heart failure with a right-to-left shunt secondary to high right-sided pressures. It is usually due to a congenital cardiac abnormality that leads to high pulmonary pressures and, over time, obliterative pulmonary vascular disease and pulmonary hypertension. Leriche's syndrome is a triad of impotence, leg atrophy, and bilateral buttock and thigh claudication due to aortoiliac occlusive disease. In Wolff–Parkinson–White syndrome an accessory conducting pathway between the atria and ventricles results in episodes of supraventricular tachycardia.

Chapter 4: Neck lump

1 **d. Feedback:** The goitre is the only midline lump; the others would all be found on the side of the neck.

2 **e. Feedback:** All of these symptoms are highly relevant as they can indicate head and neck cancer, which is your must-exclude diagnosis in a patient this age with a rapidly growing lump.

3 **d. Feedback:** Given you believe this to be a parotid mass, you must check for the integrity of the facial nerve. A facial nerve palsy is highly suggestive of an invasive and therefore malignant parotid tumour.

4 **b. Feedback:** Carbimazole causes agranulocytosis in ~0.5% of patients, thus it is extremely important to warn patients to watch out for any sign of infection. Full blood count (FBC) monitoring is less helpful as agranulocytosis can occur rapidly.

5 **a. Feedback:** There are only four types of thyroid cancer, in order of incidence: papillary, follicular, medullary, and anaplastic.

Chapter 5: Haematemesis

1 **c. Feedback:** The Rockall score is a prognostic score used in upper gastrointestinal bleeds to determine the risk of rebleeding and death. It is broken into an initial and final score. The initial score is calculated pre-endoscopy and based on age, shock (pulse and blood pressure), and the presence of certain comorbidities. The final score additionally incorporates findings on endoscopy. Although alcohol history is relevant in the context of upper gastrointestinal bleeds, it does not form part of the Rockall score.

2 **b. Feedback:** β-Blockers blunt the body's ability to mount a tachycardia in the face of low blood pressure, and can therefore mask the signs of shock. Coagulopathies, peptic ulcers, and cirrhosis are all relevant in the context of haematemesis, but none are recognized side effects of β-blockers.

3 **a. Feedback:** Spider naevi refill from the centre, are found in the distribution of the superior vena cava (SVC), and in small numbers (e.g. <5) can be normal.

4 **d. Feedback:** Factors II, VII, IX, and X are made by the liver. These are also the vitamin K dependent factors, and therefore those depleted by warfarin therapy. Note that synthesis of the anticoagulant factors protein C, protein S, and protein Z are also dependent on vitamin K. When patients are started on warfarin, levels of anticoagulant proteins C, S, and Z drop before those of the procoagulant factors II, VII, IX, and X, so the patient goes through a brief phase of being in a procoagulant phase. It is for this reason that patients started on warfarin to prevent clots are frequently covered with low molecular weight heparin until INR testing confirms the blood is in an anticoagulant state.

5 **d. Feedback:** Chronic alcohol abuse alone can cause a macrocytic anaemia by an unknown mechanism (potentially a direct toxic effect on the bone marrow). Alcoholics are also more likely to be malnourished; a vitamin B_{12} or folate deficiency would cause a macrocytic anaemia, but an iron deficiency would cause a microcytic anaemia, so together these could cause a mixed picture. Alcoholics are also at risk of developing cirrhosis, causing a coagulopathy, and oesophageal varices, which can bleed. Blood loss causes a microcytic anaemia. Thus any pattern of anaemia is possible in this patient.

Chapter 6: Dysphagia

1 **b. Feedback:** The others are globus (sensation of a lump in the throat), dysphagia (difficulty swallowing), dypsnoea (difficulty breathing), whereas there is no commonly used medical term for painful chewing.

2 **e. Feedback:** Remember that the 'E' in 'CREST' stands for 'esophageal dysmotility' (US spelling). In Plummer–Vinson syndrome, iron deficiency leads to a postcricoid web that forms an obstruction in the oesophagus. Ortner's syndrome and dysphagia lusoria are rare syndromes in which dysphagia is due to extramural pressure on the oesophagus by the cardiovascular system (usually a dilated left atrium) or an aberrant subclavian artery respectively. Ortner's syndrome is usually also associated with hoarseness due to pressure on the recurrent laryngeal nerve.

3 **c. Feedback:** Manometry is used to assess lower oesophageal sphincter pressures rather than to assess anatomical disease spread.

4 **b. Feedback:** Traditionally, squamous cell carcinoma (SCC) has been a more common histological finding in oesophageal cancers than adenocarcinoma. However, the incidence of adenocarcinoma has been growing dramatically in developed countries, such that the most recent data suggest it is now more common than squamous cell carcinoma in the UK. Small-cell carcinomas and leiomyomas are very rare forms of oesophageal cancer, and lymphoma is not an oesophageal cancer.

5 **b. Feedback:** All of the other therapies listed have a place in the management of achalasia depending on the patient's circumstances. Heller's myotomy has a high success rate in those who are fit enough to undergo the surgery. Dilatation is a reasonable alternative in those who are not fit enough for surgery but can tolerate endoscopy. Botox injections are often only effective in the short term, with high recurrence rates, but useful for those who are not fit enough for endoscopy. If all else fails, calcium channel blockers can be trialled but response rates are much lower.

Chapter 7: Cough

1 **e. Feedback:** Peripheral oedema, a raised JVP and loud P2 are all signs of right heart failure, in this case due to cor pulmonale.

2 **e. Feedback:** It is impossible to interpret information about the oxygenation of a patient without knowing the inspired oxygen (Fio_2). Thus a patient with a seemingly normal Pao_2 may have severely impaired ventilation if they are getting 15 L/min of oxygen delivered through a non-rebreathe mask. Remember to always enter this into the ABG machine or write it on the printed result.

3 **d. Feedback:** The radiograph report indicates the presence of bronchopneumonia (rather than lobar pneumonia) and an abscess. *Streptococcus pneumoniae* normally causes lobar pneumonia, i.e. localized rather than patchy infiltrates. Adenovirus causes an interstitial pneumonitis, thus the shadowing is interstitial rather than alveolar and air bronchograms would not be visible. *Mycoplasma pneumoniae* causes a bronchopneumonia but abscesses are rarely seen. Abscesses are a known complication of *Staphylococcus aureus* infection. Fluid levels are not normally seen in fungal abscesses or tuberculous granulomas.

4 **b. Feedback:** H_2 receptor antagonists, e.g. ranitidine, not H_1 receptor antagonists, are used to treat GORD. However these have now been largely superseded by PPIs. Magnesium carbonate, aluminium hydroxide, and alginates are all antacids that are good at relieving mild symptoms.

5 **e. Feedback:** All of these conditions can predispose to spontaneous pneumothorax, as can many others, most notably chronic obstructive pulmonary disease (COPD).

Chapter 8: Haemoptysis

1 **d. Feedback:** All of the conditions listed can cause a pulmonary–renal syndrome, manifest as haemoptysis and haematuria. A positive test for ANA (antinuclear antibodies) would suggest SLE. ANCA (antineutrophil cytoplasmic antibodies) positive status is consistent with granulomatosis with polyangiitis and MPA. Although either condition may have a positive cANCA or pANCA (i.e. these tests have low specificity), a positive pANCA is most likely to be seen in MPA.

2 **a. Feedback:** Silica, the mineral name of silicon dioxide which is found in stonecutter's dust, causes fibrosis. This is not the same as silicon.

3 **d. Feedback:** Remember that the skin sensitivity tests (Heaf, Mantoux) and the newer interferon-gamma release assays (IGRAs) are only useful to determine latent tuberculosis infection and tell you nothing about disease activity. As many people are infected but not diseased, these tests are of little diagnostic value. The primary application is in contact tracing.

4 **a. Feedback:** Proteins C and S and antithrombin III all have anticoagulant properties, but only proteins C and S are vitamin K-dependent. The action of antithrombin III is potentiated by heparin. Thrombomodulin is a cell surface membrane expressed on endothelial cells that, in combination with thrombin, activates protein C.

5 **c. Feedback:** CT and bone scans are investigations for staging (i.e. extent of spread) rather than grading (i.e. abnormality of cells). All cancers should be staged and graded.

Chapter 9: Chest pain

1 **c. Feedback:** Boerhaave's syndrome describes oesophageal rupture and carries a poor prognosis. Tietze's syndrome is the name given to idiopathic costochondritis. Bornholm's disease is a myalgia that can affect the intercostal muscles of the chest; it is caused by infection with Coxsackie B virus.

2 **d. Feedback:** The ECG pattern is that of an anterior infarct, i.e. affecting the anterior left ventricle, supplied by the LAD. The circumflex supplies the lateral surface of the left ventricle, picked up in leads V_5 and V_6. The RCA supplies the inferior surface, seen in leads II, III, and aVF.

3   **d. Feedback:** Normally patients with a STEMI should receive a β-blocker in the acute phase as this has been shown to reduce mortality. However, asthma is a contraindication to β-blocker use. Mild renal impairment, with a creatinine <150 micromol/L, is not a contraindication to ACE inhibitor use. ACE inhibitors should be avoided if the renal function deteriorates and creatinine rises above 150 micromol/L.

4   **d. Feedback:** Ezetimibe is a cholesterol-lowering drug that inhibits cholesterol absorption at the small intestine brush border. All the other drugs are antiplatelet agents.

5   **d. Feedback:** There is good evidence of reduced cardiovascular morbidity and mortality after coronary stenting for patients who are placed on a combination of dual antiplatelet therapy (aspirin plus another antiplatelet), an ACE inhibitor, a statin, and a β-blocker. Current evidence suggests using the second antiplatelet agent for 1 year in patients regardless of the stent being bare metal or drug eluting. If the patient is at high risk of bleeding while on a second antiplatelet, the current evidence suggests using the second antiplatelet agent for 1 month after a bare metal stent but 6 months after a drug-eluting stent (because the latter have, ironically, a greater risk of re-stenosis in the first few months).

Chapter 10: Shortness of breath

1   **d. Feedback:** Although some patients with COPD are chronic CO_2 retainers and dependent on their hypoxic drive to maintain respiration, in many hypercapnia is still the stimulus for respiration and thus giving 100% oxygen to this group will do no harm.

2   **d. Feedback:** Amiodarone can cause pulmonary fibrosis, among many other side effects (skin sensitivity, hepatotoxicity, thyroid disorder, etc.). Many other medications can also cause fibrosis (e.g. nitrofurantoin, methotrexate, bleomycin, ciclosporin), but not any of the others listed.

3   **b. Feedback:** A short course of steroids is indicated in the treatment of infective exacerbations in the context of COPD. Antibiotics should also be given for the infection, initially empirically and adjusted pending culture sensitivities, but these will rarely be gentamicin or metronidazole.

4   **e. Feedback:** First-generation calcium channel blockers (e.g. diltiazem, verapamil) are negative inotropes and therefore contraindicated. Second-generation calcium channel blockers (e.g. amlodipine, nifedipine) are however more vasoselective and not contraindicated. Aspirin is not necessarily indicated, only if there is evidence of ischaemic heart disease (which is common in heart failure), but is not contraindicated either. β-Blockers and ACE inhibitors are indicated in chronic heart failure as they bring mortality benefits, although β-blockers should not be started if the patient has acutely decompensated disease.

5   **d. Feedback:** Restrictive lung diseases cause a reduction in full vital capacity (FVC) but not forced expiratory volume in 1 second (FEV_1). Obstructive lung diseases, e.g. asthma and COPD, have the opposite effect.

Chapter 11: Breast lump

1   **b. Feedback:** Smoking is associated with duct ectasia. DCIS is often not palpable as the foci are small, and necrosis is not usually involved. Fibrocystic change includes, as the name suggests, cysts and fibrous thickening, but not necrosis. Breast-feeding leads to lactational changes but not fat necrosis.

2   **e. Feedback:** A family history of breast cancer, particularly in first-degree and/or young relatives, is a risk factor for breast cancer. Smoking, exposure to hydrocarbon compounds, and human papillomavirus are all risk factors for other cancers but there is no link to breast cancer. Fibrocystic disease is not a risk factor unless there is also atypia.

3   **d. Feedback:** Invasion of lymphatics indicates spread and is a poor prognostic sign. Smoking has no direct relevance to prognosis, but complications from any operative intervention (such as wound dehiscence) are likely to be increased. A family history makes breast cancer more likely but does not affect prognosis. Herceptin receptor positive status is a good prognostic factor as it means it will respond to herceptin. ER receptor positive tumours can be treated with various oestrogen-blocking therapies.

4   **c. Feedback:** A non-invasive lesion removed with clear margins and clear lymph nodes has a good prognosis. Some will recur locally, but many will be cured. Axillary radiotherapy and axillary node clearance are not necessary if sentinel nodes are negative. There is no benefit of tamoxifen in oestrogen receptor negative patients.

5   **e. Feedback:** This patient is complaining of gynaecomastia, a known side effect of digoxin (and also spironolactone and alcohol, among others).

Chapter 12: Epigastric pain

1   **b. Feedback:** Hypertriglyceridaemia, but not hypercholesteraemia, can cause acute pancreatitis (although it must be very elevated). Hypercalcaemia is another cause, and severe pancreatitis can cause hypocalcaemia. A positive sweat test would indicate cystic fibrosis; these patients usually present early in life with chronic pancreatic damage rather than acute pancreatitis.

2   **e. Feedback:** This is most likely to be a benign peptic ulcer. These are typically found in the gastric antrum.

3   **e. Feedback:** This is Barrett's oesophagus, due to chronic GORD. The patient is at increased risk of adenocarcinoma, not squamous cell carcinoma.

4   **a. Feedback:** Significantly elevated amylase levels are traditionally used to diagnose acute pancreatitis, although lipase levels are more sensitive and specific (but not always available). Amylase rises acutely (within 6–12 hours) and has a short half-life (~10 hours), so patients who present late may have normal amylase levels. Alcoholics may also have normal levels as their pancreas may be unable to produce amylase. In hypertriglyceridaemia, the triglycerides can interfere with the amylase assay and produce a falsely low result. Counterintuitively though, amylase levels are often low in severe/necrotic pancreatitis, and have not been found to correlate with outcome in multiple studies.

Chapter 13: Nausea and vomiting

1   **b. Feedback:** BPPV is positional and paroxysmal, as its name suggests. Motion sickness occurs only during motion (specifically when the eyes perceive a different motion to the vestibular system). Orthostatic hypotension causes light-headedness rather than vertigo (room spinning around the patient). Ménière's disease causes episodes of tinnitus, a sensation of fullness in the ear, vertigo, and progressive unilateral hearing loss. In Ménière's, though, the episodes last 30 min to 3–4 hours, thus the time course here is far too long.

2   **b. Feedback:** *Giardia* infection normally follows travel to an endemic region. *Shigella* and *E. coli* O157 cause dysentery, i.e. bloody diarrhoea. Rotavirus normally affects children under the age of 5. Norovirus is frequently reported as causing outbreaks in developed nations, including in residential homes and on cruise ships.

3   **d. Feedback:** Only the outer 'serosal' layer of the appendix is inflamed, whereas in appendicitis the inner mucosa would be inflamed. This finding suggests irritation outside of the appendix, i.e. peritonitis.

4   **d. Feedback:** Pyloric stenosis typically causes projectile vomiting, occurs in boys, and presents several weeks after birth. Gastroenteritis is also a possibility but would normally be accompanied by fever and diarrhoea, and the vomiting would not be projectile.

5 **d. Feedback:** This is linitis plastica, a diffuse, poorly differentiated gastric carcinoma, with liver metastases. Pernicious anaemia is associated with the development of this condition.

Chapter 14: Jaundice

1 **e. Feedback:** Pyruvate kinase deficiency is the second most common enzyme deficiency causing intravascular haemolytic anaemia (glucose-6-phosphate dehydrogenase (G6PD) deficiency being the most common). In thalassaemia, there is haemolysis of the unstable red cells but this occurs mainly in the spleen and liver (i.e. extravascular haemolysis).

2 **a. Feedback:** AMA is elevated in 95% of patients with primary biliary cirrhosis and in some patients with autoimmune hepatitis.

3 **c. Feedback:** This is chronic hepatitis due to hepatitis B infection. This occurs in 5–10% of those infected with hepatitis B. Of those who do develop chronic hepatitis, 20% will develop cirrhosis and 6% hepatocellular carcinoma.

4 **d. Feedback:** Ulcerative colitis is associated with numerous other conditions including primary sclerosing cholangitis (PSC), which may occur even after colectomy.

5 **e. Feedback:** This patient has painless jaundice, the classic finding in adenocarcinoma of the head of the pancreas. This causes obstruction of the common bile duct, leading to raised conjugated bilirubin (obstructive jaundice) and raised alkaline phosphatase with normal liver enzymes. Haemolytic anaemia and Gilbert's would result in an unconjugated hyperbilirubinaemia. Chronic hepatitis would be associated with a transaminitis (raised ALT/AST). Primary biliary cirrhosis is the only other diagnosis that could yield similar lab results, but usually presents with itch and lethargy rather than nausea and weight loss, and is nine times more common in women, usually in their middle years.

Chapter 15: Right upper quadrant pain

1 **b. Feedback:** a = flank bruising, c = periumbilical bruising, d = relief of epididymitis pain when elevating the testis, e = shoulder tip pain resulting from diaphragmatic irritation. Grey Turner's and Cullen's signs are (rare) signs of acute pancreatitis.

2 **d. Feedback:** A HIDA (hepatobiliary iminodiacetic acid) scan employs a radio-isotope to assess the patency of the cystic duct. It is rarely performed. MIBG (metaiodobenzylguanidine) scans are used for the investigation of phaeochromocytomas.

3 **b. Feedback:** Note that there is no D5.

4 **d. Feedback:** Anatomical variants include the a 'double cystic artery' (~15%) where the superficial and deep branches of the cystic artery arise separately (usually from the right hepatic artery). In cholecystectomies it is important to clearly identify and ligate the cystic artery (rather than a hepatic artery), hence the importance of identifying Calot's triangle intraoperatively.

5 **d. Feedback:** Both ALT and AST are markers of hepatocyte damage, but ALT is more specific. AST is also released by red blood cells, cardiac tissue, skeletal muscle, kidney, and brain tissue.

Chapter 16: Right iliac fossa pain

1 **e. Feedback:** a = deep tenderness at McBurney's point; b = pain when passively internally rotating the hip; c = pain when passively extending the hip; d = aggravation of abdominal pain by coughing. All of these are non-specific clinical signs of acute appendicitis.

2 **d. Feedback:** The rectus sheath surrounds the rectus muscles which are midline structures, located medial to the traditional incision point for an appendicectomy (McBurney's point).

3   **d. Feedback:** Intussusception is the most common cause of bowel obstruction in children, but is rare in adults. Mesenteric adenitis is also relatively common in children but rare in adults. Appendicitis and Meckel's diverticulitis may present in adults or children, >75% of colorectal carcinomas occur in the over 65s.

4   **a. Feedback:** The base of the appendix is in fact fairly uniformly located 2 cm from the ileocaecal valve. The tip, however, is retrocaecal in approximately three-quarters, with the other locations listed all possible alternatives.

5   **c. Feedback:** The other scoring systems relate to acute pancreatitis.

Chapter 17: Left iliac fossa pain

1   **e. Feedback:** The rectum has a complete coat of longitudinal muscle fibres (compared with the taenia coli of the colon) and thus is relatively resistant to pulsion diverticula.

2   **c. Feedback:** A paracolic abscess can be drained percutaneously and is not an indication for surgery in the first instance.

3   **e. Feedback:** Colonoscopy should not be performed in the acute setting as there is a risk of perforating the inflamed colon.

4   **b. Feedback:** Vancomycin is effective against *Clostridium difficile* but must be given orally as IV therapy does not achieve effective gut concentrations. The other three antibiotics listed all predispose to *Clostridium difficile*.

5   **e. Feedback:** There is no single diagnostic test for irritable bowel syndrome. Diagnosis is largely by excluding other conditions which may account for the symptoms. The Rome criteria may aid this process.

Chapter 18: Flank pain

1   **e. Feedback:** Struvite is the phosphate mineral $NH_4MgPO_4.6H_2O$. Struvite calculi are associated with bacterial infections by ammonia (NH_3)-producing organisms.

2   **c. Feedback:** By comparison, elective repair of an abdominal aortic aneurysm has a mortality of around 5%. There are a number of prognostic scoring systems for ruptured abdominal aortic aneurysms, such as the Hardman index which identifies age (>76 years), creatinine (>190 mmol/L), haemoglobin (<90 g/L), loss of consciousness, and ischaemic changes on ECG as poor prognostic factors.

3   **c. Feedback:** L4 broadly corresponds to the level of the superior iliac crests.

4   **a. Feedback:** Diabetes mellitus is a significant risk factor for atherosclerosis, but not abdominal aortic aneurysms per se.

5   **c. Feedback:** The UK Small Aneurysm Trial and the US Aneurysm Detection and Management Study both showed that aneurysms <5.5 cm are best managed non-operatively, finding no mortality benefit from surgery.

Chapter 19: Constipation

1   **e. Feedback:** Colchicine commonly causes diarrhoea whereas all the other drugs are commonly associated with constipation.

2   **c. Feedback:** Parathyroid hormone (PTH) stimulates renal uptake of calcium at the expense of phosphate, hence hyperparathyroidism results in high calcium and low phosphate. Because the normal negative feedback of calcium on PTH secretion has been lost, the PTH level will be inappropriately normal or raised.

3   **a. Feedback:** Abdominal tenderness is not a feature of uncomplicated bowel obstruction and should raise alarm bells that the bowel may be strangulated.

4   **c. Feedback:** There was no Dukes stage D (distant spread) in the original classification. Dukes stage E does not exist.
5   **c. Feedback:** The sigmoid artery is a branch of the inferior mesenteric artery.

Chapter 20: Diarrhoea

1   **d. Feedback:** Haematochezia refers to the passage of bright red blood per rectum; melaena (black, tarry) is digested blood from an upper gastrointestinal haemorrhage; a scybalum is a hard mass of faecal material in the intestine.
2   **e. Feedback:** Features a–d are typical of Crohn's disease and not ulcerative colitis.
3   **c. Feedback:** Giardia typically produces chronic malabsorptive diarrhoea rather than dysentery.
4   **a. Feedback:** This patient has coeliac disease (as evidenced by the positive antibody tests). It is most likely that the vesicular rash is dermatitis herpetiformis which is associated with coeliac disease and usually responds to a gluten-free diet.
5   **b. Feedback:** The majority of micronutrient absorption occurs in the duodenum and proximal jejunum, including iron (duodenum). Folate is primarily absorbed in the jejunum, although the distal small intestine is also capable of absorbing folate. B_{12} is absorbed in the ileum.

Chapter 21: Rectal bleeding

1   **c. Feedback:** Grade 5 haemorrhoids do not exist.
2   **b. Feedback:** In iron deficiency anaemia, the total iron binding capacity (i.e. amount of transferrin in the blood) is **high** as the body tries desperately to store as much iron as possible, but the saturation of this transferrin with iron is **low** because there is not enough iron to saturate all the transferrin.
3   **c. Feedback:** Options d and e do not enable biopsies to be taken. Proctoscopes only enable visualization of the anus, while rigid proctoscopes enable visualization of the rectum.
4   **e. Feedback:** NSAIDs are known to increase the risk of bleeds from diverticular disease.
5   **d. Feedback:** The coeliac trunk arises at T12, the superior mesenteric artery at L1, and the inferior mesenteric artery at L3.

Chapter 22: Poor urinary output

1   **d. Feedback:** Fogarty catheters are used for intravascular procedures, while Swan–Ganz catheters are used to measure pulmonary artery wedge pressure. Foley catheters are the traditional urethral catheter, but a standard Foley is unsuitable for bladder irrigation as it lacks an irrigation port. Three-way catheters have three lumens—one for urine, one for irrigation, and one for inflation of the balloon. Suprapubic bladder catheters are not suitable for this role.
2   **e. Feedback:** An enlarged prostate (BPH) can pinch the urethra, causing poor urinary output. A bladder cancer can obstruct both ureters from within the bladder. A cervical adenocarcinoma can compress both ureters by mass effect or malignant infiltration. Retroperitoneal fibrosis causes scarring around the ureters (which are retroperitoneal structures), which can pinch them off.
3   **e. Feedback:** Remember poor urinary output is most often due to prerenal causes, followed by postrenal and finally renal aetiologies (least likely).
4   **b. Feedback:** While all of the following diagnoses can lead to acute renal failure, only TTP is classically also associated with neurological disturbance. The pentad of TTP is microangiopathic haemolytic anaemia (MAHA), thrombocytopenia, fever, renal failure, and neurological symptoms.

Chapter 23: Polyuria

1   **b. Feedback:** Metformin is the first-line oral hypoglycaemic agent in patients with normal renal function (creatinine <150 micromol/L). Sulphonylureas such as gliclazide may be considered in patients who are not overweight and in those patients for whom metformin is contraindicated or not tolerated.

2   **c. Feedback:** Acarbose inhibits intestinal α-glucosidases and thus less ingested carbohydrate is converted to absorbable glucose, but more carbohydrate is consequently available to colonic bacteria, which produce copious amounts of gas.

3   **e. Feedback:** Hypernatraemia is a consequence, rather than a cause, of nephrogenic diabetes insipidus.

4   **d. Feedback:** Craniopharyngiomas, derived from Rathke's pouch, are far more likely to produce diabetes insipidus than actual pituitary tumours such as prolactinomas.

5   **c. Feedback:** Patients with HONK are prone to thromboembolism and thus should be formally anticoagulated. There is no indication for any of the other management options suggested.

Chapter 24: Groin lump

1   **d. Feedback:** The order of structure from lateral to medial is: femoral nerve, femoral artery, femoral vein. Remember NAVY: nerve, artery, vein, Y-fronts.

2   **c. Feedback:** A Spigelian hernia occurs at the lateral border of the rectus sheath; Maydl's hernia describes a W-loop strangulation with two loops of bowel in the sac and strangulation of the intraperitoneal portion; Littré's hernia involves a Meckel's diverticulum; obturator hernias occur through the obturator canal and rarely present with a palpable mass.

3   **e. Feedback:** The inferior epigastric artery (usually) arises from the external iliac artery immediately above the inguinal ligament and along the medial margin of the deep inguinal ring. It ascends from there to anastamose with the superior epigastric artery above the umbilicus. (There can be anatomical variations.)

4   **a. Feedback:** Although femoral hernias are more common in women than men, inguinal hernias are still by far more common in both men and women.

5   **c. Feedback:** Smokers are significantly more likely to develop hernias and suffer hernia recurrence. This effect appears to be independent of BMI and is most likely modulated by impaired connective tissue metabolism causing abdominal wall weakness.

Chapter 25: Scrotal lump

1   **a. Feedback:** The most common types of testicular tumours are teratomas and seminomas. Broadly speaking, teratomas are more common in men of 20–30 years age, while seminomas are more common from 30 years old upwards. You may find it easy to remember this pattern as younger 'troopers' (teratomas) and older 'sergeants' (seminomas). The other tumours listed are all testicular tumours, but are rare.

2   **e. Feedback:** Ultrasound is the most useful initial investigation, and is very sensitive for tumours when combined with clinical examination. Tumour markers and further imaging (CT chest/abdo/pelvis) are only warranted if the ultrasound detects a tumour.

3   **c. Feedback:** A gumma is a testicular granuloma caused by tertiary syphilis.

4   **e. Feedback:** There is a broad differential to scrotal lumps but careful examination is key to the diagnosis.

5   **c. Feedback:** It would be possible to get above both an epididymal cyst and a vaginal hydrocele. Femoral hernias do not extend into the scrotum. Inguinoscrotal hernias are almost always indirect.

Chapter 26: Acute limb weakness

1 **c. Feedback:** Remember the scale ranges from 0 = no movement at all (not even a flicker) to 5 = normal.
2 **a. Feedback:** Other commonly tested reflexes include the knee jerk, broadly corresponding to L3/L4 nerve roots; biceps (C5/C6); and triceps (C7/C8).
3 **c. Feedback:** The musculocutaneous nerve arises from the brachial plexus and is often damaged in brachial plexus injuries. The median and radial nerves provide the sensory innervation to the medial and posterior aspects of the forearm respectively.
4 **e. Feedback:** You must not start anticoagulant/antiplatelet treatment until a haemorrhagic stroke has been excluded by CT head.
5 **b. Feedback:** The fact that symptoms have resolved themselves 1 hour later excludes both stroke and hypoglycaemia. Epilepsy and migraine tend to be associated with 'positive symptoms' such as tingling, shaking, and disturbances of vision, whereas TIAs are usually associated with a loss of function. Furthermore, there is no warning to a TIA. Although it can be very difficult to distinguish between migraine and epilepsy, the duration of the aura in this patient is helpful. Migraine auras usually evolve over 20–30 min whereas epileptic seizures usually have their onset over seconds. Remember that migraines do not have to be associated with a headache.

Chapter 27: Acute joint pain

1 **d. Feedback:** Allopurinol must not be given during the acute phase of gout, as it can paradoxically exacerbate the condition. It is started weeks after the attack has subsided, but even then is given with colchicine to protect against relapse.
2 **d. Feedback:** You must exclude septic arthritis. The best way of doing this is by aspirating the joint.
3 **b. Feedback:** Pseudogout is due to the deposition of calcium pyrophosphate dihydrate crystals in joints. It typically affects older patients and can often be seen as calcium deposits in the knee joint on plain radiographs.
4 **d. Feedback:** These nail changes are suggestive of psoriasis—remember that psoriatic arthropathy does not have to be accompanied by psoriatic skin disease. Behçet's disease does not usually cause arthropathy.
5 **c. Feedback:** In otherwise healthy patients with native joints, *Staphylococcus aureus* is the most likely pathogen.

Chapter 28: Swollen calf

1. **e. Feedback:** The use of D-dimer to exclude venous thromboembolism is only validated in combination with a clinical probability score (e.g. Wells, Geneva, or even the clinician's 'gestalt' or impression). Always calculate the pre-test probability, and if this is moderate or high, you will not be able to rule out pathology with a negative D-dimer and should consider going directly to definitive imaging (e.g. Doppler ultrasound).
2 **c. Feedback:** The target INR range for patients presenting with a DVT is 2–3. Patients with arterial thromboembolism, or those who develop a DVT while already taking oral anticoagulants, require a higher target range of 3–4.
3 **a. Feedback:** The factor V Leiden mutation is present in ~5% of the population, and 20–30% of those presenting with venous thromboembolic disease.
4 **c. Feedback:** Most cellulitis is caused by *Streptococcus pyogenes* but it may also (less commonly) be caused by *Staphylococcus aureus*—hence flucloxacillin is used as treatment because it covers both pathogens.

5   **c. Feedback:** In a patient with a rapidly spreading redness, severe pain (which often appears out of context to the skin manifestations), and systemic signs you must consider necrotizing fasciitis. Blistering skin should always make you suspect serious pathology.

Chapter 29: Leg ulcer

1   **e. Feedback:** This history is suggestive of a Marjolin's ulcer (squamous cell carcinoma).
2   **a. Feedback:** Venous guttering is a feature of arterial disease, not venous. Venous guttering refers to delayed filling of veins during Buerger's test.
3   **c. Feedback:** The morphological features (punctuate ulcer, pale atrophic skin) are typical of an arterial ulcer. In addition, the absence of foot pulses argues in favour of this pathology.
4   **d. Feedback:** Be careful to exclude peripheral vascular disease as a cause before trying compression.
5   **e. Feedback:** Leg ulcers can be very difficult to treat, and indeed referral (ideally to a specialist leg ulcer clinic) may be warranted.

Index of cases

Index